CONTENTS

CONTRIBUTORS

M.M. Brown MD FRCP
Professor of Stroke Medicine, Institute of Neurology, University College London, and National Hospital for Neurology and Neurosurgery, London

J.H. Cross BSc PhD MRCP FRCPCH
Senior Lecturer and Honorary Consultant in Paediatric Neurology, Institute of Child Health and Great Ormond Street Hospital for Children NHS Trust, London

S. Fleminger PhD MRCP MRCPsych
Consultant Neuropsychiatrist, Lishman Brain Injury Unit, Maudsley Hospital, London

N.A. Fletcher BSC MD FRCP
Consultant Neurologist, Walton Centre for Neurology and Neurosurgery, Liverpool

T.J. Fowler DM FRCP
Consultant Neurologist, Maidstone and Tunbridge Wells NHS Trust; formerly of King's College Hospital, London

P.J. Goadsby MD PhD DSc FRCP FRACP
Professor of Clinical Neurology and Wellcome Senior Research Fellow, Institute of Neurology, University College London, and National Hospital for Neurology and Neurosurgery, London

N.P. Hirsch MB BS FRCA
Consultant Anaesthetist, National Hospital for Neurology and Neurosurgery, London

R.S. Howard PhD FRCP
Consultant Neurologist, National Hospital for Neurology and Neurosurgery, London

E.F. Hughes BSc MRCP FRCPH
Consultant Paediatric Neurologist, King's College Hospital and Guys and St Thomas' Hospital NHS Trust, London

R. Kapoor DM FRCP
Consultant Neurologist, National Hospital for Neurology and Neurosurgery, London

P.N. Leigh PhD FRCP FMedSci
Professor of Clinical Neurology, Institute of Psychiatry and Guys, King's and St Thomas' School of Medicine, London

J.G. Llewelyn MD FRCP
Consultant Neurologist, University Hospital of Wales, Cardiff

N.A. Losseff MD MRCP
Consultant Neurologist, National Hospital for Neurology and Neurosurgery and Whittington Hospital NHS Trust, London

The late C.D. Marsden FRS DSc FRCP FRCPsych
Formerly Professor of Clinical Neurology, Institute of Neurology, University College London, and National Hospital for Neurology and Neurosurgery, London

G. Neil-Dwyer MS FRCS
Honorary Emeritus Consultant Neurosurgeon, Wessex Neurological Centre, Southampton General Hospital, Southampton

D. Peterson FRCS(SN) FRCS
Consultant Neurosurgeon, Charing Cross Hospital, London

M.P. Powell FRCS
Consultant Neurosurgeon, National Hospital for Neurology and Neurosurgery, London

N.P. Quinn MA MD FRCP
Professor of Clinical Neurology, Institute of Neurology, University College London, and National Hospital for Neurology and Neurosurgery, London

J.W.A.S. Sander MD PhD
Professor of Neurology, Department of Clinical and Experimental Epilepsy, Institute of Neurology, University College London, and National Hospital for Neurology and Neurosurgery, London

J.W. Scadding MD FRCP
Consultant Neurologist, National Hospital for Neurology and Neurosurgery, London

A.H.V. Schapira MD DSc FRCP FMedSci
Professor of Clinical Neurology, University Department of Clinical Neurosciences, Royal Free and University College Medical School, London

C.E. Shaw MD FRCAP FRCP
Senior Lecturer and Consultant Neurologist, Guys, King's and St Thomas' School of Medicine, London

J.M. Stevens DRACR FRCR
Consultant Neuroradiologist, National Hospital for Neurology and Neurosurgery, London

A.J. Thompson MD FRCP FRCPI
Garfield Weston Professor of Clinical Neurology and Neurorehabilitation, Institute of Neurology, University College London, and National Hospital for Neurology and Neurosurgery, London

M.C. Walker PhD MRCP
Senior Lecturer, Department of Clinical and Experimental Epilepsy, Institute of Neurology, University College London, and National Hospital for Neurology and Neurosurgery, London

L.D. Watkins MA FRCS(SN)
Consultant Neurosurgeon and Clinical Senior Lecturer, Institute of Neurology, University College London, and National Hospital for Neurology and Neurosurgery, London

L.A. Wilson FRCP FRACP
Consultant Neurologist, Royal Free Hospital, London

The late M.J. Wood MA FRCP
Consultant Physician, Department of Infection and Tropical Medicine, Heartlands Hospital, Birmingham

N.W. Wood PhD FRCP
Professor of Clinical Neurology, Institute of Neurology, University College London, and National Hospital for Neurology and Neurosurgery, London

PREFACE

It is with great regret that we note the untimely death of David Marsden, the co-editor for the first two editions. We shall miss his wisdom, guidance and skills. He was largely responsible for the backbone of this work with a personal emphasis on history taking, relevant neurological symptoms and the art of neurological examination. This part of the text, mostly his work, remains. We dedicate this third edition to his memory.

We also are greatly saddened by the sudden death of Martin Wood, the author of the chapter on infectious diseases in all three editions. He contributed to our understanding of the important role of infections affecting the nervous system. He proved to be an editor's dream, always producing his chapter excelling in content and on time without the need for corrections. He will be greatly missed.

In this new edition fresh chapters on Neurogenetics (Professor Wood), Respiratory Intensive Care (Drs Howard and Hirsch) and Pain (Dr Scadding) have been added. New chapter authors have provided sections on Motor Neurone Disease and Spinal Muscular Atrophies (Dr Shaw), Movement Disorders (Professor Quinn), Epilepsy and Sleep Disorders (Professor Sander and Dr Walker), Headache (Professor Goadsby), Raised Intracranial Pressure (Mr Watkins), HIV Infections and AIDS (Dr Wilson), Demyelinating Diseases of the CNS (Dr Kapoor), Cerebrovascular Disease (Professor Brown and Dr Losseff) and Psychiatry and Neurological Disorders (Dr Fleminger). These authors have added a new perspective to these sections, revising and updating their contents. The previous chapters have also all been revised.

Over the last few years major progress has been made in our understanding of some of the more common neurodegenerative disorders. At the molecular level, accumulation of various proteins has been identified, e.g. tau found in the neurofibrillary tangles of Alzheimer's disease, beta-amyloid found in the amyloid plaques of Alzheimer's disease, and alpha-synuclein found in the Lewy body in Parkinson's disease and in dementia associated with Lewy bodies. In some patients there are genetic defects linked with the familial forms of these neurodegenerative diseases. In others there may be a link with some external toxin or oxidative stress.

Many of these concepts have been explored by the relevant chapter authors. New drugs have appeared to treat infections, migraine, cluster headache, epilepsy, Parkinson's disease and even dementia. These too have been included, emphasizing the appearance of new treatments for some chronic neurological disorders.

The aim of this work is to help in the education of medical students, junior doctors, and those preparing for the MRCP examination, in addition to physicians of all specialities. It is hoped that this aim is fulfilled and we thank all our contributors.

We remain indebted to our patients who continue to provide the stimulus and challenge that keep our interest in neurology.

ACKNOWLEDGEMENTS

We should like again to thank our many colleagues for all their help and advice, particularly those who have guided us, corrected our errors and furthered our education in this advancing field. We add our thanks to Dr Bidi Evans for the provision of EEG records and Dr Graham Holder from Moorfields Eye Hospital for his advice on electroretinograms and the provision of evoked potential records. Drs Christopher Penney and Martin Jeffree from the Neuroimaging Department at King's College Hospital and Dr John Stevens from the National Hospital have provided many pictures to illustrate the use of MRI and CT scans.

We should also like to thank Professor Peter Duus, Professor Joseph Furman, Professor Peter Harper, Dr David Perkin, Dr Fred Plum, Lord Walton of Detchant and Professor Charles Warlow and all their publishers for their kind permission to reproduce tables and figures from previously published work.

Dr Jo Koster, Sarah Burrows and Anke Ueberberg from Hodder Arnold also deserve thanks for their trust and patience, and their great help. Finally we should like to add our thanks to our wives and families for their support and forbearance.

CHAPTER 1

INTRODUCTION

T.J. Fowler and J.W. Scadding

Students have always found clinical neurology difficult to understand. There are many reasons for this, quite apart from the failings of their teachers. Clinical diagnosis, at least the anatomical part of it, is heavily dependent upon an adequate, if rudimentary, knowledge of human neuroanatomy and neurophysiology, which is often learnt by rote and then forgotten by the time the student enters the neurological ward. Perhaps the greatest difficulty has been that neurology is full of irrelevant facts. Like the minutiae of gross anatomy, the neurological examination and a differential diagnosis can be drawn out to such an extent that the original aim is forgotten. The student becomes confused by a wealth of irrelevant detail, and so fails to grasp the main point.

The problems of examination of sensory function illustrate the point. Armed with pin, cotton wool and tuning fork, the student approaches the patient to test sensation, but where to start? Human nature being what it is, many patients will try to help doctors by attempting to perceive minor differences in intensity of the pin or touch, and soon hapless students are confronted with a mass of apparent abnormalities that they cannot decipher. They see the experienced neurologist delicately mapping, with complete anatomical accuracy, an area of sensory loss, and wonder how they did it. The answer is simple: experienced neurologists know what they are looking for and have predicted what they will find on the basis of previous information. Sensory examination is the most difficult, so neurologists leave it until last when

they have obtained as much information as they can concerning what they expect to find!

Herein lies the clue to success in mastering clinical neurology. Students must learn to think on their feet at every moment of history taking and examination, building on a presumptive diagnosis as each new piece of information is collected, and predicting the outcome of the next series of questions or examinations. Thus neurology employs a continuous process of deductive logic to arrive at a final conclusion.

Structure of the book

The emphasis in this book is to simplify clinical neurology to manageable proportions. It is divided into three sections:

- The patient's complaints
- The doctor's examination
- The individual neurological diseases and their treatment.

This is what happens in real life. Patients tell the doctor that they cannot walk, talk, see, hear, and so on. The doctor forms an opinion as to where the trouble lies (the anatomical diagnosis). Clinical examination confirms (or refutes) the hypothesis as to the anatomical site of damage. The combination of the tempo of the patient's complaint and the site of the lesion then provide the likely pathology (pathological diagnosis). Based upon this clinical evaluation, decisions as to further investigation will be made to confirm both anatomical and pathological diagnosis. The final conclusion will dictate treatment.

In practice, the emphasis in clinical neurology is on bedside evaluation of the patient's complaints and signs. The principles of anatomical and pathological diagnosis will be discussed briefly later in this chapter. Special investigations are often not required at all for neurological diagnosis, and they can be misleading if not interpreted in the light of the history and the clinical examination. The principles of use of the major investigative techniques employed in neurology will also be discussed briefly in the ensuing chapters.

A standard joke about neurologists has been that they are 'brilliant at finding out where the trouble is, but incapable of doing anything about it'! To some extent, such comments reflect some envy, but neurology remains one of the last bastions of clinical bedside medicine, being so dependent on the vagaries of the individual patient and the examiner's skill, rather than on inanimate figures on laboratory reports, although the increasing use of magnetic resonance imaging (MRI) has greatly aided anatomical diagnosis (Figure 2.1). In fact, there are few medical disciplines that can claim to have cures for all their major diseases, but many of the commonest neurological illnesses can be treated effectively. Thus migraine, epilepsy, and Parkinson's disease are all amenable to drug therapy, while benign tumours of the head and spine can be removed successfully.

Quite apart from whether treatment exists, the doctor's role is also to relieve suffering. This is particularly important in clinical neurology, for many of its diseases produce severe physical disability. Part of the neurological apprenticeship is to learn the compassion and sensitivity to help disabled individuals to come to terms with, and surmount their problems.

Neurology thus provides a triple challenge. There is the intellectual exercise of defining the problem, the therapeutic challenge of treating it when treatment is available, and the humane responsibility of looking after those unfortunate enough to suffer from neurological diseases.

EPIDEMIOLOGY

The epidemiological study determines how often a disease occurs in the population, why it occurs and why different populations may show variable patterns. It can be readily appreciated that some neurological disorders are inherited, for example muscular dystrophy, whereas others may be determined by exposure to toxins, for example tri-ortho-cresyl phosphate neuropathy, or follow an infectious outbreak, for example the rising incidence of acquired immunodeficiency syndrome with its neurological complications. An understanding of the frequency with which different neurological disorders present both to general practitioners and to hospital clinics is a great help to the doctor concerned. Furthermore some 20% of acute medical admissions to a general district hospital arise as a result of neurological disorders. Table 1.1 gives an indication of the prevalence of some common neurological disorders and Table 1.2 an approximate annual incidence of some neurological conditions in England and Wales.

A number of surveys have provided figures for the 'top 20' and percentage of new patient consultations with neurologists in out-patient clinics in the UK (Table 1.3). It can be seen that headaches (including migraine and tension-type) and blackouts (including epilepsy) top the presenting symptom list, while at the top of the diagnostic categories are cerebrovascular disease, peripheral nerve disorders, multiple

Table 1.1 Prevalence of some neurological disorders in the UK (adapted from Warlow C (1991) *Handbook of Neurology*. Oxford: Blackwell Scientific Publications, with the permission of the author and publishers)

Disorder	Cases per 100 000	Cases per GP
Migraine	2000	40
Stroke	800	16
Epilepsy	500	10
Parkinson's disease	150*	3
Multiple sclerosis	100	2
Trigeminal neuralgia	100–150*	2
Primary tumour	46	1
Subarachnoid haemorrhage	50	1
Schizophrenia	10–50	1
Cerebral metastases	10	<1
Motor neurone disease	6	<1
Myasthenia gravis	5	<1
Polymyositis	5	<1
Friedreich's ataxia	2	<1

*Increases with age.
GP, general practitioner.

sclerosis, spine and disc problems and Parkinson's disease. Psychological diagnoses are common and may overlap with many neurological disorders. In addition there are a large number of patients who remain undiagnosed – just over one-quarter.

Modern advances in our understanding of genetics have led to better recognition of some inherited diseases. A list of more common single-gene neurological disorders is given in Table 1.4. Selected inherited disorders can now be diagnosed by laboratory testing (Table 1.5): furthermore the detection of carriers and the presymptomatic diagnosis of some conditions may occasionally prove possible; for example, the dominant inherited disorder Huntington's disease has been shown by detection of an expansion in the trinucleotide repeat sequences

Table 1.2 Approximate annual incidence of some common neurological disorders in the UK (adapted from Warlow C (1991) *Handbook of Neurology*. Oxford: Blackwell Scientific Publications, with the permission of the author and publishers)

Condition	Cases per 100 000
Dementia (<age 70 years)*	1000
Head injuries requiring hospitalization	200–300
Migraine	150–300
Stroke	200
Major depressive illness	80–200
Acute lumbar disc prolapse	150
Carpal tunnel syndrome	100
Epileptic seizures	50
TIAs	35
Bell's palsy	25
Essential tremor	25
Parkinson's disease	20
Cerebral metastases	15
Subarachnoid haemorrhage	15
Bipolar depression	10–15
Primary cerebral tumours	15
Bacterial meningitis	5
Trigeminal neuralgia	5
Multiple sclerosis	5
Motor neurone disease	2–3
Guillain–Barré syndrome	2
Meningioma	1.0–2.5
Polymyositis	1

*>age 70 years the incidence rises to c. 50%.
TIA, transient ischaemic attack.

Table 1.3 Top twenty diagnoses in a sample of 6940 patients (reproduced with permission from Perkin GD and the *Journal of Neurology, Neurosurgery and Psychiatry* 1989; **52**: 448)

Diagnosis	Proportion of sample (%)
No diagnosis	26.5
Blackouts	12.5
Epilepsy	10.4
Vasovagal attacks	2.1
Headache	12.5
Tension headache	7.5
Migraine	5.0
Cerebrovascular disease	7.4
Entrapment neuropathy	4.4
Conversion hysteria	3.8
Anatomical	3.7
Multiple sclerosis	3.5
Hyperventilation	2.0
Parkinson's disease	1.9
Post-traumatic syndrome	1.8
Dementia	1.5
Peripheral neuropathy	1.4
Depression	1.4
Non-neurological	1.3
Cervical radiculopathy/myelopathy	1.2
Lumbar spondylosis	1.0
Essential tremor	0.9

Table 1.4 Prevalence of single-gene neurological disorders in South East Wales (reproduced with permission from MacMillan JC, Harper PS and BMJ Publishing Group from *Clinical Genetics in Neurological Disease* 1995)

Disorder	Prevalence per 100 000
Neurofibromatosis I	13.3
Hereditary motor and sensory neuropathy I, II, III and V	12.9
Duchenne dystrophy*	9.6
Huntington's disease	8.4
Myotonic dystrophy	7.1
Becker dystrophy*	5.0
Hereditary spastic paraplegia	3.4
Facioscapulohumeral dystrophy	2.9
Tuberous sclerosis	1.6

*males

Table 1.5 Some inherited neurological conditions that can now be identified using laboratory tests

Duchenne/Becker muscular dystrophy
Myotonic dystrophy
Huntington's disease
Dentatorubropallidoluysian atrophy
X-linked spinobulbar muscular atrophy
(Kennedy's disease)
Spinal muscular atrophy
(autosomal recessive, proximal)
Hereditary motor and sensory neuropathy or
Charcot–Marie–Tooth disease
(aided by conduction velocity values)
Hereditary neuropathy with liability to pressure palsy
Fragile X syndrome
DYT1 dystonia
Mitochondrial encephalomyopathies
Facioscapulohumeral dystrophy
Familial motor neurone disease
Friedreich's ataxia
Spinocerebellar ataxia (SCA 1,2,3,6,7)

Screening services

Certain laboratories offer screening services:

- Limb girdle dystrophy – Newcastle
- Congenital muscular dystrophies – Hammersmith Hospital
- Muscle channelopathies – The National Hospital
- Congenital myasthenic syndromes – Oxford.

in the deoxyribonucleic acid (DNA) of the affected gene (chromosome 4). The disease can now be confirmed by blood tests and those who will develop the disease can be diagnosed before they show clinical signs. This imposes the need for provision of counselling services for individuals and their families.

ANATOMICAL DIAGNOSIS

Anatomical diagnosis

The details of the patient's complaints as the history unfolds will direct attention to the part or parts of the nervous system involved. A few very simple rules will help to focus attention on the likely site of trouble.

Seizures

Seizures (fits), disturbances of intellect and memory, and certain disorders of speech all point to disease of the cerebral cortex.

Seizures are the result of spontaneous discharges in cerebral cortical neurones, and do not occur with diseases of deep cerebral structures, the brainstem or cerebellum, unless the cerebral cortex is also involved. The faculties of intellectual prowess, reasoning and memory all depend upon the operations of the cerebral cortex, and any decline in these faculties points to damage in this zone of the brain.

Disturbances of speech fall into three categories:

1 **Dysphasia**, in which the content of speech is defective, although articulation and phonation are intact;
2 **Dysarthria**, in which articulation of speech is abnormal as a result of damage to the neuromuscular mechanisms controlling the muscles concerned with speech production;
3 **Dysphonia**, in which the larynx, the sound-box, is damaged.

Dysphasia points to a disorder of the cerebral cortex, particularly that of the dominant hemisphere (see Figure 4.7).

Disturbances of vision are common neurological problems. Loss of visual acuity points to damage to the eye itself, or to the optic nerve. Lesions behind the optic chiasm produce loss of vision in the opposite half of the visual field (hemianopia), but leave intact at least the ipsilateral half of central macular vision, and this is sufficient to provide a normal visual acuity (Figure 1.1). Patients with hemianopias complain of difficulty reading, or of bumping into objects in the blind half-field. Double vision (diplopia) occurs when the axes of the two eyes are out of alignment, that is they are not in parallel. This happens when one eyeball is displaced by some mass in the orbit, or if the ocular muscles are weak because of either primary muscle disease or damage to external ocular nerves (Figure 1.2).

Vertigo (a true sense of imbalance) is an illusion of movement and occurs with damage to the peripheral vestibular system, the vestibular nerve, or its brainstem connections. A combination of vertigo and diplopia suggests a lesion in the posterior fossa or brainstem, particularly when associated with bilateral motor or sensory disturbances.

Dysphagia and dysarthria are usually caused by either primary muscle disease, faults at the neuromuscular junction, or bilateral involvement of the neural mechanisms controlling the muscles of mastication and speech.

> **Weakness** may result from primary muscle disease or defective neuromuscular transmission, damage to the peripheral motor nerves or anterior horn cells in the spinal cord (lower motor neurone lesion), or from damage to the corticomotorneurone pathways (Figure 1.3) responsible for the cerebral control of movement (upper motor neurone lesion).

Such weakness may affect all four limbs (quadriplegia), the arm and leg on one side (hemiplegia), or both legs sparing the arms (paraplegia). A quadriplegia in an alert patient who can talk is usually a result of either primary muscle disease, a generalized peripheral neuropathy, or a high cervical cord lesion. Hemiplegia suggests damage to the opposite cerebral hemisphere, particularly if the face is involved. Paraplegia is most often the result of spinal cord damage, particularly when there is also disturbance of sphincter control. Isolated weakness of one limb (monoplegia) is frequently caused by damage to its motor nerves, although sometimes a monoplegia may arise from lesions in the cerebral cortex.

The pattern of **sensory symptoms** usually follows that of motor disturbance. Thus, a distal sensory loss in all four limbs suggests peripheral nerve disease. Sensory disturbance in a hemiplegic distribution suggests damage to the opposite cerebral hemisphere, particularly of the capsular sensory pathways, in which case the face is often involved. Hemiplegic

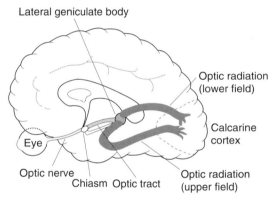

Figure 1.1 Medial sagittal view of the brain to show visual pathways; these traverse the brain from front to back.

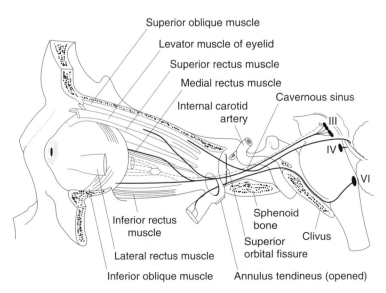

Figure 1.2 Course of the ocular motor nerves from the brainstem to the orbit (reproduced with permission from P Duus *Topical Diagnosis in Neurology*, Stuttgart: Georg Thieme Verlag).

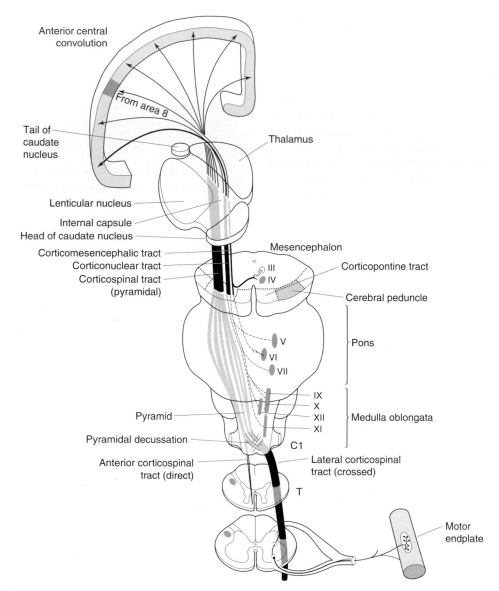

Figure 1.3 Course of corticospinal, pyramidal tract (reproduced with permission from P Duus *Topical Diagnosis in Neurology*, Stuttgart: Georg Thieme Verlag).

sensory disturbance on one side of the body with involvement of the face on the opposite side suggests damage in the brainstem (Figures 1.4, 1.5, 1.6). If the cranial nerves are not involved, sensory disturbances on one side of the body, with motor disturbances on the opposite side of the body, suggest damage to the spinal cord (Figures 1.3, 1.5). Sensory disturbance in both legs extending onto the trunk also points to a lesion of the spinal cord. Sensory loss affecting parts of one limb only is most often caused by a local peripheral nerve or root lesion.

These simple rules for interpretation of symptoms usually give the first clue to the likely anatomical site of damage responsible for the patient's complaints. Of course they are not infallible and many exceptions to such generalizations will be encountered in practice. However, they provide the easiest means of the first faltering steps in analysis of the anatomical site of the patient's lesion. The next stage is the physical examination.

Sensory   **Motor**

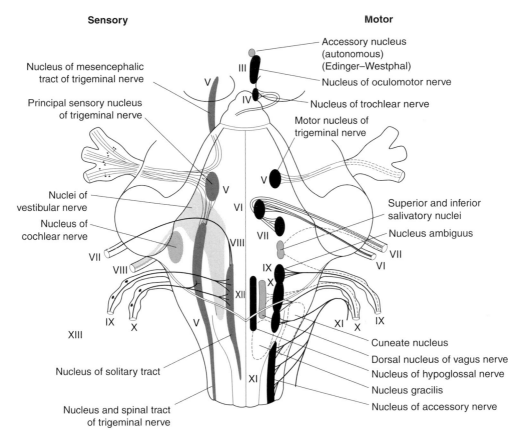

Nucleus of mesencephalic tract of trigeminal nerve

Principal sensory nucleus of trigeminal nerve

Accessory nucleus (autonomous) (Edinger–Westphal)

Nucleus of oculomotor nerve

Nucleus of trochlear nerve

Motor nucleus of trigeminal nerve

Nuclei of vestibular nerve

Nucleus of cochlear nerve

Superior and inferior salivatory nuclei

Nucleus ambiguus

Cuneate nucleus

Dorsal nucleus of vagus nerve

Nucleus of hypoglossal nerve

Nucleus gracilis

Nucleus of accessory nerve

Nucleus of solitary tract

Nucleus and spinal tract of trigeminal nerve

Figure 1.4 Cranial nerve nuclei viewed from behind. Sensory nuclei are on the left and motor nuclei are on the right (reproduced with permission from P Duus *Topical Diagnosis in Neurology*, Stuttgart: Georg Thieme Verlag).

Neurological examination will be dictated by the patient's history, which helps to determine that aspect of the nervous system requiring most detailed attention. The methods employed will be described fully later in this book, but some simple principles will be stated here.

When students approach a neurological patient for the first time, armed with a standard textbook of neurological examination, they may well find that it takes them up to 2 hours to complete the necessary bedside tests! When they see experienced neurologists completing the same task in less than 10 minutes they may think that they face an impossible apprenticeship. It cannot be stated too frequently that the secret of the art is to know what one is looking for.

In fact, neurologists divide the clinical examination conceptually into two halves. The first is a detailed evaluation of those parts of the nervous system to which attention has been drawn in the course of taking the patient's history. The second is a general screen of other sections of the nervous system which, by history, do not seem likely to be involved, but which have to be examined in every patient to ensure that nothing is missed.

To facilitate this method, neurological trainees perfect a routine of clinical examination sufficient to act as a simple screen of the nervous system, onto which they graft the extra detailed investigation of those sections to which their attention has been pointed. The routine screening examination, which can be undertaken very briefly in a matter of minutes, is learnt by repetition of the same sequence over and over again until it becomes second nature. For convenience, most start with a brief assessment of the mental faculties of the patient in the course of the interview, then move to the cranial nerves starting at

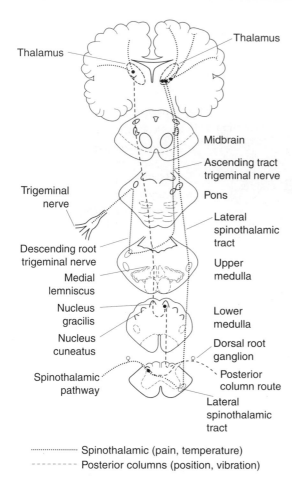

Figure 1.5 Ascending sensory pathways.

the top and working downwards. They then assess motor function of the limbs, including stance and gait, which is much easier to examine and usually is much more informative than the sensory examination, which they leave to the last. The details of this routine examination are discussed in Chapter 4.

One of the first problems that neurological beginners encounter is the ease with which apparent abnormalities are detected on careful examination. Frequently it is difficult to decide on the significance of minor degrees of apparent weakness, fleeting and inconsistent sensory signs, slight asymmetry of the tendon reflexes, slightly less facility of repetitive movements of the left hand in a right-handed patient, or a few jerks of the eyes on extreme lateral gaze. To build a neurological diagnosis on minor deficits such as these is courting disaster.

It is a useful exercise to classify each abnormality discovered as a 'hard' or 'soft' sign. 'Hard' signs are unequivocally abnormal – an absent ankle jerk even on reinforcement, a clear-cut extensor plantar response, definite wasting of the small muscles of the hand, or absent vibration sense. Any final anatomical diagnosis must provide an explanation of such 'hard' signs. 'Soft' signs, on the other hand, such as those described above, are unreliable and best ignored when initially formulating a diagnosis. Base your conclusions on the 'hard' signs, and then see if any of the 'soft' signs that you have discovered may put the diagnosis into doubt. If so, go back and repeat that section of the examination and make up your mind again whether or not the 'soft' sign is real. Students will find that neurology becomes increasingly easy the more confident they become in discarding unwanted 'soft' signs, as they become more experienced in determining the range of normal. This they will only achieve by constant repeated routine examination of the normal human nervous system.

> The interpretation of physical signs found upon clinical examination of a neurological patient depends heavily upon a practical knowledge of neuroanatomy.

This is not the place to dwell upon this aspect of neuroscience, but it is worth emphasizing which parts of neuroanatomy are of greatest value to the clinical neurologist.

The visual system spans the whole of the head from the front to back, so commonly is involved by intracranial lesions (Figure 1.1). The mechanisms controlling eye movements range from the cortex through the brainstem and external ocular nerves to the eye muscles themselves. Consequently, ocular motor function is frequently damaged by intracranial lesions. A careful anatomical knowledge of the visual and ocular motor pathways is essential to the trainee neurologist. So, too, is an understanding of the individual cranial nerves in the brainstem, their course through the basal cisterns and exits through their appointed foramina in the skull (Figure 1.6), and their distribution to their extracranial target organs.

In as far as the motor system is concerned, it is essential to be able to distinguish between the characteristics of primary muscle disease, a lower motor

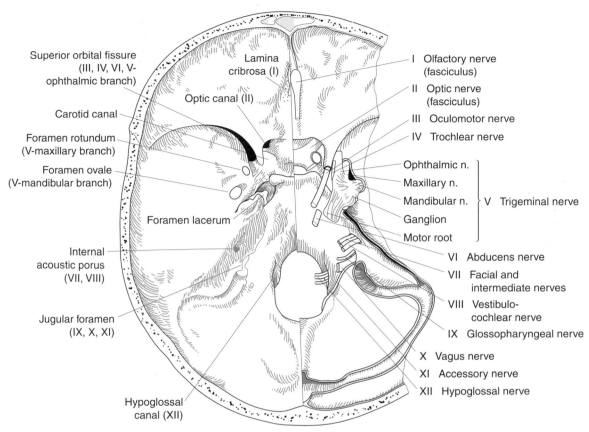

Figure 1.6 View of the skull base. On the left side are shown the exit and entry foramina and on the right side the stumps of the cranial nerves (n.) (reproduced with permission from P Duus *Topical Diagnosis in Neurology*, Stuttgart: Georg Thieme Verlag).

neurone lesion and an upper motor neurone lesion. Likewise, it is important to be able to detect the characteristic pattern of weakness in a patient with a hemiplegia, and to be able to distinguish this from the pattern of weakness that occurs with lesions affecting individual nerve roots or peripheral nerves. In the case of sensory findings, it is crucial to be able to recognize the pattern of sensory loss associated with damage to the spinal cord, or to individual nerve roots and peripheral nerves. The student should be thoroughly familiar with a cross-section of the spinal cord (Figure 1.7) in order to be able to interpret the motor and sensory consequences of spinal cord damage. Likewise, they should know the segmental distribution of motor and sensory roots, and the characteristic motor and sensory consequences of damage to individual large peripheral nerves (see Figure 4.19).

These are the minimum fundamentals of neuroanatomy required for neurological practice. Without them students will be lost trying to interpret the results of their examinations. A short period spent refreshing the memory on these basic items prior to neurological training will be time well spent. It will allow the student to enjoy that period of neurological apprenticeship in learning about neurological disease, rather than being held back through ignorance of the essential first steps that must be mastered before any sensible discussion about neurological illness can be entertained.

From this brief introduction, it will be seen that the first stage of neurological diagnosis, the anatomical site of the lesion, is deduced initially from the history, which points towards the likely parts of the nervous system to examine in detail, and from the neurological examination itself, which confirms and elaborates,

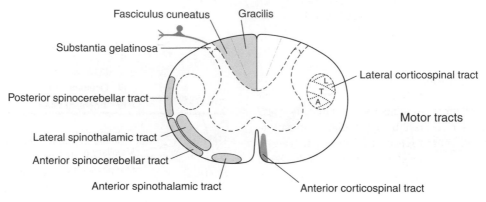

Figure 1.7 Cross-section of the spinal cord.

or refutes, the initial impression gained after hearing the patient's symptoms.

> At the end of history taking and clinical examination, neurologists should, with confidence, be able to state what portions of the nervous system are affected. They can then pass to the second stage of defining the likely pathological cause.

PATHOLOGICAL DIAGNOSIS

> The site of damage to the nervous system will obviously give some clue as to the possible pathological cause.

An example of pathological diagnosis is: evidence of a lesion affecting the optic chiasm, indicated by the presence of a bitemporal hemianopia, suggests the possibility of a pituitary tumour.

> However, the time-course of the illness gives the greatest clue to the likely pathology responsible.

Neurologists take great care to establish during history taking whether the onset of symptoms was sudden or gradual, and whether the subsequent course has been one of recovery, persistence with stable deficit, or progression of disability. Attention

to these simple points provides the best guide to the likely pathology.

> **History**
> - An illness of sudden, abrupt onset followed by subsequent gradual recovery is likely to be a result of vascular disease
> - An illness of gradual onset but relentless progression is likely to be caused by a tumour or degenerative condition
> - An illness characterized by episodes of neurological deficit lasting days or weeks, followed by subsequent partial or complete recovery, is suggestive of multiple sclerosis
> - An illness consisting of brief episodes of neurological disability lasting minutes or hours is typical of transient ischaemic attacks, migraine, or epilepsy.

Other factors that will help to define the likely pathological cause of a neurological illness are the age and sex of the patient. Thus, the sudden onset of a focal cerebral deficit lasting half an hour or so in an otherwise healthy 20-year-old woman taking the oral contraceptive pill is almost certainly migraine. A similar cerebral deficit of acute onset lasting an hour or so in a 65-year-old diabetic man who is a heavy smoker, suggests the presence of primary cerebrovascular disease as the cause.

In general, attention to these three main categories of information, the site of the lesion, its mode of onset and subsequent course, and the age and sex of the patient, will point to the likely cause of the illness.

An important rule of thumb that is worth emphasizing at this point is that any neurological illness that is progressive must be considered to be the result of a tumour until proven otherwise. One major task of neurology is to detect those benign tumours that can compress the brain, cranial nerves, or spinal cord to cause progressive neurological deficit, which can be halted or reversed by appropriate neurosurgical treatment. Thus progressive blindness not caused by local eye disease, progressive unilateral deafness, a progressive hemiparesis, or a progressive spastic paraparesis all warrant full investigation to exclude a treatable tumour or other compressive lesion as the cause.

SPECIAL INVESTIGATIONS

From the information obtained by the patient's history and examination, the neurologist will formulate a provisional anatomical and pathological diagnosis. With common neurological diseases no further investigation is required; for example, migraine is diagnosed solely on the basis of the history and the absence of any abnormal neurological signs on examination. Other patients, however, require special investigation to confirm, refute, or refine the provisional clinical diagnosis. The principles of special neurological tests will now be described, but detailed findings will be mentioned in connection with specific diseases to be described later. It is worth emphasizing at this point that neurological tests require careful evaluation in the light of the individual clinical problem. Erroneous conclusions from neuroimaging or electrophysiological investigation may arise if tests are interpreted in the absence of clinical information.

Unlike many branches of medicine, it is often difficult or sometimes impossible to obtain appropriate biopsy material to establish the diagnosis in many neurological patients. Biopsy of muscle or a peripheral sensory nerve is used routinely, but for obvious reasons the brain and spinal cord are relatively inaccessible. The special techniques that have been devised for examining these structures, which include those of neuroimaging, clinical neurophysiology, and examination of the cerebrospinal fluid (CSF), necessarily give indirect information.

ELECTRODIAGNOSTIC TESTS

Electroencephalography

The discovery that the electrical activity of the brain could be recorded through the skull using surface electrodes applied to the scalp was remarkable. The technique of electroencephalography (EEG) has now been refined into a routine method of examining brain function. Approximately 40 electrodes are secured to the scalp at standard positions, and the small electrical signals obtained between pairs of electrodes linked in standard arrays are amplified and displayed. Conventionally eight or sixteen channels are recorded. The individual signals are only a few microvolts in amplitude, so artefacts introduced by extraneous interference, eye movements, muscle contraction, or whole body movement must be scrupulously avoided or rejected.

EEG

The normal EEG is characterized by the presence of rhythmic alpha activity (at a frequency around 10 Hz) evident more in posterior channels and with the eyes shut. Abnormalities of EEG consist either of generalized changes in frequency of electrical activity, or focal abnormalities affecting specific regions.

The background EEG activity may be generally slowed into the theta (5–7 Hz) or delta (2–4 Hz) ranges by diffuse cerebral disease, such as that caused by inflammatory or metabolic encephalopathies, for example, drug intoxication or liver failure. Local areas of cerebral abnormality resulting from infarction, trauma or tumour, may be indicated by a focal area of slowing of EEG activity. However, it is worth remembering that the EEG cannot explore all areas of the brain so a normal EEG by no means excludes cerebral damage. The surface EEG reflects the electrical activity of the underlying cerebral cortex so that extensive lesions of the deeper structures, such

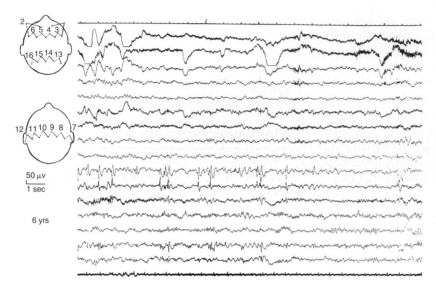

Figure 1.8 Electroencephalogram of a boy with a benign focal epilepsy. Focal spike discharges are seen in the right sylvian region (channels 10 and 11).

50 μv
1 sec

6 yrs

as thalamus and basal ganglia, and of the posterior fossa regions may not cause any EEG abnormality. Even lesions of the temporal lobes may not be evident in the surface EEG; these structures are on the undersurface of the brain. Special techniques such as placement of electrodes in the nasopharynx or via sphenoidal needles inserted in front of the ears, or needles through the foramina ovale, may be required to detect temporal lobe abnormalities.

Another problem in interpreting the presence of an abnormality of brain function indicated by the EEG, is that it does not suggest the pathological cause. In general, neuroradiological studies, especially computerized tomography (CT) and, better still, MRI scanning, are more appropriate for patients suspected of having focal lesions of the brain, for they will give further information on the probable cause. In contrast, CT and MRI scanning and other neuroradiological techniques may reveal no abnormalities in patients with severe metabolic or inflammatory brain disease, which produce profound changes in EEG activity.

> The EEG finds its greatest use in the investigation of patients with epilepsy, in whom it can detect a wide range of abnormalities, including frank seizure discharges.

An EEG of an epileptic patient may consist of either focal spike or sharp wave discharges (Figure 1.8) arising in relation to an irritative lesion affecting the cerebral cortex, or of generalized spike and wave abnormalities that occur in primary generalized epilepsies such as petit mal (Figure 1.9). The details of such EEG changes will be discussed in Chapter 15, but it is important to note at this point that the EEG cannot diagnose epilepsy. A small proportion of those with undoubted seizures, particularly those arising in the temporal lobe, have normal surface EEG recordings, and a small proportion of the normal population who have never had a fit may show EEG abnormalities similar to those found in patients with epilepsy. A repeat EEG, and a sleep record, will increase the chances of finding an abnormality in patients with epilepsy. More detailed EEG studies are also a very important part of the work-up in epileptic patients being screened for a possible focus amenable to surgical excision. The EEG using prolonged recordings and accompanied by video-telemetry has proved a most important test in diagnosing both unusual forms of epilepsy, particularly seizures with a frontal lobe origin, and in the diagnosis of non-epileptic seizures.

The EEG is also a very important diagnostic aid in a number of uncommon diffuse encephalopathic processes, such as spongiform encephalopathies (Creutzfeldt–Jakob disease Figure 1.10), herpes encephalitis, sub-acute sclerosing panencephalitis, where a more specific diffuse EEG disturbance is present, sometimes accompanied by periodic lateralized epileptiform discharges. The EEG may also be very helpful in the diagnosis of some types of

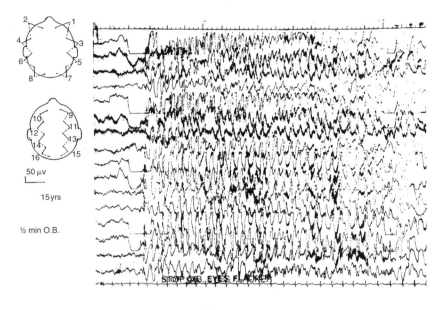

Figure 1.9 Electroencephalogram of a 15-year-old girl with absence seizures. Bursts of symmetrical spike-wave activity are seen during hyperventilation (O.B.) lasting several seconds and accompanied by loss of awareness with eyelid flickering (O.B., overbreathing).

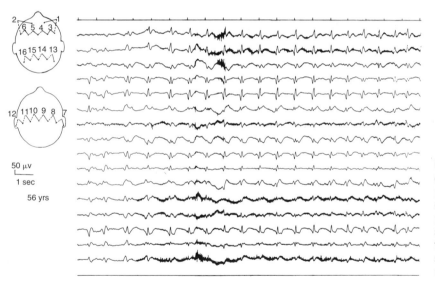

Figure 1.10 Electroencephalogram of a 56-year-old patient with Creutzfeldt–Jakob disease. The record shows periodic 1-second-long duration sharp waves in all areas. At this time the patient was mute, spastic and showed frequent myoclonic jerks.

epileptic status, particularly if minor seizures have been recurring serially. The EEG may show changes preceding clinical features in certain disturbances such a hepatic encephalopathy.

Evoked potential studies

Standard electroencephalographic recordings have been supplemented by the addition of evoked potential investigations. Early on it was discovered that abnormal discharges could be provoked in a proportion of epileptic patients by repetitive photic stimulation with flash stimuli. This principle has been extended to computerized averaging of the electrical activity generated by individual sensory stimuli repeated hundreds of times to generate an averaged evoked potential signal. In the visual domain, the stimulus now used most widely is that of a black and white chequer-board that is moved in front of the

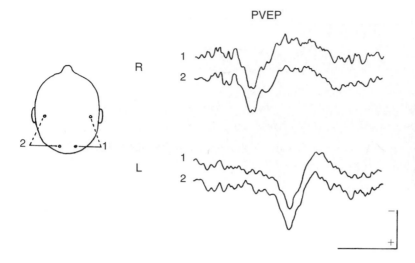

PVEP

R

L

Figure 1.11 Pattern visual evoked potential (PVEP). Patient with optic neuritis in the left eye: visual acuity right 6/5, left 6/9. Traces (1) from right and (2) left hemisphere. Upper pair of traces from the right eye are normal showing a major positive component with a latency of 100 ms. Lower pair of traces from left eye showing gross delay with major positive component's latency of 160 ms with preservation of amplitude. Calibration: amplitude 5 mV; latency 100 ms.

eyes. Each movement of the chequer-board is used to trigger the recording of electrical activity from the surface of the scalp over the occipital cortex. The average of a series of several hundred such responses is computed after stimulation of each eye separately. The latency of this **visual evoked response** can be measured to, say the first major positive peak following the movement of the pattern, and the size of such a component of the visual evoked response can be recorded (Figure 1.11). It has been found that demyelinating lesions of the optic nerve may reliably produce delays in such a visual evoked response, indicating the presence of an optic nerve lesion even in the absence of any clinical symptoms or signs of such damage. This technique now is widely used in the investigation of patients suspected of having multiple sclerosis. The method of evoking visual responses to pattern stimulation can be adapted to half-field or even quarter-field stimulation in patients suspected of hemianopic or other visual disturbances. Pattern visual evoked potentials (PVEPs) can also prove useful in following patients with parachiasmal lesions, and can be very helpful in assessing non-organic visual loss.

Electroretinograms (ERGs) using a flash stimulus enable the study of retinal function. Using a dark-adapted eye it is possible to look at rod function, whereas white flicker stimulation under photopic conditions examines cone function. Pattern ERGs using a chequer-board stimulus test both central retinal and retinal ganglion cell functions. By combining ERGs with PVEPs it is now possible to obtain a very accurate electrophysiological assessment of the anterior visual pathways, including the macula, retinal ganglion cells, rods and cones, and optic nerves. The findings in a patient with an ischaemic optic neuropathy differ from those found in the case of a demyelinating optic neuritis.

Similar principles underlie the use of **brainstem auditory evoked potentials (BSAEP)** to investigate the auditory pathways. The electrical activity recorded from the lateral surface of the scalp, in response to a standard click stimulus delivered through headphones to one or other ear, is averaged for a few hundred responses (Figure 1.12). The resulting auditory evoked response consists of a whole series of components, each one of which has been carefully established by neurophysiological experiments to arise from activity in different segments of the auditory pathway. Thus cochlear activity can be distinguished from that of a number of brainstem nuclei and fibre tracts, which can be distinguished from activity in the auditory cortex. The BSAEPs are useful in measuring brainstem function, to screen for the presence of an acoustic neuroma, and in the evaluation of patients with prolonged depressed conscious levels.

Averaged **somatosensory evoked potentials (SSEPs)** can be recorded from electrodes placed over the sensory cortex and over the spinal cord, in response to electrical stimulation of the contralateral digits or peripheral nerves of the arms or legs. The SSEPs give information about conduction proximally in the roots and centrally in the sensory pathways ascending via the dorsal column and

BSAEP

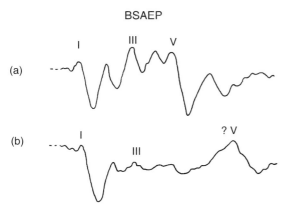

Figure 1.12 Brainstem auditory evoked potentials (BSAEP). (a) Normal trace: wave I probably arises from the cochlear nerve, that is, peripheral function; wave III probably arises from the superior olive, that is, in the lower pons; wave V probably arises from the inferior colliculus, that is, more centrally. (b) Patient with multiple sclerosis showing grossly increased central conduction and loss of waveform (note the different latencies from I to V (a) and (b)). Calibration: amplitude 0.3 mV; latency 2 ms.

medial lemniscus to relay through the thalamus and reach the parietal cortex. For example in upper limb studies, recordings are usually made over Erb's point, over C2 or C7 and the contralateral parietal cortex. Prolongation of latency measurements would support the presence of damage specific to that site; for example, a delay from Erb's point to C2 or C7 occurs with a spinal cord lesion.

Transcranial magnetic stimulation

Over the past 10 years it has become possible to stimulate the motor cortex using a magnetic coil and to record the motor response in a distal muscle in a contralateral limb. Stimulation at other sites such as the motor roots at the level of the spinal cord, and the peripheral motor nerves, allows measurement of the latencies in these various pathways. Central delay in the corticomotorneurone pathway may occur for example in demyelination, and there is often a reduction in amplitude of the evoked muscle response in motor neurone disease. This still remains largely a research tool but its use is spreading into diagnostic clinics. It again has proved helpful in assessing functional motor disturbances.

Electromyography and nerve conduction studies

In the same way that electrical activity of the brain can be recorded by the EEG, the electrical activity of contracting muscles can be recorded either by surface electrodes or through needles inserted directly into the muscle itself.

Surface recordings pick up and average activity from many individual motor units, while needle recordings can detect the activity from single motor units or even single muscle fibres if the recording surface is made small enough. Needle recordings of electromyographic activity in weak muscles may be used to decide upon the cause of muscle weakness. Motor unit action potentials in primary muscle disease (myopathies) are characteristically reduced in size and shortened in duration. Spontaneous activity in the form of fibrillation potentials occurs in muscles denervated by damage to peripheral nerves, nerve roots, or anterior horn cells. Muscle action potentials become abnormally large as a result of collateral re-innervation in anterior horn cell disease. The normal picture of electromyography (EMG) activity that occurs on muscle contraction when recorded with needle electrodes (the interference pattern) is distorted in upper motor neurone disease in a manner distinctive from that seen in denervation or primary muscle disease. Single fibre recordings may reveal instability of neuromuscular transmission ('jitter') in a variety of conditions, but particularly in myasthenia gravis. In the latter condition, the muscle is incapable of responding to repetitive nerve stimulation, showing characteristic electrical and contractile fatigue.

The function of peripheral nerves may also be assessed by electrical techniques.

Motor nerve conduction can be studied by stimulating a mixed nerve containing motor fibres, and recording the resulting compound action potential from the muscle activated by surface or needle electrodes. Motor nerve conduction velocity can be calculated by stimulating the motor nerve at two sites

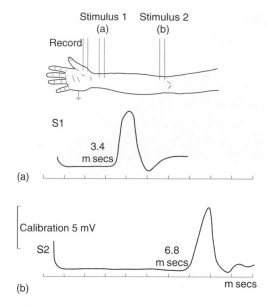

Figure 1.13 Motor conduction measured in the median nerve by stimulation (S1) at the wrist and (S2) at the elbow, recording from abductor pollicis brevis. The distance between S1 and S2 can be measured and the velocity calculated, as the difference in the two latencies is known (6.8−3.4 = 3.4 ms).

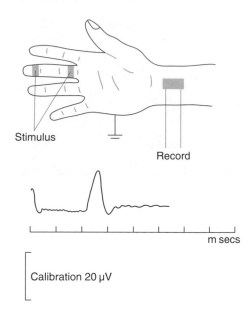

Figure 1.14 Sensory conduction measured in the median nerve stimulating the middle finger and recording from the nerve at the wrist.

proximally and distally (Figure 1.13), measuring the difference in latency to the onset of the muscle action potential, and the distance between the two sites of stimulation. Motor conduction through a particular region, for example, in the ulnar nerve across the elbow, may be calculated by measuring conduction velocity in response to stimulation above and below the site of interest. Sensory nerve conduction can be studied by stimulating pure sensory nerves, such as those of the digits with ring electrodes, and recording the nerve action potential with surface or needle electrodes applied close to the appropriate nerve trunk (Figure 1.14). For sensory studies, it is usually necessary to average many responses to obtain a reproducible wave form. Sensory nerve conduction may also be measured by recording somatosensory cortical evoked potentials in response to stimulation of peripheral nerves at different proximal and distal sites, calculating the difference in latency and the distance between the two sites in the usual manner.

The most sensitive test for detecting a generalized peripheral neuropathy is the measurement of the amplitudes of sensory and nerve action potentials in an arm and leg, together with the conduction velocities.

Most nerve conduction studies are undertaken on peripheral segments of nerves, and it is more difficult to study proximal nerve roots. However, certain electrical reflexes may be employed to investigate their function, including the H reflex, which is elicited on stimulation of a mixed nerve with low intensity electrical shocks. These selectively activate spindle afferent fibres to produce an electrical analogue of the tendon jerk. Likewise, the activity in proximal segments of motor nerves may be assessed by recording the F wave, which results from retrograde stimulation of motor fibres invading the anterior horn cell to produce a descending volley which is subsequently detected from the surface or needle EMG.

Routine nerve conduction studies look at conduction in large calibre, fast conducting fibres. Modern techniques enable conduction in the small fibres, relaying pain and temperature, to be measured in the same way by estimating thermal thresholds quantitatively using specially designed instruments.

CEREBROSPINAL FLUID

Samples of CSF may be obtained with relative ease at the bedside by lumbar puncture. The technique requires some practice, but once mastered is simple and usually painless.

> However, when there is an intracranial or intraspinal mass lesion, lumbar puncture carries a serious risk of causing rapid deterioration in function as a result of shifts of intracranial or intraspinal contents.

Because of the risks involved, lumbar puncture is not an investigation to be considered if a patient is suspected of harbouring an intracranial or intraspinal tumour.

Indications for brain imaging prior to lumbar puncture
- Signs or symptoms of raised intracranial pressure
- Focal neurological deficit
- A fixed dilated or poorly reactive pupil
- Coma or a rapidly deteriorating consciousness level
- Signs of posterior fossa lesion (e.g. dysarthria, ataxia).

Lumbar puncture is also contraindicated in the presence of local skin sepsis in the lumbar region. Lumbar puncture is essential to the diagnosis of meningitis and subarachnoid haemorrhage, and is a valuable adjunct to the diagnosis of a number of inflammatory conditions such as multiple sclerosis (MS) or encephalitis.

For **lumbar puncture** the patient is best positioned lying on the side, flexed and with the spine horizontal (Figure 1.15a). The needle is usually introduced at the L3/4 interspace, which is indicated by a line drawn joining the tips of the iliac crests (Figure 1.15a). It is worth recalling in adults that the spinal cord usually ends at the lower border of L1 so a needle inserted into the subarachnoid space below this level will enter the sac containing the cauda equina floating in CSF. Local anaesthetic is used for the skin and immediate tissues. After allowing time for this to be effective, a sharp, disposable fine lumbar puncture needle (22 gauge) with stilette in position is introduced through the skin and advanced through the space between the two spinous processes. The needle point usually needs to be directed slightly forwards (anteriorly). At a depth

of about 4–7 cm firmer resistance may be encountered as the ligamentum flavum is reached. Beyond this there is a slight 'give' as the needle punctures the dura. The stilette is then removed and clear CSF will drip out of the needle if this has been correctly positioned. If no fluid appears or bone is encountered, it is probable that the needle is not in the correct place. The stilette should be re-inserted, the needle partially withdrawn and then advanced at a slightly different angle. The commonest causes of failure are that the needle is not in the midline, or is at too great an angle with the skin (Figure 1.15b).

Complications of lumbar puncture
- Low pressure headache – postural, worse erect occurs in approximately 20%
- Backache
- Introduced infection
- Precipitation of pressure cone with a cranial or spinal mass lesion
- Subarachnoid or epidural haemorrhage (anticoagulants, bleeding disorder)
- Cranial nerve palsies – diplopia from CN VI
- Dermoid formation.

The CSF findings characteristic of specific conditions will be discussed later in this book, but a few general principles will be mentioned now. It is crucial always to obtain the maximum information from examination of the CSF.

Normal cerebrospinal fluid (CSF) values
Clear colourless fluid

Pressure	40–180 mm
Cells	0–5 lymphocytes/mm^3
Sugar	2.5–4.4 mmol/l
	(>60% of blood glucose)
Lactate	<2.8 mmol/l
Protein	0.2–0.5 g/l
IgG	<14% of total protein
	(70% of serum globulin)
Volume (adult)	150 ml

If the presence of blood is suspected, three sequential tubes of CSF should be collected to establish whether the fluid is uniformly and consistently bloodstained, or whether the initial bloody CSF gradually clears, as occurs as a result of a traumatic

(a)

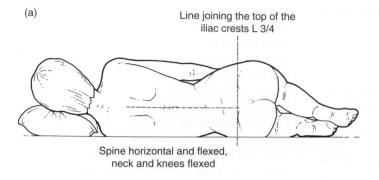

Line joining the top of the
iliac crests L 3/4

Spine horizontal and flexed,
neck and knees flexed

(b)

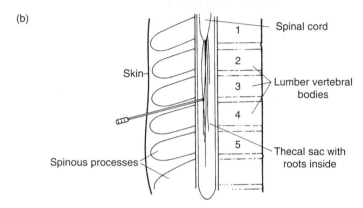

Skin

Spinous processes

1 — Spinal cord

2

3 — Lumber vertebral
bodies

4

5

Thecal sac with
roots inside

Figure 1.15 (a) Position of patient for lumbar
puncture. (b) Diagram to show correctly
positioned needle within the subarachnoid space.

tap. Likewise, when haemorrhage is suspected, the sample should be centrifuged and the supernatant examined for the presence of xanthochromia, which indicates pathological bleeding rather than the consequences of trauma at the time of lumbar puncture. If infection is suspected, the CSF sugar may be an invaluable guide to the presence of bacterial or fungal inflammation. However, the CSF glucose can only be interpreted in the light of the blood level obtained at the same time. Thus, bacterial or fungal meningitis is suggested if the CSF contains an excess of cells in the presence of a glucose concentration of 2 mmol/l or less than 40% of the blood glucose concentration (Table 1.6). If there are red cells in significant numbers resulting from a traumatic tap, a rough guide suggests that about 10 white cells may be allowed for every 7000 red cells.

Specific abnormalities of CSF protein content may be invaluable in diagnosis, particularly the excess gammaglobulin found in many patients with MS, who also commonly exhibit the presence of oligoclonal bands of gammaglobulin on electrophoresis. Nowadays, these are most reliably demonstrated by isoelectric focusing. The synthesis of immune globulins in the central nervous system

is not pathognomonic of MS and may occur in a number of inflammatory/infective disorders, for example sarcoidosis, syphilis, Behçet's disease. The CSF immunoglobulin G (IgG) index is a means of evaluating the rate of IgG synthesis in the CSF. The CSF IgG index = (IgG CSF × albumin serum)/(albumin CSF × IgG serum). Normally the value ranges from 0 to 0.77. Higher values suggest increased IgG synthesis, as in MS.

The CSF may also give useful information in a number of disorders: for example the CSF angiotensin-converting enzyme levels may be raised in neurosarcoidosis or the measurement of 14-3-3 protein in patients suspected of having Creutzfeldt–Jakob disease. In patients with pineal region germ cell tumours markers may be found in the CSF, such as alpha-fetoprotein in yolk sac tumours, beta-human chorionic gonadotropin in choriocarcinoma and human placental alkaline phosphatase in germ cell tumours.

Examination of CSF for specific bacteria or fungi, such as the tubercle bacilli or cryptococcus, or for malignant cells requires considerable care and experience. The immunodetection of specific bacterial antigens and antibodies has also aided diagnosis

Table 1.6 Abnormal cerebrospinal fluid findings

Finding	Interpretation

Elevated polymorph count low glucose	meningitis:
	     bacterial
	     TB early
	     fungal
	     viral (uncommon)
	 parameningeal infection

Elevated lymphocyte count low glucose	meningitis:
	     partially treated bacterial
	     TB
	     listeriosis
	     fungal
	     viral
	 carcinomatous meningitis
	 sarcoidosis

Elevated lymphocyte count normal or low glucose	meningitis:
	     partially treated bacterial
	     TB
	     listeriosis
	     spirochaetal – syphilis, *Borrelia burgdorferi*
	     Mycoplasma pneumoniae
	     viral – mumps, enterovirus, HIV, HSV
	     fungal – cryptococcus

Atypical aseptic meningitis	sarcoidosis SLE vasculitis drug-induced – NSAIs (ibuprofen, naproxen, sulindac) post-traumatic lumbar puncture post serial major epileptic seizures

TB, tuberculosis; HIV, human immunodeficiency virus; HSV, herpes simplex virus, NSAIDs, non-steroidal anti-inflammatory drugs.

of infections, particularly in some patients who have already been started on an antibiotic prior to examination of their CSF. Latex agglutination tests for bacterial antigens may detect *Haemophilus influenzae* B, *Streptococcus pneumoniae* and *Neisseria meningitidis* in over two-thirds of patients. Polymerase chain reactions to detect bacterial DNA may also be useful, for example in tuberculous meningitis or neurological Lyme disease.

It will be apparent that thought must be given before lumbar puncture to what information is to be sought from the material obtained, and care must be exercised in ensuring that the samples are delivered to the appropriate laboratories and individuals. Finally, lumbar puncture provides an opportunity to record CSF pressure using simple manometry, which should be undertaken routinely.

Muscle and nerve biopsy

Muscle biopsy is undertaken routinely in most patients suspected of primary muscle disease, the sample being removed from a weak muscle that has not previously been subjected to electromyographic needling. Routine histology is supplemented by histochemistry, to type muscle fibre populations, and by biochemical investigation of muscle energy metabolism. Electron microscopy may also be necessary.

Special staining with immunolabelling may also add information: for example, the use of dystrophin in Duchenne muscular dystrophy. Muscle biopsy also affords the opportunity to examine small blood vessels in patients suspected of inflammatory diseases such as polyarteritis nodosa. In patients thought to have giant cell arteritis, however, it is usual to biopsy the temporal artery directly.

Nerve biopsy is used less frequently, but it is simple and safe to remove the cutaneous branch of the sural nerve at the ankle, which leaves no motor deficit and only a small patch of sensory loss. In a few patients there may be complaints of pain from the biopsy site. Examination of nerve biopsy in patients with peripheral nerve disease may confirm the presence of axonal damage, demyelination, or a combination of these. The tissue examined may also reveal evidence of an arteritis, or of infiltration by substances such as amyloid or lymphoma. Quantitative studies can be undertaken, which look at the size and type of the nerve fibres present, and teased fibre preparations may show the presence of segmental or generalized demyelination. Special staining techniques may be useful in evaluating certain patterns of neuropathy in association with dysproteinaemias or immune-mediated diseases.

Other investigations

Many other investigations are employed in individual patients with neurological disease; for instance, skin, liver, rectal, or marrow biopsy may be required for the diagnosis of a number of storage diseases that cause progressive encephalopathy in childhood. Biopsy of lymph glands may be useful in the diagnosis of a number of disorders, particularly in lymphomas, in carcinomatosis and in sarcoidosis. Occasionally biopsy of the brain itself or the meninges is required to establish the diagnosis in progressive obscure cerebral disorders. Image-linked stereotactic brain biopsies now allow very precise sampling of areas of abnormal signal within the brain substance.

Many metabolic and hormonal diseases may affect the nervous system, so that a wide range of biochemical tests, such as examination of serum electrolytes, liver, renal and bone function, may be required, as will tests of thyroid, parathyroid, pancreas, adrenal and pituitary function. Neurosyphilis, Lyme disease and now AIDS are the great mimics of neurological disorders so that serological tests such as a *Treponema pallidum* haemagglutination test, tests for IgG antibodies for *Borrelia* and human immunodeficiency virus titres are essential to exclude these disorders. A wide range of immunological tests may also be used to assess a variety of connective tissue disorders and an increasing number of neurological conditions where antibodies may be detected to aid diagnosis; for example, anti-acetylcholine receptor antibodies are found in most patients with generalized myasthenia gravis (sero-positive) and muscle specific kinase antibodies may be found in many sero-negative myasthenic patients. IgG antibodies to P- or Q-type voltage-gated calcium channels may be found in patients with the Lambert–Eaton syndrome.

REFERENCES AND FURTHER READING

Aminoff MJ (1992) *Electrodiagnosis in Clinical Neurology*, 3rd edn. New York: Churchill Livingstone.

Binnie CD, Prior PF (1994) Neurological investigations: electroencephalography. *Journal of Neurology, Neurosurgery and Psychiatry*, **57**:1308–1319.

Duus P (1998) *Topical Diagnosis in Neurology*, 3rd revised edn. Stuttgart: Georg Thieme.

Fishman GA, Birch DG, Holder GE, Brigell MG (2001) *Electrophysiologic Testing in Disorders of the Retina, Optic Nerve, and Visual Pathway*, 2nd edn. Ophthalmology Monograph 2. San Francisco: The Foundation of the American Academy of Ophthalmology.

Greenstein B, Greenstein A (2000) *Color Atlas of Neuroscience – Neuroanatomy and Neurophysiology*. Stuttgart: Georg Thieme.

MacMillan JC, Harper PS (1995) Clinical genetics in neurological disease. In: Wiles GM (ed.) *Management of Neurological Diseases*. London: BMJ Publishing Group.

Mills KR (1999) *Magnetic Stimulation of the Human Nervous System*. Oxford: Oxford University Press.

Perkin GD (1989) An analysis of 7835 successive new out-patient referrals. *Journal of Neurology, Neurosurgery and Psychiatry*, **52**:447–448.

Warlow C (1991) *Handbook of Neurology*. Oxford: Blackwell Scientific Publications Ltd.

CHAPTER 2

NEUROIMAGING

J.M. Stevens

INTRODUCTION

Of all diagnostic tests in neurological disease, imaging often has the most decisive influence on management. Nowadays the most useful imaging modalities are harmless to patients, and imaging equipment generally has been appropriately prioritized and is widely available. In most situations, the only modality to consider is magnetic resonance imaging (MRI), and in patients for whom MRI cannot be performed, X-ray computerized tomography (CT) is usually satisfactory. The latter still has great utility, and is the test of first choice to exclude surgical emergencies. Angiography is rarely indicated for diagnostic purposes, and such diagnostic applications that remain are best implemented by non-invasive methods. Myelography is indicated only in patients who cannot undergo MRI. Plain X-rays of the skull are rarely helpful, but a limited role for plain X-rays of the spine remains.

PLAIN X-RAYS

Skull

Several textbooks are devoted to the interpretation of skull X-rays. However, it was recognized that diagnostic changes were either too infrequent or too non-specific to be of real help. Notable exceptions, however, were the investigation of visual failure and hearing loss, where specific changes diagnostic of the commonest surgical causes were present in around 90% of cases. However because MRI or CT was required anyway in order to plan treatment, skull films became redundant.

Identification of skull fractures is now the commonest reason for performing a skull X-ray. Although patients with skull fractures are more likely to have intracranial haemorrhage than those without, the risk is predicted more reliably by clinical criteria.

Spine

Trauma

Plain X-rays probably remain the most appropriate test in the initial investigation. **X-rays of the cervical spine are indicated after head injury if the patient is unconscious or unable to be assessed, or when there is clinical evidence of neck injury.** Considerable variability in reporting of post-traumatic spine films has been recorded. Attention needs to be paid to the soft tissues as well as to vertebral alignment and separation, especially the pre-vertebral soft tissues above the cricoid cartilage of the larynx, which should be no more than 2–3 mm thick in adults, and slightly thicker in children, but never convex anteriorly. Instability may be excluded by careful flexion and extension views after pain and muscle spasm has subsided. Delayed instability is a problem especially in two situations: after unrecognized fractures of the odontoid and following easily reducible or self-reducing rotatory subluxation of the cervical spine with unilateral locked facets.

Instability

Plain X-rays remain the best modality to demonstrate spinal instability in conditions not linked to trauma, such as rheumatoid arthritis and other disorders, and in the variety of connective tissue disorders, which are often hereditary, where spinal instability is common, such as Down's syndrome. Carefully performed flexion and extension views to the extremes of tolerable movement demonstrate subluxation, and establish whether it is reducible.

Spinal cord and root compression

Spondylotic spinal stenosis may be deduced by the presence of osteophytes or inferred by a degenerative spondylolisthesis, but not with sufficient sensitivity to be used as a realistic screening test. Similarly spinal metastases and other tumours that destroy and erode bone need to remove 50–70% of bone mass before it becomes apparent on plain X-rays.

Tumours of the spinal cord and cauda equina

Tumours of the spinal cord and cauda equina may result in reasonably characteristic focal or regional expansion of the canal, but only in about 30% of children with such tumours (or syringomyelia) and in about 12% of adults.

Osteomyelitis

Plain X-ray is still frequently the first investigation that alerts physicians to the possibility of spinal osteomyelitis. The most important sign is progressive loss of the vertebral end-plates. Unusual forms of osteomyelitis are usually misdiagnosed as metastases, even on CT and MRI.

Congenital abnormalities

Most congenital abnormalities are occult incidental findings, but some, which involve neural structures, can have a characteristic appearance on plain X-ray, such as diastematomyelia and lipomyelomeningodysplasia. These too may be incidental findings.

Other causes

Symptoms such as headache, occipital neuralgia, and dizziness have been attributed to disease in the cervical spine, usually cervical spondylosis. Many plain X-rays of the cervical spine are requested with this in mind, but the significance of any abnormalities shown is, at best, doubtful. Cervical ribs are most easily recognized on plain X-rays and are sometimes implicated as a cause of arm pain.

Chest X-ray

Chest X-ray remains a quick, cheap and generally easily interpreted method of suggesting or excluding many systemic diseases that may present neurologically. These include sarcoidosis, tuberculosis, myasthenia and other paraneoplastic syndromes.

> A chest X-ray is more likely to provide helpful positive or negative information than a plain X-ray of the skull.

CT AND MRI

Despite its eclipse by MRI (Figure 2.1), CT (Figure 2.2) retains its place as a highly useful imaging modality. A recent development has been volumetric data acquisition in times compatible with a single breath-hold, achieved by the patient being moved through the gantry during scanning, often referred to as helical or spiral CT. Whole regions such as the head or the thoracic spine can be imaged in seconds, but there is a time penalty involved for increasing image quality and also a reduction in the area covered. There are still clinical advantages of CT over MRI; there are no contraindications as there are to MRI; the configuration of the gantry is generally far less **claustrophobic** and life-support systems are not incompatible,

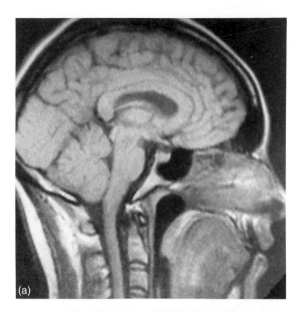

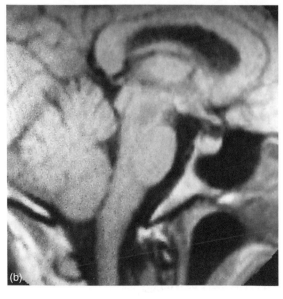

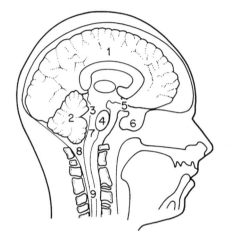

Figure 2.1 (a) MRI brain scan, sagittal view. (b) Magnified view of the posterior fossa: (1) cerebral hemisphere; (2) cerebellum; (3) fourth ventricle; (4) pons; (5) pituitary stalk with chiasm anteriorly; (6) sphenoid sinus; (7) medulla; (8) craniocervical junction; (9) cervical spinal cord.

provided they are portable. A major constraint of both CT and MRI is that the patient has to be transported to the instrument. Although MR-compatible life-support equipment is available, it is considerably more expensive and may be underused. This, combined with poor patient access, makes MRI logistically more difficult than CT in the critically ill patient. Although X-ray radiation dose should be considered, risks should be far outweighed by diagnostic benefit.

The main contraindications to MRI are cardiac pacemakers and other implanted electronic devices such as cochlear implants, heart valves and intracranial aneurysm clips. Not every device in each of these cases is an absolute contraindication, and lists defining the MRI compatibility are available. A common misconception is that orthopaedic metal implants and haemostatic vascular clips in the dura are a contraindication. Most implants do not move in the magnetic fields, and if they do, they are sufficiently embedded in tissue not to loosen, although generally a period of 6 weeks after insertion is preferred before exposure to MRI. Heating effects induced by electric currents are negligible.

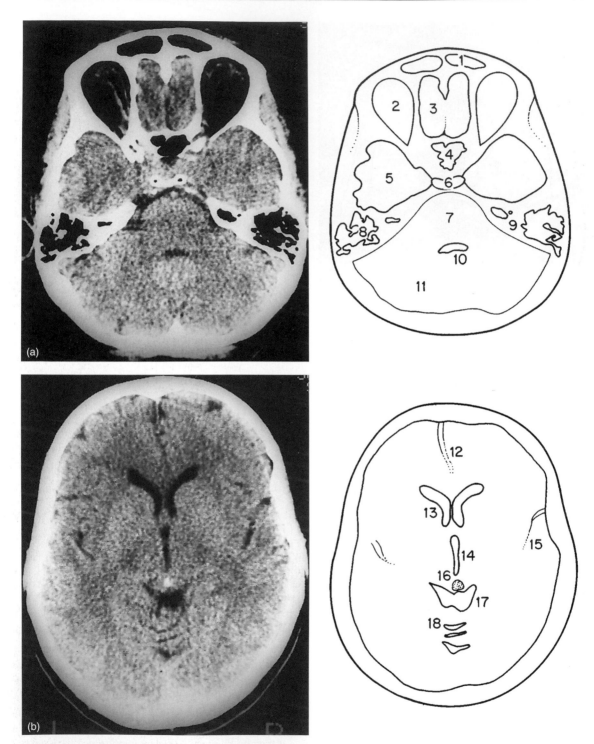

Figure 2.2 (a–d) CT brain scan at four levels moving up from the orbitomeatal line: (1) frontal sinus; (2) orbit; (3) ethmoid sinus and nasal cavity; (4) sphenoid sinus; (5) middle fossa; (6) dorsum sellae; (7) pons; (8) mastoid air cells; (9) petrous ridge; (10) fourth ventricle; (11) cerebellum, lateral lobe; (12) interhemispheric fissure; (13) lateral ventricles; (14) third ventricle;

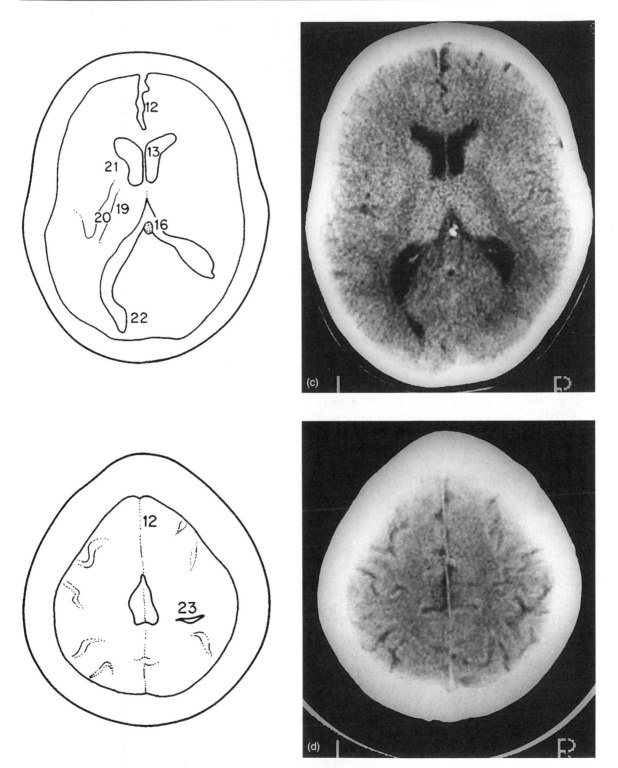

Figure 2.2 (*Continued*) (15) sylvian fissure; (16) pineal; (17) quadrigeminal cistern; (18) vermis; (19) thalamus; (20) pathway of pyramidal tract; (21) caudate nucleus; (22) occipital horns; (23) surface sulci.

Contrast mechanisms

In CT, the most important physical property of brain tissue that determines X-ray absorption is electron density, which is reflected by physical density.

There are many contrast mechanisms in MRI, and most are still not fully understood. The signal from the brain comes from protons in water molecules. T1 relaxation time reflects the rate at which tissue gives back absorbed radio frequency (RF) energy, T2 relaxation time reflects the rate at which resonance is lost by phase dispersal, and proton (spin) density, the amount of magnetism induced (Figure 2.3).

T1 and T2 contrast mechanisms remain the most important for detecting most disease states in the brain and for demonstrating normal anatomy. Some others are finding their way into routine practice and are available as options on most modern equipment.

Diffusion-weighted contrast is generated by applying an additional strong magnetic gradient to induce phase dispersal as a result of molecular motion. In the brain diffusion is markedly anisotropic, being greater in the direction of major white matter tracts. Diffusion-weighted images (DWI) generally are acquired rapidly (seconds rather than minutes),

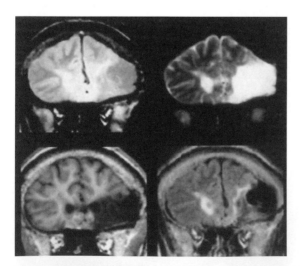

Figure 2.3 Coronal MRI showing post-traumatic left frontal lobe brain damage – a cavity plus surrounding gliosis. Four MR contrast mechanisms are selectively emphasized, one on each image: top left, proton density; top right, T2; bottom left, T1; bottom right, T2 with suppression of cerebrospinal fluid signal (FLAIR).

and usually can be processed to produce apparent diffusion coefficient (ADC) maps. Restricted diffusion results in increased signal on DWI and decreased signal on ADC maps; T2 contrast effects can intrude to produce increased signal on DWI, but not on ADC maps. There is increased clinical use of DWI in assessing early cerebral infarction.

Susceptibility-weighted contrast is caused by magnetic fields induced in tissue as a result of the presence of paramagnetic substances such as endogenous iron or injected gadolinium, and is emphasized by generating signal by magnetic gradient reversal (field echo imaging). It is sometimes referred to as T2* ('T2 star') weighted imaging, T2* referring to the effects of local magnetic field inhomogeneity. This is used clinically mainly to detect haemosiderin in tissues which, it has been found, often is not visible on imaging with mainly T1 or T2 contrast, and hence is good for detecting old intracerebral haemorrhage. Many patients with extensive ischaemic damage in the brain caused by diabetes or hypertension show multiple small old haemorrhages on T2* weighted images.

Perfusion-weighted imaging can be performed with both MRI and CT, although these days more often with MRI. It requires a bolus injection of intravenous contrast medium, and the phases of vascular enhancement over time are followed by a series of rapidly acquired images, usually in a single plane. Quantities, such as mean transit time, time to peak contrast, and derivatives, such as regional cerebral blood flow and blood volume, can be displayed as maps. Although widely used in some centres, especially in evaluating early stroke, most applications (including stroke) remain research tools.

Flow-related contrast results from bulk fluid flow and is generated by two main effects, time-of-flight and phase contrast. These are exploited in MR angiography and cerebrospinal fluid (CSF) dynamic studies.

Functional MRI is a term mainly used to refer to changes that can be detected in cerebral activation experiments, the origins of which still remain controversial. Regional cerebral blood flow can be estimated by dynamic MRI or CT performed with injection of an intravenous bolus of contrast medium (haemodynamically weighted imaging).

Magnetization transfer contrast reflects signal loss induced by applying a preparatory broad-spectrum off-resonance pulse thought to saturate water tightly bound to macromolecules (membranes).

It has had little impact on clinical practice as yet, generally because of disappointing sensitivity.

Contrast enhancement

Iodine photoelectrically absorbs X-ray wavelengths used in diagnostic radiology, and nearly all X-ray contrast materials contain iodine. **Gadolinium** is a strongly paramagnetic substance, which induces powerful T1 and T2 relaxation enhancement, the toxicity of which is eliminated by chelation. These water-soluble compounds are injected intravenously during CT or MRI to induce transient sequential contrast enhancement of arteries and veins, and less transient contrast enhancement of extracellular fluid in tissues with no blood–brain barrier or when broken down by disease.

Rarely, an abnormality is visible only after intravenous contrast injection, but in most cases contrast enhancement does not increase sensitivity significantly (the Imaging Commission of the International League against Epilepsy does not recommend routine use of contrast enhancement, even in patients with recent onset of focal seizures) and enhancement when it occurs conveys little or no direct information about the nature and actual extent of the disease process. In the UK, about 10 deaths a year are attributed to intravenous contrast agents, and the risk of death is estimated at one in 40 000.

Intrathecal enhancement of CT using water-soluble myelographic contrast material can be useful in evaluation of a CSF leak (provided it is leaking or can be induced to leak at the time) and very occasionally in evaluation of cystic lesions in the cisterns, or as an alternative to myelography.

Brain imaging

> **CT versus MRI**
> Areas in which CT generally is either approximately equivalent or superior to MRI are:
> - Subarachnoid haemorrhage
> - Acute head injury
> - Lesion of orbits, paranasal sinus and petrous bones

> - Exclusion of neurosurgical emergencies in critically ill patients
> - Acute stroke (exclusion of intracerebral haemorrhage).

Head injury

> **Head injury**
> Clinical criteria (impaired or fluctuating consciousness, the unassessable patient with previous craniotomy, clinical deterioration or failure to improve, neurological signs or seizure) are more reliable guides to risk of intracranial haemorrhage than the presence of a skull fracture, and should indicate urgent CT.

Serial CT in the absence of sustained clinical deterioration is not recommended, but an examination on discharge is desirable.

Abnormalities that may be shown are:

1 Intracranial haemorrhage. **Clotted blood appears white on CT**. It may be extradural or subdural, where urgent neurosurgery is often indicated, or subarachnoid, intraventricular or superficial intracerebral where neurosurgical intervention is rarely if ever required.
2 Intracranial air. This may be extradural, subdural, subarachnoid or intraventricular, and indicates a compound fracture and CSF leak, which is usually transitory.
3 Cerebral infarction. This occurs within 1–14 days post-injury; the posterior cerebral artery territory is most often involved. Mortality is high.
4 Diffuse axonal injury (DAI). Both CT and MRI may show small marker lesions, MRI being more sensitive. Typical sites are high convexity white matter adjacent to the falx, posterior part of corpus callosum, junction of callosum and corona radiata, postero-lateral aspect of upper brainstem. The number and distribution of lesions correlate less well with extent of DAI than was originally thought. Diffuse vascular injuries manifest as haemorrhages in the basal ganglia, a severe form of DAI. Outcome is perhaps best predicted on MRI several weeks after the injury.

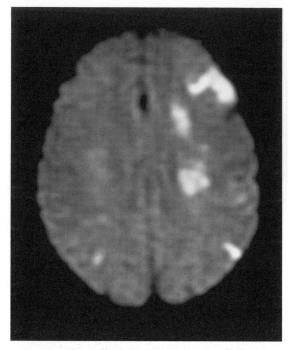

Figure 2.4 Acute cerebral infarction shown by diffusion-weighted imaging. Only a small part of this extensive damage was visible on conventional spin echo imaging. The clinical onset was 14 hours previously.

Cerebrovascular disease

With careful attention to subtle changes in grey matter (cortex and basal ganglia), most acute cerebral infarcts are visible on both CT and MRI within 24 hours, but in up to 20% of patients with acute stroke no causative infarct is ever shown.

Diffusion-weighted imaging may show early infarcts as areas of increased signal on MRI before any changes are visible on any other imaging; the corresponding area appears of low signal on ADC maps. This is a result of restricted diffusion, which generally is present only in acute infarcts, a feature usually lost within about 3 days (Figure 2.4).

In acute intracerebral haemorrhage CT is easiest to interpret. The electron-dense clot is surrounded by a halo of low density; the high density melting away from the periphery over days as mass diminishes. Occasionally transitory vasogenic oedema develops and mass may increase. After intravenous contrast medium, a thin rim of enhancement is usually evident for a few days within the low density halo. Extravasated blood has a highly variable appearance on MRI. Very acute haemorrhage presents a non-specific appearance. Acute haematomas present low signal on T2-weighted images, which gradually rises over days. On T1-weighted images the signal becomes markedly increased from the periphery inwards over days.

After 2 weeks, MRI appearances of intracranial haemorrhage are more sensitive and specific than CT. Very low signal appearing in the brain may persist around a haematoma cavity for months or years and represent haemosiderin. Haemosiderin is more sensitively detected by susceptibility (T2*) weighted images.

Infarct-like lesions are shown in the brain on MRI in 36% of patients over 65 years old, rising to 43% in the over 85 s.

These lesions are both more common and numerous in patients with past history of stroke or risk factors, especially hypertension. The deep and superficial cerebral white matter is involved in 80%, the basal ganglia in 40%, thalami and ventral pons in 10%. These features usually allow distinction from other white matter diseases such as multiple sclerosis.

Subarachnoid haemorrhage
In patients with subarachnoid haemorrhage, blood will be visible in the basal cisterns on CT in over 90% within 3 days of the ictus but in only 40% after 5 days (Figure 2.5). Up to 50% may be detected on MRI within 3 days but perhaps over 80% after 3 days, although only when non-routine acquisitions are used.

However, sensitivity of MRI is not well established and CT is preferred. Haemorrhage confined to the midline basal cisterns is less likely to be associated with aneurysm. Cerebral infarction usually complicates cases with extensive rather than localized cisternal blood.

Venous infarction is most characteristic when bilateral and parafalcine. The thalami are selectively involved in deep venous thrombosis, and the temporal lobe in transverse sigmoid sinus thrombosis. Venous infarcts are frequently haemorrhagic. A

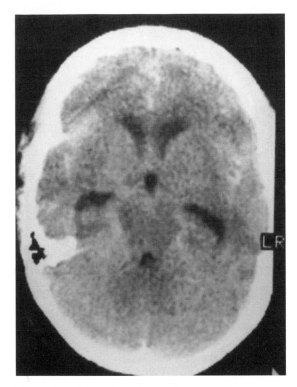

Figure 2.5 Subarachnoid haemorrhage plus mild hydrocephalus. CT 2 days after ictus. Blood is present in the basal cisterns and interhemispheric tissues (see also Figure 16.1).

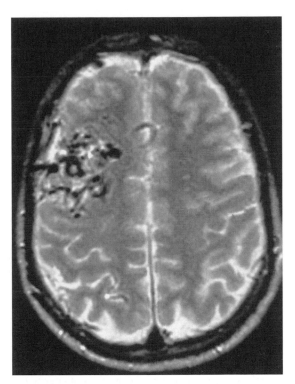

Figure 2.6 Arteriovenous malformation in the right frontal lobe. MRI with T2-weighted contrast. The low signal (black) structures are dilated draining veins.

recent study has suggested that unenhanced CT is at least as good as MRI for diagnosis of acute sinus thrombosis, but MRI is better for excluding it. The involved sinuses are distended with electron-dense or high signal blood clot. Subacute and chronic thrombosis can be difficult to diagnose, even with angiography.

Thrombosis of the internal carotid artery is usually diagnosed reliably by routine head MRI but may be mimicked by slow flow. **Acute dissection of the internal carotid artery** is best diagnosed by routine head MRI provided the subpetrous carotid is visualized, and angiography is unnecessary and should be avoided. **Vertebral artery dissection** is more difficult to diagnose.

Angiomas are of two broad types: (i) arteriovenous shunts or fistulas, recognizable by enlarged draining veins and sometimes feeding arteries; (ii) cavernous angiomas (cavernomas), recognized as sharply circumscribed areas of signal change surrounded by a dark rim on MRI, or as a dense,

often partly calcified area on CT. MRI is both more sensitive and more specific than CT (Figure 2.6).

Aneurysms

Most aneurysms larger than about 5 mm will be correctly diagnosed on routine head MRI or contrast-enhanced CT. Large aneurysms usually have a characteristic appearance on MRI, even when extensively thrombosed.

Inflammatory conditions

Multiple sclerosis (MS) remains a clinical diagnosis (see Chapter 21), however, in the appropriate clinical setting, MRI can be sufficiently suggestive to remove the need for further tests (Figure 2.7).

Suggestive features are discrete ovoid lesions around the lateral ventricles especially posteriorly, in the corpus callosum, tegmentum of the pons,

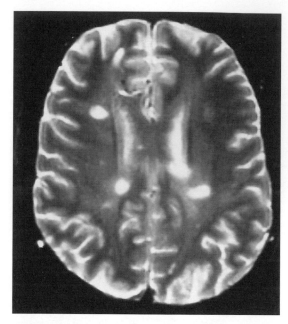

Figure 2.7 Multiple sclerosis. MRI with T2-weighted contrast.

middle cerebellar peduncles and cerebellar white matter. One may be enough, but in excess of six is more suggestive. Acute lesions can be quite large; they shrink over time and show central contrast enhancement only for about 8 weeks, not beyond. Serial MRI reveals new lesions much more frequently than clinical relapses, and there is generally a poor correlation between MRI abnormalities and clinical status. **In patients with clinically isolated syndromes, such as optic neuritis, the presence of multiple brain lesions implies a markedly increased chance of progression to MS in the next 1–5 years, which is about 70% of such patients.** CT has no role other than to exclude alternative diagnoses such as optic nerve compression.

Other conditions can mimic MS:

1 **Acute disseminated encephalomyelitis** – lesions generally are larger and disappear over days or weeks, whereas MS lesions persist; however, new lesions may appear for up to 14 months.
2 **Sarcoidosis** – usually distinguishable by evidence of meningeal disease and superficial enhancing granulomas.
3 **Systemic lupus erythematosus (and other arteritides)** can be very similar indeed; lesions tend to be more superficial, and additional

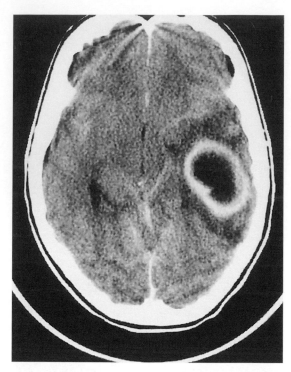

Figure 2.8 Abscess in the left temporal lobe. CT after intravenous contrast enhancement.

infarct-like lesions in the grey matter or the brainstem can be discriminatory.
4 **Infections** such as human T-cell lymphotropic virus-associated myelopathy and progressive multifocal leukoencephalopathy are distinguished clinically.
5 **Neoplasms**, especially gliomas can be confused with acute lesions of MS; serial MRI should distinguish such cases without the need for immediate biopsy.
6 **Ischaemic lesions** in non-inflammatory arteriopathies, and in metabolic disorders such as mitochondrial cytopathy, where frequent involvement of basal ganglia should discriminate.

The marked reduction in mortality from suppurative intracranial infection, particularly **brain abscess and empyema** can probably be attributed as much to CT (Figure 2.8) as to advances in surgery or antimicrobial therapy. With the possible exception of some AIDS-associated infections, CT and MRI are broadly comparable in their sensitivity and specificity.

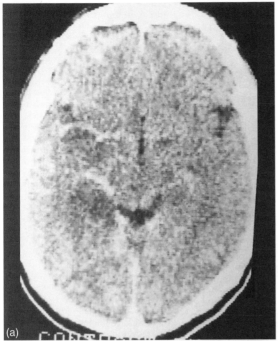

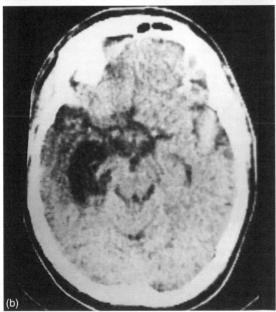

Figure 2.9 Herpes simplex encephalitis. (a) CT 10 days into illness; disease affects medial part of right temporal lobe; (b) CT 4 months later, showing severe unilateral brain damage.

Intracranial tuberculosis is more sensitively diagnosed, and monitored on post-contrast images.

Encephalitis, as distinct from acute disseminated encephalomyelitis, is suggested in the appropriate

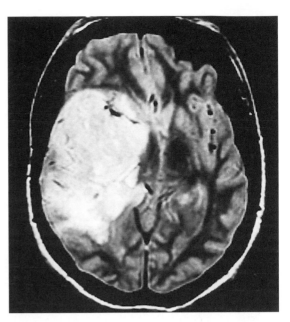

Figure 2.10 Glioma, right temporal lobe. MRI with mainly T2-weighted contrast.

clinical setting by predominant grey matter involvement. Herpes simplex (type I) often yields early changes in mesial temporal lobes and insula, usually becoming bilateral; haemorrhages can occur in this and in other necrotizing types (Figure 2.9).

Meningitis does not require brain imaging unless there are focal neurological signs, deterioration or failure to improve. Infarcts, empyemas, cerebritis, abscesses and hydrocephalus then may be shown.

Cerebral mass lesions

> **Cerebral mass lesions**
> Sensitivity to MRI and CT is high, nearly all lesions being detected, but specificity of diagnosis is only about 90% or less (Figure 2.10), and biopsy is frequently desirable.

Raised intracranial pressure
When ventricles are 'slit-like', and brain substance appears normal, the interpretation 'generalized brain oedema' is nearly always incorrect. Cytoxic oedema, as in hypoxic ischaemic brain damage, changes the imaging characteristics of grey matter compared to that of adjacent white matter, whether normal or abnormal.

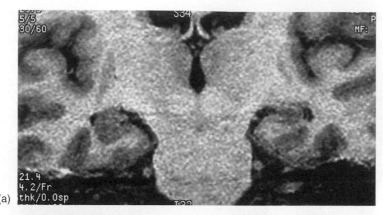

(a)

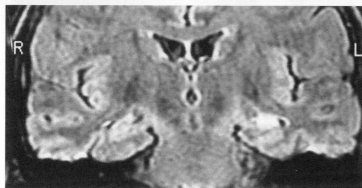

(b)

Figure 2.11 Left hippocampal sclerosis. Coronal MRI (a) T1-weighted contrast and (b) T2-weighted contrast showing the left hippocampus (on the right of the figure) to be small and yielding abnormally high signal on appropriate images.

Modern imaging has made it clear that most pressure cones (herniations) are not lethal and often are asymptomatic. Imaging has little role to play in the diagnosis of brain death, which remains a clinical diagnosis, save to help establish its cause.

Intracranial mass and lumbar puncture

The presence of an intracranial mass or demonstration of progressive obliteration of basal cisterns, or compression of brainstem, indicates probable raised intracranial pressure. However, at least 30% of patients who clinically cone after lumbar puncture have an entirely normal brain CT.

Epilepsy

Epilepsy

Patients with recent seizure onset require either CT or MRI, and intravenous enhancement is not generally recommended if the brain appears normal.

Early repeat studies may be appropriate if seizures persist or neurological signs develop because some neoplasms grow rapidly. In the investigation of chronic intractable epilepsy, especially if functional neurosurgery is contemplated, MRI is clearly superior to CT, but is best carried out at epilepsy centres with surgical programmes. The major advance in recent years has been the reliable diagnosis of hippocampal sclerosis, found in over 60% of patients with intractable temporal lobe epilepsy (Figure 2.11).

Cranial nerve lesions

Some lesions of the optic nerve in the orbit are more sensitively detected by CT than by MRI (drusen, optic nerve sheath meningioma), because of calcification (Figure 2.12). Magnetic resonance imaging is preferable for lesions of the optic chiasm and other cranial nerves, including the ocular motor and vestibulo-acoustic (Figures 2.13 and 2.14). Intravenous contrast is not essential for diagnosis of neurinomas but may help to distinguish inflammatory from some neoplastic lesions, such as meningiomas, especially

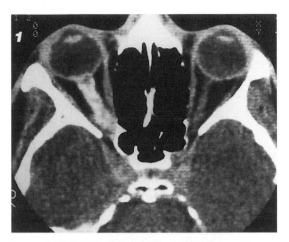

Figure 2.12 Right optic nerve sheath meningioma, CT orbits showing a thickened and heavily calcified optic nerve sheath.

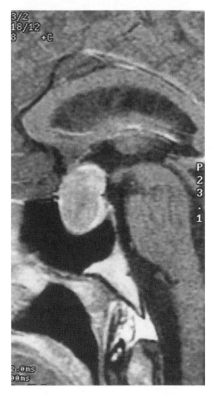

Figure 2.13 Pituitary macroadenoma compressing the optic chiasm. Sagittal MRI with T1-weighted contrast made after gadolinium enhancement.

in the region of the cavernous sinuses. Aneurysms causing oculomotor palsy should be reliably excluded by targeted MRI (or CT with contrast injection) without recourse to angiography.

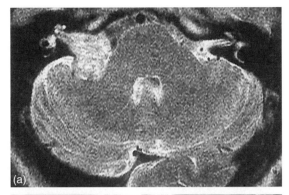

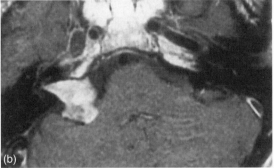

Figure 2.14 Large right acoustic neuroma. (a) Axial T2-weighted MRI. (b) T1-weighted MRI after gadolinium enhancement.

Spinal imaging

The obligatory limitation of CT to axial slices reduced its clinical utility in the spine because of reduced coverage, but spiral CT, and fast acquisition techniques with multiplanar reformatting, have reduced this disadvantage. Results with CT are about as good as MRI in diagnosing lumbar disc herniations and lumbar canal stenosis; it is less useful elsewhere where sensitivity to intradural disease is much lower than MRI. Cervical radicular syndromes remain a problem for MRI as well as CT, because only (infrequently found) large lesions show good clinical correlation (Figures 2.15, 2.16 and 2.17).

> MRI is the first and usually the only choice when investigating suspected lesions of the spinal cord.

The identification of signal change in cord substance seems the best correlate of definite clinical myelopathy; the degree of compression correlates poorly. There are a wide variety of causes of signal

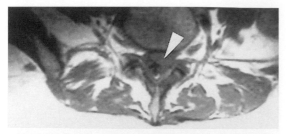

Figure 2.15 Large left L5–S1 posterior disc herniation (arrowed). Axial MRI, T1-weighted contrast.

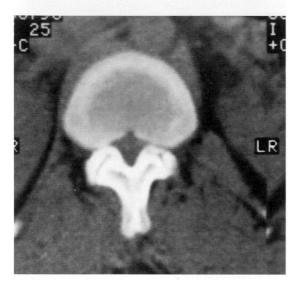

Figure 2.16 Congenital lumbar canal stenosis. Axial CT.

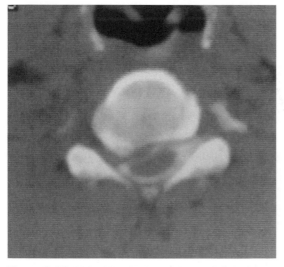

Figure 2.17 Right-sided C5–6 disc protrusion. Axial CT with intrathecal contrast; the patient only had a C6 radiculopathy, but the spinal cord is also compressed.

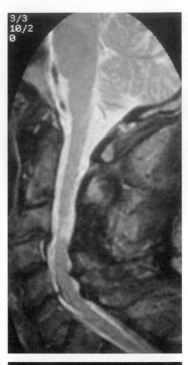

(a)

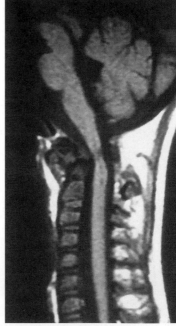

(b)

Figure 2.18 Signal change in the spinal cord as a result of compressive damage. (a) Sagittal MRI, T2-weighted contrast, showing focal signal change in the spinal cord at C3 where there has been a localized laminectomy. (b) Sagittal T1-weighted image showing focal signal change in the cord at C1, where there is atlantoaxial subluxation caused by an os odontoideum.

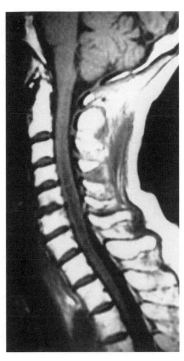

Figure 2.19 Extensive signal change in the spinal cord with swelling as a result of a glioma. T1-weighted sagittal MRI after completing a course of radiotherapy, which has destroyed the red marrow in the vertebrae, hence replacement by high signal fatty marrow.

change: compression (trauma, spondylosis), arteriovenous malformations and dural fistulas, neoplasms, infarction and inflammation (Figures 2.18, 2.19, 2.20). Where necessary the use of intravenous enhancement, or serial examinations, may help to distinguish some of the aetiologies without recourse to biopsy.

Extradural metastatic disease is shown best by MRI, including neural compression. In some skeletal conditions, however, the treatment plan may be influenced by the estimation of structural integrity of bone displayed by high resolution CT. Local practices based on the preferences of the surgeons involved will dictate precise indications.

ANGIOGRAPHY

The increase in the range and quality of less invasive ways of imaging the cerebral arterial tree have removed nearly all the indications for catheter (intra-arterial) arteriography for purely diagnostic purposes. It is still generally used to demonstrate intracranial aneurysms but then **only when it is planned to treat**, and there is no effective non-invasive alternative to spinal angiography. It is also necessary to

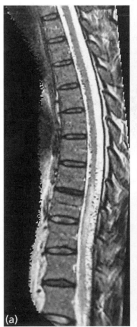
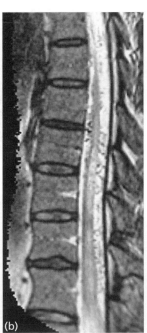
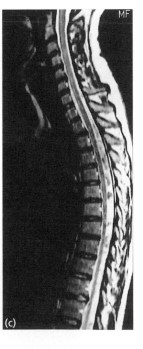

Figure 2.20 Spinal dural arteriovenous fistula with clinical myelopathy. (a) Sagittal T2-weighted MRI. (b) Magnified view of (a), showing multiple serpiginous low signal vessels and high signal cord substance. (c) A normal sagittal MRI for comparison showing focal dark areas in the cerebrospinal fluid (CSF) posterior to the spinal cord caused by turbulent motion of CSF not to be confused with enlarged veins.

demonstrate the anatomy of arteriovenous malformations, but then again only when there is intention to treat. Gone are the days when a house officer simply sent a request for angiography down to an X-ray department and expected it to be done with no questions asked.

MR Angiography

The spins of moving protons behave differently in magnetic field gradients than stationary spins, and the behaviour of coherent or bulk flowing spins can be selectively enhanced to produce images of flowing blood in both arteries and veins. This is achieved without injecting any contrast medium and is therefore non-invasive. Two motion effects are exploited: (i) time-of-flight (TOF), which exploits differences in radio frequency saturation between moving and stationary spins; and (ii) phase contrast (PC), which exploits phase shifts that occur as a result of motion. The PC effect is most dependent on flow velocity and direction, and TOF is more widely used. Single slice (two-dimensional) and volumetric (three-dimensional) acquisitions are choices, three-dimensional or multi-slab strategies generally being most commonly employed for intracranial vessels, and two-dimensional strategies for the cervical vessels. Display is usually by maximum intensity pixel ray projections, although reporting usually involves review of raw data also. Contrast-enhanced MR angiography is increasingly used these days to increase vascular contrast in aneurysms, carotid stenosis and to demonstrate large vessels like the aorta and branches, all being structures in which flow enhancement may be insufficient. This requires a timed intravenous bolus of contrast into a peripheral vein (Figure 2.21).

In patients requiring diagnostic angiography who cannot have MRI, **CT angiography** is usually a very satisfactory alternative. This always requires an intravenous bolus of contrast medium (usually about 90 ml), and the resultant images can be processed in a similar way to MR angiograms and look very similar.

Limitations

Spatial resolution is low relative to other forms of angiography, and small arteries, including third- or

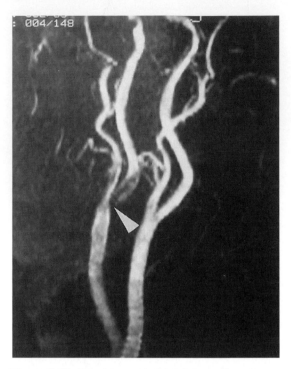

Figure 2.21 Bilateral carotid sinus atheroma shows on an intravenously contrast-enhanced magnetic resonance angiogram, using a vascular coil giving field of view, which includes the aortic arch.

fourth-order branches and beyond, are poorly seen, if seen at all. Plug flow is displayed best; turbulent and very slow flow may not be visualized. Image is sensitive to patient motion, and suboptimal studies are relatively common.

Carotid stenosis

The convenience of simply adding MRA to brain imaging when investigating stroke patients is an overwhelming recommendation.

Obsessional 'measurers' of percentage stenosis are not comfortable with MRA; but if the only tenable criterion on which to offer carotid endarterectomy is greater than 70% stenosis, then MRA is entirely satisfactory. Problems with slow and turbulent flow require cautious interpretation; most workers recommend adding another non-invasive test, carotid sonography, when MRA suggests a significant stenosis (Figure 2.21). Tests giving normal or near normal results on MRA need no further imaging.

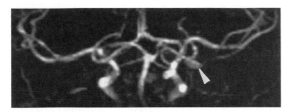

Figure 2.22 Left posterior communicating artery origin aneurysm (arrowed), pointing mainly laterally and about 1 cm in size. Magnetic resonance angiogram, three-dimensional time-of-flight image, frontal maximum intensity pixel ray projection.

Carotid artery dissection does not require even MRA, as static brain MRI is more specific. The dissections are usually transient, and initial imaging is most likely to be positive. Vertebral artery dissection is more difficult and MRA may play a role.

Aneurysm

Aneurysms greater than 4 mm in diameter are reliably shown – less than 3 mm unreliably–MRA seems adequate to screen for incidental aneurysms, but subarachnoid haemorrhage is more controversial because small aneurysms may be involved. Many patients are now having aneurysms clipped on the basis of MRA alone (Figure 2.22).

Arteriovenous malformations

Approximately the same amount of information is obtained from MRI as from MRA, and MRA is not recommended. Vascular relationships to tumours are just as well appreciated by MRI.

Arteritis

Brain MRI with intravenous enhancement may show mural thickening when larger vessels are involved, which may be more specific than flow imaging.

Dural sinus thrombosis

Selective imaging of the dural sinuses and cerebral veins by MRI is possible and advocated by many as the test of choice. Slow flow can be better imaged after intravenous gadolinium. However non-visualization of a sinus is common in normal

tests, and does not mean thrombosis, so utility is doubtful.

Angiography

Angiography is an invasive test and serious questions need to be asked about how essential it is to management. It is uncomfortable and carries significant risk: around 5% complications at the arterial puncture site, and 1–2% risk of stroke or death.

It cannot be overemphasized that the patient needs to have accepted these risks before reaching the angiography department. Most angiography is performed using digital subtraction techniques (DSA), but it is a misapprehension that this increases safety, nor does non-selective aortic arch injection of contrast medium.

Angiography is still widely employed to investigate subarachnoid haemorrhage, to evaluate arteriovenous malformations, and as a preliminary to endovascular treatment delivery.

In the author's opinion it should be regarded as contraindicated in the investigation of carotid artery dissection, and, more controversially, may also be contraindicated in carotid stenosis. However, for many vascular surgeons formal angiography is still the 'gold standard'. Arteritis remains a problem because the most specific abnormalities occur in distal vessels not shown by MRA, and positive data from biopsy, or perhaps angiography, are much to be desired before considering immunosuppressive therapy. Recent studies have indicated that nothing is to be gained from angiography if MRI of the brain is normal, and it should be appreciated that even when present, angiographic abnormalities usually are too non-specific to be definitive or even particularly supportive of the diagnosis.

Intravenous DSA is a reasonable alternative to MRA in patients, who cannot have MRI. It is minimally invasive, but systemic complications are minor and occur in less than 0.5% and there is no risk of stroke. Similarly helical CT angiography can be performed after intravenous contrast injection, which also is often an entirely satisfactory alternative to angiography.

MYELOGRAPHY

The introduction of water-soluble intrathecal contrast material is rarely indicated, but in patients with suspected spinal neurological disease who cannot have MRI it may be the only alternative. Today it commonly is carried out by CT, supplemented by multiplanar reformatting. Spiral CT is particularly helpful in obtaining adequate coverage in reasonable periods of time. However if modern MRI is negative or unhelpful in other ways, no form of myelography is likely to make a contribution. The higher resolution provided by conventional myelography has been used to demonstrate pial vein enlargement in dural arteriovenous fistulas, when all other investigations including MRI are negative. However the range of normal variation is wide, dural fistulas can be incidental findings, and recent reviews suggest that patients who warrant treatment are readily diagnosable by MRI (Figure 2.20).

DOPPLER SONOGRAPHY

Doppler sonography is a reasonably accurate and reliable technique for non-invasive investigation of carotid artery stenosis. Colour flow mapping provides spatially oriented velocity data, colour indicating direction of flow, as well as two-dimensional reference anatomy. Pulsed and continuous-wave sonography are methods by which blood velocity in a sample volume (pulsed) or volume along a cursor (continuous-wave) are mapped over time. Stenosis is estimated from peak flow velocities, and two-dimensional real-time grey scale display permits characterization of plaques. Unilateral severe stenosis or occlusion can increase flow in the contralateral vessel and lead to overestimation of stenosis, and cursor orientation to flow direction is critical. Comparisons between sonographic and angiographic estimates of carotid stenosis usually yield significant discordance in about 10% of cases, which is generally regarded as acceptable. Fortunately

concordance is best when stenosis exceeds 75% where the scope for variation sharply narrows.

Sonography of the carotid arteries is not as easy to perform or subsequently to interpret as MRA, but it is used most widely as a screening test, probably dictated as much by availability as by an impression of greater precision in estimating percentage stenosis.

> Many stroke units worldwide use MRA and sonography as complementary investigations, and consider invasive angiography prior to carotid endarterotomy only when there is doubt about distinguishing carotid occlusion for severe stenosis.

INTERVENTIONAL NEURORADIOLOGY

Recently neuroradiologists have been involved with increasing frequency in interventional procedures. Most often these involve treatment of vascular lesions:

- Aneurysms
- Arteriovenous malformations
- Dural fistulas
- Stenosed arteries.

A variety of techniques have been employed to 'close' or block off aneurysms, including the insertion of platinum coils and of balloons. To close fistulas and arteriovenous malformations coils, injections of 'super glue', or synthetic embolic particles have been used. Vessel expanders to open a tight arterial stenosis may be employed, and stents inserted to maintain patency. All these techniques rely on the skilful insertion of fine catheters, usually threaded from the femoral artery so their tip is close to the lesion. Risks do arise from such measures, but these are often less than with open operation and stays in hospital are shorter. These interventional procedures represent a currently expanding field of treatment.

CONCLUSIONS

'If in doubt as to whether an investigation is required or which... is best, it makes sense to ask a suitable radiologist... who will know more about the speciality than those whose primary interest is in another field' (Royal College of Radiologists, 1996). This is particularly true at the present time when imaging options are multiplying faster than therapeutic options, and changes in clinical management are being dictated as much by changes in technology as by new knowledge about disease.

REFERENCES AND FURTHER READING

Black WC (1994) Intracranial aneurysms in adult polycystic kidney disease: is screening with MR angiography indicated? *Radiology*, 191:18–20.

Bryan RN, Wells SW, Miller TJ *et al.* (1997) Infarct-like lesions in the brain: prevalence and anatomic characteristics of MR imaging of the elderly – data from the cardiovascular health study. *Radiology*, 202:47–54.

Harris KG, Tran DD, Sickels WJ, Cornell SD, Alsanjari N, Stevens JM (1995) High resolution magnetic resonance imaging in adults with partial or secondary generalised epilepsy attending a tertiary referral unit. *Journal of Neurology, Neurosurgery and Psychiatry*, 59:898–904.

Katz DA, Marks MP, Napel SA, Bracci PM, Roberts SL (1995) Circle of Willis: evaluation with spiral CT angiography; MR angiography and conventional angiography. *Radiology*, 195:445–449.

Ketonen LM, Berg MJ (1997) *Clinical Neuroradiology 100 Maxims in Neurology*, Vol. 5. London: Edward Arnold.

Miller DH, Albert PS, Barkhof F *et al.* (1996) Guidelines for the use of magnetic resonance techniques in monitoring the treatment of multiple sclerosis. *Annals of Neurology*, 39:6–16.

Moseley IF (1986) *Diagnostic Imaging in Neurological Disease*. London: Churchill Livingstone.

Moseley IF (1995) Imaging the adult brain. *Journal of Neurology, Neurosurgery and Psychiatry*, 58:7–21.

Royal College of Radiologists (1996) Making the best use of a Department of Clinical Radiology. In: *Guidelines for Doctors*, 3rd edn. London: Royal College of Radiologists.

Savy LE, Stevens JM, Taylor DJ, Kendall BE (1994) Apparent cerebellar ectopia: reappraisal using volumetric MRI. *Neuroradiology*, 36:360–363.

Stevens JM (1994) Imaging patients with TIAs. *Postgraduate Medical Journal*, 70:604–609.

Stevens JM (1995) Imaging the spinal cord. *Journal of Neurology, Neurosurgery and Psychiatry*, 58:403–408.

Stevens JM, Mandel C (1997) Imaging the CNS. In: Webb AW, Shapiro MJ, Singer M, Suler P (eds) *Oxford Textbook of Critical Care*. Oxford: Oxford University Press.

Stevens JM, McAllister V (1996) The imaging of spinal pathology. In: Granger RG, Allison DJ (eds) *Diagnostic Radiology: A Textbook of Medical Imaging*, 3rd edn. London: Churchill Livingstone.

Tofts PS (1995) Novel MR image contrast mechanism in epilepsy. *Magnetic Resonance Imaging*, 13: 1099–1106.

Yah WT, Simonson TM, Wang AM *et al.* (1994) Venous sinus occlusion disease: MR Findings. *American Journal of Neuroradiology*, 15:309–316.

CHAPTER 3

SYMPTOMS OF NEUROLOGICAL DISEASE

T.J. Fowler, C.D. Marsden and J.W. Scadding

INTRODUCTION

In this chapter the common symptoms a patient may present with in the neurological clinic are discussed. The first step is to decide on the broad category of the disorder that the patient is trying to describe. The discovery that the patient's complaint is one of headache, a blackout, difficulty in walking, or a disturbance of memory, immediately sets in train an established thought process that includes the probable differential diagnosis of the causes of such a complaint, and the questions necessary to ask at some stage of the interview to establish which diagnosis is likely to be correct. In other words, specific complaints act as triggers to the neurologist's diagnostic process, selecting programmes of enquiry and differential diagnosis for each complaint.

The commonest symptoms encountered in neurological practice are shown in Table 3.1. This list is by no means exhaustive, but it does account for the majority of complaints encountered.

In addition to the patient's presenting complaint, it is important to obtain the answers to a series of routine questions, the purpose of which is to disclose the possibility of disease in other parts of the nervous system (Table 3.2).

It is not our purpose here to describe in detail the individual diseases causing the various symptoms discussed. We will concentrate on the approach to the differential diagnosis of each symptom, and upon the practical management of such patients.

HEADACHE

Headache is one of the commonest symptoms encountered in general practice, and certainly is the commonest complaint of patients attending the neurologist. It is estimated that approximately one in five of the general population may suffer from headache of sufficient severity to consult a doctor. The majority of these patients will have no abnormal physical signs on examination, and diagnosis depends entirely on the history. The most important distinction is how long the patient has suffered headache.

The diagnosis and management of someone with the acute onset of their first severe headache, 'first and worst', is entirely different from that of someone who has suffered from chronic daily headache for a matter of many years.

Table 3.1 Common symptoms in neurological disorders

Pain
    Headache
    Facial pain
    Spinal pain – cervical, lumbar
    Limb pain – often accompanied by weakness
      and tingling
Loss of consciousness
    Epileptic seizures
    Syncope
    Impaired cerebral perfusion – cardiac causes
    Non-epileptic seizures
Disturbances of the senses
    Visual upsets – impaired acuity, blurred,
      double vision
    Deafness
    Giddiness
    Impaired smell, taste
Motor
    Weakness
      limbs – often with pain and tingling
      bulbar muscles – swallowing, speech
      respiratory muscles – breathless
    Stiffness – spasticity and rigidity
    Clumsiness – incoordination and ataxia
    Imbalance and walking problems
    Tremor
    Involuntary movements
Sensory
    Loss of feeling – numbness
    Distorted – tingling, paraesthesiae,
      bizarre sensations, hyperaesthesiae
    Loss of position sense – sensory ataxia
Autonomic
    Disturbances of bowel, bladder, sexual function
    Faintness – postural hypotension
Disturbances of higher functions
    Memory impairment – dementia
    Confusion
    Changes in mood, behaviour
    Changes in speech – aphasia
    Visuo-spatial disturbance
    Disordered thinking – psychiatric

Table 3.2 Symptoms to aid neurological diagnosis

A suitable range of ten routine neurological questions is:
1. Have you noticed any change in your mood, memory or powers of concentration?
2. Have you ever lost consciousness or had a fit or seizure?
3. Do you suffer unduly from headaches?
4. Have you noticed any change in your senses: (i) smell; (ii) taste; (iii) sight; (iv) hearing?
5. Do you have any difficulty in talking, chewing or swallowing?
6. Have you ever experienced any numbness, tightness, pins and needles, tingling or burning sensation in the face, limbs or trunk?
7. Have you noticed weakness, stiffness, heaviness or dragging of arms or legs?
8. Do you have any difficulty in using your hands for skilled tasks, such as writing, typing or dressing?
9. Do you have any unsteadiness or difficulty in walking?
10. Do you ever have any difficulty controlling your bladder or bowels?

for this may be the presenting symptom of intracranial haemorrhage or infection.

Most patients with subarachnoid haemorrhage (SAH) from aneurysm or angioma present with a sudden dramatic, and explosive onset of devastating headache, which rapidly becomes generalized and is accompanied by neck stiffness. They might complain, 'It was as if I had been kicked by a mule.'

Many patients with SAH lose consciousness and some may develop mild focal neurological signs. Patients with primary intracerebral haemorrhage often complain of headache and vomiting, and then rapidly lose consciousness. Commonly they are hypertensive. They may also exhibit a dense neurological deficit resulting from brain destruction, and often do not have a stiff neck.

If SAH is suspected, an early computerized tomography (CT) scan must be undertaken (Figure 3.1) and this will detect blood in the majority of patients scanned within the first 48 hours.

Acute sudden headache

The sudden onset of severe headache over a matter of minutes or hours often poses a medical emergency,

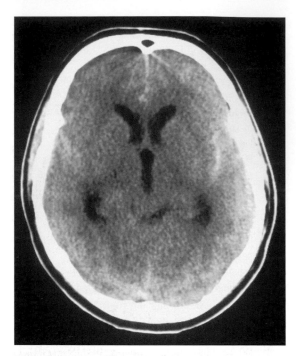

Figure 3.1 CT brain scan of a patient presenting with an acute severe headache following a subarachnoid haemorrhage. There is blood in the sylvian fissure and slight enlargement of the ventricles.

Table 3.3 Causes of headache

Acute
   Subarachnoid haemorrhage
   Intracerebral haemorrhage
   Migraine
   Meningitis
   Encephalitis
   Sudden rise in intracranial pressure
   Non-specific – infective – secondary to
     septicaemia, influenza, psittacosis
   Drugs, alcohol – vasodilators, statins, 'hangover'
Sub-acute
   Raised intracranial pressure
     Abscess, subdural empyema
     Tumour
     Hydrocephalus
     Subdural haematoma
   Giant cell arteritis
   Arterial dissection
Chronic
   Persistent
     Tension-type
     Psychological – depression, anxiety,
      hypochondriasis
     Post-traumatic
   Intermittent
     Migraine
     Episodic tension-type
Referred
   Neck, sinuses, eyes, teeth – often acute or
     sub-acute

If the scan is negative, then the cerebrospinal fluid (CSF) should be examined to confirm the diagnosis in the 15% of patients where blood has not been shown on the scan. Xanthochromia of the spun supernatant of the CSF is present for about 10 days after a bleed. Patients who have bled from an intracranial aneurysm, which is the commonest cause of SAH, are at serious risk of a second bleed in the next few weeks, which is often lethal. Surgical clipping of the aneurysm, or other obliterative methods, can prevent repeat bleeding.

Those in whom SAH is confirmed by lumbar puncture or CT scanning should be referred urgently to a neurosurgical centre for further treatment.

The commonest condition that may be confused with SAH is the acute onset of a migraine headache (Table 3.3). Migraine usually builds up over minutes or hours, but on occasion may apparently start sufficiently abruptly to suggest a subarachnoid bleed.

Such patients also may have mild photophobia and neck stiffness as part of their severe migraine, but examination of the CSF and a CT brain scan will reveal no blood or other abnormality.

The headache of meningitis and encephalitis does not start with such a dramatic acute onset, but builds up over a matter of hours. Such patients also are likely to have fever and in the case of meningitis, severe neck stiffness.

In some elderly patients, the very young or the very sick, meningitis may be present without neck stiffness. In the case of encephalitis, neck stiffness is less conspicuous, but confusion, early coma and seizures are characteristic. Any patient suspected of having meningitis or encephalitis requires lumbar puncture to establish the diagnosis and the cause. Systemic infections may cause acute headache, for example, influenza, mumps, psittacosis.

Subacute headache

Headache that has been present for a few weeks or months in an individual not previously prone to this complaint must always be taken seriously. In fact, such a complaint usually turns out not to be sinister, but to be the beginning of a much more chronic problem such as tension-type headache or migraine. However, the possibility of other more serious conditions should always be considered in those with the recent onset of disabling headache.

In the elderly patient, or in anyone aged over about 55 years, **cranial or giant cell arteritis** should be considered (see p. 478)

Such patients are usually unwell, with systemic symptoms of malaise, weight loss, and generalized aches and pains. Their main symptom, however, is persistent headache with tenderness of the scalp, as when brushing the hair. The cranial arteries, particularly the superficial temporal arteries, may be visibly enlarged, tortuous, and tender to the touch, and there may be obvious reddening of the overlying skin. Patients with giant cell arteritis are at risk of losing their vision as a result of ischaemic damage to the optic nerves, so suspicion of the condition should lead to urgent action. The erythrocyte sedimentation rate almost invariably is raised above 40 mm/h and a biopsy of a temporal artery is frequently diagnostic. Such patients should be urgently started on steroids to suppress further complications of the illness, particularly sudden visual loss.

The headache of raised intracranial pressure (ICP) of whatever cause, be it tumour, subdural haematoma, or obstructive hydrocephalus, characteristically has been present for a matter of some weeks or months. Frequently it may wake the patient from sleep and is made worse by coughing, sneezing, bending or straining at stool, all of which increase

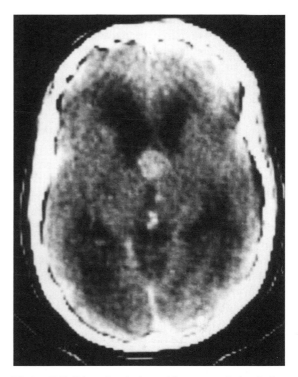

Figure 3.2 This patient had a sudden crescendo headache. This was the result of the colloid cyst shown in the third ventricle causing an intermittent obstructive hydrocephalus, as shown on this CT scan.

ICP. The headache of raised ICP may be accompanied by effortless vomiting. Frequently, papilloedema is evident on examination and there may be signs suggesting a focal intracranial mass lesion. Occasionally there may be an acute crescendo headache as may occur with an intermittent obstructive hydrocephalus (Figure 3.2).

However, patients with intracranial space-occupying lesions producing severe headache may not have papilloedema and may exhibit no focal neurological signs, yet the history may be sufficient to warrant further investigation.

The majority of patients with isolated cough headache, or isolated headache at the peak of sexual excitement (coital cephalgia or orgasmic headache) do not have brain tumours. The mechanisms responsible for these benign conditions are not known.

Persistent headache after minor concussive head injuries (post-traumatic headache) is a common complaint, often accompanied by other symptoms such as postural dizziness, impaired memory and concentration, fatigue and depression. The post-traumatic syndrome is well recognized in the law courts as one of the common sources of claims for compensation for injury. Often after settlement occurs, which unfortunately may take many years, such symptoms may disappear slowly. However, a true post-traumatic (post-concussional) syndrome, with all the symptoms mentioned, may occur in otherwise stable individuals in whom no thought of compensation exists. It is now apparent that minor head injuries may cause cerebral damage, slowing of some cognitive functions and also lesions of the vestibular system, which may be responsible for some of the troublesome symptoms that occur in a proportion of patients in such circumstances. Very prolonged symptoms may be linked with psychological processes.

Chronic headache

> **Chronic headache**
>
> The commonest causes of chronic headache are migraine and tension-type headache. It is a useful working rule that patients who have been complaining of headache for 3 years or more without any other sinister symptoms or physical signs on examination nearly always turn out to have one of these two conditions.

Migraine is exceedingly common and approximately 20% of the population is likely to suffer one or more migrainous episodes in their life. Characteristic of migraine is that it is a periodic disorder, with episodes of headache separated by periods in which the subject is entirely normal. Migraine with aura (classical migraine) is instantly recognizable because of the presence of characteristic warning symptoms in the half-hour or so prior to the onset of headache. The commonest of these are visual, in the form of flashing lights or zigzags caused by ischaemia or spreading depression in the occipital cortex (see p. 327). Other warning symptoms are hemisensory

disturbances, alarming dysphasia, and diplopia with dysarthria and ataxia. These warning symptoms may occur in the absence of subsequent headache. The headache may be hemicranial or, more often, generalized. During the period of headache, the patients feel ill, nauseated, anorectic, photophobic and drowsy. Frequently they vomit, following which the headache often subsides and the patients sleep. The headache usually lasts several hours but may persist for 2–3 days. Once the headache disappears, the patient soon returns to normal and remains so until a further episode occurs. Migraines usually appear at intervals of a few weeks or months, and some more fortunate sufferers may experience only one or two attacks in their lifetime.

The intermittency of migraine contrasts with the persistent, continuous headache characteristic of **tension-type headache**. Such patients claim that they are never free from pain, day in and day out for months or years. Nothing appears to help the pain, which commonly is blamed for causing disturbance of sleep and depression. In fact, tension-type headache is a common symptom of an underlying depressive illness, the latter being responsible for early morning waking, loss of appetite, and malaise. In other patients, tension-type headache appears to be a symptom of long-standing anxiety states, often precipitated by marital discord, other family tensions or job dissatisfaction. The patient usually describes tension-type headache as a constant aching or pressure sensation, which may be generalized or confined to the vertex, or acting like a band around the head. Prodromal symptoms do not occur and vomiting is not a feature. The pain may be exacerbated or may occur only at times of obvious stress, and few of us have not experienced the typical tightening sensation in the scalp when under considerable external pressure. Tension-type headache is associated in some instances with excessive sustained contraction of the muscles of the scalp and neck. Tension-type headaches may be episodic or chronic. In the latter there is a recurring daily headache over a period of more than 6 months. Chronic daily headache describes recurring headaches for more than 15 days each month. There may be an overlap between migraine and tension-type headache and it may sometimes be difficult to differentiate between the two. These may be aggravated by medication-overuse headaches. The recent concept of new daily persisting headache is described in Chapter 16.

Uncommon causes of headache

Typical tension-type headache is frequently blamed on other common conditions such as constipation, dental caries, hypertension, sinusitis, cervical spondylosis, and eye strain. Few of these conditions cause headache, and the majority of patients suffering from them do not complain of this symptom.

Headache does occur in patients with malignant hypertension, or during paroxysmal hypertension provoked by phaeochromocytoma, but is not a symptom of lesser degrees of high blood pressure. Constipation never causes headache, and dental caries causes pain in the face rather than in the head. There is no doubt that straining to read with defective vision in a poor light may cause muscle contraction/tension-type headache, eased by appropriate prescription of spectacles, but such patients are aware of the cause of their head pain. Acute sinusitis undoubtedly causes intense pain and local tenderness over the affected sinus. In contrast, chronic sinusitis is not a cause of headache unless there is intermittent obstruction to drainage from the affected sinus, which then causes the typical features of acute sinus disturbance. Cervical spondylosis causes pain in the neck, which may radiate up to the occiput, and typically is made worse by neck movement. A rare cause of occipital pain, sometimes accompanied by paraesthesiae in the side of the tongue, is sudden trapping of the upper cervical roots on neck movement.

PAIN IN THE FACE

As in headache, patients complaining of pain in the face frequently exhibit no neurological signs and the diagnosis must be made solely on the history. When confronted with a patient complaining of pain in the face, it is useful to keep in mind that this may arise from local structures such as eyes, sinuses, teeth or jaw; referred pain resulting from fifth nerve involvement, in which case there are

likely to be signs of sensory loss in trigeminal territory; and in disorders with no abnormal physical signs such as trigeminal neuralgia, post-herpetic neuralgia, migrainous neuralgia, migraine variants (lower-half headache), and atypical facial pain.

Local causes

Disease of teeth, sinuses, the parotid glands, and the eyes can, of course, cause pain in the face, but nearly always also causes obvious symptoms resulting from damage to these structures. Pain caused by dental caries is precipitated by extremes of temperature and sweets, as is familiar to everyone. A dental abscess causes throbbing pain and marked local tenderness, particularly to percussion of the affected tooth. Acute maxillary sinusitis causes severe, explosive, throbbing pain in the cheek, increased by lying flat, coughing or sneezing, and accompanied by considerable local tenderness. Eye disease, such as acute glaucoma or iritis, causes intense local pain and tenderness in the affected eye, with disturbances of vision and evident reddening of the eye itself. Salivary calculi cause pain in the appropriate salivary gland on eating or on anticipation of good food. Arthritis involving the temporomandibular joint may cause pain in the face and neck, provoked by chewing or opening of the mouth. Pain on chewing may also occur in giant cell arteritis as a result of claudication in ischaemic jaw muscles.

Referred pain

Pain referred into the face may be provoked by compression or infiltration of the trigeminal nerve by posterior fossa tumours, tumours invading the base of skull, or extracranial tumours involving the sinuses or salivary glands. Such referred pain typically is constant, sometimes with superimposed spontaneous jabs of discomfort, and is accompanied by signs of sensory loss in the distribution of the affected nerves. The acute onset of pain in the forehead and eye, associated with a third nerve palsy involving the pupil, is a not uncommon presentation of an aneurysm of the internal carotid at the origin of the posterior communicating artery. Acute third nerve palsies caused by arteritis or vascular disease in hypertension and diabetes mellitus also may result in pain in and around the eye.

Facial pain with no signs

Trigeminal neuralgia (tic douloureux) is a common cause of intermittent pain in the face in the second half of life. Pain, which is unilateral, is usually confined to the second or third division of the fifth nerve, and possesses two absolute characteristics. First, the individual spasms of pain are extremely brief, like a knife jabbing into the cheek or jaw. Second, these spasms are triggered by at least two of the following events: talking, eating, washing the face, brushing the teeth, blowing the nose, touching the face, cold wind on the face, or attempting to put on make-up. The paroxysm triggered by these stimuli lasts a few seconds to several minutes, during which the patient may clutch the side of the face in agony. Commonly, the pain shoots from a characteristic site of onset, in the cheek or side of the nose or gums, to another part of the face, for example, to the ear or jaw. The illness is intermittent with bouts lasting days or weeks followed by long periods of freedom, which tend to become shorter as the patient ages (see p. 196).

Glossopharyngeal neuralgia is analogous to trigeminal neuralgia in that the pain is paroxysmal and very severe. It is felt at the back of the throat or tongue, or deep in the ear, and is triggered by swallowing (see p. 205).

The ophthalmic division of the trigeminal nerve is a common site for involvement by herpes zoster, and a proportion of such patients, usually the elderly, are left with the distressing aftermath of **postherpetic neuralgia**. Such pain is felt in the eye and forehead, where typical scarring and sensory loss is evident. The pain is continuous and often has a burning quality, superimposed on which are occasional jabs of pain, which may be triggered by light touch to the affected area.

Patients with otherwise typical migraine may also experience pain of similar calibre and character in the face **(facial migraine)**. As with migraine headache, the pain lasts for a few hours to a day or so, is often accompanied by nausea, vomiting and prostration, and is intermittent, leaving the patient normal between attacks. Part of the trigeminal autonomic cephalgias is **migrainous neuralgia or cluster headache**, which produces a different history (see p. 333). The sufferer is usually male and, during a bout, is often awoken from sleep by the onset of a severe continuous pain in or around one eye, building up over 45–120 minutes. One, two or three attacks may occur within 24 hours, both while asleep and in the day. At the height of the pain, the eye frequently reddens and waters, the nostril may become blocked and the eyelid may droop. Such pain recurs daily for a matter of weeks and then disappears for long periods until another bout starts. These features of migrainous neuralgia are quite different from those of migraine, and the condition may respond to specific therapy (see p. 334).

A similar continuous pain in the eye accompanied by progressive ptosis rarely may be caused by a structural lesion, sometimes malignant or granulomatous, at the base of the skull involving the paratrigeminal region with fifth cranial nerve signs (Raeder's neuralgia). **Chronic paroxysmal hemicrania** bears some resemblance to migrainous neuralgia. It affects women more than men, and consists of repeated, short-lived (10–20 minutes) attacks of knife-like excruciating pain in one side of the head, occurring 1–30 times a day; it responds dramatically to indometacin.

Short-lasting unilateral neuralgiform headache attacks with conjunctival injection and tearing are a further rare form of trigeminal autonomic neuralgia. Intense stabbing pain in and around one eye lasting 5–250 seconds (usually about 60 seconds) is described (see p. 337). The pain may be triggered by touch. Attacks vary in frequency from one per day to several per hour. Lamotrigine is probably the treatment of choice.

Finally, there is a group of patients complaining of pain in the face whose description accords with none of the entities outlined above, and who have no abnormal physical signs on examination. Such patients are said to suffer **atypical facial pain**. Most complain of continuous pain in the face unrelieved by any medication and present unaltered for months or years. These features have much in common with tension-type headache, and a proportion of those with atypical facial pain also have clinical symptoms of depressive illness, including sleep disturbance, diurnal mood fluctuation, anorexia and weight loss. Others, however, are not depressed, although they may exhibit a long-standing anxiety state. Frequently the intensity of their atypical facial pain is related to the stresses of everyday living, in the same way as occurs in patients with tension-type headache. The latter group of patients is sometimes said to suffer psychogenic facial pain. Antidepressants are probably the best treatment.

BLACKOUTS, FITS AND FAINTS

Patients commonly use the word blackout to describe loss of consciousness, when it really means loss of vision.

In a faint, caused by a drop in systemic blood pressure, vision goes black before consciousness is lost; the retinal circulation is also compressed by intraocular pressure, so it fails before the supply to the brain.

The doctor rarely has the opportunity to be present when a patient has an attack of loss of consciousness, and the diagnosis nearly always has to be established on the history. Naturally, if the patient passes out without warning, they will be unaware of the circumstances or of what happened during the attack.

Accordingly, a **description** of events from an independent **witness** is absolutely essential in coming to the correct conclusion about the cause of many such episodes.

The circumstances in which the attack occurred must be determined, and the details of exactly what happened during the attack, and afterwards, must be obtained. Eye-witnesses often describe what they think they saw, for example by concluding that the patient had a fit, but are not trained to distinguish between epilepsy, syncope and hysteria. Precipitants are also important, such as prolonged standing, flickering lights.

Epilepsy

The majority of patients presenting with sudden, unexplained episodes of loss of consciousness will be found to have epilepsy, but many other causes can provoke such events.

Epilepsy itself takes many forms, some of which do not cause loss of consciousness.

Major epileptic seizures
A major seizure consists of a period of tonic muscle contraction during which the subject becomes anoxic, followed by repetitive generalized whole body jerking in the clonic phase. The whole event lasts less than 5 minutes, when the subject stops fitting and either drifts into sleep or recovers.

Focal or simple partial epileptic seizures arising in one temporal lobe or in some other cortical area, may not cause loss of consciousness. More extensive focal discharges may cause loss of awareness, as in complex partial seizures, which may then propagate to involve both hemispheres to become generalized (secondary generalization). Then the patient will go into a typical tonic-clonic or grand mal seizure.

If such grand mal fits are caused by secondary generalization from some primary focal cortical source, then they may be prefaced by an aura that the patient remembers.

The aura is appropriate to the focal source of the seizure; for example, a discharge arising in the sensorimotor cortex will provoke contralateral motor and sensory phenomena for a short period prior to the loss of consciousness and the commencement of the generalized fit. Details of the characteristics of focal or partial seizures occurring in different parts of the cerebral cortex will be found in Chapter 15.

However, many patients with idiopathic epilepsy develop major grand mal seizures without any focal onset or aura. They are said to have primary generalized epilepsy of grand mal type.

Another form of epilepsy that causes temporary loss of consciousness, occurring in children, is also a form of primary generalized seizure discharge causing a brief **absence attack**, called **petit mal**. For a few seconds or so, the child ceases to speak or move, appears stunned with open flickering eyes, and then rapidly recovers back to normal. Similar absence attacks also may occur during brief focal seizures arising in the temporal lobe structures, often accompanied by purposeless movements of chewing, or fumbling with clothing. Such temporal lobe attacks frequently are accompanied by highly complex distortions of thought, sensation and emotion to produce a typical psychomotor or complex partial seizure.

> The old term temporal lobe seizure has largely been replaced by complex partial seizure as a significant number of such attacks arise in other areas of the brain, such as the frontal lobes.

In **complex partial seizures** there is impairment of awareness during attacks. By contrast in **simple partial seizures**, a focal discharge may occur without loss of awareness so that in a simple partial motor seizure there may be contralateral jerking of the thumb, spreading into the arm and perhaps the corner of the mouth on the same side, without loss of awareness. After such a focal motor attack there may be a temporary weakness in the affected limb – a Todd's paresis.

Sometimes, following grand mal seizures, particularly those caused by generalization from temporal lobe foci, or after complex partial seizures, the patient may enter into a period of **automatic behaviour** for up to about an hour or so, but usually much shorter (minutes). During this phase of post-epileptic automatism, the patient may undertake relatively co-ordinated action for which they subsequently have no memory, amnesia. In such a state, epileptic patients may travel some distance and arrive at their destination with no idea as to how they got there.

Diagnosis of epilepsy

The criteria that contribute to a confident diagnosis of epilepsy are:

1   The sudden, unexpected onset in an otherwise apparently healthy individual of a brief period of loss of consciousness not exceeding 5 minutes.
2   The episode of loss of consciousness may be prefaced by a characteristic aura in which the same events occur in every attack.
3   If the seizure is of grand mal type, witnesses will say that the patient fell, went stiff and blue, and shook. The patients may find afterwards that they have injured themselves, bitten their tongue, or been incontinent.
4   If it was an absence seizure, as a result of either petit mal or a complex partial seizure, witnesses will remark that the patient suddenly lost contact with the world and was inaccessible for a short period, during which they may have undertaken simple crude motor automatisms.
5   The attacks are always brief (unless the patient goes into repeated attacks as in status epilepticus), and the patient returns to normal between the episodes.

Table 3.4 Causes of epilepsy

Focal, partial seizures, often symptomatic of a primary brain lesion, e.g:
  Tumour – benign, malignant; metastatic
  Infections – meningo-encephalitis, abscess, subdural empyema
  Trauma
  Vascular
    Thromboembolic infarct, haemorrhage
    Cortical venous thrombosis, angioma, cavernoma
    Hypertensive encephalopathy
  Degenerative – Alzheimer's disease
  Miscellaneous – multiple sclerosis
Generalized seizures, often idiopathic
  Includes major tonic-clonic, absence (petit mal), myoclonic, atonic
Systemic disorders
  Anoxic
  Metabolic – uraemic, hepatic failure, hypoglycaemia,
  Drugs
    Amphetamines, cocaine, baclofen, isoniazid
    High dose penicillin (intrathecal)
  Alcohol – include withdrawal

Finally, it should be noted that many patients complaining of 'blackouts' may be suspected of suffering from epilepsy, but the evidence initially is insufficient to be certain of that diagnosis. As already has been stated, the electroencephalogram cannot be used to establish a certain diagnosis of epilepsy. In this situation, it is usually best to avoid a firm diagnosis and to await subsequent events. To label someone as epileptic on insufficient evidence may be catastrophic for the patient's livelihood and there is little risk in seeing what happens.

If the patient's attack of loss of consciousness is confidently diagnosed as being a result of epilepsy, the next stage is to determine its cause (Table 3.4).

The cause of epilepsy changes with age

A simple but important principle is that the aetiology of epilepsy changes with age. Epilepsy in the infant indicates some serious metabolic, infective or structural cause. Epilepsy in the child usually is of unknown cause (idiopathic) or a result of some static cerebral pathology, such as that produced by a birth injury or head trauma. Epilepsy beginning in the younger adult often is the first sign of a cerebral tumour (Figure 3.3). Epilepsy commencing for the first time in the elderly frequently is caused by vascular or other degenerative disease.

Focal (partial) epilepsy usually has a structural cause

A second useful simple principle is that focal (partial) epilepsy commonly is a result of some identifiable structural lesion (Figure 3.4), while primary generalized grand mal or petit mal frequently appears idiopathic in origin.

These principles guide the subsequent management of the patient whose episodes of loss of consciousness are diagnosed as being caused by epilepsy, which is discussed in greater detail in Chapter 15.

Epilepsy must be distinguished from other causes of loss of consciousness, in particular from fainting (syncope), sleep attacks of narcolepsy, hypoglycaemia, cerebrovascular disease, and psychogenic illness.

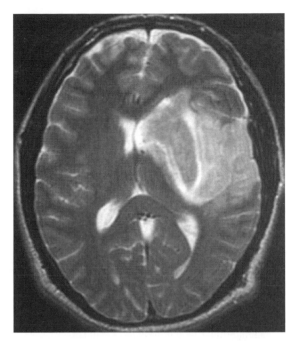

Figure 3.3 T2-weighted axial view MRI scan showing a left frontal tumour. This patient presented with complex partial seizures with secondary generalization.

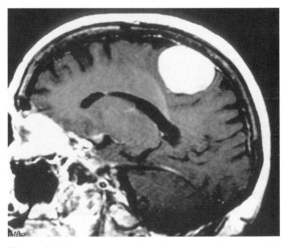

Figure 3.4 Sagittal view MRI scan showing a large convexity meningioma. This was causing simple partial seizures with a focal onset in the face and arm on the opposite side.

Syncope (Table 3.5)

Syncope is defined as transient loss of consciousness caused by an acute decrease in cerebral blood flow.

Table 3.5 Causes of syncope

Vasovagal, vasodepressor
Simple faint
Cough
Micturition
Orthostatic, postural hypotension
Autonomic neuropathy, dysautonomia, spinal
cord lesions
Drugs
Hypotensive – β-blockers, ACE inhibitors
Vasodilators
Antipsychotics
Antidepressants
Endocrine
Hypopituitarism
Addisonian
Cardiac
Arrhythmias – too fast, too slow
Outflow obstruction – aortic stenosis, obstructive
cardiomyopathy, left atrial mobile mass
Cardiomyopathy
Hypovolaemic – blood loss, dehydration
Vascular
Carotid sinus sensitivity, vertebrobasilar TIAs
Anaemia
Metabolic – hypoglycaemia, hyperventilation
Psychogenic
Anxiety, panic
Non-epileptic attack disorder
ACE, angiotensin-converting enzyme; TIAs, transient ischaemic attacks.

Fainting provoked by the sight of blood, needles, prolonged standing in church or on parade, or intense emotion and pain (reflex, vasodepressor or vasovagal syncope) is commonplace. The term vasovagal indicates two components of reflex fainting – vagal slowing of the heart rate and peripheral vasodilatation. Such patients 'come over queer', feel dizzy and 'swimmy', their eyesight dims and hearing recedes, the face goes pale, and they slump forward or fall to the ground. Provided they are laid flat, consciousness soon returns, although patients may feel sick and break out into a heavy sweat.

This sequence of events is precipitated by a profound drop in systemic systolic blood pressure, below about 60 mmHg, resulting in a combination of sudden bradycardia and peripheral vasodilatation in skeletal muscle and internal organs. A similar sequence of events may be triggered in men getting up at night to pass water **(micturition syncope)**, or by pressure over the carotid bifurcation in the occasional older patient with excessive sensitivity of the carotid sinus **(carotid sinus syndrome)**. Repeated coughing in those with chronic lung disease also may provoke fainting by causing obstruction of venous return to the heart and perhaps by baroceptor stimulation **(cough syncope)**. A similar mechanism is probably responsible for the syncope seen in trumpet playing and weight-lifting.

Another cause of fainting is damage to peripheral or central autonomic pathways **(areflexic, orthostatic or paralytic syncope)**. In this situation, patients faint when they stand upright, because they are unable to adjust heart rate and the resistance of peripheral blood vessels to cope with the rapid shift of blood to the legs and viscera that occurs when suddenly standing up. Such postural syncope occurs in any type of peripheral neuropathy affecting the autonomic nervous system, but particularly in those with diabetes. In addition, drugs such as hypotensive agents, alcohol, barbiturates, dopamine agonists and phenothiazines may all interfere with the operation of normal baroceptor reflexes to cause postural faintness. Ageing itself leads to some loss of efficiency of baroceptor reflexes, and many elderly patients experience transient dizziness on rising quickly from a bed or chair. Such patients are particularly sensitive to relatively small doses of hypotensive agents.

Fainting caused by cardiac disease **(cardiac syncope)** is also relatively common in the elderly and may account for some 25% of patients presenting with 'syncope' as an emergency. Symptoms typical of a faint may occur in those with cardiac dysrhythmias (conduction defects), aortic stenosis or congenital heart disease. However, many patients with heart block lose consciousness abruptly (Stokes–Adams attack) probably as a result of cardiac arrest. Cardiac causes of syncope carry a worse prognosis, particularly in the elderly.

In general, a careful history will distinguish syncope from epilepsy, but a complication arises if failure of cerebral perfusion during a syncopal attack persists for longer than a minute, for in these circumstances the patient who faints may go on to have a fit. This situation may occur if someone faints in a position where they are unable to lie with the head lower than their heart, as may happen on the stairs, in the lavatory or if the patient is supported upright by well-wishers. If unconsciousness lasts longer than 20 seconds, convulsive features may occur (convulsive syncope). In addition, if the bladder is full during a faint, incontinence may occur.

Other causes of episodic loss of consciousness

Other conditions that may be confused with epilepsy, or with syncope, are much less common. **Spontaneous hypoglycaemia** certainly can lead to loss of consciousness and many patients with this condition do not recall the premonitory symptoms of anxiety, palpitations and sweating (see p. 486). The only definitive way of confirming the diagnosis is to obtain a blood sugar estimation during an attack: a value of <2 mmol/l is diagnostic. Any patient found unconscious for no apparent reason must have blood withdrawn for estimation of sugar and insulin levels, and 50 g of glucose should be given intravenously; it can do no harm but may save a life. Fortunately, spontaneous hypoglycaemia (which usually is caused by an islet cell pancreatic tumour) is rare, but should be considered in any patient with episodes of altered behaviour or loss of consciousness for which there is no other ready explanation.

Cerebrovascular disease also can cause episodic loss of consciousness without other obvious neurological symptoms, particularly when transient ischaemia occurs in the territory of the vertebrobasilar arterial system. However, such patients usually suffer other symptoms such as diplopia, dysarthria and ataxia, indicating brainstem ischaemia. Some patients with cerebrovascular disease affecting the posterior cerebral arterial territory, which supplies the medial portions of the cerebral hemispheres, may experience prolonged periods of loss of awareness. Such **transient global amnesia** may last minutes to hours. During such an episode the patients are disorientated, unable to recall what they are doing, where they are, or when it is, but can undertake simple automatic tasks, such as washing, dressing or cooking. Subsequently they have no memory for the event, that is, they are amnesic. Likewise, patients with **migraine** in whom there is profound ischaemia in the vertebrobasilar territory (basilar artery

migraine) occasionally may also complain of episodes of loss of awareness for up to 30 minutes, although they too usually describe other symptoms of brainstem ischaemia and severe occipital headache. Rarely transient global amnesia may arise in the context of a form of complex partial seizure.

Patients with intense vertigo also may complain of loss of consciousness. The diagnosis of vertigo will be considered in a later chapter, but it should be noted here that some patients with epilepsy have a vertiginous aura to their seizures, while other patients with intense vertigo as a result of labyrinthine disease may complain of loss of consciousness at the height of an attack. The sleep attacks characteristic of **narcolepsy** should not be confused with either epilepsy or syncope. Such sufferers describe lapsing into otherwise typical sleep, from which they can be awoken, at quite inappropriate moments.

Occasionally, patients with obstructive hydrocephalus, may suddenly lose consciousness, often at the height of a bout of severe headache. Head injuries sometimes may present with a complaint of loss of consciousness, if the blow was unexpected and there is residual amnesia for the events surrounding the incident.

Prolonged overbreathing, **hyperventilation**, may produce a respiratory alkalosis with symptoms of paroxysmal tingling in the extremities and around the mouth. These are usually accompanied by giddiness, and, rarely, loss of consciousness. If the attack persists, carpopedal spasm and muscular twitching may appear. A proportion of these patients complain of headache and visual upset. Many are young women and a trial of overbreathing may provoke similar symptoms.

Finally, it will rapidly become apparent to the student attending neurological out-patients that many patients complaining of blackouts cannot be easily allocated to one of the diagnostic categories described above. Frequently this is because there is insufficient information on the circumstances of the attack, particularly if a witness is not available. However, many of these patients describe attacks of altered awareness occurring in relation to emotional provocation. As usual, marital discord, family tensions, job dissatisfaction, and other such stresses may provoke acute episodes of phobic anxiety in which the subject is distraught, breathless and incoherent, a state of affairs for which they claim subsequent amnesia. Often it is obvious that such patients have an underlying severe anxiety state, and careful enquiry may unearth the usual precipitating circumstances. Other patients may actually feign epileptic attacks (**non-epileptic attacks**, sometimes called pseudoseizures) to attract attention. Such patients, frequently adolescent females, exhibit other hysterical features and careful enquiry into the circumstances and character of their attack will indicate a hysterical origin; for example, sexual abuse may sometimes be the provocation. Unfortunately, some individuals (approximately 10–15%), who also suffer from epilepsy, may be prone to hysterical attacks as well. In such individuals, it may take prolonged observation and careful searching through every facet of the history to establish the true situation. As a general principle, it is best not to commit oneself to a certain diagnosis in those with bizarre attacks of uncertain origin. Non-epileptic attack disorder (NEAD) is the term increasingly used to describe some of these episodes of uncertain origin. If these episodes are frequent (several weekly), then video-telemetry with electroencephalography (EEG) may establish a clear diagnosis.

LOSS OF VISION

The patient complaining of disturbance of vision either may have disease of the eye, or may have damage to the optic nerve or posterior parts of the visual pathways.

Local eye disease is common, and it is necessary to exclude refractive errors, corneal damage, cataract, glaucoma, and obvious retinal lesions by appropriate ophthalmological techniques. These will not be considered in detail here, but most refractive errors are a result of short-sightedness (myopia), which can be corrected with a pin-hole. This simple test should be employed in all complaining of visual loss, before considering other causes. A neurological cause of visual failure can only be assumed if vision cannot be improved to normal by correction of refractive error, the ocular media are clear, and there is no gross retinal abnormality.

Visual sensitivity or acuity depends upon intact central or macular vision.

Lesions of the optic nerve cause loss of central macular vision (scotoma) and reduced visual acuity.

However, lesions placed further back in the visual pathways, in the optic chiasm, or radiations, or in the occipital cortex, only produce loss of vision in one half of the visual field (hemianopia; see later). Visual acuity is normal in patients with such posteriorly placed lesions because, although they have lost vision in the opposite half-field, the remaining intact half of central macular vision is sufficient to preserve normal acuity. Patients with visual failure caused by anteriorly placed lesions of the optic nerve complain of loss of visual perception of detail of distant objects or of reading print, and can be demonstrated to have a reduced visual acuity, which cannot be improved by correcting refractive error. In contrast, patients with posteriorly placed visual pathway damage complain of difficulty in perceiving objects in the affected opposite field of vision, but retain sensitivity in the remaining intact visual field so that they can still make out detail and read print, and show a normal visual acuity on formal testing. Patients with posteriorly placed lesions do complain of difficulties with reading, but they are of a different character. Those with loss of the right half of vision have difficulty seeing the next word in a sentence, while those with loss of the left half of vision have difficulty moving from one line to the next. The significance of such hemianopic field defects will be discussed later. Here the problem of visual failure as a result of a reduced visual acuity that cannot be attributed to local eye disease, is considered.

The most valuable aid in distinguishing different causes of neurological visual failure is the tempo of the illness (Table 3.6).

Visual deficit may be: present from early life and static (amblyopia); sudden and transient; sudden but persistent; or progressive. Usually it is possible to distinguish between these patterns of visual loss, but one problem is that of the patient who discovers visual impairment in one eye accidentally when rubbing the other, whereupon the onset is thought to be acute. In fact, many patients with progressive

Table 3.6 Causes of persistent visual loss

Acute
  Ophthalmic
    Retinal vein occlusion
    Retinal artery occlusion
    Retinal detachment
    Glaucoma
    Vitreous haemorrhage
    Acute maculopathy
    Inflammatory – uveitis
  Neurological
    Optic neuritis
    Ischaemic optic neuropathy (include giant
      cell arteritis)
    Optic nerve compression
    Pituitary apoplexy
    Bilateral occipital lobe infarction
Sub-acute/progressive
  Ophthalmic
    Glaucoma
    Macular degeneration
  Neurological
    Leber's optic neuropathy
    Optic nerve compression
      Pituitary tumours, gliomas, meningiomas
      Aneurysms, orbital masses
    Metabolic – diabetic retinopathy
    Toxic – tobacco/alcohol, methanol
    Drugs – chloramphenicol, ethambutol,
      chloroquine
    Vitamin B12 deficiency

unilateral visual failure are not aware of their problem until, for some reason or another, they occlude the vision of the opposite intact eye.

Amblyopia

Ocular defects in early life, particularly muscle imbalance, cause suppression of visual acuity in one eye to prevent continuing double vision. Such visual suppression is known as amblyopia, which is not progressive after about 6–8 years of age, and which does not affect perception of colour or pupillary responses. Amblyopia as a cause of reduced visual acuity is suggested by visual loss since early childhood, evidence of a squint, or obvious refractive error.

Sudden transient visual loss

Sudden but temporary loss of vision occurs in a number of circumstances. **Obscurations of vision**, as a result of raised intracranial pressure, consist of episodic visual loss affecting one or both eyes and lasting for a few seconds to one-quarter of a minute. Obscurations may be provoked by any manoeuvre that increases intracranial pressure, such as straining, coughing, sneezing or bending. Examination will reveal swollen optic discs, and further investigation and treatment are a matter of some urgency, for obscurations threaten impending permanent visual loss. **Amaurosis fugax** refers to episodic unilateral visual loss caused by vascular disturbance in ophthalmic artery territory. The patient commonly describes a curtain ascending or descending to occlude the lower or upper half of vision resulting from involvement of the superior or inferior branches of the ophthalmic artery. These field defects respect the vertical meridian. Such episodes may last for minutes to hours, but sooner or later the curtain gradually disappears and the vision returns to normal. Amaurosis fugax thus is a transient ischaemic attack in ophthalmic artery distribution and, in the middle-aged or elderly subject, is likely to indicate the existence of cerebrovascular disease. Uhtoff's phenomenon describes dimness or loss of vision provoked by a rise in body temperature, such as occurs when taking a hot bath or on vigorous exercise, and is a feature of optic nerve demyelination produced by multiple sclerosis.

Sudden persistent visual loss

Sudden persistent visual loss is nearly always a result either of acute optic neuritis (most commonly caused by multiple sclerosis) in the younger subject, or a vascular cause (ischaemic optic neuropathy) in the middle-aged or elderly.

Occasionally a tumour or cyst compressing the optic nerve expands suddenly to cause abrupt visual failure.

Progressive visual loss

> **Progressive visual loss**
> In the absence of any ocular pathology, a history of progressive visual loss in one or both eyes must be taken to suggest compression of the anterior optic pathways until proven otherwise by appropriate investigations.

Many compressive lesions turn out to be benign tumours, such as pituitary adenomas or suprasellar meningiomas, which can be surgically removed with subsequent restoration of sight. Toxic damage to the optic nerve by drugs and alcohol/tobacco, and hereditary optic neuropathies, are less common than compressive lesions, which must always be excluded in a patient with progressive visual failure.

In practice, patients complaining of visual loss must be assessed by an ophthalmologist and, if the eyes are found to be normal, by a neurologist. Acute loss of vision must be treated as an emergency, and progressive loss of vision must always be investigated fully to establish the cause.

GIDDINESS

Patients use the words 'giddiness', 'dizziness', 'light-headedness' and 'unsteadiness' to describe a great variety of sensations with many causes. Thus patients with postural syncope will say that they become giddy when standing up, while patients with cerebellar ataxia of gait may say they are dizzy and unsteady.

> Vertigo refers to a sensation of unsteadiness or disequilibrium that is felt in the head.

Patients with a cerebellar ataxia know that they are unsteady when trying to walk, but the sensation of disequilibrium is not felt in the head so it is not vertigo.

The sensation of vertigo is one of disequilibrium, whatever its nature; it may be a sensation of rotation, a sensation of falling, a sensation as if on a pitching boat moving up and down, or a sensation of swaying. All are sensations of disequilibrium which, if felt in the head, may be described as vertiginous. Thus vertigo is an illusory movement of oneself or one's surrounds. It implies a defect of function of the vestibular system, either of the labyrinthine end-organ or of its central connections, particularly those in the brainstem. Lesions of the cerebral hemispheres rarely cause vertigo, although it may form an uncommon symptom in occasional patients with temporal lobe epilepsy.

> The first step in diagnosis of a patient with vertigo is to decide whether the cause lies peripherally in the labyrinth, or centrally in the brainstem (Table 3.7).

Peripheral lesions causing vertigo also commonly cause intense nausea, vomiting, sweating and prostration. Because of the proximity of auditory to vestibular fibres in the eighth cranial nerve, deafness often accompanies vertigo. Conductive deafness caused by middle ear disease suggests a peripheral lesion, but perceptive deafness, resulting from damage to the cochlear end-organ or vestibular nerve may be caused by peripheral or central lesions. If peripheral, perceptive deafness is often less severe with loud sounds (loudness recruitment), and also causes severe speech distortion. Central lesions of the eighth nerve rarely show loudness recruitment, but exhibit auditory fatigue in that the intensity of sound has to be increased progressively to maintain a constant noise level. Vertigo caused by vestibular damage is also often accompanied by evidence of nystagmus on examination, which consists of to-and-fro movements of the eyes because of interrupted visual fixation. Different types of nystagmus will be described later.

> Suffice it to say here that peripheral vestibular lesions causing vertigo are usually accompanied by horizontal jerk nystagmus in one direction which becomes worse with loss of fixation (as in the dark), while central lesions produce nystagmus that changes direction depending upon the patient's gaze, and which is often rotatory and vertical as well as horizontal.

Table 3.7 Causes of dizziness

Peripheral
    Acute labyrinthine failure
        Vestibular neuronitis
        Vascular
    Benign positional vertigo
    Ménière's disease
    Post-traumatic vertigo
    Local infection – bacterial, viral
Central
    Brainstem
        Ischaemia, infarction
        Demyelination
    Tumours – primary, secondary
    Cerebellopontine angle tumours
    Seizures (rare)
Systemic
    Drugs
        Vestibulotoxic – aminoglycosides, streptomycin
        Hypotensives, hypnotics, alcohol, tranquillizers
        Analgesics, anticonvulsants
    Hypotension
    Cardiac arrhythmias
    Endocrine – myxoedema, diabetes mellitus
    Vascular – vasculitis, SLE, giant cell arteritis,
        PRV, anaemia
    Infective – systemic infection, syphilis
    Sarcoidosis
Psychogenic

SLE, systemic lupus erythematosus; PRV, polycythaemia rubra vera.

Acute single attack of vertigo

An acute episode of vertigo may be provoked by sudden loss of unilateral labyrinthine function, or by sudden brainstem damage.

Either may cause the sudden onset of acute severe vertigo, nausea, vomiting, and great distress because the patient is unable to move without provoking further severe vertigo. The patient with acute vestibular failure will usually lie with the affected ear uppermost. The acute episode commonly lasts days, sometimes as long as 2–3 weeks, and then gradually eases because adaptation to vestibular failure occurs. During the recovery phase, which may last 3–4 weeks, any sudden head movement may cause brief vertigo and unsteadiness. Acute vestibular failure resulting from sudden unilateral labyrinthine damage may develop in the course of middle ear disease when infection gains access to the labyrinth. Such a course of events must be treated as an emergency. If the middle ear is normal, acute peripheral vestibular failure may be attributed to a virus infection (vestibular neuronitis) or to ischaemia in the distribution of the internal auditory arteries. However, in many such cases, the cause is uncertain. Acute brainstem lesions that may provoke an attack of vertigo include a plaque of demyelination as a result of multiple sclerosis, or a vascular lesion such as infarction or haemorrhage in the brainstem or part of the cerebellum. Such lesions may cause diplopia, dysarthria, weakness, ataxia and sensory disturbances.

Differential diagnosis of vertigo

The differential diagnosis of causes of vertigo is aided by considering the time-course of the symptoms. The duration of the actual sensation of spinning is important. Benign positional vertigo lasts seconds, that of vertebrobasilar ischaemia or migraine minutes, that of Ménière's disease hours and that of acute vestibular failure days. Some diseases produce a single acute episode of vertigo, others produce recurrent attacks (and, of course, any single episode may be the first of such attacks), while others produce persistent vertigo.

Recurrent attacks of vertigo

If the patient describes repeated attacks of acute vertigo with recovery between episodes, they may be suffering from peripheral vestibular disease such as Ménière's syndrome, or from repeated brainstem ischaemia.

The latter occurs as basilar artery migraine in the younger subject, or as vertebrobasilar transient ischaemic attacks in the middle-aged and elderly. Such recurrent episodes of vertigo may, very rarely, indicate epilepsy. More commonly patients may describe recurrent fleeting episodes of vertigo provoked by some critical position. This is usually most striking when lying down at night, or when moving the head suddenly. Such benign paroxysmal positional vertigo may be a result of damage arising from otoconia being displaced from the utricle and ending in the posterior semicircular canal. Positional testing will establish the diagnosis (see p. 97). Positional vertigo may follow trauma to the head or infections but often is of undetermined origin. It may also arise from central causes as a brainstem disturbance.

Persistent vertigo

Chronic persistent vertigo is uncommon because of the rapid compensation that occurs with vestibular deficits. Those patients complaining of persistent dizziness usually are not really describing vertigo proper, but are drawing attention to minor degrees of true instability or a sense of insecurity. However, drug damage to the vestibular nerves (streptomycin, gentamicin), brainstem demyelination or infarction, and occasionally posterior fossa tumours, all may cause a persistent vertigo, although this often proves to be ataxia. Many of those with complaints of persistent vertigo may have a phobic anxiety state, with fear of falling. This can be triggered by an episode of true vertigo, by insecurity as a result of ataxia, or even by a fall or trip. Such patients may become housebound (agarophobic) or unable to leave the security of walls or furniture (space phobia).

PAIN IN THE ARM

The painful, tingling or weak arm

Acute pain in the arm, of course, is most commonly caused by trauma or local disease of muscle, joint or bone. Only after these are excluded can neurological causes be considered (Table 3.8). Damage to the peripheral nerves, brachial plexus, or cervical roots causes sensory disturbance and muscle wasting with weakness in a characteristic distribution, which

Table 3.8 Neurological causes of acute pain in the arm

Peripheral nerve
Carpal tunnel syndrome
Peripheral neuropathy
Diabetic, amyloid, paraneoplastic, ischaemic, drug-induced e.g. metronidazole
Brachial plexus
Trauma
Malignant infiltration
Cervical rib
Inflammatory – neuralgic amyotrophy
Cervical roots
Trauma – avulsion
Compression – disc, bony spur, malignancy
Post-herpetic
Cervical cord
Intramedullary tumour
Syrinx
Central causes
Thalamic lesion
Extrapyramidal disorder

must be learnt (see later) in order to diagnose the site of damage to these structures. Pain resulting from lesions of peripheral nerves, plexus or spinal roots, however, often does not follow exact anatomical distribution: for example, pain caused by compression of the median nerve at the wrist (carpal tunnel syndrome) often spreads up to the elbow or even to the shoulder; the pain resulting from damage to a spinal root is felt in the myotome and not in the dermatome, for example, a lesion of C7 causes pain in the *triceps*, forearm extensors, and *pectoralis*, while paraesthesiae occur in the middle finger. Pain in the arm also may be felt occasionally by patients with cerebral disease; for example, pain and clumsiness in one arm may be the first signs of Parkinson's disease.

Paraesthesiae, which describes positive sensory symptoms such as pins and needles or tingling, may be a result of damage to peripheral sensory neurones from the peripheral nerve itself to the spinal root, or result from lesions of the central sensory pathways in spinal cord, brainstem or internal capsule.

Cortical lesions generally do not produce positive paraesthesiae. Sensory disturbances, whether paraesthesiae or sensory loss, are often difficult to put into words, and terms such as pins and needles, tingling, numbness, stiffness, constriction, wrapped in tight bandages, or like going to the dentist, all may be used to describe sensory deficit.

> Weakness of the arm may be caused by primary muscle disease (rare), lesions of peripheral nerves, brachial plexus or cervical roots, or by damage to central motor pathways.

The latter causes signs typical of upper motor neurone lesions (weakness without wasting, spasticity, and enhanced tendon reflexes). Lesions of peripheral nerves, plexus or roots cause the signs of a lower motor neurone lesion (weakness with wasting, normal or diminished tone, reduced or absent tendon reflexes).

Acute pain in the arm

Acute disease of the shoulder joints or adjacent structures is a common cause of pain in the arm. A variety of conditions are responsible for the clinical syndrome of **'frozen shoulder'**, which causes acute severe pain, restriction of joint movement, and later wasting of the surrounding shoulder muscles. The frozen shoulder sometimes is accompanied by a curious sympathetic disturbance of the hand which becomes swollen, painful, shiny and weak, for reasons that are not understood (see p. 520). This shoulder – hand syndrome occurs in some patients with a hemiplegia caused by a stroke and, occasionally, after myocardial infarction.

Primary muscle disease confined to the arm is very unusual, but giant cell arteritis may affect the muscles around the shoulder girdles and cause the syndrome of **polymyalgia rheumatica**. This illness affects middle-aged or elderly patients who develop increasing pain and stiffness symmetrically in the muscles of both shoulder girdles, which become tender to palpation and painful to move. The erythrocyte sedimentation rate is high, as in cranial arteritis, which may coexist in a few patients with polymyalgia rheumatica.

Neuralgic amyotrophy is another mysterious condition, probably a brachial plexopathy from patchy demyelination. This presents as acute, very severe pain affecting one upper limb and shoulder girdle, and accompanied by subsequent rapid wasting of the muscles of the arm, usually those around the shoulder, winging of the scapula being a common feature. Sensory disturbance is minimal, but there is often a patch of altered sensation over the deltoid corresponding to the circumflex nerve distribution.

A **cervical disc prolapse** may present with acute pain and stiffness of the neck, with referred pain in the distribution of the cervical root involved, usually C5, C6 or C7. In addition, there may be paraesthesiae and weakness of the arm in the distribution of the affected nerve root. The neck is fixed or extremely painful to move, and coughing and sneezing also frequently provoke impulse pain referred into the arm. When lateral flexion or rotation of the neck aggravates pain on the same side in the arm or shoulder (ipsilateral) this is suggestive of nerve root irritation.

Herpes zoster may cause pain in the arm, even before the appearance of the characteristic skin rash, if the cervical roots are affected.

The acute pain of neuralgic amyotrophy, cervical disc prolapse, and herpes zoster usually resolves in a matter of weeks or months.

Chronic pain in the arm

A number of entrapment neuropathies affecting peripheral nerves in the arm are common causes of chronic pain.

> The carpal tunnel syndrome is by far the commonest cause of chronic arm pain, particularly in women.

A complaint of pain at night accompanied by paraesthesiae in the fingers, particularly the thumb, index and middle finger, relieved by moving the hands about or hanging them out of bed is quite characteristic. Signs often are minimal. Occasionally, the carpal tunnel syndrome may be symptomatic (see Table 8.2).

In men, it is usually the ulnar nerve that is affected, particularly at the elbow.

Previous damage to the elbow joint causing osteoarthritis, or entrapment of the ulnar nerve in the cubital tunnel causes local pain, paraesthesiae in the little and ring fingers, and weakness and wasting of the small muscles of the hand.

The **lower cord of the brachial plexus** may be compressed by a cervical rib, or infiltrated by malignant disease extending from an apical lung carcinoma (Pancoast's syndrome), or by local spread from a breast carcinoma. Such lesions cause pain referred down the inner side of the arm, paraesthesiae on the medial aspect of the forearm, and weakness of the small muscles of the hand. Cervical ribs compressing the brachial plexus may also compress the subclavian artery to cause vascular disturbances in the arm.

Cervical spondylosis, degenerative disease of the cervical spine is very common with advancing years and sometimes causes chronic pain in the arm, accompanied by paraesthesiae and weakness in the distribution of affected root or roots. Such chronic pain may follow acute cervical disc protrusions or, more commonly, may result from compression of cervical roots by osteophytes narrowing the spinal exit foramina through which the nerves enter the neck. The C5, C6 and C7 vertebrae are most commonly involved.

Spinal tumours may present with pain in the arm. Malignant disease of the cervical vertebrae, usually from breast or lung, may lead to compression of cervical roots. Benign neurofibromas and occasional intrinsic cervical cord tumours such as gliomas may present with chronic arm pain. So too, may **syringomyelia**, which also causes characteristic dissociated sensory loss, absent tendon jerks and wasting of the hand muscles.

The wasted hand

Wasting of the small muscles of the hand either with or without pain, is a common clinical problem. These muscles are innervated predominantly by the ulnar nerve (the median nerve only supplies muscles of the thenar eminence), the inner cord of

Table 3.9 Neurological causes of wasted small hand muscles

Peripheral nerve
Ulnar, median (thenar pad)
Peripheral neuropathy
Diabetic, amyloid, paraneoplastic, ischaemic, toxic, e.g. alcohol
Brachial plexus
Lower cord compression
Malignancy
Cervical rib, fibrous band
Irradiation fibrosis
Neuralgic amyotrophy
Cervical root C8/T1
Spondylotic degenerative changes, disc prolapse
Compression by tumour
Trauma
Cervical cord
Syrinx
Intramedullary tumour
Motor neurone disease
Poliomyelitis
Disuse associated with arthritis
Rheumatoid
Osteoarthritis

the brachial plexus, the T1 spinal root, or the equivalent group of anterior horn cells.

Obviously, lesions of the ulnar nerve, the inner cord of the brachial plexus, the T1 root or that part of the spinal cord may all produce wasting of small hand muscles (Table 3.9).

However, wasting of the hand is also one of the commonest presenting features of **motor neurone disease**, which also causes fasciculation and signs of upper motor neurone damage, but no sensory loss.

Wasting of the muscles around the shoulder occurs in the frozen shoulder syndrome, neuralgic amyotrophy, cervical spondylosis affecting the C5 roots, and motor neurone disease. Symmetrical wasting around the shoulder may also be a sign of primary muscle disease, including thyrotoxicosis.

BACK PAIN

Low back pain is very common, probably affecting 60–70% of the population at some time in their life. Most episodes are of short duration but they often recur. There appears to be a link with the physical demands of work, and a previous history of back problems is an adverse risk factor. Simple back pain centred on the lumbosacral region and upper buttocks is probably **mechanical** in origin and carries a good outlook, with some 90% of patients recovering within approximately 6 weeks. If there is associated nerve root pain which often radiates down the back of the leg into the foot and toes with sometimes sensory symptoms, the outlook is less good, with only about 50% recovering by 6 weeks. If the pain appears more severe, progressive, not helped by rest and accompanied by more widespread neurological signs or those of systemic upset, these are considered 'red flags', marking the need for special investigation (see p. 187).

PAIN IN THE LEG

The painful, tingling or weak leg

As in the arm, the commonest cause of pain in the leg is local bone or joint disease. The speed with which the quadriceps muscle wastes after a knee injury may amaze the young sportsman, while the commonest cause of pain in the thigh and wasting of the quadriceps in later life is osteoarthritis of the knee. The commonest neurological cause of acute leg pain is sciatica, but a number of conditions may cause chronic pain in the lower limb.

Acute sciatica

Traditional terms such as lumbago and sciatica describe syndromes of acute pain in the back and acute pain radiating into the leg, respectively.

Acute lumbago probably has many causes including: tears of paraspinal muscles, or spinal ligaments; acute damage to hypophyseal joints of the spine; and acute ruptures of lumbar discs. Radiation of pain into the leg may be caused by hip disease, however, when it is **unilateral and extends below the knee it is most usually a result of irritation of the corresponding lumbosacral nerve root by a lateral disc protrusion**. Musculoskeletal pain of lumbar origin often radiates widely and into both legs. Sciatica is commonly accompanied by lumbago, but may occur by itself; lumbago often occurs without sciatica. Typically the onset is sudden during physical activity, particularly when lifting weights with the back flexed. Excruciating back pain, with or without radiation into the leg, is accompanied by spasm of the back muscles so that the spine 'locks', and any slight movement causes exquisite agony. Coughing, sneezing, or straining at stool all aggravate pain. The sciatica is in the distribution of the nerve root involved, down the back of the leg to the heel in the case of S1, or down the lateral surface of the leg to the instep in the case of L5, these being the **two roots most commonly affected by disc degeneration at the L4/5 (L5 root) and L5/S1 (S1 root) disc spaces respectively**. Root compression also gives rise to typical sensory symptoms of numbness or paraesthesiae and motor weakness in the appropriate distribution. When the onset is acute in the setting of physical exercise, the diagnosis of acute sciatica is rarely in doubt. However, disc protrusions not uncommonly may cause a more gradual onset of pain without any obvious precipitating cause. In this situation, alternative diagnoses have to be considered (Table 3.10).

Chronic leg pain

Pain referred into the leg may be caused by pelvic carcinoma spreading from the uterus, cervix, prostate or rectum to infiltrate the lumbar or sacral plexus. Such pain is insidious in onset and gradually becomes more severe and constant. A rectal examination, which is essential in all patients with unexplained persistent leg pain, will usually reveal the cause.

Meralgia paraesthetica is caused by an entrapment neuropathy of the lateral cutaneous nerve of

Table 3.10 Neurological causes of acute leg pain

Peripheral nerve
　　Tarsal tunnel, interdigital neuroma
　　Peripheral neuropathy
　　　　Diabetic, ischaemic, amyloid, paraneoplastic
Lumbosacral plexus
　　Diabetic plexopathy
　　Malignancy
　　Haematoma – excess anticoagulants
Roots
　　Prolapsed disc
　　Malignancy
　　Arachnoiditis
Lumbosacral cord (often bilateral leg symptoms)
　　Tumour
　　Myelitis

the thigh as it passes through the lateral end of the inguinal ligament. This causes pain, often of burning quality, and tingling or numbness on the lateral aspect of the thigh down to, but not below the knee.

Diabetic amyotrophy or plexopathy is another common cause of pain in the leg. This complication of diabetes presents as subacute severe pain in the thigh accompanied by wasting of the quadriceps and minor sensory changes in the distribution of the femoral nerve. It is usually a result of an acute vascular lesion affecting the femoral nerve. The femoral nerve also may be compressed acutely by haemorrhage into the *iliopsoas* muscle in those with a bleeding diathesis or on anticoagulant therapy.

The **tarsal tunnel syndrome** is a rare cause of pain in the foot. It is directly analogous to the carpal tunnel syndrome in the arm, being caused by an entrapment neuropathy of the tibial nerve beneath the flexor retinaculum of the ankle. This causes pain, numbness and tingling of the medial plantar surface of the foot, aggravated by standing and walking, and often worse at night.

Foot drop

Foot drop
Paralysis of the dorsiflexors of the ankle may be attributable to lesions of the common peroneal

nerve, the sciatic nerve, the L5 root, or occasionally the motor cortex.

The common peroneal nerve is extremely vulnerable as it travels around the neck of the fibula, where it may be compressed by external pressure, or stretched by prolonged bending or sitting with the knees fully flexed. Apart from the foot drop, such patients also exhibit numbness on the dorsum of the foot, but the ankle jerk is preserved. The sciatic nerve is vulnerable to misplaced injections into the buttocks or thigh, which leave not only a foot drop, but also weakness of plantar flexion of the foot, sensory loss extending onto the sole of the foot, and loss of the ankle jerk. L5 root lesions are difficult to distinguish from common peroneal palsies, but presence of lumbago and extension of weakness to involve the knee flexors will point to this proximal lesion. *Extensor hallucis longus* has an almost pure L5 innervation. Motor cortex lesions affecting the foot area may present with a foot drop but the plantar response will be extensor and there may be other upper motor neurone signs.

Cramps in the legs

Many patients use the word cramp to describe pain in the legs caused by vascular insufficiency, or nerve damage. However, genuine cramp consists not only of pain but also intense and involuntary muscle contraction affecting the calf muscles in particular. Such cramps are the plague of the untrained athlete, and are well known to occur in hot climates as a result of salt depletion. Muscle cramps occur in those recovering from sciatica and in motor neurone disease, but other findings will point to these diagnoses. Occasionally, isolated muscle cramps may be found to result from primary metabolic muscle disease, but in the majority of such patients no obvious cause can be discovered and they are extremely difficult to treat.

True muscle cramps are electrically silent on electromyographic study. In contrast flexor spasms of leg muscles that occur in those with damage to corticospinal pathways are associated with intense electromyographic activity and, of course, with the signs of an upper motor neurone lesion (weakness without wasting, spasticity, and exaggerated tendon reflexes).

Restless legs

Some patients will complain of discomfort in the legs that is not caused by pain, cramp or paraesthesiae. They find it impossible to put into words the quality of the intense discomfort that they feel, but describe relief from movement. Such patients cannot sit still because of the discomfort, and may be forced to get out of bed at night to walk around to gain relief from this distressing complaint. The cause for this bizarre symptom, know as Ekbom's syndrome, is not known, although some patients are found to have an iron-deficient anaemia or uraemia.

Intermittent claudication

> Pain in the calves or buttocks on exercise, relieved rapidly by rest, is, of course, the characteristic feature of arterial insufficiency in the legs.

However, this syndrome of intermittent claudication occasionally may be mimicked by disease of the lumbar spine, particularly in those with a narrowed spinal canal from congenital lumbar stenosis or from degenerative lumbar spondylosis. Such patients also complain of pain in the legs on exercise, but the pain is in the distribution of one of the spinal roots, and is accompanied by neurological symptoms, including foot drop or paraesthesiae. Rest relieves the pain, but usually after a longer period of time than is required in the case of vascular intermittent claudication.

> This neurological syndrome, because it mimics vascular claudication, has been called intermittent **claudication of the cauda equina**.

DIFFICULTY IN WALKING

Difficulty in walking is one of the commonest neurological complaints. First it is necessary to distinguish the different anatomical causes that may provoke difficulty in walking. It is convenient to work mentally from muscles up to cerebral cortex (Table 3.11).

Difficulty with walking with wasted legs

Primary muscle disease (myopathy) often presents with an abnormality of gait, because it affects proximal muscles of the hip girdle symmetrically at an early stage. Similar symmetrical proximal muscle weakness around the shoulder girdle usually occurs later. **Characteristically the gait is waddling** because of failure to stabilize the pelvis on the femur when the opposite leg is lifted from the ground. In addition, patients with primary muscle disease frequently complain of difficulty in rising from a low chair, and of climbing stairs or stepping onto the platform of a bus, because of weakness around the hips. When the arms are affected, an early symptom often is difficulty raising the hand above the head to brush the hair. Other characteristics of primary muscle disease are that sensation is normal and sphincter function is not affected. There are many causes for myopathy including hereditary muscular dystrophy, inflammatory myositis, thyrotoxicosis, steroid therapy and metabolic myopathies. A family history suggests muscular dystrophy, which causes painless progressive wasting of muscles in characteristic distribution. Pain and systemic disturbance suggest polymyositis. Many endocrine and electrolyte disturbances may cause metabolic myopathies.

> The physical signs of primary muscle disease are those of muscle wasting and weakness, symmetrical and proximal, with normal or reduced tendon jerks, and no evidence of sensory deficit.

Defects of neurotransmission resulting from **myasthenia gravis**, or from the much rarer myasthenic **(Lambert-Eaton)** syndrome often associated with carcinoma, may also present with difficulty in walking because of proximal leg weakness. However, the legs are not wasted in myasthenia. As in primary muscle disease, sensation is not affected. **The characteristic feature of myasthenia is muscle fatigue**. Patients may not complain of feeling tired, but of weakness of muscle action on exercise. Thus,

Table 3.11 Causes of walking difficulty

Site	Pathology
Muscle	Myopathy (proximal)
Neuromuscular junction	Myasthenia gravis (fatigue)
Peripheral nerve (LMN)	Neuropathy (distal)
Roots (LMN)	Disc protrusion, compressive, cauda equina (+ sphincters)
Spinal cord (UMN)	Compression (tumours, discs)
	Demyelination, inflammatory
	Vascular, degenerative (MND), intrinsic damage (syrinx, tumour)
Brain, brainstem (UMN)	Vascular, demyelination, tumours (intrinsic, extrinsic)
	Abscesses, degenerative
Cerebellar (ataxic)	Vascular (acute), tumour, degenerative (slow)
Extrapyramidal	Parkinsonian
Sensory loss (JPS loss)	Locomotor ataxia
Psychogenic	Functional, chronic fatigue states
Joint disease	Painful arthritis, Charcot's joints
Weakness (general)	Systemic disease, cachexia, hypotensive, malnutrition

LMN, lower motor neurone; UMN, upper motor neurone; MND, motor neurone disease; JPS, joint position sense.

they may start the day walking strongly, but as time goes on and as exercise continues, they become weaker and weaker. Rest restores strength, but further exercise leads to further weakness.

Peripheral nerve disease may also cause difficulty in walking. This may arise either as a result of damage to an isolated peripheral nerve (a mononeuropathy), such as a common peroneal palsy or femoral nerve palsy, or from damage to a number of peripheral nerves but sparing some (mononeuritis multiplex), or damage to generalized peripheral nerve disease (peripheral neuropathy). In all such conditions, the signs will be those of a lower motor neurone lesion (wasting with weakness, normal or reduced tone, and normal or depressed tendon reflexes). In addition, there will be appropriate sensory disturbance in the distribution of the affected peripheral nerves. In the case of a generalized peripheral neuropathy, symptoms commence in the feet symmetrically, with paraesthesiae and numbness which spread upwards into the legs, and bilateral foot drop resulting from distal weakness. Generalized peripheral neuropathies usually affect the legs before the arms, because long axons are affected first. Sphincter function, however, is normal. Subacute peripheral neuropathy, with onset and progression rapidly over a matter of a few days or weeks, most commonly is a result of the acute idiopathic inflammatory polyneuritis known as the Guillain-Barré syndrome. More rarely, similar subacute generalized peripheral neuropathy may occur in glandular fever, acquired immunodeficiency syndrome (AIDS), acute intermittent porphyria, or result from toxicity of heavy metals and industrial agents. Diphtheria now is exceedingly rare, but the early palatal palsy and paralysis of accommodation is characteristic. There are many causes for chronic peripheral neuropathy, but the commonest in the UK would be diabetes, with alcohol and malignancy close behind. Worldwide, the most common cause is leprosy.

Proximal lesions of the lumbosacral roots (cauda equina lesions) may present with difficulty walking caused by weakness of the legs associated with sensory disturbance which characteristically is focused around the perineum (the patient 'sits on their signs'), and early disturbances of sphincter function.

Motor neurone disease, too, may present with painless wasting, weakness and fasciculation of leg muscles, usually asymmetrically, and without sensory or sphincter disturbance.

Difficulty in walking with spastic legs

Lesions of the corticomotorneurone pathways bilaterally will cause a **spastic paraplegia**, which manifests as a characteristic disturbance of gait. **The patients walk with stiff straight legs, scuffing the toes and outer border of the feet along the ground**. Physical examination will confirm the signs of an upper motor neurone lesion (weakness without wasting, spasticity, exaggerated tendon reflexes and extensor plantar responses). The next stage is to decide on the anatomical level and the cause of such a spastic paraplegia (Table 3.11).

Acute paraplegia

Acute damage to the spinal cord by trauma, inflammatory disease (acute transverse myelitis) or vascular lesion, as may occur with spinal angioma, produces an acute paraplegia, but initially the signs are not those characteristic of spasticity. Immediately after such an acute insult the segment of spinal cord below the lesion is in a state of shock, when it is unresponsive to peripheral input.

> **Acute spinal cord lesion**
> Immediately after an acute spinal cord lesion the legs are flaccid, the tendon reflexes absent and the plantar responses often unobtainable. Spasticity, exaggerated reflexes, and extensor plantar responses gradually emerge over a matter of some weeks following the acute insult.

> An acute flaccid paraplegia, or quadriplegia if the arms are also affected, may be difficult to distinguish from a subacute peripheral neuropathy or even from severe acute metabolic myopathies such as that resulting from hypokalaemia, at least in the early stages.

The presence of sensory loss obviously will exclude primary muscle disease, and urinary retention points to spinal cord damage rather than a peripheral neuropathy. In those with an acute paraplegia thought to be the result of spinal cord damage, it is crucial to exclude spinal cord compression, for example by dorsal disc protrusion or extradural abscess (Table 3.12), for the longer the delay before surgery the less the chance of useful recovery. All such patients demand immediate neurological assessment and imaging of the spinal cord if a compressive lesion is to be excluded. This is best undertaken by magnetic resonance imaging (MRI) or, where this is not available, by myelography.

Acute quadriplegia

> Sudden or rapid paralysis of all four limbs may be a medical emergency if breathing is threatened.

Respiratory failure occurs when arterial oxygen tension falls below 8.0 kPa (60 mmHg), or if arterial carbon dioxide tension rises above 6.6 kPa (50 mmHg). However, patients with neurological disease causing respiratory distress may be in

Table 3.12 Neurological causes of cord compression

Trauma - fracture dislocations, burst fractures of vertebral body
Infection - epidural abscess, tuberculosis
Vascular
Arteriovenous malformations
Epidural haemorrhage
Anticoagulant excess, bleeding diathesis
Tumour
Primary
Intramedullary - glioma, ependymoma
Extramedullary - meningioma, neurofibroma
Metastatic deposits
Degenerative
Disc prolapse, spondylotic changes
Osteoporotic collapse
Paget's disease
Atlanto - axial subluxation
Congenital
Craniocervical junction abnormalities
Inflammatory
Acute swollen cord - myelitis, arachnoiditis

severe difficulty long before the blood gases are compromised.

> A rising respiratory rate and breathlessness indicate impending respiratory failure, which may require assisted respiration. The best index of respiratory reserve is the vital capacity (VC), which is the volume of maximal expiration following a maximal inspiration.

In an adult, a falling VC with a value of less than 50% of the predicted normal is a warning of impending crisis, and an action is undoubtedly required if the VC falls to 1.0 l or less. Peak expiratory flow rate is a measure of obstructive respiratory defects and is an inappropriate and dangerously misleading measure of respiratory function in patients with neuromuscular disease.

Causes of acute quadriplegia

The common causes of acute or subacute (with onset over days) quadriplegia are polymyositis, myasthenia gravis, acute inflammatory polyneuritis (Guillain–Barré syndrome), and high cervical cord lesions resulting from trauma, inflammation or vascular damage. Rarer conditions include hypokalaemic paralysis, acute porphyria, poliomyelitis, tetanus, and other causes of high cervical cord damage, such as subluxation of the odontoid peg (as occurs in rheumatoid arthritis) or cord tumours. Brainstem lesions may also cause a quadriplegia, but bulbar muscles are involved to cause diplopia, dysphagia and dysarthria.

Chronic spastic paraparesis

> The most common cause of a chronic spastic paraparesis in the young adult is multiple sclerosis, and in the elderly individual it is cervical spondylosis.

However, it is crucial to exclude other treatable causes of spinal cord disease in both age groups before accepting either diagnosis.

> In particular, any patient with a chronic progressive spastic paraparesis requires imaging of the spinal cord to exclude a spinal tumour or other causes of cord compression,

unless there are obvious signs or symptoms of multiple sclerosis elsewhere, or some other clear evidence to establish an alternative diagnosis. To carry out a few unnecessary imaging studies is much better than to miss treatable benign spinal tumours, such as neurofibromas or meningiomas, until the damage is too severe to remedy by surgical treatment. Unfortunately, in the older age group metastatic deposits in the spine, usually from breast, lung or prostate cancer, are more often than not the cause of spinal cord compression. Rarer causes include dorsal disc prolapse, arachnoiditis, intramedullary cord tumours and syringomyelia. It is also essential to exclude subacute combined degeneration as a result of pernicious anaemia and vitamin B12 deficiency, neurosyphilis, and in patients particularly from abroad, infection with the human T-cell lymphotropic virus type I, as causes of chronic spastic paraparesis. Subacute combined degeneration nearly always presents with paraesthesiae first in the feet, because of the associated peripheral neuropathy, and the ankle jerks will be lost. The picture of a spastic paraplegia but with absent ankle jerks also may be seen in patients with hereditary spinocerebellar degenerations, and as a remote complication of a primary neoplasm. Motor neurone disease also may present as a spastic paraparesis before evidence of lower motor neurone damage with wasting and fasciculation is evident.

Spastic weakness of one leg

Stiffness and dragging of one leg is a common presenting complaint in neurology.

> The difficulty is always to decide whether the lesion lies in the spinal cord or in the brain.

Full investigation would include MRI imaging of the spine and brain. If not available, a CT brain scan and myelography could be undertaken, although they provide less information. Examination of the CSF may be helpful to support or refute a diagnosis of multiple sclerosis. Progression to involve the arm does not necessarily help to decide between spinal cord and brain, while spread to the opposite leg does not always indicate that the lesion is in the spinal cord. The notorious parasagittal meningioma may produce upper motor neurone signs in both legs.

Unsteadiness of gait

> **Ataxia of gait**
> An unsteady, uncertain gait may be caused by sensory loss (sensory ataxia), cerebellar disease (cerebellar ataxia), hydrocephalus or extrapyramidal disease such as Parkinson's disease or chorea.

In **sensory ataxia** the patient characteristically walks unsteadily with the feet wide apart and lifted high off the ground to slap into the floor. In addition, the patient with sensory ataxia is much worse in the dark when vision cannot be used to compensate. The patient with **cerebellar ataxia** again walks with the feet wide apart and reels from side to side as if drunk. The patient with **Parkinson's disease** slowly shuffles with small steps and a bent posture. The patient with **chorea** unexpectedly dances and lurches as the balance is disturbed by unpredictable involuntary movements.

Gait disturbance with small shuffling steps may arise from a number of disorders. In Parkinson's disease there is a tendency to festination with a flexed posture and impaired balance. In patients with a frontal lobe disturbance (often a gait apraxia) there may be no weakness and often preserved movements on the bed. However there may be difficulty turning over in bed. Examination may show a degree of leg spasticity without sensory loss but walking using short shuffling steps on a wide base. There may be perseveration of some actions. Often there is a degree of dementia and sometimes urinary urgency and even incontinence. One such cause may be widespread vascular disease with multiple lacunar infarcts resulting in the *marche a petits pas.*

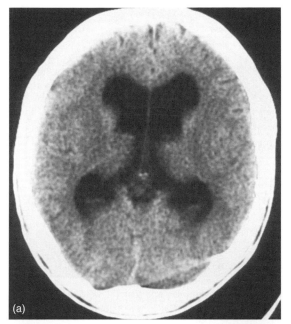

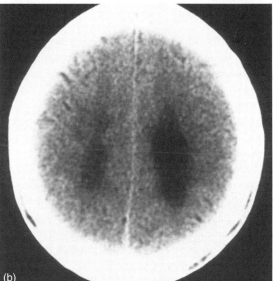

Figure 3.5 (a) Axial view CT brain scan to show triventricular enlargement and (b) absence of cortical sulci in a patient with normal pressure hydrocephalus. The patient presented with dementia, a gait with short shuffling steps and incontinence.

In patients with a normal pressure hydrocephalus again there may be a gait with short shuffling steps and a wide base (Figure 3.5). Commonly there is an associated dementia and incontinence of urine. A patient who is unsteady will walk with a wide base using small steps.

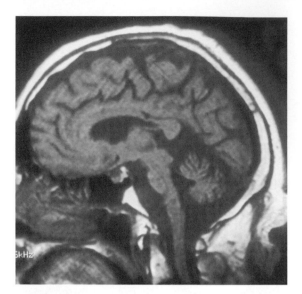

Figure 3.6 Sagittal view MRI scan (T1-weighted) to show cerebellar and brainstem atrophy in a patient with progressive unsteadiness.

Extensive sensory loss in the legs may be caused by a profound sensory peripheral neuropathy or by degeneration of the posterior columns as in tabes dorsalis. In both conditions the tendon jerks are absent; in peripheral neuropathy there are likely to be distal motor signs, while in tabes dorsalis there is likely to be urinary retention with overflow and abnormal pupils.

Progressive cerebellar ataxia occurs in diffuse diseases of the central nervous system, such as multiple sclerosis, when it is often accompanied by a spastic paraparesis to produce a typical spastic-ataxic gait. Isolated progressive cerebellar ataxia may be the result of a cerebellar tumour, hereditary spinocerebellar degeneration (Figure 3.6), alcohol, endocrine disturbance such as myxoedema, or a remote effect of a primary neoplasm elsewhere. Patients who are ataxic sitting and standing are likely to have a midline cerebellar fault. A cerebellar syndrome in childhood most frequently is caused by a posterior fossa tumour, which may present without symptoms suggesting raised intracranial pressure. In adults this is seldom so, and most isolated progressive cerebellar ataxias without headache and vomiting are found to be degenerative in origin.

Extrapyramidal diseases are discussed in the next section.

MOVEMENT DISORDERS

The term 'movement disorders' has come to be applied to those diseases of the nervous system, mostly of the basal ganglia, that cause disturbances of movement that cannot be attributed to sensory loss, weakness or spasticity, or obvious cerebellar ataxia.

Movement disorders fall into two main categories:

- Those characterized by a poverty (hypokinesia) and slowness (bradykinesia) of movement, the so-called akinetic-rigid or parkinsonian syndrome
- Those characterized by excess abnormal and uncontrollable involuntary movements, otherwise known as dyskinesias.

Idiopathic Parkinson's disease, associated with a characteristic pathology including the presence of Lewy bodies in affected pigmented nerve cells and loss of nigro-striatal neurones, is the commonest cause of an akinetic syndrome in middle or late life. A similar condition could be produced as an aftermath of encephalitis lethargica (post-encephalitic parkinsonism), and occurs commonly nowadays as a result of intake of neuroleptic drugs such as phenothiazines or butyrophenones **(drug-induced parkinsonism)**. Rarer causes include **multiple system atrophy** and **progressive supranuclear palsy** in the older age group, while in juveniles or young adults **Wilson's disease** and the rigid form of **Huntington's disease** have to be considered. An important distinction is between Parkinson's disease, or the other conditions mentioned that may cause parkinsonism, and the akinetic-rigid features that occur in patients with many diffuse cerebral degenerations. In the latter conditions, which include diffuse cerebrovascular disease and Alzheimer's disease, the akinetic-rigid features are only part of a much greater disorder of higher mental function, which produces profound disturbances of memory, intellect and cognitive function.

Abnormal involuntary movements

Abnormal involuntary movements (dyskinesias) are a feature of many diseases of the nervous system, but most can be included within five main categories – tremor, chorea, myoclonus, tics and torsion dystonia. These are not diseases, but clinically identifiable syndromes with many causes. In some patients such dyskinesias are accompanied by other neurological deficits, but in others the involuntary movements occur in isolation and constitute the illness.

Tremor is a rhythmic sinusoidal movement, which may occur at rest (rest tremor) or on action (action tremor), when it may be present while maintaining a posture (static or postural tremor), or on executing a movement (kinetic or intention tremor). Rest tremor is characteristic of Parkinson's disease. Postural tremor often is no more than an exaggeration of physiological tremor by anxiety, drugs, alcohol, or thyrotoxicosis. Intention tremor is a distinctive sign of cerebellar disease.

Chorea is characterized by continuous, randomly distributed and irregular-timed muscle jerks. The limbs, trunk and facial features are continually disturbed by brief, unpredictable movements; walking is interrupted by lurches, stops and starts (the dancing gait); hand movements and fine manipulations are distorted by similar unpredictable jerks and twitches; while speech and respiration also deteriorate. Strength is usually normal, but the patient is unable to maintain a consistent force of contraction so that the grip waxes and wanes (milkmaid's grip), while the protruded tongue pops in and out of the mouth (flycatcher's tongue). The limbs are hypotonic and tendon jerks brisk and often repetitive. The chief causes of chorea are shown in Table 11.4 (see p. 236). Sydenham's chorea and Huntington's disease are the commonest causes of generalized chorea, but this may be the presenting feature of a number of general medical illnesses or may occur as a side-effect of drug therapy. Hemichorea or hemiballism describes unilateral chorea most apparent in proximal muscles, so that the arm and leg are thrown widely in all directions.

Myoclonus consists of brief, shock-like muscle jerks, similar to those provoked by stimulating the muscle's nerve with a single electric shock. Myoclonic jerks may occur irregularly or rhythmically, and they often appear repetitively in the same muscles. In this respect myoclonus differs from chorea, which is random in time and distribution. The chief diseases causing myoclonus are shown in Table 11.5 (see p. 236).

Tics resemble myoclonus for they too consist of brief muscle contractions, but they differ in a number of respects. The movements themselves are repetitive and stereotyped, can be mimicked by the observer, and usually can be controlled through an effort of will by the patient, often at the expense of mounting inner tension. Tics typically involve the face, such as blinking, sniffing, lip smacking or pouting, and the upper arms, such as shoulder shrugging. In fact tics occur in at least one-quarter of normal children, but disappear with maturity. A number of normal adults also display persistent motor tics as part of their personality. The chief causes of pathological tics are shown in Table 11.6 (see p. 237).

Torsion dystonia differs from the other movements that are mentioned in that it is caused by sustained spasms of muscle contraction that distort the body into characteristic postures for prolonged periods of time. The neck may be twisted to one side (torticollis) or extended (retrocollis); the trunk may be forced into excessive lordosis or scoliosis; the arm is commonly extended and hyperpronated with the wrist flexed and the fingers extended; the leg is commonly extended with the foot plantar flexed and in-turned. Initially these muscle spasms may occur only on certain actions (action dystonia), so that patients walk on their toes or develop the characteristic arm posture on writing. In progressive dystonia, however, such abnormal muscle spasm and postures soon become apparent at rest and cause increasing dystonic movements and deformity. The term athetosis is also used to describe similar dystonic movements, although originally it was employed to describe wavering movements of the fingers and toes. The chief causes of torsion dystonia are shown in Table 11.7 (see p. 238).

DECLINE OF MEMORY, INTELLECT AND BEHAVIOUR

A global loss of all higher intellectual function, memory and cognitive function, accompanied by disintegration of personality and behaviour forms the clinical syndrome know as dementia, which usually is caused by diffuse cerebral cortical disease.

The syndrome of dementia may occur acutely, as after head injury or cerebral anoxia resulting from cardiac arrest, or may commence insidiously and be progressive, as in the various presenile and senile dementing illnesses of which **Alzheimer's disease** is the commonest. However, there are other causes of a progressive dementia that are reversible, including certain treatable brain tumours and metabolic diseases such as myxoedema or vitamin B12 deficiency (Table 3.13).

Diagnosing dementia

When faced with a patient, or their relatives, complaining of memory difficulty, intellectual decline, or changes in personality, three questions have to be answered:

1 Is this really caused by a true dementia as a result of organic brain disease, or are these symptoms those of a pseudodementia resulting from a psychiatric illness such as depression?
2 Are these symptoms those of a true global dementing illness, or are they caused by a focal cortical syndrome as the result of damage to one part of the cerebral cortex, rather than diffuse disease?
3 If they are the result of a true global dementia, then is there any treatable cause for the condition?

Pseudodementia

Impairment of memory with change in personality and behaviour, of course, are typical symptoms of **depression**, which also produces sadness, sleep disturbance, diurnal mood swing, loss of libido, anorexia and weight loss. Difficulty arises because a considerable proportion of patients with true organic dementing illnesses experience a reactive depression in the early stages of their illness. Accordingly, in a patient who exhibits decline of memory and intellect with alteration of personality and behaviour accompanied by depression, it can be exceedingly difficult to distinguish a primary depressive illness from a dementing process with reactive depression. Careful assessment by experienced psychologists may assist,

Table 3.13 Causes of dementia

Primary degenerative
Alzheimer's disease, dementia with Lewy bodies, frontotemporal dementia
Huntington's chorea, Parkinson's disease, corticobasal degeneration
Prion disease
Creutzfeldt–Jakob disease–sporadic and variant
Infective
Chronic meningitis, neurosyphilis
AIDS dementia complex
Progressive multifocal leukoencephalopathy
Post-meningo-encephalitis
Metabolic, endocrine
Uraemia, hepatic encephalopathy, myxoedema
Hypopituitarism, hypoglycaemia
Hypercalcaemia, hypocalcaemia
Deficiencies – thiamine, vitamin B12, multiple nutritional
Vascular – multi-infarct, Binswanger's subcortical leukoariosis
Drugs
Alcohol
Barbiturates
Trauma
Head injury, 'punch-drunk' boxers
Subdural haematoma
Tumours
Primary – glioma, meningioma,
Secondary – metastatic
Obstructive hydrocephalus
Normal pressure hydrocephalus
Depression – pseudo-dementia

but often does not resolve the matter. If in doubt, it is prudent to treat the illness as a depression and to await events. Other psychiatric conditions that may produce a pseudodementia include hysteria and malingering, but these are rare.

Focal cortical syndromes

Bilateral damage to the temporal lobes, particularly to their medial structures including the hippocampus, or to the hypothalamus may produce a pure **amnesic**

syndrome, consisting of dense loss of memory for recent events with inability to retain new information, but with preserved intelligence and personality. Such amnesic syndromes are seen most commonly in Korsakoff's psychosis as a result of thiamine deficiency in alcoholics, but occasionally may occur as a result of parapituitary tumours or bilateral temporal lobe damage secondary to head injury or encephalitis. A **transient global amnesia** also occurs as one of the manifestations of transient cerebral ischaemia in posterior cerebral territory. Here patients usually have a marked short-term memory loss extending for some hours, during which they may repeatedly ask the same questions. It has also been proposed that such symptoms may arise with migraine and even, rarely, as part of a complex partial seizure. An amnesic syndrome may persist for some time after head injury (post-traumatic amnesia), or after an epileptic seizure (post-epileptic amnesia).

Dysphasia (see p. 84) may be mistaken for dementia. The severe disturbance of the content of speech that occurs in Wernicke's dysphasia resulting from damage to the posterior temporal region of the dominant hemisphere may consist of such nonsensical language and jargon that the inexperienced observer may mistake the behaviour for that caused by dementia.

Damage to the frontal lobes by tumour, which is often a benign meningioma, by syphilis, as in general paralysis of the insane, or by myxoedema may produce a remarkable change in personality and behaviour, without deterioration of intellect or memory. Such a focal frontal lobe syndrome is often mistaken either for primary psychiatric illness or global dementing disease.

Causes of dementia

If the conclusion is that the patient's symptoms are those of a diffuse global dementing illness, the next stage is to decide on the cause (Table 3.13).

> In about 10% of patients, some potentially treatable condition will be discovered on careful examination and full investigation, the yield being greatest in those under the age of 70 years.

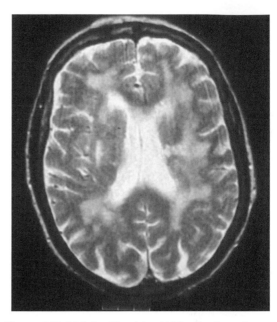

Figure 3.7 Axial view T2-weighted MRI scan of a patient with widespread small vessel disease and multi-infarct dementia.

The commonest cause of dementia is Alzheimer's disease, which becomes increasingly frequent with age. (Previously the term 'presenile dementia' was used for the syndrome with onset prior to the age of 65 years, while 'senile dementia' was applied when the illness commenced after the age of 65 years. Senile dementia became equated with Alzheimer's disease, which, in fact, can occur at any age, and accounts for over 80% of those exhibiting dementia in later life). Cerebrovascular disease is a less common cause of dementia, and usually is suggested by the presence of established hypertension and a history of repeated stroke-like episodes **(multi-infarct dementia)**, with often diffuse small vessel damage (Figure 3.7). Less common causes include **dementia with Lewy bodies**, frontotemporal dementias, Huntington's disease (which is suggested by the typical chorea and family history), and **Creutzfeldt–Jakob disease (CJD)**, which is a prion encephalopathy producing a subacute, rapidly progressive dementia, often with characteristic myoclonus, sometimes marked cerebellar signs, and EEG findings. In younger patients variant CJD should be considered and the **human immunodeficiency virus-associated dementia** complex is also seen regularly in AIDS patients with immune compromise.

Potentially reversible causes of dementia

Reversible causes of dementia include not only unexpected cerebral tumours (particularly frontal and non-dominant temporal lobes in site) and other mass lesions, such as giant aneurysms, but also obstructive or communicating hydrocephalus, neurosyphilis and various metabolic conditions, such as vitamin B12 deficiency, chronic drug intoxication, myxoedema and disturbances of calcium metabolism. Full investigation is required to exclude such treatable causes and should be undertaken in every patient under the age of 75 years, and in all those over that age in whom the cause of dementia is not established.

REFERENCES AND FURTHER READING

Bradley WG, Daroff RB, Fenichel GM, Marsden CD (2000) *Neurology in Clinical Practice*, 3rd edn. Boston: Butterworth-Heinemann.

Brazis PW, Masdeu JG, Biller J (2001) *Localization in Clinical Neurology*, 4th edn. Philadelphia: Lippincott Williams & Wilkins.

Bronstein AM, Brandt T, Woollacott M (1996) *Clinical Disorders of Balance, Posture and Gait*. London: Arnold.

Marshall RS, Mayer SA (2001) *On Call Neurology*, 2nd edn. Philadelphia: WB Saunders.

Victor M, Ropper AH (2001) *Adams & Victor's Principles of Neurology*, 7th edn. New York: McGraw-Hill.

CHAPTER 4

EXAMINATION OF THE NERVOUS SYSTEM

T.J. Fowler and C.D. Marsden

NEUROLOGICAL EXAMINATION

A full examination of the nervous system could occupy a whole day but, in practice, it must be completed in half-an-hour or less. A routine screening examination has to be undertaken in 5–10 minutes. Accordingly, the neurological examination has to be highly selective. What actually is carried out on each individual patient will be determined by their history, which will focus attention on that aspect of the nervous system that needs the most detailed investigation.

When approaching each neurological patient, it is helpful to have in one's mind two simple plans:

1 The routine basic scheme of examination that is to be conducted in every neurological patient – the screening examination.
2 Those special tests required in this patient because of the history of their complaint – the specific examination.

This plan will be followed in this chapter. First, the basic routine examination will be described. Details of individual tests will not be elaborated, because they are best learned at the bedside. Second, more specific detailed examinations required in patients with certain problems will be discussed.

The basic scheme of neurological examination
This consists of:

1 Assess higher mental function:
   (a) Intellect, memory, personality and mood
   (b) Speech and cognitive function.
2 Test the cranial nerves.
3 Test motor functions.
4 Test sensory functions.
5 Test autonomic function.
6 Examine related structures.

Higher mental function

Intellect, memory, personality and mood

The clarity with which a patient presents their story and answers questions, and their cooperation during examination, will convey a picture of their intellectual capacity and of their personality and mood. Compare your own estimate with what might be expected from the patient's type of work and scholastic record. A patient's mood and insight may be further demonstrated by their reaction to the illness; while their power of memory may be indicated by the coherence and ease with which symptoms and past history are recalled and dated. Whenever there is doubt about a patient's higher mental function, it is crucial to obtain the story and observations of an independent witness who can testify to the patient's intellectual competence.

If history taking does not suggest any defect of higher cerebral function, then no further testing is required. However, if a decline in higher mental function is suspected, more extensive examination is necessary (see later).

Speech and cognitive function

The content and articulation of speech will be evident while taking the history. Always note whether the patient is right-handed or left-handed and, if speech difficulty is apparent, it is also worth checking which eye and which leg are dominant. Abnormalities of speech may include the following:

1 **Dysphonia**, in which the content of speech is normal and articulation preserved but basic voice production is disturbed by mechanical abnormality of the organs of speech, including the vocal cords and resonating sound boxes. The hoarse voice of laryngitis and the nasal speech of the common cold are examples of dysphonia.
2 **Dysarthria**, which describes abnormal articulation resulting from damage to the nervous pathways or muscles responsible for speech production, with intact language content. Lower motor neurone paralysis of the soft palate produces nasal escape of air and the characteristic nasal speech of a paralytic dysarthria. Spasticity of the tongue, palate and mouth produces a monotonous, stiff, slurred type of speech known as a spastic dysarthria, which sounds as if the patient is talking with a plum in their mouth. Incoordination of muscular action responsible for speech because of cerebellar disease results in irregular, staccato and explosive speech known as scanning or cerebellar dysarthria. The akinetic-rigid syndrome of parkinsonism produces a characteristic slow, soft, monotonous speech known as an extrapyramidal or hyphonic dysarthria. Edentulous patients show a degree of dysarthria.
3 **Dysphasia**, which describes impairment of language, is either difficulty of understanding the spoken or written word, or of speaking or writing itself. The various types of dysphasia that may be encountered with

lesions affecting the dominant hemisphere are described later.

Cognition refers to the capacity to know and perceive one's surroundings and one's self in relationship to those surroundings. The inability to recognize objects in space, colours, faces or even one's own body parts is known as **agnosia**. Inability to undertake a skilled motor act despite intact power, sensation and coordination is known as **apraxia**. (Different types of agnosia and apraxia will be described later.)

Cranial nerves

I Olfactory nerve

The sense of smell should always be tested if there are complaints of disturbance of taste or smell, after a head injury, if there is suspicion of a lesion involving the anterior fossa or of dementia. It is important to realize that patients complaining of loss of taste are usually describing the effects of damage to the olfactory nerve, which results in loss of appreciation of subtleties of good food or wine. Such patients can still recognize the elementary four tastes – sweet, sour, salt and acid – but cannot appreciate flavour. The sense of smell may be tested by the ability to identify and distinguish the odours of common objects, such as coffee, peppermint or orange peel, with each nostril in turn. Unilateral anosmia suggests a lesion of the olfactory nerve, but bilateral anosmia is usually the result of local nasal disease, such as that following a common cold or head injury.

II Optic nerve

The function of the optic nerve can be tested by examining visual acuity, the visual fields and the optic fundus. This requires an acuity chart, a large red-headed (5 mm) hatpin and a grid card, and an ophthalmoscope.

The *visual acuity* tests the integrity of central macular vision. The distance acuity should be measured in each eye using the standard Snellen chart at 6 m with the patient wearing spectacles to correct any refractive error. If no spectacles are available,

Any refractive error can usually be corrected by asking the patient to look through a pinhole aperture.

The normal distance acuity is 6/6, the numerator representing the distance of the patient from the chart (6 m) and the denominator the distance in metres at which a normal person is able to read that line (Figure 4.1). Decreasing acuity is recorded as 6/9, 6/12, 6/18, 6/24, 6/36, 6/60, and then as the ability to count fingers, perceive hand movements or, finally, perceive light. Near acuity is tested by asking the patient to read test type, again correcting any refractive error. Near vision is a less accurate assessment of acuity. Most patients with an acuity of 6/18 for distance can read N5 or N6 size test type. For driving in the UK it is necessary to read a number plate at 75 feet (22.9 m), which is an acuity between 6/9 and 6/12.

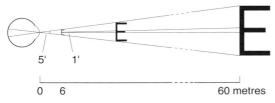

Figure 4.1 Distance visual acuity – the angles subtended by test type on a standard Snellen chart at 6 m.

Colour vision may be affected by optic nerve damage and is tested with standard Ishihara plates. Some 8% of the male population may be colour-blind, most often with red–green impairment.

The *visual fields* may be tested at the bedside by the confrontation technique, where the patient's field is compared with that of the tester.

Lesions of the posterior visual pathways cause defects in the opposite half of the peripheral fields (hemianopias).

With one eye covered, the patient faces the examiner and is asked to fix their pupil on that of the examiner. Using a 5 mm red pin the target is brought into each of the four quadrants to detect any impairment. First the patient is asked to say when they first see the pin (often described as dark) and after this to repeat the test asking them to say when they first perceive the pin as red. Each eye is tested separately and any peripheral defect is often matched in the initial peripheral field (dark) and that of the smaller field to red. Peripheral defects as hemianopias, quadrantanopias, and altitudinal defects should be recognized by this technique. Visual fields should be recorded in the notes with the right-eye field on the right and the left-eye field on the left (Figure 4.2).

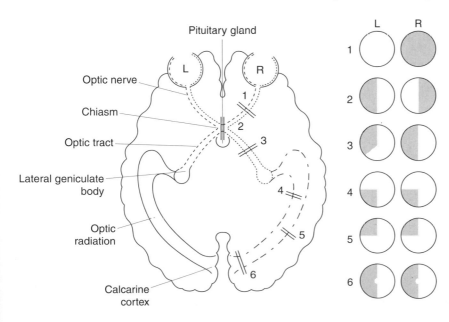

Figure 4.2 Common visual field defects.

More accurate visual field testing is now carried out using automated perimeters with a computer print-out, for example, the Humphrey visual field analyser. In a subsequent examination both eyes should be tested together to look for any visual inattention or neglect (see later). Here small finger movements can be used as targets.

> Central field loss occurs most often with lesions of the anterior visual pathways, particularly the macular area of the retina and the optic nerve.

Patients commonly show a depressed acuity and may complain of blurred vision or a central impairment (central scotoma). This can be confirmed using a 5 mm red hatpin or by checking central macular vision using an Amsler chart (Figure 4.3). This is a 'grid' printed on paper and the patient is asked to look at the central spot and point out any fault. It tests the central 10 degrees of the field. It is also often useful to look for colour desaturation in the central part of the field comparing the intensity of the red colour of the target between the two sides at the centre of the field.

Examination of the optic fundi with an ophthalmoscope is an art that can only be learnt by practice. Good illumination is essential and modern instruments with halogen bulbs and long-life batteries provide excellent light (Plate 1a).

Optic fundus examination
It is helpful to pursue a routine in fundus examination, concentrating initially on the optic disc, looking for swelling (papilloedema) or optic atrophy when a disc is unusually pale, then exploring

Amsler recording chart
A replica of Chart No. 1, printed black on white for convenience of recording

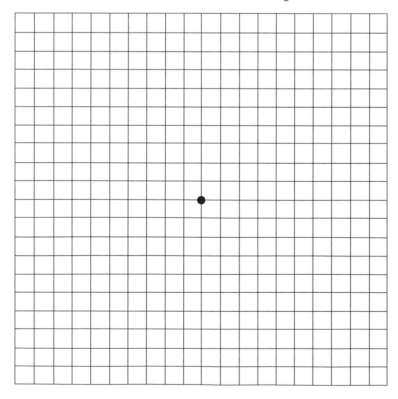

Figure 4.3 Amsler grid for recording central field of vision. When held at a reading distance of 14 in, 1/3 m, this tests the central 10 degrees of the visual field, that is 10 degrees in all directions from the fixation point.

the four quadrants of the retina looking for haemorrhages or exudates and examining the retinal arteries, which should be about two-thirds of the diameter of veins, the latter often being pulsatile at least as they emerge from the optic disc.

Visible venous pulsations in the vessels entering the optic cup in the disc indicate there is no papilloedema. Venous pulsation is best seen if the patient is standing or sitting. It is important to distinguish between swelling of the optic nerve from local disease (optic neuritis) and papilloedema resulting from raised intracranial pressure.

Optic neuritis vs papilloedema

In optic neuritis, there will be an obvious and often profound drop in visual acuity accompanied by a central scotoma, while in papilloedema as a result of raised intracranial pressure the visual acuity remains normal, and the only field defect initially is an enlarged blind spot. Later effects of damage to the optic nerve or chiasm lead to a pale, clearly demarcated disc – optic atrophy (Plate 1b).

III, IV and VI Oculomotor, trochlear and abducens nerves

Examination of the three nerves innervating the muscles of the eyes involves assessment of pupillary function and of eye movement.

The size, shape and equality of the pupils should be recorded. Their reaction to a bright light should be tested both directly, by shining the light into the eye under observation, and consensually, by shining the light into the opposite eye, both of which should produce brisk pupillary constriction. The 'swinging light' test is a particularly sensitive method of detecting optic nerve lesions. The light is alternately focused on one pupil then the opposite. The pupil of the affected side will dilate slightly when the light is directed onto it because the optic nerve lesion reduces the direct light response, while the consensual response from the opposite eye is preserved.

The pupillary response to accommodation or near-vision, should be tested by asking the subject to focus upon a finger or object, which is carried towards the nose: again, the pupils will constrict on convergence. The position of the upper eyelid should be noted, looking particularly for the presence of drooping (ptosis). Defects of pupillary function are described later (see p. 89).

Eye movements should be tested in two ways. The **saccadic system** is examined by asking the patient to look voluntarily to right and left, and up and down. The **pursuit system** is examined by asking the patient to follow an object moved to right and left, and up and down. Note the range of movement of each eye in all directions, and whether the movements of the two eyes are yoked together (conjugate eye movements). Note whether saccadic movements are carried out rapidly to the extremes of gaze in each direction, and whether pursuit movements are carried out smoothly without interruption.

Ask whether the patient sees double at any point (diplopia); this is the most sensitive index of defective ocular movement and may be evident to the patient even when the examiner can see no abnormality of gaze.

Assessment of diplopia

1 Is it constant, intermittent or variable?
2 Note the direction of separation of images – horizontal, vertical or tilted.
3 Note the direction of gaze in which there is maximal separation.
4 By 'cover' testing, check which is the most peripheral image. The weak muscle gives the more peripheral image.
5 Note the presence of any head tilt, and whether this improves or worsens the diplopia
6 Any associated features:
   (a) pupillary size and reactions
   (b) ptosis
   (c) weakness of eye closure
   (d) proptosis
   (e) peri-orbital changes.

Look for any **nystagmus**, which is a repetitive drift of the eyeball away from the point of fixation, followed by a fast corrective movement towards it.

Nystagmus – peripheral vs central

Peripheral vestibular lesions cause horizontal nystagmus away from the side of the lesion, which enhances if fixation is lost. Central lesions causing nystagmus tend to produce a more coarse nystagmus towards the side of the lesion. It may also be multidirectional, vertical and rotatory, and may change direction with gaze.

V Trigeminal nerve

Both the sensory and motor divisions of the trigeminal nerve should be examined.

The most sensitive index of impairment of the sensation in the trigeminal nerve is usually loss of the corneal reflex.

The reflex is elicited by touching the cornea with a wisp of cotton wool, which evokes an afferent volley in the ophthalmic division of the trigeminal nerve to cause a bilateral blink, which is mediated by motor impulses in the facial nerve. Sensation in all three divisions of the trigeminal nerve should be examined with pin and cotton wool to test pain and light touch, respectively. Remember the anatomical confines of the trigeminal territory, which extends back to meet the zone innervated by the C2 sensory division well past the crown of the head behind the ears (Figure 4.4). Also the mandibular division of the trigeminal nerve supplies the skin over the jaw, but spares that portion over the angle of the jaw, which again is supplied by C2. These landmarks are of value in distinguishing true trigeminal sensory loss from false claims of facial numbness. Another useful point is that fibres of the trigeminal nerve supplying the cornea travel with the nasociliary branch of the ophthalmic division so that depression of the corneal reflex is almost always accompanied by impairment of pinprick sensation at the root of the nose next to the eye. The lining of the inner nostril is also supplied by the ophthalmic division of the trigeminal nerve.

The motor functions of the trigeminal nerve are examined by comparing the size of the masseter and temporalis muscles on each side by palpation while the teeth are clenched. Look for unilateral wasting of these muscles on the side of a trigeminal nerve lesion. Then ask the patient to open their mouth; normally the jaw does not deviate from the midline on mouth opening. In a unilateral trigeminal nerve lesion, the jaw will deviate towards the side of damage, because of weakness of the pterygoid muscles, which normally protrude the jaw. However, a common cause of jaw deviation is subluxation of one temporomandibular joint, so before diagnosing a trigeminal nerve lesion, always check by palpation that the mandibular condyle has not flipped out of its socket. Finally, test the jaw jerk by a brisk tap applied to a finger placed on the point of the half open jaw.

VII Facial nerve

Test facial movements by asking the patient to wrinkle the forehead, screw up the eyes, show the teeth and whistle. Asking a patient to whistle often makes them laugh, which will give you the opportunity to assess facial weakness around the mouth.

Facial nerve lesions – upper motor neurone vs lower motor neurone

Lesions of the facial nerve, or of its nucleus, produce weakness of the whole side of the face, including the forehead. In contrast, a unilateral lesion of the supranuclear corticobulbar pathway for facial movement [an upper motor neurone (UMN) lesion] only affects the lower half of the face, sparing the forehead. The facial nerve also supplies a small branch to the stapedius muscle.

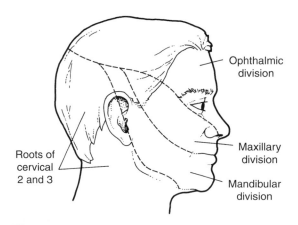

Ophthalmic division

Maxillary division

Mandibular division

Roots of cervical 2 and 3

Figure 4.4 Trigeminal sensory innervation.

The facial nerve itself has no important sensory component. However, fibres originating in the lingual nerve, which carry a sensation of taste from the anterior two-thirds of the tongue, join the facial nerve via the chorda tympani branch in the petrous temporal bone. Rarely, it is necessary to test the sensation of taste. To do so, ask the subject to protrude the tongue, and keep it out, while a test substance is applied to one side of the tongue tip. There are four tastes – salt, sweet, bitter (quinine) and acid or sour (lemon). The facial nerve also supplies the lacrimal gland.

VIII Auditory or vestibulocochlear nerve

> The auditory nerve has two divisions, one conveying impulses from the cochlea subserving hearing, and the other conveying impulses from the labyrinth responsible for vestibular function.

Hearing can be tested quickly by asking the patient to repeat whispered words or numbers with the eyes shut and one ear occluded by the examiner's forefinger. Alternatively, a wristwatch may be brought towards the ear and the distance at which the subject hears the ticking is noted for each side. A watch ticking is a high frequency sound and useful for detecting nerve deafness. If deafness is detected, define whether it is as a result of middle ear disease **(conductive deafness)** or a nerve lesion **(perceptive deafness)**. To do this, compare the noise of a tuning fork (256 Hz or, better, 512 Hz) held close to the ear (air conduction) with that when the fork is placed on the mastoid (bone conduction): this is called Rinne's test. In normal subjects, and in those with perceptive deafness, air conduction is better than bone conduction. In patients with conductive deafness, the reverse is true. Weber's test also may help to distinguish between unilateral conductive and perceptive deafness. A tuning fork is placed on the centre of the forehead; in the normal subject this is heard equally well in both ears. In conductive deafness it is usually heard loudest in the deaf ear, whereas in perceptive deafness it is heard loudest in the normal ear. These bedside tests, however, are crude: deafness is more accurately assessed by formal audiometric investigation, which will provide a quantitative measure of auditory acuity at different frequencies of sound.

The vestibular nerve carries impulses from the semicircular canals: these sense head rotation (angular acceleration). It also carries impulses from the utricle and saccule, which are the sensors of linear motion (acceleration) and static tilt of the head. Apart from examining for nystagmus it is not necessary to test vestibular function routinely. In patients with vertigo or imbalance, special tests are required which will be described later.

IX and X Glossopharyngeal and vagus nerves

The glossopharyngeal nerve supplies sensation to the posterior pharyngeal wall and tonsillar regions. The vagus nerve, apart from supplying autonomic fibres to thoracic and abdominal contents, supplies motor fibres to the muscles of the soft palate. Interference with glossopharyngeal and vagus nerve function causes difficulty with talking and swallowing.

Vagus function can be examined easily by watching the uvula rise in the midline when the patient says 'Aah'. A unilateral palatal palsy causes drooping of the affected side and, on phonation, the palate deviates to the opposite side, pulled in that direction by the intact muscles. A unilateral vagal lesion will also paralyse the ipsilateral vocal cord to cause a typical hoarse voice and 'bovine' cough. Watch and listen while a patient drinks sips of water.

It is not necessary to test glossopharyngeal sensation routinely, because this involves eliciting the 'gag' reflex, which is unpleasant. When required, the 'gag' reflex is obtained by touching the posterior wall of the pharynx with an orange stick, which causes the patient to 'gag'; both sides of the pharynx should be tested.

XI Accessory nerve

The accessory nerve innervates the sternomastoid and trapezius muscles. Its fibres are derived from the lower brainstem and the upper cervical cord segments. The sternomastoid turns the head to the opposite side, while the trapezius is activated by shrugging the shoulders. Bilateral weakness raises the possibility of muscle disease.

If a patient sustains a hemispheric stroke, then it is the sternomastoid muscle contralateral to the hemiparesis that is affected (i.e. ipsilateral to the cerebral lesion). This will result in weakness of head-turning towards the side of the hemiparesis.

XII Hypoglossal nerve

The hypoglossal nerve innervates the muscles moving the tongue. Normally the tongue is held in the floor of the mouth by activity in the tongue retractors. A unilateral hypoglossal lesion therefore will cause the tip of the tongue to deviate away from the affected side when lying in the floor of the mouth. On protrusion, the tip of the tongue will deviate towards the affected side. Wasting of the tongue can be appreciated in lower motor neurone lesions, often accompanied by fasciculation. In bilateral upper motor neurone lesions, the tongue may be small and spastic. Spasticity is elicited by asking the subject to attempt rapidly to protrude the tongue in and out, or move it from side to side.

Motor functions

It is convenient to screen for motor deficits by examining coordination first. Any type of motor abnormality will impair the capacity to execute rapid fine arm and finger movements, or the ability to walk normally.

Motor function screen
- Hold arms outstretched
- Rapid finger movements, finger/nose testing
- Stance, observe balance
- Gait, observe walking and on tiptoe and heels.

Screen of muscle strength

C5	deltoid	shoulder abduction
C6	biceps	elbow flexion
C7	triceps	elbow extension
C8	finger flexors	grip
T1	dorsal interossei	finger abduction
L1	ilio-psoas	hip flexion
L2	adductors	hip adduction
L3	quadriceps	knee extension
L4	tibialis anterior	foot dorsiflexion
L5	ext. hallucis longus	big toe dorsiflexion
S1	tibialis posterior	foot plantar flexion

Ask the patient to hold the arms outstretched, with fingers spread and with the eyes shut. Look for a tendency: for the arm to drop, which suggests weakness of the shoulder; for the forearm to pronate, which suggests mild upper motor neurone deficit or dystonia; for the fingers to waver uncertainly (pseudoathetosis), which suggests sensory loss; or for abnormal movements, such as tremor, to develop. Then ask the patient to touch their nose rapidly with the point of the forefinger and then the examiner's finger, going to and fro as fast and accurately as possible. Such 'finger–nose testing' examines the skill of large proximal arm movements. Look particularly for kinetic or intention tremor, an oscillation that appears during movement and becomes worse as the point of aim is reached. Also note if the finger overshoots or undershoots its target (dysmetria). Then test the capacity for rapid finger movement by asking the patient to approximate the pulp of the thumb to the pad of each finger in turn rapidly and accurately. This 'five finger exercise' directly tests the integrity of the 'true pyramidal' pathway, which controls fine manual skills, and also detects parkinsonism, which causes slowness, reduced amplitude and fade of such repetitive movements. Finally ask the patient to pronate and supinate the outstretched arms rapidly. Such alternating movements are impaired in cerebellar disease (dysdiadochokinesis) and in parkinsonism.

Gait should always be examined, either as patients walk into the consulting room, or before they undress. Patients who are in bed should always be asked to get up and walk at some stage of the examination. It is also useful to observe stance, to make the patient stand on one leg alone and to walk on their toes and then on their heels. Many defects of motor control of the legs can be rapidly deduced from watching the patient walk; for example, a foot drop as a result of a peroneal nerve palsy or L5 root lesion will cause the patient to lift the foot high to help the toes clear the ground, and the affected foot 'slaps' onto the floor as it is returned to the ground. There is also difficulty walking on the heels. Spastic legs drag as they are moved, with the foot plantar flexed and inverted, the toes scuffing the ground. The small-stepped, shuffling gait of parkinsonism is unmistakable. The wide-based unsteady reeling gait of someone with cerebellar disease or sensory ataxia is also diagnostic. Ataxia of gait can be exaggerated by asking the patient to walk heel-to-toe along a straight line. If ataxia is caused by sensory loss, it becomes much worse with the eyes closed (Romberg's sign). Incoordination of the legs is best detected by watching a patient walk, but also may be brought out on the bed by asking the patient to run the heel carefully up and down the front of the opposite shin, or by asking them to touch the examiner's finger with the big toe.

During the examination for coordination of the arms and legs, look out for the presence of **wasting and involuntary movements**. Muscle wasting implies either primary muscle disease (myopathy) or a lower motor neurone lesion. It can be difficult, particularly in the elderly or in those with joint disease, to decide whether apparent thinning of muscle bulk is merely a result of disuse or whether it indicates neurological deficit.

> Muscle wasting is only of significance if it is accompanied by definite muscle weakness.

The characteristics of the typical abnormal movements of tremor, chorea, myoclonus, tics and dystonia have been described earlier (see p. 67). Other abnormal movements that may be observed include fasciculation, which is a random involuntary twitching of large motor units that occurs as a result of denervation and re-innervation. The characteristic of pathological fasciculation is that twitches of muscle fascicles occur randomly in time and site.

Rapidly test **muscle tone** by noting the resistance of the limbs to passive movement. In the arms, this can be studied by shaking the shoulders with the subject standing, looking for the ease with which the limp arms swing from side to side, or by pronation/supination movements of the forearm. In the legs, tone can be assessed by rolling the thigh to and fro, or by passive flexion of the leg onto the abdomen. Muscle tone must be assessed with the subject

attempting to relax. Resistance to passive movement may take one of three forms.

Muscle tone

Spasticity is a resistance to attempted stretch of the muscle that increases with applied force until there is a sudden give at a certain tension, the 'clasp-knife' or 'lengthening' reaction. Rigidity is a resistance to passive movement that continues unaltered throughout the range of movements, and so has a plastic or 'lead pipe' quality. Gegenhalten describes a curious intermittent resistance to movement in which the patient seems to be unknowingly attempting to oppose efforts to displace the limb.

Muscle power is tested by asking the patient to exert force against resistance imposed by the examiner.

> In a simple screening examination of the nervous system, all that is necessary is to test the strength of two critical muscles, one proximal and one distal, in both arms and legs.

The reason for choosing a proximal and distal muscle to examine is that primary muscle disease will be detected by proximal muscle weakness, while the impact of peripheral nerve disease will be apparent in distal muscle weakness. The proximal and distal muscles chosen to test can be selected also to detect weakness resulting from an upper motor neurone lesion. The latter has a quite distinctive distribution, which can be remembered by recalling the posture of a patient rendered hemiplegic by a stroke. The stroke victim carries the arm held to the side, the elbow flexed and the wrist and fingers flexed onto the chest. The leg is held extended at both hip and knee, with the foot plantar flexed and inverted. This characteristic posture is the result of a selective distribution of spasticity working against a selective distribution of weakness. Hemiplegic weakness in the arm affects the shoulder abductors, elbow extensors, wrist and finger extensors, and small hand muscles. Hemiplegic weakness in the leg affects hip flexors, knee flexors, and dorsiflexors and evertors of the foot. Accordingly, the critical muscles to test in a screening motor examination are: (i) in the arm, proximally the shoulder abductors and distally the small muscles of the hand, which spread the fingers; and (ii) in the leg, proximally the hip flexors and distally the dorsiflexors and evertors of the ankle.

The reflexes (Table 4.1)

Elicit the following reflexes

The deep tendon reflexes of the biceps, triceps, supinator, and finger flexors in the arms, and of the knee and ankle in the legs. When eliciting such 'tendon jerks' always compare the two sides, taking care to have the limbs in comparable positions. When hyper-reflexia is present, try to elicit **clonus** (a repetitive self-sustaining reflex contraction) by rapid passive dorsiflexion of the ankle, and by downward thrust of the patella. Also routinely elicit the superficial reflexes known as the **plantar responses** by firmly stroking the outer border of the sole of each foot upwards. This normally produces plantar flexion of the big toe (a flexor plantar response). The abnormal response consists of upwards movement of the big toe, often accompanied by fanning of the toes; this is known as an extensor plantar response or Babinski's sign. If there is doubt as to the presence of hyper-reflexia or Babinski's sign, elicit the abdominal reflexes by gently stroking the skin of the abdomen in each quadrant in turn. This normally

Table 4.1 Reflexes

Arm	Biceps	C5/6
	Supinator	C5/6
	Triceps	C7
	Finger flexors	C8
Abdominal	Upper	T8–10
	Lower	T10–12
	Cremasteric	L1/2
	Anal	S4/5
Leg	Knee	L3/4
	Ankle	S1

causes a twitch contraction of the appropriate quadrant of the underlying muscles, tending to pull the umbilicus in that direction. The abdominal reflexes are lost in an upper motor neurone lesion. They may also be absent after extensive abdominal surgery or with very lax stretched muscles.

Sensory functions

The student will soon learn that testing sensation is difficult and frustrating. It is crucial to have some clear idea of what is being looked for before embarking on this part of the neurological examination. In a routine screening of the nervous system, sensory examination may be brief, providing the patient has no sensory complaint and there is no other good reason for extensive sensory testing.

> **Spinal cord sensory pathways**
> The three main sensory systems entering the spinal cord are:
>
> • Pain and temperature travelling via the spinothalamic tracts
> • Vibration and position sense travelling via the posterior columns
> • Light touch, which travels through both these other pathways.

The anatomical pathways are outlined in Figure 4.5, where it is shown that all the sensory modalities pass via the dorsal root ganglion into the spinal cord. **Pain and temperature sense** cross to the other side of the spinal cord within one or two segments of entry and then ascend in the spinothalamic tracts to reach the thalamus, while **vibration and position sense** after entry, ascend in the posterior columns (fasciculus gracilis and cuneatus) of the same side of the spinal cord to reach the lower brainstem where the pathway crosses to ascend on the opposite side in the medial lemniscus to reach the thalamus and to relay to the cortex.

Test appreciation of pinprick and light touch on the tips of the fingers and the toes. Pinprick should always be tested with a disposable pin; syringe needles may draw blood and should not be used. Also examine the ability to appreciate joint movement in the distal interphalangeal joints of a finger and the big toe. Remember joint position sense is extremely sensitive, such that small movements of only a few degrees may be perceived accurately. Finally, examine vibration by applying a standard tuning fork (128 Hz) to the tips of the fingers and the big toes. Some estimate of quantitative sensory appreciation of vibration may be obtained by checking whether the patient has ceased to recognize vibration after a standard 'tweak' when

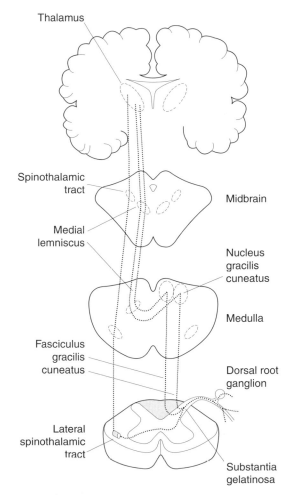

Figure 4.5 Ascending sensory pathways. Posterior columns – position sense, vibration, tactile sense, discrimination. Lateral spinothalamic tract – pain, temperature, tactile sense, tickle, itch.

compared to the application of the same stimulus to the examiner.

Autonomic functions

The autonomic nerves innervate the viscera, bowel, bladder and sexual organs and are responsible for control of circulatory reflexes, sweating and pupillary reactions (Figure 4.6). Symptoms of autonomic failure may include constipation with impaired bowel motility, incomplete bladder emptying from a hypotonic bladder, which may lead to urinary incontinence, and impotence in the male. Failure of the circulatory reflexes may cause postural hypotension with feelings of faintness or dizziness on standing, sometimes syncope, and often a fixed relatively rapid heart rate. There may be impaired sweating with difficulties in temperature regulation, occasionally patchy hyperhidrosis, dry eyes and oral mucous membranes. The pupils may become non-reactive.

The easiest simple tests of autonomic function include measurement of the blood pressure (BP), when the patient is standing and when lying, and the measurement of the pulse rate at rest, during the Valsalva manoeuvre, when deep breathing and on standing.

With autonomic failure the BP will fall by more than 30 mmHg on standing. Orthostatic hypotension is defined as a fall in systolic BP of >20 mmHg and a fall in the diastolic BP of >10 mmHg on standing upright. The pulse rate normally rises on standing: in autonomic failure this may not occur. With a Valsalva manoeuvre, during the strain the BP normally falls and the pulse rate rises. With release the BP rises and the pulse rate falls. With autonomic failure there is no change in pulse rate. Normally the pulse rate varies with deep breathing, but again with autonomic failure this may not occur. Measuring the R-R interval on an electrocardiogram during such tests is a useful way of measuring such heart rate changes. More detailed tests of urodynamic function, penile plethysmography, and pharmacological tests for sweating and pupillary reactions may also be used.

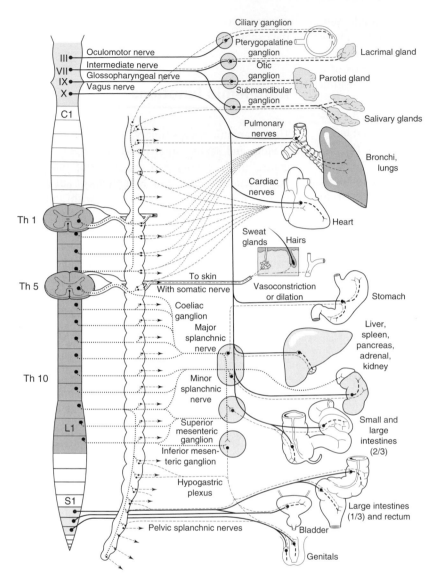

Figure 4.6 The autonomic nervous system and the organs supplied by this. Sympathetic pathways are shown in black. Parasympathetic pathways in grey. Only the left trunk is shown. (Reproduced with permission from P. Duus (1998) *Topical Diagnosis in Neurology*. Stuttgart: Georg Thieme Verlag.)

Examination of related structures

> **The neurological examination is completed by looking at:**
> - The skeletal structures enclosing the central nervous system
> - The extracranial blood vessels
> - The skin
> - A general physical examination.

Check the size and shape of the skull, noticing any palpable lumps. Bruits over the skull and neck may indicate arterial narrowing or the presence of an arteriovenous malformation. Check the skin for any birth marks or stigmata of cutaneous disease, for example neurofibromatosis (Plate 2a).

Look for **meningism** by flexing the head and neck onto the chest. Normally the chin will reach the chest but if the meninges are irritated by blood or infection, such movement is limited by painful spasm of the neck extensors. In severe instances there may be actual head retraction.

Meningeal irritation can also be found in the lumbar region, where spasm of the hamstrings causes limitation of leg movement so that when the thigh is at 90 degrees to the trunk, the knee cannot be straightened (Kernig's sign).

In the case of spinal lesions, examine the spine for any local tenderness or deformity and test spinal movements. Straight-leg raising, by flexing the thigh at the hip with the knee extended, will cause stretching of the sciatic nerve and if the contributing nerve roots are compressed or irritated, results in limitation of the movement with accompanying pain. The pain may be in the back or territory of the sciatic nerve and may be accentuated by dorsiflexing the foot while the leg is raised in the test.

Add a general physical examination for all patients. In particular the pulse rate and rhythm and the BP should be recorded. Check for any signs of heart disease, especially valvular damage. Any enlargement of lymph glands, liver or spleen should be noted and the presence of any mass. This examination is to screen for possible sources of clues to neurological complications of systemic diseases.

Interpretation of abnormal findings

Anatomical site
As discussed in the introduction, the first object of history taking and clinical examination is to find the anatomical site of damage to the nervous system. Every abnormality discovered on physical examination suggests that a particular group of neurones is damaged. By defining the pathways involved, the likely site or sites of the disease may be deduced.

This exercise in applied neuroanatomy is hampered by the ease with which minor insignificant abnormalities may be discovered on examination. Even normal findings sometimes may be misinterpreted as indicating a disease process; for instance, the helpful patient will manufacture sensory abnormalities as fast as you suggest that they may be present!

To overcome this problem, it is a useful exercise to classify each abnormality discovered as a 'hard' or 'soft' sign.

'Hard' signs are unequivocally abnormal – an absent ankle jerk, even on reinforcement; a clear-cut extensor plantar response; definite wasting of the small hand muscles. Any final anatomical diagnosis must provide an explanation for such 'hard' signs. 'Soft' signs are frequently found in the absence of any definite abnormality and are, therefore, unreliable. Examples of such 'soft' signs are a slight asymmetry of the tendon reflexes, slightly less facility of repetitive movements of the left hand in a right-handed person, and a few jerks of nystagmus of the eyes on extreme lateral gaze. When in doubt, it is best to ignore such findings in the initial assessment.

The importance of 'hard' signs
Base your first attempt at diagnosis on the 'hard' signs only. Having taken each of these into account in your final conclusion, then review the 'soft' signs that you discovered on the way, and just make certain that none of them raises doubts about your conclusion.

Another point of neurological examination must be emphasized. The speed and precision with which the site of the lesion may be established depends upon continual deduction throughout the process of history taking and examination. In these first few chapters, emphasis has been laid on the way the findings at one stage in the diagnostic process determine the pattern of the succeeding phases of history taking and examination. Whenever an abnormality has been detected, either in the history or on physical examination, its implications must be followed up to the full; for example, the discovery of a bitemporal hemianopia demands a careful search for evidence of pituitary dysfunction. If a patient with headache is discovered to have such a physical sign, then the examiner may immediately return to ask more questions on this history, such as whether a man still shaves regularly or whether a woman's menstrual periods remain regular. This is the true art of neurology. Each clue that emerges during history taking or examination should prompt new thought. Previous provisional conclusions should be re-examined and new questions or physical tests considered. In other words, to arrive at the correct final conclusion requires a constant alert mental processing of every scrap of information that is available.

SPECIFIC ABNORMALITIES

Having described briefly a basic scheme for examination of the nervous system, one to be undertaken in every neurological patient, we will now turn to the more detailed examinations that may be required when certain abnormalities are discovered. The topics chosen by no means cover all the abnormalities that may be found on clinical examination, but they represent the commonest problems, which will require further exploration.

Dementia

If the patient's complaint is one of memory difficulty or impairment of intellectual processes, or if a relative or acquaintance suggests that this may be the case, then extensive investigation of higher mental function will be required. Likewise, a detailed examination of the mental state is necessary if, in the course of history-taking and physical testing, the patient's intellectual processes seem impaired. Detailed analysis of intellect, reasoning and powers of memory can be a very time-consuming business, requiring the expertise of trained clinical psychologists. They will undertake a formal psychometric assessment of the patient's current level of intellectual performance, using tools such as the Wechsler Adult Intelligence Scale (WAIS), Raven's progressive matrices, and other standardized test batteries. The WAIS test is used most widely, and consists of a number of subtests which assess both 'verbal' and 'performance' abilities. Details of such complex investigations are beyond the scope of this book. Here we are concerned with simple bedside testing of mental powers. However, once the need for formal examination of the mental state has been decided upon, it is best to proceed to gather information in a standard fashion.

An appropriate, standardized, bedside tool for evaluating higher mental function is the Mini-Mental State Examination (MMS; Table 4.2). The tests included in the MMS have been devised to examine most aspects of mental activity briefly but reproducibly. The whole test takes no longer than 5 minutes to complete, and will be a reliable index of intellectual function. In younger patients a score of 28–30 is expected: this may fall to 24 in older patients. Its weakness is perhaps too much emphasis on language functions and too little on recent memory.

Aphasia

Once a defect of the use of language has been detected, either on history-taking or examination, a more extensive evaluation of speech function is required. A great deal of detailed information is available on the way in which human speech and the use of language can break down in neurological disease, but much of this is irrelevant to routine neurological practice.

> Disorders of language with faulty speech may arise from damage to the dominant hemisphere and are important localizing signs. The left hemisphere is dominant in right-handed subjects, but also in some 70% of left-handers.

Much of our understanding of language disorders results from the study of patients who have sustained dominant hemisphere damage. More recently, positron emission tomography and magnetic resonance imaging (MRI) have added to our understanding of the anatomical localization of certain faults and in the production of 'normal' speech. Strictly, aphasia implies a severe or total loss of speech; dysphasia being a milder deficit.

A **global aphasia** describes the impairment of all functions – comprehension, expression, problems in naming, reading, writing and in repetition. These should all be tested. A global aphasia arises from extensive damage.

Two particular speech areas are recognized. Broca's area lies in the posterior frontal region (Figure 4.7), which is close to the motor regions

Table 4.2 The mini-mental state examination

Assessing	Questions	Points (max.)
1 Orientation	Ask the date, the day, the month, the year and the time: score one point for each correct answer	(5)
	Ask the name of the ward, the hospital, the district, the town, the country: again score one point each	(5)
2 Registration and calculation	Name three objects and ask the patient to repeat these: score three for all correct, two if only two	(3)
	Ask the patient to subtract seven from 100 and repeat this five times (93,86,79,72,65)	(5)
	Recall: ask for the three objects to be named again	(3)
3 Language	Name two objects shown to the patient (e.g. pen, watch)	(2)
	Score one point if they can repeat 'No, ifs, ands or buts'	(1)
	Ask the patient to carry out a three-stage command, e.g. 'Take a piece of paper in your right hand, fold it in half and put it on the table'	(3)
	Reading: write in large letters 'Close your eyes' and ask the patient to read and follow this	(1)
	Write: ask the patient to write a short sentence: it should contain a subject, a verb and make sense	(1)
4 Visuo-spatial	Copying: draw two intersecting pentagons, each side about one inch and ask the patient to copy this	(1)
Total		(30)

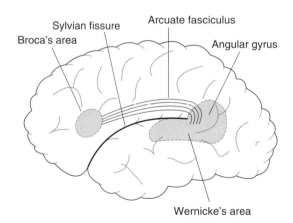

Figure 4.7 Speech areas of the brain.

concerned with articulation. **Broca's aphasia** causes expressive difficulties with non-fluent speech with telegrammatic utterances. Short connecting words may be missing (agrammatic speech) and there may be difficulty with 'ifs, ands or buts'. Sometimes there is perseveration and there may be writing difficulties. Comprehension is good.

The second area lies in the posterior part of the superior temporal gyrus, Wernicke's area, which is close to the region of the brain concerned with auditory input. In **Wernicke's aphasia** there are comprehension difficulties with fluent speech, which exhibits many errors of content. Words and phrases may be incorrect and often repeated – paraphasia. Writing is abnormal and commonly there is difficulty understanding the written word, dyslexia.

The speech areas are connected by the arcuate fasciculus (Figure 4.7). A lesion in this pathway may separate the two sites, allowing fluent paraphasic speech with preserved comprehension, **conduction aphasia**. In such patients repetition is highly abnormal. In some aphasic patients the deficit appears to be one of naming, word finding, anomic aphasia. This may occur with lesions in the left temporoparietal region, including the angular gyrus, when it may be associated with alexia and agraphia. A rare symptom complex also arising from lesions in the region of the angular gyrus is Gerstmann's syndrome. This combines agraphia, acalculia, right–left disorientation, and finger agnosia. In general,

Table 4.3 Aphasia

Broca's aphasia	Wernicke's aphasia	Conduction aphasia	Anomic aphasia
Speech non-fluent telegrammatic	Fluent speech poor content, paraphasic errors	Fluent speech, paraphasic errors	Fluent speech
Comprehension good	Comprehension poor, both verbal and written	Comprehension good	Comprehension good
Repetition good	Repetition poor	Repetition very poor	Repetition normal
Object naming poor	Object naming poor	Object naming poor	Object naming poor
Often hemiparesis arm > leg	Absent or mild hemiparesis, ±hemianopia	Cortical sensory loss	Usually no hemiparesis

Global aphasia – large lesions affect all functions

Although strict divisions are made, in nearly 60% of aphasic patients there appears to be a mixture of problems.

cortical lesions in the dominant hemisphere disrupt spontaneous speech and repetition. Subcortical lesions **(transcortical aphasia)** leave repetition intact, although understanding may be impaired (Table 4.3).

> **Examination of language functions can be tested by observing six basic abilities:**
> - Spontaneous speech (fluent versus non-fluent, errors of content)
> - Naming of objects
> - Repetition
> - Comprehension
> - Reading
> - Writing.

explore the object. Such defects reflect parietal lobe damage.

Visual agnosia is the inability to recognize what is seen when the eye, optic nerve and main visual pathway to the occipital cortex are preserved. Affected patients can often describe the shape, colour or size of an object without recognizing it. **Prosopagnosia** is the inability to recognize a familiar face. Parieto-occipital lesions are responsible.

Anosognosia is a term used to describe the lack of awareness or realization that the limbs on one side are paralysed , weak or have impaired sensation. It is most often seen in patients with right-sided parietal damage who may seem to be unaware of their faulty left limbs.

Agnosia

Agnosia is the failure to recognize objects when the pathways of sensory input from touch, sight and sound are intact. This sensory input cannot be combined with the ability to recall a similar object from the memory areas of the brain, a sort of 'mind-blindness'. Such deficits can be tested by asking patients to feel, name and describe the use of certain objects.

Tactile agnosia, astereognosis, is the inability to recognize objects placed in the hands. There must be no sensory loss in the fingers and sufficient motor function and coordination for the patient's fingers to

Apraxia

Apraxia is the inability to perform purposeful willed movements in the absence of motor paralysis, severe incoordination or sensory loss. It is the motor equivalent of agnosia. Patients should also be able to understand the command, although it is quite common for some dysphasia to be present. To test for apraxia patients may be asked to perform a number of tasks, such as to make a fist, to pretend to comb their hair, lick their lips, to pretend to light a cigarette or to construct a square with four matches. In **ideomotor apraxia** patients cannot perform a movement to command, although they may do this automatically, for example, lick their lips. In **ideational apraxias** there is difficulty in carrying out a complex series of movements, like taking a match from a box to light a cigarette.

Gait apraxias create problems walking, although patients may show good leg movements when tested on the bed. In **dressing apraxias**, patients cannot put their clothes on correctly. **Constructional apraxias** produce problems in copying designs or arranging patterns on blocks.

In most instances apraxias are caused by dominant parietal lobe damage with breakdown in the connections via callosal fibres with the opposite hemisphere, and in the links between the parietal lobes and the motor cortex.

Visual field defects

Light from an object on the left-hand side of the body falls on the right-hand half of each retina after passing through the narrow pupillary aperture. The temporal or outer half of each retina eventually is connected to the cerebral cortex on that side by nerve fibres, which never cross the midline. The inner, or nasal, half of the retina is connected to the cortex on the opposite side by fibres which cross the midline of the optic chiasm. It follows that the right-hand halves of both retinae are connected to the right occipital cortex, which views objects on the left side of the body. Analysis of visual field defects follows from these simple anatomical principles.

The visual field defect may be caused by a lesion affecting the eye, the optic nerve, the optic chiasm, the optic tract between the chiasm and lateral geniculate bodies, the optic radiation, or the occipital cortex. The resulting patterns of visual field defect are illustrated in Figure 4.2.

Optic nerve lesions

In the case of optic nerve lesions the macular fibres are often damaged first as these are most sensitive to pressure or ischaemia. Accordingly, the initial symptoms of an optic nerve lesion are a loss of visual acuity accompanying a central visual field defect (a central scotoma). Degeneration of optic nerve fibres

can be seen with the ophthalmoscope as optic atrophy, in which the disc becomes unnaturally white. As an optic nerve lesion progresses, visual acuity falls further and the size of the central scotoma enlarges. Eventually, a complete optic nerve lesion will lead to blindness in that eye (Figure 4.2). However, the patient will still be able to see clearly and to either side with the remaining opposite intact eye. The pupil of the blind eye will not react to light shone directly into it, but will react briskly when the light is shone in the opposite eye to evoke the consensual reaction.

Afferent pupillary defect

The **'swinging light test'** (see p. 75) employs the principle that there is a difference in the direct and consensual pupillary reactions to light when there is a fault on the afferent visual pathway, the optic nerve or a severe degree of retinal damage. If a light is flashed from one eye to the other, the direct response on the side of the affected optic nerve will be less powerful than the consensual response evoked from the normal eye. As a result, when the light is shone in the affected eye, the pupil will dilate. In normal subjects the response is symmetrical. When there is an asymmetry in the response this is called the afferent pupillary defect or Marcus Gunn phenomenon.

Chiasmal lesions

The optic chiasm contains both non-crossing fibres from the outer halves of the retina, which lie laterally, and decussating fibres from the inner halves of the retina. The decussating fibres are arranged with those from the upper part of the retina above and posteriorly, and those from the lower part below and anteriorly. Macular fibres also lie in the posterior part of the chiasm.

Another anatomical peculiarity is that fibres from the lower part of the nasal retina, having passed in the chiasm, may loop anteriorly into the optic nerve before passing posteriorly into the optic tract. Accordingly, a posteriorly placed lesion of the optic nerve will cause not only a central scotoma on that side, but also an upper temporal quadrantic defect in the visual field of the opposite eye, the so-called 'junctional scotoma'.

A lesion dividing the optic chiasm in the midline interrupts fibres from the inner half of each retina and results in the loss of the temporal field of vision in each eye, the bitemporal hemianopia (Figure 4.2).

It is important to realize that the visual fields of the two eyes overlap binocularly when they are both open. The extent of overlap is almost complete except for a few degrees at each temporal crescent. Accordingly, it is possible to miss entirely a total bitemporal hemianopia when examining the visual fields to confrontation, unless each eye is tested separately. The details of the anatomical arrangement within the optic chiasm dictate the pattern of visual defects caused by different lesions in this region.

Pressure on the chiasm from behind and below, such as by a pituitary tumour, often affects the decussating macular fibres first to produce bitemporal paracentral scotomas.

As such a tumour enlarges, the scotomas extend out to the periphery to cause the characteristic bitemporal hemianopia. Pressure on the chiasm from one side first affects the non-crossing fibres from the outer half of the retina, to cause a unilateral nasal hemianopia.

Posterior lesion

Lesions of the optic tract

Lesions in the optic tract will damage all fibres conveying vision from the opposite side of the patient to cause a homonymous hemianopia, in which the field defects of the left and right eyes will be the same (Figure 4.2).

However, such lesions also often impinge upon the posterior part of the chiasm, thereby damaging fibres from the upper inner quadrant of the ipsilateral retina before they cross to the opposite side. This results in the addition of an ipsilateral lower temporal field defect to the contralateral hemianopia, so that optic tract lesions commonly are incongruous.

Lesions in the region of the optic nerve, optic chiasm and optic tract lie close to, and may arise from, the pituitary, and to the adjacent hypothalamus above. Accordingly, such parapituitary lesions often produce disturbances other than visual field defects, including abnormalities of eye movement, hypopituitarism and diabetes insipidus. The effect of damage to the optic nerve on the pupillary reaction to light was described earlier, and any lesion in this region causing damage to central vision may produce an afferent pupillary defect. However, if the field defect is a hemianopia, sufficient vision remains in the intact half of the macular region to preserve visual acuity as normal, and the pupillary reaction likewise will be normal.

Lesions of the optic radiation

The fibres of the optic radiation leave the lateral geniculate body to pass via the posterior limb of the internal capsule to the visual cortex. In their course, fibres carrying impulses from the homonymous upper portions of the retinae pass via the parietal lobe to the supracalcarine cortex. Fibres representing the lower portions of the retinae pass over the temporal horn of the lateral ventricle, where they lie in the posterior portion of the temporal lobe before reaching the infracalcarine cortex.

Optic radiation damage
Destruction of the whole optic radiation produces a contralateral homonymous hemianopia (see Figures 1.1 and 4.2) without loss of visual acuity, without optic atrophy (because optic nerve fibres have synapsed in the lateral geniculate body), and without alteration in the pupillary light reflex. Partial lesions of the radiation are common. Parietal lobe lesion will produce predominantly an inferior homonymous quadrantic field defect, while temporal lobe lesions produce superior homonymous quadrantic defects.

When dealing with hemianopic field defects, it is important to test both eyes simultaneously to confrontation.

COLOUR PLATES

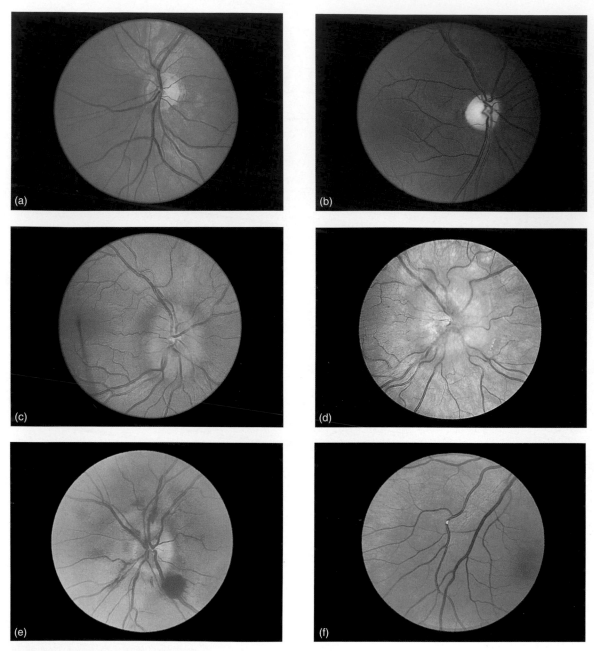

Plate 1   (a) Normal optic disk; (b) Optic atrophy – the pallor of the disc appears accentuated because the patient was pigmented (Indian); (c) Acute papilloedema; (d) More chronic and more severe papilloedema; (e) Haemorrhagic lesions in a patient with acute leukaemia; (f) Cholesterol embolus in a retinal artery branch.

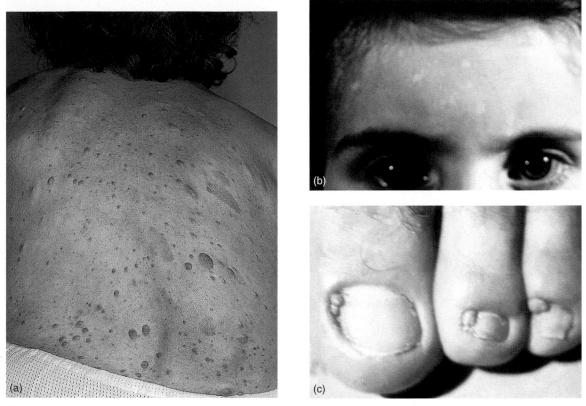

Plate 2 (a) Typical widespread skin changes in a patient with type I neurofibromatosis. Note there is also a scoliosis; (b) Depigmented skin lesions on a child's face with tuberous sclerosis; (c) Subungual fibroma in patients with tuberous sclerosis.

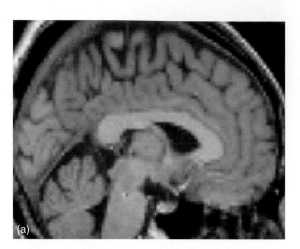
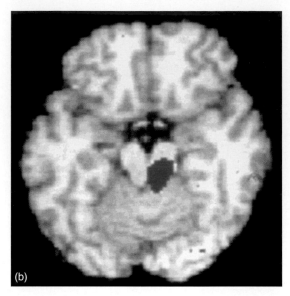

Plate 3 (a) Activation on positron emission tomography (PET) in a patient with cluster headache and migraine, who experienced a migraine without aura during the scan and demonstrated activation in the rostral ventral pons; (b) Similarly, PET activations are shown in 11 patients with migraine without aura who were scanned during an attack and who demonstrated activations in the dorsal midbrain.

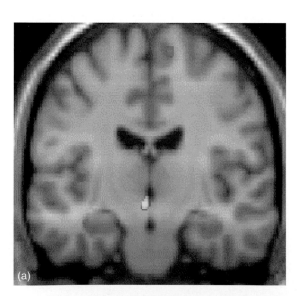
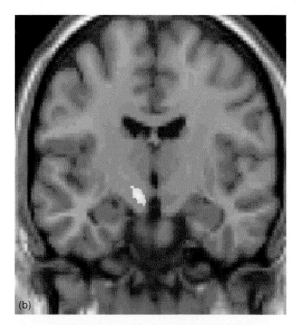

Plate 4 (a) Activation on positron emission tomography (PET) in the posterior hypothalamic grey matter in patients with acute cluster headache. The activation demonstrated is lateralized to the side of the pain; (b) When comparing the brains of patients with cluster headache with a control population using an automatic anatomical technique known as voxel-based morphometry that employs high-resolution T1-weighted MRI, a similar region is demonstrated and has increased grey matter.

The earliest sign of a hemianopia may be the inability to perceive an object in the affected field of vision when the corresponding portion of the normal field is tested at the same time; this is called an **inattention hemianopia**.

Lesions of the occipital cortex

The characteristic field defect resulting from a lesion of the occipital cortex is a contralateral homonymous hemianopia (Figure 4.2) without loss of visual acuity and with preserved pupillary responses. However, local anatomical arrangements of visual representation in the occipital cortex and of blood supply to this area may cause a variety of other field defects. The macula is extensively represented in the cortex of the tip of the occipital pole, an area sometimes supplied by the middle cerebral artery. Compressive lesions at this site, or middle cerebral arterial insufficiency, may produce **contralateral homonymous paracentral scotomas** (Figure 4.2). The remainder of the occipital cortex is supplied by the posterior cerebral arteries, which, because they derived from a common stem, the basilar artery, often are occluded simultaneously. If the occipital tip is supplied by the middle cerebral artery in such patients, then bilateral occlusion of posterior cerebral artery flow will cause **grossly constricted visual fields with preservation of small tunnels of central vision**. These central 'pinholes', the size of which will depend upon the extent of the middle cerebral supply to the occipital cortex, may be sufficient to preserve normal visual acuity. It is important to distinguish such constrictive visual fields from those seen in some patients with hysterical visual loss. It is a physical fact that the size of the central pinhole must increase, the further away from the patient one moves. In contrast, hysterical 'tunnel' vision commonly takes the form of preservation of a central area of vision, the size of which remains the same whether one is 1 foot (0.31 m) or 10 feet (3.1 m) from the patient's face – this is physically impossible. Finally, if the whole of the occipital cortex is supplied by the posterior cerebral arteries, and both are occluded, then the patient will develop **cortical blindness**, in which the patient can perceive nothing yet pupillary responses are preserved and the optic discs appear normal. Because damage often also involves adjacent areas of cortex in some patients, many of them may exhibit other cognitive deficits, including even **denial of blindness – Anton's syndrome**.

Pupillary abnormalities

The size of the pupil is controlled by the influence of the two divisions of the autonomic nervous system, which act in response to the level of illumination and the distance of focus. The sphincter muscle makes the pupil smaller (miosis), and is innervated by cholinergic parasympathetic nerves; the dilator makes it larger (mydriasis), and is innervated by noradrenergic sympathetic fibres.

The parasympathetic fibres, which control both pupillary constriction and contraction of the ciliary muscle to produce accommodation, arise from the Edinger–Westphal nucleus. They travel by the IIIrd nerve to the ciliary ganglion in the orbit; postganglionic fibres from the ciliary ganglion are distributed by the ciliary nerve. A lesion of the parasympathetic nerves produces a dilated pupil, which is unreactive to light or accommodation. The parasympathetic fibres to the eye are nearly always damaged by lesions affecting the IIIrd nerve, which also produce ptosis and a characteristic loss of ipsilateral eye movement (see later).

Adie's tonic pupil

Adie's tonic pupil is a rare cause of damage to the parasympathetic fibres within the ciliary ganglion, presenting usually with a large pupil (Figure 4.8). The condition commonly presents in young women with the sudden appreciation that one pupil is much

(a)
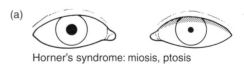
Horner's syndrome: miosis, ptosis

(b)
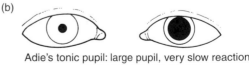
Adie's tonic pupil: large pupil, very slow reactions, reacts to weak pilocarpine

(c)
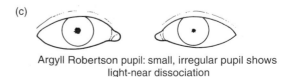
Argyll Robertson pupil: small, irregular pupil shows light-near dissociation

Figure 4.8 Abnormal pupils.

larger than the other. The dilated pupil does not react immediately to light, but prolonged exposure in a dark room may cause slow and irregular contraction of the iris. Likewise, accommodation on convergence is very slow to take place. With time, the dilated tonic pupil gradually constricts and may end up eventually smaller than the other. Inspection of the affected pupil with a slit-lamp may show irregular wormlike movements of the iris border. Pharmacological testing will confirm the label by showing denervation hypersensitivity to weak pilocarpine (0.125%) or methacholine (2.5%) eye drops. These drugs will cause a tonic pupil to constrict but have no effect on the normal pupil. Some patients with a tonic pupil, or tonic pupils, also lose their tendon jerks in the so-called Holmes–Adie syndrome.

Argyll Robertson pupils

The pupillary response to light depends on the integrity of the afferent pathways. As already described, the direct light response is impaired, with damage to the retina or optic nerve, and this can be shown by the presence of an afferent pupillary defect. The relevant optic nerve fibres responsible for the light reaction leave those responsible for the perception of light to terminate in the pretectal region of the midbrain, from whence a further relay passes to the Edinger–Westphal nucleus. Damage to this pretectal region is believed to be responsible for the Argyll Robertson pupil classically seen in neurosyphilis. The characteristics of these pupils are that they are small, irregular and unequal, and exhibit **light–near dissociation** (Figure 4.8). Light–near dissociation refers to the loss of pupillary reaction to light, with preservation of that to accommodation. Pupils resembling those of Argyll Robertson also occur occasionally in diabetes and in other conditions with autonomic neuropathy. Large pupils exhibiting light–near dissociation are characteristic of damage in the region of the superior colliculi, as may be produced by tumours of the pineal gland. These cause **Parinaud's syndrome** in which there is pupillary light–near dissociation, with paralysis of upgaze and convergence.

Horner's syndrome

The sympathetic fibres supplying the eye arise from the eighth cervical and the first two thoracic segments of the spinal cord. They synapse in the cervical

ganglia and pass via the carotid plexus to the orbit. The activity of these fibres is controlled by hypothalamic centres, from which central sympathetic pathways pass to the spinal cord (Figure 4.9b). A lesion of the ocular sympathetic pathways anywhere along this route will produce a Horner's syndrome (Figure 4.8).

Horner's syndrome (Figure 4.9a,b)
The pupil on the affected side is constricted. It reacts to light and accommodation, but does not dilate normally in response to shade or pain. In addition, denervation of the smooth muscle of the upper eyelid leads to ptosis, which can be overcome by voluntary upgaze, enophthalmos, and denervation of the facial sweat glands causes loss of sweating on the affected side of the face.

As indicated, a Horner's syndrome may appear as a result of lesions affecting the hypothalamus, brainstem or spinal cord, or as a result of damage to the

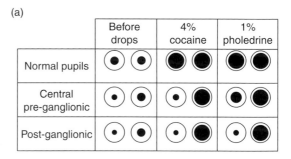

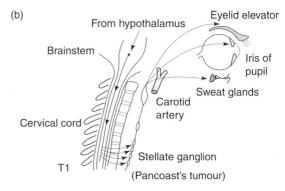

Figure 4.9 Horner's syndrome. (a) Pharmacological testing of the pupil with 4% cocaine and 1% pholedrine (*N*-methyl hydroxyamphetamine) to show the site of the lesion. (b) Anatomical pathways of sympathetic innervation of the eye and pupil.

emergent T1 root and cervical ganglion containing sympathetic nerve output, or to the sympathetic plexus on the carotid artery anywhere from the neck to the head. Pharmacological testing may help to establish the anatomical level of the sympathetic damage. Nearly all post-ganglionic lesions are 'benign': preganglionic or central lesions may affect the brainstem, cervical cord, and particularly lesions at the lung apex or lower neck. With preganglionic and central lesions, application of 4% cocaine eye drops will cause slight dilatation of the affected pupil. With post-ganglionic lesions, 1% hydroxyamphetamine or 1% pholedrine eye drops will cause no reaction, while preganglionic and central lesions show dilatation. Phenylephrine (1%) will also cause dilatation of the affected pupil in post-ganglionic but not in preganglionic or central lesions (Figure 4.9a).

Defects of ocular movement and diplopia

Abnormalities of eye movement may arise at one of three levels in the nervous system: in the muscles, in the brainstem and more centrally.

Primary muscle disease may impair ocular motility (ocular myopathy), when eye movements usually remain conjugate, or in myasthenia gravis, in which fatigue is typical. Lesions of individual muscles or their nerve supply, caused by damage of the IIIrd, IVth or VIth cranial nerves or their nuclei, will impair specific individual movements of the eye. This will result in a breakdown of conjugate gaze to cause double vision (diplopia). Within the brainstem, complex pathways link together centres for conjugate gaze to the individual ocular motor nuclei; for example, horizontal gaze to one side demands conjugate activation of one VIth nerve nucleus and the portion of the opposite IIIrd nerve nucleus innervating the medial rectus. These two nuclear regions are linked by fibres passing in the medial longitudinal bundle (Figure 4.10). Damage to such pathways produces dysconjugate gaze known as an internuclear ophthalmoplegia. Finally, conjugate gaze to either side and up and down, is controlled by pathways from the cerebral hemispheres arising in frontal and occipital eyefields. Damage to these pathways will cause defects of conjugate eye movements known as supranuclear gaze palsies.

Infranuclear lesions

Each eye is moved by three pairs of muscles. The precise action of these depends upon the position of the eye, but their main actions are as follows:

1 The lateral and medial recti, respectively, abduct and adduct the eye.
2 The superior and inferior recti, respectively, elevate and depress the abducted eye.
3 The superior and inferior obliques, respectively, depress and elevate the adducted eye.
4 The superior oblique also internally rotates, and the inferior oblique externally rotates the eye.

Weakness of an individual muscle will cause limitation of movement of one eye in a characteristic direction, and diplopia will occur as a result of misrepresentation of the object on the retina. The term **squint** describes a misalignment of ocular axes, but is sufficiently great as to be obvious to the observer. When the misalignment is present at rest and equal for all directions of gaze (concomitant squint) it is not caused by a local weakness of the ocular muscles.

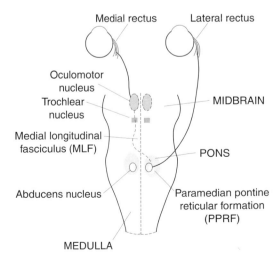

Figure 4.10 Pathway of medial longitudinal fasciculus yoking the abducens and oculomotor nuclei for conjugate horizontal eye movements.

Concomitant squint develops during childhood because of failure to establish binocular vision. The abnormal image from the squinting eye is suppressed, so there is no diplopia. In contrast, a misalignment of the eye that is more apparent when gazing in a particular direction indicates weakness of the muscle acting in that direction (paralytic squint), and diplopia. It should be noted that slight muscle weakness will produce diplopia before any defect of movement can be observed by the examiner.

Diplopia assessment

A scheme to examine the eyes in patients complaining of diplopia has been outlined on page 75. Three cardinal points should be emphasized:

1 The diplopia may consist of images that are side by side (horizontal), or one above the other (vertical), or both. Horizontal diplopia must be a result of weakness of a lateral or medial rectus muscle. Vertical diplopia, or diplopia in which the two images are at angles to one another, can result from weakness in any of the other muscles.

2 Separation of the images is maximal when the gaze is turned in the direction of action of the weak muscle; for example, maximal separation of images on looking to the right, with horizontal diplopia, indicates weakness of the left medial or right lateral rectus.

3 When the gaze is directed to cause maximal separation of the images, the abnormal image from the lagging eye is displaced further in the direction of gaze; for example, if horizontal diplopia is maximal on looking to the right, and the image furthest to the right comes from the right eye (tested by covering each eye separately), the right lateral rectus is weak. Conversely, diplopia is minimal when the gaze is directed in such a way as to avoid the use of the weak muscle. Patients sometimes make use of this fact to prevent double vision, by adopting a convenient head posture. Thus the patient with a right lateral rectus palsy will maintain the head deviated to the right so as to be gazing slightly to the left, when the image will be single.

Although these rules sound simple, in practice it can often be difficult to analyse complex diplopia at the bedside. The use of red and green spectacles to identify two images, and the use of Hess charts to plot their position, may sometimes be required to make analysis easier and to follow progress.

Disorders of function of individual eye muscles, and the diplopia so produced, may be caused by disorder of the eye muscles themselves, or by lesions of the nerves controlling them. Lesions of the eye muscles occur in two situations. **Primary ocular myopathy** occurs in the group of disorders known as chronic progressive ophthalmoplegia. Such patients have profound defects of all forms of eye movement, but the ocular axes remain parallel so that diplopia does not develop. In contrast, **myasthenia gravis**, which commonly affects the eyes, causes loss of conjugate gaze and inevitable diplopia.

Characteristic of myasthenia is fatigue of eye muscle contraction with exercise, so that diplopia occurs towards the end of the day, or on sustained gaze in a particular direction. Ptosis is also often present and there may be weakness of eye closure (orbicularis oculi).

Lesions of the nerves to the ocular muscles may result from disorders affecting the nuclei in the brainstem, or from damage to the nerves themselves in their course to the orbit. Such lesions inevitably produce diplopia (unless the patient is blind in one eye), for conjugate gaze is destroyed.

Oculomotor (IIIrd nerve) lesions produce ptosis because the levator palpebrae is paralysed. On lifting the lid it will be apparent that the eye is deviated outwards and downwards, because of the respective actions of the intact lateral rectus and superior oblique (which are supplied by the VIth and IVth nerves) (Figure 4.11). The pupillomotor fibres lie towards the outside of the nerve so compressive lesions cause the pupil to be dilated and unresponsive to light, and accommodation may be paralysed. Partial lesions of the IIIrd nerve are common, however, and in these the parasympathetic fibres to the pupil may either be spared or selectively involved.

Trochlear (IVth nerve) lesions paralyse the superior oblique muscle, producing inability to look downwards and inwards. Such patients commonly present

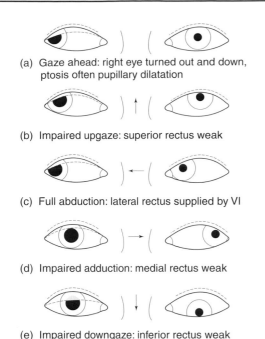

(a) Gaze ahead: right eye turned out and down, ptosis often pupillary dilatation

(b) Impaired upgaze: superior rectus weak

(c) Full abduction: lateral rectus supplied by VI

(d) Impaired adduction: medial rectus weak

(e) Impaired downgaze: inferior rectus weak

Figure 4.11 Right oculomotor palsy.

with a complaint of diplopia when walking downstairs. The presence of intact IVth nerve function can be demonstrated by showing the eye intorts, that is, it rolls inwards about an anterior–posterior axis, when the patient is asked to look at the root of their nose (Figure 4.12). Many patients may show a head tilt to the side opposite to that of the defective eye.

Abducens (VIth nerve) lesions paralyse the external rectus, producing inability to abduct the eye (Figure 4.13).

Internuclear lesions

The complex details of interconnection between ocular motor nuclei and pontine gaze centres (see below and Figure 4.10) are beyond the scope of this book. The important point is the critical role played by the medial longitudinal bundle linking the VIth nerve nucleus in the pons with the IIIrd nerve nucleus in the midbrain.

A unilateral lesion of the medial longitudinal bundle causes the characteristic features of an internuclear gaze palsy **(internuclear ophthalmoplegia)**. These consist of difficulty in adducting the ipsilateral eye on horizontal gaze, with the development of coarse jerk nystagmus in the contralateral abducting eye (Figure 4.14).

The syndrome is sometimes called ataxic nystagmus of the eyes. Lesser degrees of internuclear ophthalmoplegia may be evident simply as a relative slowness of adduction compared with abduction on horizontal gaze. The adducting eye is seen to lag behind the abducting eye. Diplopia does not occur in an internuclear ophthalmoplegia, but oscillopsia,

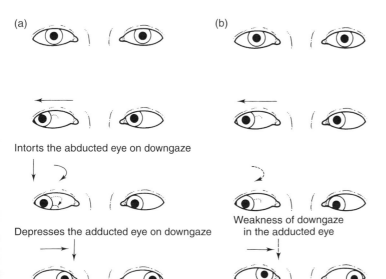

(a)

(b)

Intorts the abducted eye on downgaze

Depresses the adducted eye on downgaze

Weakness of downgaze in the adducted eye

Figure 4.12 (a) Actions of normal superior oblique muscle. (b) Right superior oblique palsy.

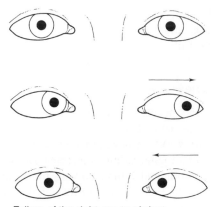

Failure of the right eye to abduct

Figure 4.13 Right abducens palsy.

that is, a tendency for the outside world to bob up and down, often occurs with brainstem lesions. Bilateral internuclear ophthalmoplegia is almost always the result of multiple sclerosis, although vascular disease and brainstem tumours occasionally may produce unilateral internuclear lesions.

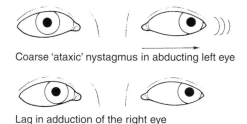

Coarse 'ataxic' nystagmus in abducting left eye

Lag in adduction of the right eye

Figure 4.14 Right internuclear ophthalmoplegia. Lesion of the medial longitudinal fasciculus.

Supranuclear lesions

Supranuclear lesions

Four separate mechanisms exist for eliciting conjugate ocular gaze in any direction:

1 The saccadic system allows the subject voluntarily to direct gaze at will, even with the eyes shut. The pathways responsible for saccadic gaze arise in the frontal lobe and pass to the pontine gaze centres.
2 The pursuit system allows the subject to follow a moving object. The pathways responsible for pursuit gaze arise in the

parieto-occipital region and pass to the pontine gaze centres.
3 The optokinetic system restores gaze, despite movements of the outside world. The operation of the optokinetic system is seen in the railway train, where the eyes of the subject gazing out of the window are seen to veer slowly as the train moves, to be followed by rapid corrections back to the primary position of gaze.
4 The **vestibulo–ocular reflex (VOR)** system corrects for movements of the head to preserve the stable visual world. Inputs from the labyrinths and from neck proprioceptors are directed to the brainstem ocular mechanisms to achieve stabilization of the visual image, despite head movements.

These systems for controlling conjugate gaze may be interrupted in many different ways. Lesions of the frontal lobes commonly disrupt voluntary saccadic gaze, while pursuit, optokinetic and vestibulo-ocular mechanisms remain intact. Diffuse cerebral disease, of whatever cause, may interfere with both saccadic and pursuit systems. Saccadic movements become slowed and hypometric, while smooth pursuit is broken up into small jerky steps. Optokinetic nystagmus, as tested with a hand-held drum bearing vertical black and white stripes, is also disrupted in such patients. In fact, optokinetic nystagmus tested in this way is frequently disturbed before evidence of interruption of the pursuit system is apparent. Patients with such supranuclear gaze palsies for saccadic and pursuit movements, often have preserved VOR movement. This is tested by the doll's head manoeuvre, the **oculocephalic reflex**. The patient is asked to fixate on the examiner's face, and the head is briskly rotated from side to side or up and down. Patients unable voluntarily to direct their gaze to either side, and unable to follow a moving object in the same directions, may exhibit a full range of ocular movement to the doll's head manoeuvre. It is this preservation of VOR eye movement in the absence of voluntary saccadic or pursuit movements that is diagnostic of a supranuclear gaze palsy. Caloric tests may also demonstrate preserved VOR function in the brainstem (see p. 98). The VOR may also be assessed at the bedside by the **head impulse** test. The patient is asked to fixate on a nearby target and then the head is turned briskly by the examiner's hands, first to one side and then to the other, rotating the head by about 30 degrees. The test is abnormal if the eyes have to make a few saccadic jerks before refixing on the target. With an intact VOR the patient can maintain fixation despite the head movements. This test is sensitive in detecting a unilateral peripheral vestibular fault.

Despite defects in gaze, the eyes remain conjugate in supranuclear palsies, so diplopia does not occur.

The centres in the cerebral hemispheres responsible for saccadic and pursuit movement control deviation of the eyes conjugately towards the opposite side of the body.

> Thus, a unilateral hemisphere lesion will cause weakness of conjugate deviation of the eyes away from the side of the lesion. As they descend towards the brainstem, these pathways cross before they reach the pons. Accordingly, damage to the region of the pontine gaze centres will cause weakness of deviation of the eyes towards the side of the lesion.

The combination of damage to the pontine paramedian horizontal gaze centre with involvement of the ipsilateral medial longitudinal bundle (internuclear ophthalmoplegia) may produce the **one-and-a-half-syndrome** (Figure 4.15).

The centres for conjugate vertical gaze in the brainstem lie in the midbrain. Lesions at that site cause difficulty in conjugate upgaze. The centres responsible for downgaze are less well localized, and

lesions both in the midbrain and at the level of the foramen magnum can produce defects of voluntary downgaze. **Downbeat nystagmus strongly suggests a lesion at the craniocervical junction or in the cerebellum** (Figure 4.16).

Defects of vestibular function and nystagmus

The **vestibular system** is responsible for maintaining balance, and the direction of gaze, despite changes in head and body positions. Its components provide information on the static position of the head in space (from the otolith organs in the utricle and saccule), and on the character of dynamic changes in head position (from the semicircular canals). The information is correlated from that arising in neck proprioceptors, which provide data on the relationship of the head to the body. The integration of these various data on posture occurs in the brainstem and cerebellum. The information is used to adjust postural muscle activity to maintain balance, and eye position to maintain gaze. Damage to the vestibular

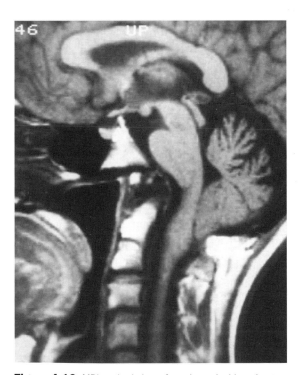

Figure 4.16 MRI sagittal view of craniocervical junction to show basilar impression in a patient who presented with slight ataxia and showed downbeat nystagmus.

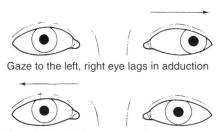

Gaze to the left, right eye lags in adduction

Gaze to the right, gaze paresis

Figure 4.15 Right 'one-and-a-half' syndrome. This is a combination of an internuclear ophthalmoplegia and an ipsilateral gaze paresis on the same side.

system, whether it be in the labyrinth or in the brainstem/cerebellum, inevitably leads to imbalance and defects of eye movement control.

> Each labyrinth at rest exerts tonic influence tending to deviate the eyes to the opposite side.

The effects from the two sides counterbalance each other, thereby maintaining a forward gaze. Sudden destruction of one labyrinth produces a forced drift of the gaze to the affected side because of the unopposed action of the normal labyrinth, followed by a rapid correction in an attempt to restore visual fixation. The jerk nystagmus provoked by such unilateral labyrinthine destruction (**'canal' vestibular nystagmus**) has the following characteristics: the slow phase is always directed to the abnormal ear; it is most marked when the gaze is directed away from the abnormal ear; it is predominantly horizontal or rotatory; it is independent of vision, for it persists or is enhanced when the eyes are shut or defocused using strong plus lenses (Frenzel's lenses); and it is frequently accompanied by vertigo and evidence of damage to the cochlear portion of the middle ear in the form of deafness or tinnitus. Peripheral vestibular damage causes intense vertigo, accompanied by all the other symptoms associated with 'sea-sickness' including nausea, sweating and vomiting. These symptoms are accompanied by fear. In addition, the patient is severely ataxic, and often can only move around by crawling on the floor.

Compensation rapidly occurs after loss of one vestibular apparatus. The remaining intact labyrinth adapts to the new conditions so that balance is restored and vertigo disappears over a matter of a few weeks. Indeed, even when both labyrinths are destroyed, the patient soon can walk and even dance, provided the floor is even, because visual, cutaneous and proprioceptive sensations provide the necessary alternative information.

> In contrast to the dramatic and explosive symptoms caused by peripheral vestibular damage, lesions of the vestibular nerve or its brainstem connections produce fewer symptoms.

Vertigo and ataxia may be evident, but dramatic nausea and vomiting are unusual. Such brainstem damage causes **'central' vestibular nystagmus** (Table 4.4), which differs from 'canal' vestibular nystagmus in certain important characteristics: frequently it is vertical as well as horizontal; its direction changes with the direction of gaze, such that the jerk is to the right on right lateral gaze and to the left on left lateral gaze; compensation occurs but slowly; and it is improved or abolished by eye closure.

Lesions of the brainstem may cause nystagmus, not only by compromising vestibular connections, but also by interfering with the mechanisms responsible for gaze. Gaze nystagmus, which is analogous to the oscillatory movement that may occur in a weak limb when the patient attempts to maintain it in a given position against gravity, occurs when the eyes are deviated in the direction of weakness of gaze. Because the pontine gaze centres are responsible for drawing the eyes towards that side, damage to this region will cause nystagmus on looking towards the lesion. In contrast, as noted above, damage to the vestibular system causes nystagmus, which is maximal on looking away from the side of the lesion. As a consequence, a lesion in the cerebellopontine angle, such as an acoustic neuroma, may initially cause nystagmus on gaze away from the affected side because of damage of vestibular fibres in the VIIIth nerve, but subsequently the nystagmus changes and becomes maximal on looking towards the side of the lesion when it has grown large enough to impinge upon the brainstem.

The semicircular canals are the sensors of dynamic changes (angular acceleration) of head position, while the otolith organs, the utricle and saccule, are the sensors of linear acceleration and gravity changes (including head tilt). The hair cell is the basic sensory cell. In each semicircular canal there is a mound

Table 4.4 Characteristics of nystagmus

Peripheral	Central
Unidirectional	Directional
Fast phase away from side of lesion	Fast phase towards the site of lesion
	May include vertical, rotatory
Fixation inhibits	No change with fixation
Darkness, defocus enhances	Darkness, defocus may reduce

of hair cells, the ampulla, with a divider, the cupula. These hair cells either increase or decrease their firing rate depending on the direction of fluid displacement. In the otolith organs the hair cells are situated in the maculae and are covered by a crystal-laden gelatinous membrane. These crystals are particles of calcium carbonate, the otoconia. Movements of the head by tilting or by linear acceleration may displace the otoconia and stimulate the otolith hair cells.

Benign paroxysmal positional vertigo is the most common cause of vertigo and reflects dislocation of otoconia from the utricle that have migrated into the posterior semicircular canal causing abnormal stimulation. The Dix–Hallpike manoeuvre is the diagnostic test to show whether this is so. With the patient sitting on the couch, their head is turned slightly to one side and the neck extended. The eyes of the patient should be fixed on the examiner's eyes. The patient is then lain supine quickly, the head still being supported by the examiner's hands and their eyes still fixed on those of the examiner (Figure 4.17). In a normal patient there is no nystagmus or distress. In patients suffering with positional vertigo there is a brief latent period of 2–6 seconds, then usually a torsional upbeating nystagmus lasting 20–30 seconds which is accompanied by intense vertigo.

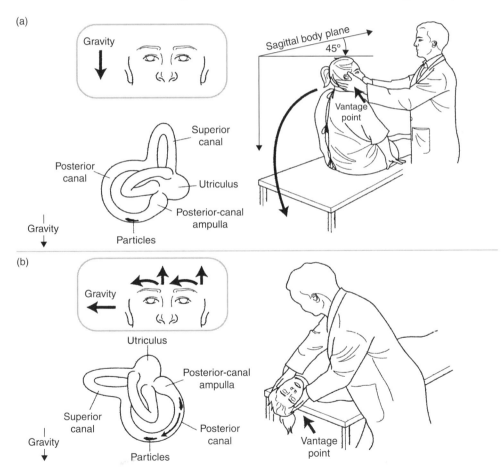

Figure 4.17 Dix-Hallpike manoeuvre to test for paroxysmal positional vertigo arising from the right posterior semicircular canal. (a) The patient's head is held in the examiner's hands and turned some 45 degrees to the right with the neck slightly extended. The patient is then lain supine with the instructions that they should fix their eyes on the eyes of the examiner. (b) If the test is positive, the patient will notice brief intense vertigo accompanied by nystagmus. The latency, direction and duration of that nystagmus should be noted. The arrows in the inset show the direction of that nystagmus in a fault arising from the right posterior semicircular canal. The presumed location of the free-floating debris in the canal is also shown. If the patient then sits up, there may be a further brief spell of vertigo and nystagmus, although to a lesser degree. (Redrawn, with permission, from J Furman, S Cass (1999) *New England Medical Journal* **341:** 1590–1596. Copyright © 2003 Massachusetts Medical Society.)

The rotatory nystagmus is directed to the undermost ear. The signs and symptoms settle only to reappear, but to a lesser degree, on sitting up again. If the test is then repeated it fatigues – that is, it is much less or has largely disappeared.

A similar complaint, but usually less severe, may occur in patients with brainstem lesions causing vertigo, **central positional vertigo**. This is accompanied by persistent positional nystagmus without any latent period and which does not show fatigue.

Many of the vestibular defects described here may be deduced from careful clinical examination at the bedside. However, full assessment of vestibular function requires specialized neuro-otological investigation. This would include caloric testing, in which air 7°C above and below body temperature is blown into the external auditory canal. With the patient lying supine and the head flexed to 30 degrees from the horizontal, this stimulates the horizontal semicircular canals to produce nystagmus, often with vertigo. Damage to the semicircular canals or to the vestibular nerve may abolish caloric-induced nystagmus, **canal paresis**. Damage to the vestibular apparatus in the brainstem often produces a lesser degree of abnormality on caloric testing, in which the response to one direction is reduced to produce a directional preponderance. Other more detailed tests of vestibular function are available, such as posturography.

Muscle weakness

Muscle weakness

Weakness of muscles may be from disease of the muscle itself (myopathy), defects in the transmission of the neuromuscular impulse at the muscle end-plate (myasthenia), damage to the motor nerve or anterior horn cell that gives rise to it [lower motor neurone (LMN) lesion], or damage to the corticomotor neurone pathway [upper motor neurone (UMN) lesion]. The characteristic findings that enable these different lesions to be distinguished are shown in Table 4.5. The critical differences are in the presence or absence of muscle wasting, changes in muscle tone and stretch reflexes, and in the distribution of weakness.

Table 4.5 Differences between upper and lower motor neurone lesions (UMN and LMN)

UMN	LMN
Weak	Weak
	Wasted
	Fasciculation
Hypertonic, spastic	Hypotonic, flaccid
Clonus	
Reflexes exaggerated	Reflexes depressed or absent
Plantar responses extensor	Plantar responses flexor

Muscle wasting

The integrity of muscle fibres depends not only on their own health, but also on an intact nerve supply. Muscles waste either because they themselves are damaged (myopathy), or because of lesions of the LMN. The more proximal the damage to the LMN, the greater is the opportunity for collateral re-innervation from adjacent nerve fibres, in an attempt to overcome the consequences of denervation. Such collateral re-innervation produces abnormally large motor units, which are responsible for the involuntary twitching **(fasciculation)** that occurs in denervated muscles.

Muscle tone and the stretch reflex

Our understanding of the functions of the nervous system were built upon Sherrington's discovery of the stretch reflex. Muscle tone and the tendon jerks are believed to represent operation of stretch reflex mechanisms, but still there is considerable ignorance about their exact relationship.

Delivery of a tendon tap produces a transient sudden stretch of muscle, which excites primary endings wrapped around the central portion of the muscle spindles. The resulting afferent volley is rapidly conducted to the spinal cord via large group IA fibres, which synapse with anterior horn cells of both the same muscle and of synergistic muscles. The number of anterior horn cells discharged by this synchronous afferent volley depends upon excitability of the anterior horn cell pool and the size of the afferent volley. The sensitivity of the muscle spindle endings is controlled by the pre-existing tension exerted on the central portion of the spindle muscle fibres by the contractile pull of the intrafusal fibres. Contraction of the intrafusal fibres increases the tension exerted on the central receptor and, hence, increases its sensitivity to stretch. The intrafusal fibres are innervated by fusimotor nerves originating in small anterior horn cells (gamma motor neurones). Alteration of fusimotor activity therefore will change the 'bias' of the muscle spindles. It follows that the amplitude of a response to a tendon tap depends on:

- The integrity of the spinal reflex
- The sensitivity of the muscle spindles as determined by pre-existing activity of fusimotor neurones
- The excitability of the appropriate alpha motor neurone pool.

> Peripheral nerve lesions decrease the size of the tendon jerk. This is much more evident with sensory lesions than with pure motor abnormalities.

Damage to sensory nerve fibres, which desynchronizes the afferent volley, soon abolishes tendon jerks. In contrast, quite extensive muscle wasting by itself may be insufficient to remove the response to a tendon tap. The tendon jerks are exaggerated (hyper-reflexia) in damage to the UMN pathway, as a result of enhanced anterior horn cell excitability. The latency of the tendon jerk is more difficult to judge at the bedside, but slow muscle relaxation may be evident in patients with myxoedema, and certain other metabolic disorders that delay muscle relaxation time.

Although Sherrington considered the tendon jerk to be a fractional manifestation of the stretch reflex, the basis of muscle tone as appreciated by the clinician at the bedside is unclear. Muscle tone is defined as the resistance to passive movement imposed by the examiner. Such resistance must comprise both passive elements of viscosity and elasticity arising in muscle, tendons and joints, as well as the active response of the muscle itself. Probably, muscle tone involves the combined effect of activation of both primary and secondary muscle spindle endings, both of which cause reflex muscle contraction.

Decreased muscle tone and depression of tendon jerks occur physiologically during sleep, including rapid eye movement sleep, and in anaesthesia or deep coma. In all these situations, fusimotor activity and anterior horn cell excitability are likely to be decreased. Muscle tone is also diminished in cerebellar disease, perhaps as a result of decreased fusimotor spindle drive.

> Increased muscle tone is characteristic of lesions of the descending motor pathways from the brain to the spinal cord.

Spasticity is a resistance to attempted stretch of the muscle that increases with the applied force, until there is a sudden give at a certain tension, the 'clasp knife' or 'lengthening' reaction. **Rigidity** is a resistance to passive movement that continues unaltered throughout the range of movement, and so has a plastic or 'lead-pipe' quality. Both types of hypertonia are the result of excessive alpha-motor neurone discharge in response to muscle stretch. In spasticity, the tendon jerks are also exaggerated (hyper-reflexia), but in rigidity the tendon jerks are usually of normal amplitude and threshold.

The distribution of spasticity and rigidity differs. The spastic posture of the patient after a stroke, with flexed arm and extended leg, indicates that tone is increased mainly in the adductors of the shoulder, the flexors of the elbow, the flexors of the wrist and fingers, the extensors of the hip and knee, and the plantar flexors and invertors of the foot. By contrast, the posture of generalized flexion in Parkinson's disease illustrates that rigidity is maximal in all flexor muscles in the body, although it is appreciated in extensors as well.

The complete picture of damage to UMN pathways includes not only spasticity and hyper-reflexia, but also absence of the abdominal reflexes and an extensor–plantar response. However, different corticoneurone pathways may be involved in the expression of these various manifestations of a UMN lesion. A lesion restricted to the 'pyramidal' pathway in the medulla, thereby sparing all other corticomotor neurone systems, only causes loss of abdominal reflexes and an extensor plantar response. Spasticity and hyper-reflexia appear when the alternative nonpyramidal corticomotor neurone pathways are interrupted. Such damage liberates overactive stretch reflex mechanisms to produce the increased muscle tone and exaggerated reflexes.

Distribution of muscle weakness

Careful analysis of the distribution of muscle weakness in a patient discovered to have motor signs may be invaluable. It is much easier to examine the motor than the sensory system, and deductions based upon motor deficit may dictate the pattern of subsequent sensory examination.

The distribution of UMN weakness

The distribution of weakness resulting from a UMN lesion can be recalled. The hemiplegic patient has the arm flexed across the chest and the leg extended with the toes scraping the ground. Accordingly, UMN weakness selectively involves shoulder abduction, elbow extension, wrist and finger extension, and the small muscles of the hand, and in the leg, hip flexion, knee flexion, dorsiflexion and eversion of the foot.

Damage to the **motor roots or anterior horn cells** also causes distinctive patterns of weakness, depending upon the level involved (see Figures 1.3 and 4.18). Likewise, lesions of a peripheral nerve containing motor fibres also produce a distinctive pattern of weakness. Careful attention to detail allows the

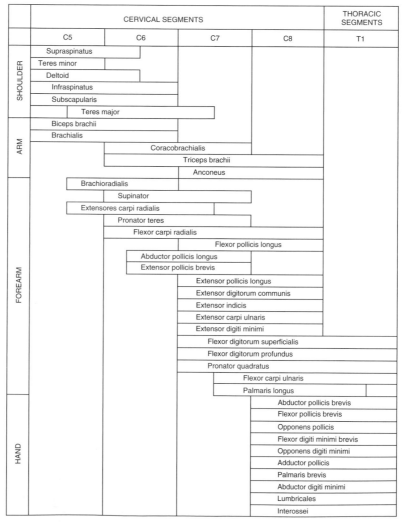

(a)

Figure 4.18 Segmental innervation of (a) arm muscles; (b) leg muscles. (Courtesy of Lord Walton of Detchant and Oxford University Press, *Brain's Diseases of the Nervous System*, 8th edn.)

examiner to distinguish weakness resulting from a UMN lesion from that caused by root or peripheral nerve damage. The following examples will illustrate the point.

Weakness of shoulder abduction may be the result of a UMN lesion, a C5 root lesion, or from damage to the circumflex nerve. In a UMN lesion, elbow extension and wrist and finger extension will also be weak; in a C5 root lesion, the biceps will be weak and the biceps jerk will be lost; in a circumflex nerve lesion, weakness will be restricted to shoulder abduction and the biceps jerk will be normal.

Region	Muscle	T12	L1	L2	L3	L4	L5	S1	S2
HIP	Iliopsoas		X	X	X				
	Tensor fasciae latae					X	X	X	
	Gluteus medius					X	X	X	
	Gluteus minimus					X	X	X	
	Quadratus femoris					X	X	X	
	Gemellus inferior					X	X	X	
	Gemellus superior						X	X	X
	Gluteus maximus						X	X	X
	Obturator internus						X	X	X
	Piriformis							X	X
THIGH	Sartorius			X	X				
	Pectineus			X	X				
	Adductor longus			X	X	X			
	Quadriceps femoris			X	X	X			
	Gracilis			X	X	X			
	Adductor brevis			X	X	X			
	Obturator externus				X	X			
	Adductor magnus			X	X	X			
	Adductor minimus			X	X	X			
	Articularis genus				X	X			
	Semitendinosus					X	X	S1	
	Semimembranosus					X	X	X	X
	Biceps femoris						X	X	X
LEG	Tibialis anterior					X	X		
	Extensor hallucis longus						X	X	
	Popliteus					X	X		
	Plantaris					X	X		
	Extensor digitorum longus					X	X	X	
	Soleus						X	X	X
	Gastrocnemius						X	X	X
	Peroneus longus						X	X	
	Peroneus brevis						X	X	
	Tibialis posterior						X	X	
FOOT	Flexor digitorum longus						X	X	X
	Flexor hallucis longus						X	X	X
	Extensor hallucis brevis						X	X	
	Extensor digitorum brevis						X	X	
	Flexor digitorum brevis						X	X	
	Abductor hallucis						X	X	
	Flexor hallucis brevis						X	X	X
	Lumbricales						X	X	X
	Adductor hallucis							X	X
	Abductor digiti minimi							X	X
	Flexor digiti minimi brevis							X	X
	Opponens digiti minimi							X	X
	Quadratus plantae							X	X
	Interossei							X	X

Column headers: THORACIC SEGMENT (T12); LUMBAR SEGMENTS (L1, L2, L3, L4, L5, S1, S2).

(b)

Figure 4.18 (*Continued*)

Elbow extension may be weak because of a UMN lesion or because of damage to the radial nerve. In a UMN lesion, shoulder abduction will also be weak.

Weakness of one hand may result from a UMN lesion, from damage to the T1 motor root or anterior horn cells, or to an ulnar nerve lesion. If a UMN lesion is responsible, there will also be weakness of wrist and finger extension, and elbow extension, and of shoulder abduction. If the ulnar nerve is involved, the thenar eminence is not wasted and the abductor pollicis brevis is strong because these are innervated by the median nerve. If the ulnar nerve is involved at the wrist, only the hand muscles will be weak. If the ulnar nerve is involved at the elbow, there will be weakness of the long finger flexors (flexor digitorum profundus) of the ulnar two digits, which flex the top joints of the fingers.

Weakness of hip flexion may be from a UMN lesion, damage to the L1/2 motor roots, or result from a femoral nerve lesion. If a UMN lesion is responsible, then knee flexion and dorsiflexion and eversion of the foot will be weak. If the L1/2 roots are involved, then hip adduction will also be weak, but knee flexion and dorsiflexion of the foot will be normal.

A **foot drop** may be caused by a lesion of the UMN, of the L4/5 root or the peroneal nerve. If a UMN lesion is responsible, hip flexion and knee flexion will also be weak. If the L4/5 roots are involved, then hip extension and knee flexion will be weak. If the peroneal nerve lesion is responsible, then hip movements and knee flexion will be normal.

In addition to the very distinctive patterns of weakness caused by UMN lesions, root lesions, and peripheral nerve lesions, diffuse generalized peripheral neuropathies and primary muscle disease (myopathy) also produce characteristic patterns of muscle weakness. A **generalized peripheral neuropathy** usually affects the longest nerve fibres first, so that the distal parts of the limbs are most affected, and the legs before the arms. Accordingly, weakness around the feet in dorsiflexion and plantar flexion with wasting of the lower limb are the commonest earliest signs of a peripheral neuropathy, to be followed by wasting and weakness of the small muscles of the hand.

In contrast, **primary muscle disease** selectively involves the more proximal muscles, to cause weakness and wasting around the hip and shoulder girdle.

In both peripheral neuropathy and primary muscle disease, flexors and extensors are involved more or less equally. UMN lesions, root lesions, and peripheral nerve lesions usually preferentially affect flexors or extensors, with relative sparing of antagonists.

Bulbar and pseudobulbar palsy

Bilateral LMN lesions affecting the nerves supplying the bulbar muscles of the jaw, face, palate, pharynx and larynx cause **a bulbar palsy**. Speech and swallowing will be impaired. In particular, speech develops a nasal quality caused by escape of air through the nose. The paralysed soft palate no longer can occlude the nasopharynx. Swallowing of liquids is badly impaired, with a tendency to regurgitate fluids back through the nose and to cough because fluids spill over into the trachea. Paralysis of affected muscles will be evident, and the tongue appears wasted.

A **pseudobulbar palsy** results from bilateral damage to corticomotorneurone pathways innervating the bulbar musculature. In other words, a pseudobulbar palsy is the result of a UMN lesion affecting corticobulbar systems. A unilateral UMN lesion produces only transient weakness of many of the muscles supplied by the cranial nerves. Thus after a stroke, there is no loss of power in the upper part of the face, and weakness of the muscles of the jaw, palate, neck and tongue is transient.

Bilateral damage to the corticobulbar tracts causes persistent weakness and spasticity of the muscles supplied by the bulbar nuclei. As a result, there is slurring of speech, known as a spastic dysarthria, and difficulty in swallowing (dysphagia). The jaw jerk is abnormally brisk, and movements of the tongue are reduced in velocity and amplitude as a result of spasticity. In addition, patients with a pseudobulbar palsy exhibit emotional incontinence. This describes a loss of voluntary control of emotional expression such that the patient may laugh or cry without apparent provocation.

The differential diagnosis of bulbar and pseudobulbar palsies is shown in Table 4.6.

Sensory defects

The assessment of sensory function starts with the history, because symptoms may precede any

Table 4.6 Differentiation between bulbar and pseudobulbar palsies

Bulbar	Pseudobulbar
Weakness of muscles (LMN) from motor brainstem nuclei V–XII	Bilateral corticobulbar (UMN) lesions
Tongue: atrophic, fasciculating	Tongue, small, spastic, difficulty with rapid movements, protrusion
Speech: monotonous, hoarse, nasal	Speech: spastic slurring dysarthria
	Exaggerated reflexes: jaw jerk, snout, pout
Gag may be depressed	Brisk gag reflex
Lips, facial muscles may be weak	Stiff, spastic facial muscles
Saliva may pool and dribble out	Trouble chewing, food may stay in mouth or spill
Spill-over of fluids, occasional nasal regurgitation	May choke
Weak cough	Emotional incontinence
	Often bilateral corticospinal tract signs in limbs

LMN, lower motor neurone; UMN, upper motor neurone.
Motor neurone disease, which is the commonest cause of a bilateral wasted tongue, may also show UMN signs.

demonstrable abnormality of simple sensation as tested by standard bedside techniques.

> The patient's symptoms will suggest which area of the body, or which type of sensory function, needs the most detailed attention. The examination of the motor system will also direct attention to the appropriate sensory testing.

Sensory symptoms are of two types.

Defects of sensation

If there is impairment of all forms of cutaneous sensation, the patient may complain of numbness or freezing feelings. Many liken it to the sensation that follows dental treatment under local anaesthesia. If there is more specific sensory loss, it may only come to attention indirectly. Thus, inability to perceive pain usually is detected because unexpected painless injuries occur, such as burns of the fingers on cooking utensils or by cigarettes. Loss of temperature appreciation may be recognized by inability to perceive the heat of bath water.

Abnormal sensations

Abnormal sensations may be qualitative changes in an existing sensation (dysaesthesiae), or spontaneous sensations (paraesthesiae). Paraesthesiae may take the form of burning, coldness, wetness or itching (all of which suggest a lesion of pain pathways), or they may consist of feelings of pins and needles, vibration, electric shock, or tightness as if wrapped in bandages (all of which suggest a lesion of the posterior column sensory pathways). Two other types of distorted sensation may occur: hyperpathia refers to exaggeration of pain to a painful stimulus; allodynia refers to pain evoked by a non-painful stimulus.

The anatomical arrangements of sensory pathways are such that the signs on physical examination usually make it possible to distinguish between lesions at the following sites; a peripheral nerve or trunk of a nerve plexus, a spinal root, the spinal cord, the brainstem, the thalamus, and the cerebral cortex (see Figure 1.5). The distribution of the resulting sensory signs is illustrated in Figures 4.19–4.22.

A lesion of the peripheral nerve or of one trunk of a plexus usually causes both sensory and motor loss in its area of distribution, although one may strikingly precede the other. The sensory loss involves all sensory functions, and its site roughly corresponds with the anatomical distribution of the nerve (Figure 4.19).

and to make judgements based upon crude sensory appreciation from the opposite half of the body. Cortical damage does not impair the ability to be able to appreciate simple touch, pain, temperature, or vibration. However, the patient cannot utilize such information to make sensory judgements. Thus, appreciation of joint position and two-point discrimination is impaired. The ability to identify familiar objects placed in the hand (stereognosis), and the ability to judge the comparative size and weight of different objects placed in the hand, are compromised by cortical lesions. Another useful test of cortical sensory function is the ability to perceive two simultaneous sensory stimuli applied with equal intensity to corresponding sites on opposite sides of the body. A unilateral cortical lesion may lead to failure to perceive the contralateral stimulus, even though it is easily detected when administered by itself. Such sensory inattention or neglect, when severe, may extend to an apparent unawareness of the contralateral limb or even one whole half of the body, a form of agnosia.

Coma

Impairment of cerebral function may cause depression or clouding of consciousness leading to coma. Consciousness or the maintenance of the alert state relies on an intact ascending reticular activating system. This starts in the brainstem in the pons, ascending through the midbrain to end in the hypothalamus and thalamic reticular formation (Figure 4.23). Any structural damage in this pathway will cause a depressed conscious level so that infarcts, haematomas or mass lesions at this site may be responsible. These may be relatively small in size. In the supratentorial compartments, bihemisphere lesions, bilateral thalamic infarcts or a massive unilateral lesion causing significant shifts or distortion (see p. 111) may also cause a depressed conscious level. Other important causes include:

- Metabolic upsets – such as, uraemia, hepatic failure, hypoglycaemia or hyperglycaemia
- Infective processes – meningitis, encephalitis
- Hypoxic/ischaemic disturbances – cardiac/respiratory arrests
- Poisoning – from drugs or alcohol overdosage.

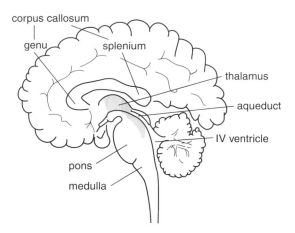

Figure 4.23 Sagittal section to show ascending reticular activating system in the brainstem and diencephalon (shaded).

Many terms are used to describe various levels of depression of consciousness. **Comatose** patients are unconscious and unable to respond to verbal command, although they may show motor responses to painful stimuli. **Stuporose** patients are unconscious but can be roused by verbal command or painful stimuli for short periods to produce a verbal response. When stimulation ceases, they lapse back into coma. **Confused patients** are alert, but disorientated for time, place, and even person. Delirious patients are confused, but also restless and overactive. Another way to describe delirium is a **toxic confusional state**.

Such grades of depression of consciousness are difficult to define and a valuable method of recording data is the international Glasgow Coma Scale (Table 4.7), which has proved easy to administer by doctors and nurses. The scale describes the best verbal, motor and eye responses to stimulation, either by verbal command or pain. Each of the three categories of response is graded on a scale ranging from normal (the patient is orientated, obeys command, and shows spontaneous eye opening – a score of 15) to deep coma (the patient exhibits no verbal response to stimulation, no motor response to pain, and never spontaneously opens the eyes – a score of 3). In addition it is essential to record the pupillary responses to light, the reflex eye movements in both vertical and horizontal plane to oculocephalic (doll's head manoeuvre) and/or caloric stimulation, the blood pressure, respiration, pulse and temperature in every unconscious patient.

Table 4.7 Glasgow coma scale (adults and children)

Assessment of conscious level	Adults	Children	Score
Eye opening	Spontaneous	Spontaneous	4
	To speech	To sound	3
	To pain	To pain	2
	None	None	1
Best motor response	Obeys command	Appropriate for age	6
	Localizes to pain	Localizes to pain	5
	Flexion to pain	Flexion to pain	4
	Spastic flexion	Spastic flexion	3
	Abnormal extension	Abnormal extension	2
	None	None	1
Best verbal response	Orientated	Appropriate for age	5
	Confused	Cries	4
	Monosyllabic	Irritable	3
	Incomprehensible sounds	Lethargic	2
	None	None	1

After Teasdale and Jennett (1974).

Other terms are used to describe the level of consciousness and physical state of patients surviving coma. A **vegetative state (VS)** is defined as a 'clinical condition of unawareness of self and environment in which the patient breathes spontaneously, has a stable circulation and shows cycles of eye closure and eye opening, which may simulate sleep and waking'. Such patients survive coma, but do not speak or exhibit any purposeful response to the outside world. They may show periods of wakefulness, groan and grunt, and exhibit stereotyped primitive movements in response to external stimuli, but they have no intelligent communication. This state has also been called the apallic syndrome. The term continuing vegetative state is applied when the state continues for more than 4 weeks and the term **persistent (permanent) vegetative state** is best used when the diagnosis of an irreversible state can be made with a high degree of clinical certainty. No absolute timescale has been established, although the term persistent VS may reasonably be made in patients stable some 12 months after a head injury or 6 months after other causes of brain damage. Akinetic mutism may also refer to a patient with a continuing vegetative state, although not all such patients are akinetic.

The **'locked–in' syndrome** refers to patients who have sustained extensive damage to the pons, causing complete loss of speech and a quadriplegia. However, because the midbrain is intact such patients are alert and give normal results on electroencephalography (EEG). Their only means of communication is by eye movements. The pontine damage paralyses horizontal gaze, but eyelid movements and vertical gaze are preserved. These patients can see, hear and think normally.

Causes of coma

The causes of coma are shown in Tables 4.8 and 4.9. Loss of consciousness is caused by diffuse brain disease affecting both cerebral hemispheres, large supratentorial lesions causing considerable shifts or distortions, or by relatively focal upper brainstem lesions. Diffuse brain disease may be the result of some generalized extrinsic condition, whose primary cause lies outside the brain, or of diffuse intrinsic disease of the brain itself. Extrinsic conditions include metabolic disturbances and poisoning with drugs or alcohol; intrinsic causes include meningitis and encephalitis. Focal lesions causing coma are most

Acute medical treatment of raised intracranial pressure

Assisted ventilation will reduce cerebral blood volume to give more space, and cerebral oedema around infarcts, haemorrhages or tumours may be reduced by the use of intravenous mannitol. Critically ill patients may be intubated and hyperventilated. The head of the bed should be elevated to 30–45 degrees. Mannitol, a hyperosmolar agent, withdraws oedema fluid out of the brain and causes a brisk diuresis. Intravenous infusion of 100–200 ml of 20% mannitol will rapidly reduce intracranial pressure and may stop or reverse the process of coning long enough to allow further investigation and definitive treatment to be undertaken. Patients with a depressed conscious level should have a urinary catheter inserted. Steroids also reduce cerebral oedema, but their effect is slower in onset. Dexamethasone 5–10 mg intravenously followed by 4 mg 6-hourly may help to control cerebral oedema around tumours. If a mass lesion is present, a neurosurgical consultation should be made.

Examination of the unconscious patient

Because the unconscious patient cannot cooperate, a different system of examination must be employed to assess coma. A suitable sequence (Table 4.10) should include the investigations detailed in the following paragraphs.

Respiration and circulation: the first and most urgent need is to make sure that the **airway, breathing and circulation (ABC)** are adequate to sustain life. If these are compromised, emergency action should be taken to ensure an airway with assisted ventilation, and an adequate cardiac output. Once emergency resuscitation has been completed, further examination can continue.

Blood pressure, the pulse rate and rhythm, and temperature are recorded. The character of respiration is noted.

Damage to the respiratory neurones produces a variety of abnormalities of breathing. **Cheyne–Stokes breathing** refers to periodic cycles of hyperventilation

Table 4.10 Examination of the unconscious patient

A	**A**irway
B	**B**reathing – respiratory rate, rhythm
C	**C**irculation – pulse rate, rhythm, blood pressure, cardiac output

Temperature
Meningism
Conscious level – Glasgow Coma Scale
    Best verbal response
    Best motor response
    Eye opening
Appearance – jaundice, rashes, fetor (ketotic, ethanol), bruising, needle marks (addicts), blood from nose, ears, bitten tongue
Pupils – size, symmetry, reactions
Fundi
Eye movements
    Spontaneous, conjugate, dysconjugate, abnormal
    Doll's head
    Cold calorics
Corneal, lash reflexes
Facial movements – grimaces
'Gag', cough reflexes
Spontaneous limb movements
Abnormal movements – myoclonus
Response to pain
    Decorticate rigidity
    Decerebrate rigidity
Reflexes, plantar responses
General examination

alternating with apnoea in a waxing and waning pattern. Each cycle lasts about a minute. The patient ceases respiration, then begins to breathe again, the rate and depth increasing to a peak, and then dying away again. This respiratory drive is linked to the carbon dioxide level: when this is high it stimulates the medullary respiratory centre and a number of deep breaths follow, the level then falls and the drive is lowered and the breaths diminish. The commonest cause is circulatory failure but it may also arise with metabolic disturbances, such as with uraemia, and with bihemisphere cortical lesions and supratentorial herniation. A similar pattern with a shorter cycle length of about half a minute, occurs in some patients with midbrain and internal capsule lesions. **Central neurogenic hyperventilation** is associated with destruction of the reticular formation in the pons and midbrain. It causes respiratory alkalosis. **Apneustic breathing** describes a prolonged pause after each inspiration and before the next expiration occurs. It results from damage to the lower half of the pons. **Ataxic breathing** is completely irregular in amplitude and frequency. It indicates damage to the medullary respiratory neurones. **Gasping respiration** is characterized by an abrupt inspiration followed by expiration, then a long pause before the next breath. It occurs shortly before death.

Progressive transtentorial herniation of the brainstem thus may produce an orderly sequence of changes in respiration. As coning occurs, central neurogenic hyperventilation may give way to apneustic breathing, followed by ataxic breathing, gasping respiration and then death.

Assess the level of consciousness: take note of the patient's spontaneous verbal, motor and ocular responses, and observe how they react to external circumstances and your commands.

The aim will be to place the patient in the appropriate category on the Glasgow Coma Scale in due course.

Suitable graded stimuli are spoken commands, shouted commands, pinprick, pressing on the sternum or supraorbital notch, which causes pain. While watching the response of the patient to stimuli, always look for asymmetric motor reactions, or apparent neglect of such stimuli on one half of the body.

Examine the head and skull: palpate the skull for signs of fracture and for bruising. Note any bruising or discharge of blood or CSF from the ears, nose or mouth. This might suggest a basal skull fracture. Check the skin for any rash, such as the purpuric changes of a meningococcal septicaemia, or for jaundice or extensive bruising, the last suggesting a haemorrhagic state.

The neck: flex the neck on the head and note any resistance to movement suggesting meningeal irritation from either blood or infection. Obviously this test should not be carried out if there is a suspicion that cervical vertebrae may have been fractured.

The eyes: the visual fields may be examined in such patients either by advancing a bright light in each quadrant, or by making threatening movements of the hand towards the eye. Patients whose level of consciousness allows reaction to such stimuli, will turn the head and eyes away, or blink.

Examine the optic fundi to check for disc swelling, retinal haemorrhages or other retinal changes.

Note the size of **the pupils and their response to light**. The midbrain contains the IIIrd nerve, parasympathetic and pretectal nuclei, so that midbrain lesions produce obvious pupillary abnormalities.

The pupils, therefore, are invaluable in indicating the presence of a focal brain lesion responsible for coma.

Pupillary changes in coning

A unilateral supratentorial mass lesion causing transtentorial coning, leads to a IIIrd nerve palsy as the process evolves. The pupil on the side of the lesion dilates, becomes unreactive to light and accommodation, ptosis develops and the eye turns down and out. Bilateral supratentorial mass lesions, or diffuse brain swelling, which produces a central transtentorial herniation, tend to affect pupillary pathways in the diencephalon and brainstem in an orderly sequence. At first, damage to the sympathetic fibres causes the pupils to become small but reactive. Then, as the process evolves, the pupils begin to dilate and eventually become dilated and unreactive to light. Primary pontine lesions spare the parasympathetic pupillary systems causing disruption only of the sympathetic mechanisms. As a result, the pupils are constricted and may become very small ('pinpoint pupils'). Lesions of the lateral part of the medulla affect the descending sympathetic fibres to produce a unilateral Horner's syndrome.

Some specific poisons also affect the pupillary responses, e.g. atropine and gluthemide cause dilatation, opiates cause constriction.

The pupillary responses are, perhaps, the single most important guide to the cause of coma.

'Metabolic coma'

It can be stated that an unconscious patient showing no focal motor deficit, who has equal, normal-sized and reactive pupils is in coma because of diffuse brain disease. The absence of a history or signs of cerebral trauma, and a normal computerized tomography (CT) brain scan and CSF examination in such patients will exclude intrinsic causes of diffuse brain disease. In such circumstances a confident diagnosis of extrinsic diffuse brain disease or 'metabolic' coma can be made.

Examine the eye movements: provided the patient is capable of some response to command, the range of eye movements can be assessed simply. However, many stuporose and/or comatose patients will not obey verbal commands, so eye movements must be tested in other ways. Two techniques can be used. Eye movement may be provoked by the **oculo-cephalic reflexes** elicited by the **doll's head manoeuvre**. Brisk rotation of the head from side to side, or flexion and extension of the neck, will produce conjugate eye movements in the opposite direction to the head movement. This gives the impression that the patient's gaze is focused on an object straight in front. Such oculocephalic responses are attributed to the effect of vestibular input combined with proprioceptive impulses from the neck. This information eventually ascends via the medial longitudinal bundle in the brainstem to the ocular motor nuclei.

Preservation of horizontal and vertical eye movement in response to the doll's head manoeuvre implies that the brainstem is intact.

Loss of reflex conjugate upgaze indicates damage to the midbrain. Loss of reflex conjugate horizontal gaze indicates damage to the pons. Dysconjugate eye movements may be provoked by the doll's head manoeuvre, or may occur spontaneously in the comatose patient. Failure of lateral deviation of one eye when gaze is reflexively provoked in that direction indicates a VIth nerve palsy. Failure of adduction of the eye with normal abduction suggests an internuclear ophthalmoplegia. If the doll's head manoeuvre is insufficient to provoke eye movement, then caloric responses may be employed to elicit **VOR**

(vestibulo–ocular reflex), which again depend upon an intact brainstem. Ice-cold water is syringed into each ear in turn, making sure that the ear drum is normal before doing so. If brainstem function is intact, there will either be nystagmus in the direction away from the irrigated ear, or conjugate deviation of the eyes to the irrigated side. Again, patients with specific ocular motor palsies may show a dysconjugate response to caloric stimulation. In addition to examination of voluntary or reflex eye movements, spontaneous eye movements should be carefully recorded in the unconscious patient.

Tonic ocular deviation

Tonic deviation of the eyes conjugately to one side suggests a focal lesion, either of the cerebral hemisphere or of the brainstem. With a hemisphere lesion, the opposite limbs will be paralysed and the eyes look away from them towards the side of the lesion. In a brainstem pontine lesion, the opposite limbs will be paralysed, but the eyes will look towards them, that is, away from the side of the lesion.

Other abnormalities of spontaneous eye movements are described in coma; these include ocular bobbing, repetitive divergence and nystagmoid jerking of one eye.

The face: look for signs of a unilateral facial paralysis (drooping of one side of the mouth which is puffed out with each breath). Test the corneal and lash reflexes with a wisp of cotton wool, and the facial response to pinprick or supraorbital pressure. Both of these stimuli should cause screwing up of the same side of the face.

The ears: examine the ear drums with an auroscope, looking for evidence of middle ear infection, such as an opaque, bulging drum, or a ruptured drum with purulent discharge. With trauma, there may be blood behind the drum or in the external canal.

The mouth: smell the breath for alcohol, ketones, or other distinctive odours. Look for lacerations of the tongue, which suggest a recent epileptic fit. Check for the presence of a 'gag' reflex.

Examine the limbs: establish whether all four limbs move, either spontaneously or in response to painful stimuli. Squeezing the Achilles tendon or a finger nail, or rubbing the sternum are useful means of provoking reflex movement. Such stimuli should always be applied at various sites to allow for local anaesthesia. Failure to move an arm or leg on one side in response to stimuli to each side, indicates a hemiplegia. Absence of any limb movement in response to strong stimuli occurs with bilateral severe damage to the brainstem, as in the 'locked-in' syndrome, but also occurs in very deep coma without any focal brain damage.

Provided the limbs are not paralysed, stimuli may provoke appropriate or inappropriate reflex responses. When there is no motor deficit, painful stimuli will cause withdrawal of the limb, attempts to remove the source of pain with the opposite limb, screwing up of the face, and even verbal responses. An early motor sign of severe focal cerebral damage is the appearance of stereotyped limb movements in response to painful stimuli. Destructive lesions involving the internal capsule cause **decorticate rigidity**. A painful stimulus provokes flexion and adduction of the arm with extension of the leg on the affected side. Damage to the upper brainstem causes **decerebrate rigidity** in response to a painful stimulus. The neck retracts, and the teeth clench. The affected arm extends, adducts and the forearm pronates. The affected leg extends and the foot plantar flexes. Spontaneous spasms of decerebrate rigidity may occur with severe brainstem lesions, often accompanied by shivering, hypertension and hyperpyrexia.

Muscle tone can be assessed in the unconscious patient by passive manipulation of the limbs, or by noting the response to dropping the limb to the bed. Lift the arms and legs, individually or together, and note the speed with which they fall to the bed when dropped. Hemiplegic limbs, which are flaccid in the acute stage, fall harder and faster than normal limbs.

Examine the tendon jerks and plantar responses. However, remember that it may take some days for hyper-reflexia and Babinski's sign to appear after an acute lesion of corticomotorneurone pathways. In the stage of shock following an acute hemiplegia, the limbs are flaccid, the tendon jerks are normal or absent, and the plantar response may be unresponsive.

General examination: examine the heart, lungs and abdomen.

Always test the urine for protein, glucose and ketones, and examine it with a microscope for pus cells and casts.

Measure the glucose in all unconscious patients

If the cause of coma is not apparent at this stage, *always measure the blood glucose* concentration and administer glucose intravenously. Most casualty departments have an absolute rule that blood glucose must be measured in all unconscious patients. In addition, give thiamine by injection. Many unconscious patients admitted to casualty departments are victims of chronic alcoholic abuse, and may have Wernicke's encephalopathy.

The differential diagnosis of coma

The important features distinguishing diffuse brain disease and focal brain lesions causing coma are shown in Table 4.11. The important features distinguishing a supratentorial focal brain lesion from an

Table 4.11 Differentiation of diffuse and focal brain lesions leading to coma

Diffuse
Absence of focal or lateralizing signs: motor or sensory
May be bilateral changes in tone, reflexes and extensor plantar responses
Brainstem functions often preserved initially, especially ocular movements and pupillary responses
Often self-poisoning, metabolic causes, infection, bleeding or epilepsy, so CT brain scan often negative
Focal
Focal or lateralizing signs usually present to suggest hemisphere or brainstem damage
Include flaccid weakness and loss of response to pain on one side
Reflex asymmetry, including plantar response
Tonic deviation of eyes to one side
Derangements in ocular motility and pupillary responses
Often supratentorial mass (abscess, tumour, haematoma) or infratentorial mass (haematoma, infarct, tumour), so CT brain scan positive.

4 There is an absent 'gag' reflex or no response to a suction catheter in the trachea.

5 No purposeful movements should be elicited, nor facial grimaces to painful stimuli applied to the limbs, trunk or face.

6 The patient's medullary respiratory centre will not respond to a rise in arterial carbon dioxide ($PaCO_2$) of greater than 6.65 kPa (50 mmHg) if the patient is disconnected from the ventilator, that is, to an adequate chemical stimulus for that centre.

Such tests should be repeated after an interval to ensure that the signs remain absent.

REFERENCES AND FURTHER READING

Acheson JF, Sanders MD (1997) Common Problems in Neuro-ophthalmology. In: *Major Problems in Neurology*. Philadelphia: WB Saunders.

Brandt T (1999) *Vertigo, its multisensory syndromes*, 2nd edn. Berlin: Springer Verlag.

Devinsky O (1992) *Behavioural Neurology: 100 Maxims*. (100 Maxims in Neurology Series). London: Arnold.

Duus P (1998) *Topical Diagnosis in Neurology*, 3rd revised edn. Stuttgart: Georg Thieme.

Folstein MF, Folstein SE, McHugh PR (1975) Mini-mental state – a practical method for grading the cognitive state of patients for the clinician. *Journal of Psychiatric Research*, 12:189–198.

Gilman S (2000) *Clinical Examination of the Nervous System*. New York: McGraw-Hill.

Goebel JA (2001) *Practical Management of the Dizzy Patient*. Philadelphia: Lippincott, Williams & Wilkins.

Haerer AF (1992) *De Jong's the Neurological Examination*, 5th edn. Philadelphia: JP Lippincott.

Hodges JR (1994) *Cognitive Assessment for Clinicians*. Oxford: Oxford University Press.

McCarthy RA, Warrington EK (1990) *Cognitive Neuropsychology – a Clinical Introduction*. San Diego: Academic Press.

Plum F, Posner JB (1980) *Diagnosis of Stupor and Coma*. 3rd edn. Philadelphia: FA Davis Coy.

Teasdale G, Jennett B (1974) Assessment of coma and impaired consciousness: a practical scale. *Lancet*, ii:81–84.

Working Party of the Royal College of Physicians (2003) The Vegetative State: guidance on diagnosis and management. *Clinical Medicine*, 3: 249–254.

CHAPTER 5

NEUROGENETICS

N.W. Wood

INTRODUCTION

Over the past decade there has been dramatic progress in our understanding of the genetic basis of disease. Unsurprisingly as the majority of genes are expressed in the nervous system, neurology has seen the greatest developments. A decade ago only a handful of disease-causing nervous system genes were known. Now it would be the work of a large textbook to do justice to the developments and implications of this new knowledge. As we near the completion of the full human genome sequence the possibilities for exploiting this landmark achievement are huge. Initially the benefits are being seen in the rapidity and number of 'simple' Mendelian genes and mutations being found and described. As the basic structure of the genome and how it is transmitted is understood in finer detail the major impetus will be to use these technologies to find 'susceptibility' genes for common disorders. However, the techniques used to find such genes can also be used to find any genetic factor that has a biological effect; for example, the new field of pharmacogenomics is based on this approach. It is very likely that over the coming years we will understand much more about variable drug response and idiosyncratic side-effects. This approach holds great promise for the future, as no longer will we as clinicians just have to use a trial and error approach to selection of the right drug but rather we will, using genetic testing, be able to select a drug that a patient is likely to respond to but also is unlikely to provoke serious side-effects. In addition to this 'personalized medicine' it can also be predicted that if an investigator knew beforehand something about the metabolic profile of the patients in a study, the design of drug trial could be greatly facilitated. This could lead to huge economies: decreasing the size of the treated groups; decreasing the risk of adverse reactions; and shortening the time of drug development. This, in turn, should decrease the cost of drug development.

GENETICS FOR THE NEUROLOGIST

Fortunately, despite the jargon, the genetic principles (Mendel, etc.) that were learnt at medical school still apply, only the technology and our capability to investigate genetic factors have changed.

In brief, deoxyribonucleic acid (DNA) is a double-stranded helical molecule, which provides the molecular basis for the genes that encode the proteins made by the cell. There are two genomes: the large nuclear genome encompassing 3 billion basepairs and encoding approximately 30 000 genes; and the much smaller and compact mitochondrial genome, which is only 16 500 basepairs and encodes a minority of the subunits of the respiratory chain complex. The nervous system demands a large amount of energy production. It therefore bears the brunt from disease resulting from mutations in mitochondrial DNA. This is discussed at the end of the chapter.

Much of the nuclear genome does not yet appear to have a discernable role and only a fraction of it appears to be involved in the production of functional protein. The human genome project produced many surprises, one of the biggest being the fact that humans only have approximately 30 000 genes – far less than predicted. However, we produce many more proteins than this and this is achieved in part by alternative splicing. **Most genes are encoded in blocks (exons); the intervening blocks of basepairs are called introns.** Therefore, for example, one can see that for a simple gene made up of three exons there are a number of possibilities: A-B-C; A-B; A-C; and so on. Many genes have much greater numbers of exons than this. After proteins are produced, most undergo some form of modification (so-called post-translational modification) whereby they are phosphorylated, glycosylated or some other change is made. The factors controlling these latter steps are only poorly understood. In fact the new fields of genomics and proteomics are based on furthering our understanding of basic gene/protein structure, function and regulation.

The DNA strands are packaged into chromosomes, 22 autosomes and two sex chromosomes. Therefore for autosomal genes we have two copies, one paternal the other maternal. If a mutation on one copy is sufficient to cause a disease, this is known as **autosomal dominant**; if both copies of the genes (also called alleles) need to be mutated to give rise to disease, then this is called **autosomal recessive**. It takes only the simplest of mathematics to work out that

the recurrence risk is simply a function of this, namely 50% for other siblings if autosomal dominant and 25% if autosomal recessive. Moreover, the offspring of the patient with autosomal dominant disease will still be at 50% risk, whereas the offspring in the autosomal recessive case will be related to the carrier frequency in the population. Thus the offspring must be a carrier of one copy of the mutation as that is the only form of gene the patient can transmit, and the risk to the offspring is determined by the chance that the other parent also carriers a mutation in the same gene. This is usually very unlikely, so a low recurrence risk estimate can be given. Exceptions to this rule include consanguineous marriages and diseases with a high carrier frequency (e.g. cystic fibrosis).

A similar situation exists for **mutations** in genes on the X chromosome, excepting that women have two copies and thereby are somewhat protected from a single mutation, whereas for men the Y chromosome cannot 'rescue' a single mutant on the single X chromosome. **Therefore for X-linked recessive conditions, women carry and men express.** Men must transmit the mutation to their daughters and cannot transmit it to their sons (to be male they must have received the Y chromosome). If one sees male–male transmission, this excludes X-linked inheritance. Some conditions, such as Charcot–Marie–Tooth disease (CMT-X) resulting from mutations in connexin-32 are dominant and therefore manifest in females as well as males, although the phenotype may be slightly different.

Mitochondrial DNA (mtDNA) is entirely maternally derived but can affect males and females. Therefore consistent evidence of only maternal transmission could point towards a mtDNA abnormality.

In addition to these basic recurrence risk estimates, there are a number of other factors one needs to take into account. The presence of a disease-causing mutation is not always the only determinant of disease. In some cases, such as dystonias caused by mutations in the *DYT1* gene, there is reduced penetrance, thus in this situation only ~40% of gene carriers manifest the disease. The cause of **reduced penetrance** is not known. It is also worth the clinician being aware of the **variable expression** of a given mutation; for example, CMT type 1a resulting from a duplication on chromosome 17 can vary from a severe childhood neuropathy to presentation in late life with pes cavus. Both of these factors need to be taken into account when counselling patients.

It is not possible to cover all the areas in any detail in this chapter so only the major developments and their place in a clinical context will be given and, where appropriate, details of recent review articles and chapters. As this is the most rapidly changing field in neurology a list of useful websites is given at the end. Included in this list are databases that give clinical summaries, available gene tests and so forth.

This chapter provides a brief outline of the simple Mendelian disorders, a list of suggested further reading is provided at the end. The approach here follows an anatomical path starting at the cortex and moving 'down' the nervous system ending with muscle diseases. Clearly some disorders cannot be approached in such a simplistic way. In these cases discussion takes into account the predominant feature. This seems a more clinically rational approach than choosing mode of inheritance or any other equally arbitrary system.

THE DEMENTIAS

The overwhelming factor emerging from genetic studies of the dementias and other central nervous system neurodegenerative conditions is abnormalities of protein handling.

The first gene to be isolated for familial dementia was the amyloid precursor protein (APP) on chromosome 21. The amyloid cascade hypothesis has gained ground with the numerically much more important finding of mutations in *presenilin 1*, which is intimately involved with APP processing, in a number of early onset familial dementia families and is certainly common enough to consider testing in the cases with possible autosomal dominant inheritance. *Presenilin 2*, a closely related molecule, is also implicated in a very rare form of familial dementia: this is so rare it is not usually included in a genetic screen. There are still other genes to be found for familial dementia. *Apoe-4* has also been shown to be important in sporadic, late onset Alzheimer's disease (see p. 281). It appears to be most important as a factor determining age of onset.

Much as the finding of APP mutations and subsequent work brought attention to the amyloid pathway, scientists working on the other major protein deposition found in Alzheimer's disease, tau filaments, have been rewarded with the demonstration that mutations in the *tau* gene (sometimes involving splice variants and thereby influencing which exons are spliced in or out) have been found in a variety of complicated dementia–parkinsonian overlap syndromes. Not only are primary pathogenic mutations in *tau* responsible for autosomal dominant **frontotemporal dementias** but also there is an established association with **progressive supranuclear palsy**. The causal variant within the *tau* gene region is not known.

A rarer but important dementing process to consider is **familial prion disease**. In the UK, there is a national laboratory for screening this gene. This diagnosis should be considered even in the absence of a clear family history in any 'unusual' dementia, especially if rapidly progressive and/or associated with the presence of a movement disorder.

THE EPILEPSIES

Although amongst the most common disorders seen by a neurologist and certainly known to have a relatively high heritability, no gene tests for the primary epilepsies are currently available. This is not because of a lack of genetic data but rather is because of the complexity and, in part, quantity of data that has emerged in the past 5 years. There are now over 30 loci identified for the primary epilepsies (if all the syndromes of which epilepsy were a part were included this list would exceed 250). Of these loci, over 10 genes are known. However, in all cases to date they are either single families or exceedingly rare. Nevertheless they are clearly pointing the way forward, as virtually all are **ion channel mutations**. This is hardly surprising and does allow molecular, cellular and animal models for all forms of epilepsy to be developed and investigated. In terms of gene testing some of the rare forms of 'complicated' epilepsy such as Unverricht-Lundborg are available but at present no gene test is available for the commoner primary epilepsies.

MOVEMENT DISORDERS

Such has been the pace of progress in the area of movement disorders that it is only possible to detail some of the major developments.

The following is an overview and new discoveries are frequently being made. It is now inconceivable to think of movement disorders and genetics as completely unrelated disciplines.

The dystonias

The dystonias are a genetically very heterogeneous group of disorders. The commonest **generalized dystonia** (see p. 241), with onset in childhood, is caused by a mutation in the *torsin A* gene (also called *DYT1*). It appears that over 99% of patients with abnormalities caused by this gene carry the same mutation, a GAG deletion. It is therefore a relatively simple analysis. This test should be considered in all dystonias if onset occurs before the age of 26 years, and in others if the phenotype is compatible or if there is a significant family history. The typical appearance is of childhood onset in the foot spreading up the body and most typically sparing the head and neck. There are exceptions.

It is always worth considering whether a **dystonia could be dopa-responsive** (see p. 243). If there is a dramatic improvement on dopa, then abnormalities in the biosynthetic pathway for dopamine should be considered. Most commonly this is a result of mutations in GTP-cyclohydrolase 1, the rate-limiting enzyme in the biopterin pathways. Tetrahydrobiopterin is required for the functioning of a number of monoamine hydroxylases, including tyrosine hydroxylase. Mutations in the gene have been reported in a small number of families.

There are a large number of *DYT* (dystonia) genes appearing in the databases and there are still many genes to be found. Moreover the nomenclature is complicated by the use of *DYT* loci for paroxysmal dystonic and choreic movement disorders, and in some cases for which the loci are yet to be identified.

Although the gene for **Wilson's disease** (see p. 234) was cloned some years ago, direct testing of copper, caeruloplasmin and urinary copper are most widely used for diagnosis.

Parkinsonism and related disorders

Parkinson's disease

At the time of writing there are now 10 different gene loci identified for Mendelian parkinsonism. Of these, in only two cases is the gene proven to cause Parkinson's disease. **Alpha-synuclein** produces a rare autosomal dominant form of the disease and **parkin** accounts for the majority of very early onset disease (occurring before the age of 20 years). They may also produce the disease with onset in the sixth decade. A third gene, *UCHL1* – an enzyme involved in the ubiquitination process – has been implicated in a single small family; this observation needs further investigation.

Progressive supranuclear palsy (see p. 233)

Although not overtly a genetic disease, progressive supranuclear palsy is of late onset and almost always has no family history, yet there is an established robust association with the *tau* gene. The pathogenic process is still being elucidated but it does fit neatly into the known pathology of progressive supranuclear palsy, namely *tau* deposition.

It is highly likely that there are other loci and genes yet to be located and the clinical investigation of the parkinsonian patient will, at least in part, be genetic in the very near future.

Ataxias

The dominantly inherited ataxias are given the acronym **spinocerebellar ataxia (SCA)**. There is a long list of loci and several genes. Numerically important are *SCA* 1, 2, 3, 6 and 7, numbered in the order in which the loci were found. These tests are widely available and should be considered in dominant ataxia families and patients in whom a genetic explanation is suspected. The yield from testing singleton late-onset cases of degenerative ataxia is low but not zero and often there is no option but to test for these genetic mutations. Interestingly, all of these genes share the same mutational mechanism, an **expanded CAG repeat** (similar to Huntington's disease). This is discussed below (see box p. 128). There is a rare group of disorders that produce episodic ataxias. In these families there is often an excess of epilepsy, migraine and other paroxysmal movement disorders. These are caused by **ion channel mutations** as in epilepsies. The most common are the result of abnormalities in the voltage-gated calcium channel on chromosome 19 (the same gene is implicated in *SCA6* and familial hemiplegic migraine).

Early-onset ataxias (at less than 20 years of age) are usually recessively inherited and the majority of cases are caused by mutations in the gene encoding frataxin and result in **Friedreich's ataxia**. This is another repeat expansion disorder but this time the repeat is in the intron and appears to work by somehow reducing the mitochondrial ribonucleic acid (mtRNA) and protein levels, that is, it is a loss-of-function mutation. In addition to the classical phenotype of progressive ataxia, pyramidal signs and sensory neuropathy, one should consider gene testing in all cases of early onset and any cases that are of later onset but have many or most of the typical features. The author has seen a case with onset in a patient aged over 60 years.

There is a long list of very rare early-onset ataxias and in most cases the genes remain unidentified, but this situation is likely to change over the next few years.

Myoclonus

Myoclonus (see p. 240) is most frequently found as part of a more widespread movement disorder. On occasions it can be seen as the sole or predominant abnormality. A recent discovery of a sarcoglycan gene in families with dystonia myoclonus (also called myoclonic dystonia) has provided the first insights into this movement disorder. The gene for 'essential myoclonus' remains unknown.

Choreiform disorders

The classic choreiform disorder is **Huntington's disease**, which is caused by an **expanded CAG** repeat in the huntingtin gene. It presents typically in the third and fourth decades of life, although earlier and later onsets can be seen (see p. 239). It should be considered in all cases of unexplained chorea, even in the absence of a family history. There is a much rarer but clinically similar disorder, dentatorubropallidoluysian, which can also be tested (see box p. 128).

Tremors

Essential tremor is the commonest familial movement disorder seen yet no genes have currently been identified.

Tics

Tourette's syndrome presents with a combination of multiple motor and vocal tics and obsessive-compulsive behaviour abnormalities. Although known to run in some families, linkage studies have been singularly unsuccessful in identifying a locus.

Miscellaneous movement disorders

There is potentially a long and complex catalogue of miscellaneous movement disorders. Although the list above implies that movement disorders can be readily sorted into those categories on the basis of the sole or predominant feature, dystonia, myoclonus, and so on, in reality, in many usually rare conditions, a mixture of movement disorders can be seen. Many of these disorders start early in life and often detailed descriptions are to be found in the larger paediatric neurology textbooks; for example, **ataxia telangiectasia**, an autosomal recessive disorder caused by mutations in the gene *ATM* (ataxia telangiectasia mutant), produces, in addition to the ataxia, a combination of dystonia and myoclonus with an oculomotor apraxia. **Neuro-acanthocytosis** can be inherited as an X-linked or autosomal dominant disorder and in both cases the genes are now identified. Classically this produces dystonia, chorea (especially oro-buccal), myoclonus and occasionally ataxia. **Hallervorden–Spatz disease**, most well known perhaps because of its characteristic MRI appearance of the 'eye of the tiger' sign caused by iron deposition in the striatum, produces a combination of movement disorders with dystonia and parkinsonism chief amongst them. The gene *PANK-2* has recently been identified.

HEREDITARY SPASTIC PARAPLEGIAS

The hereditary spastic paraplegias are clinically classified into pure and complicated (see p. 259). Both are genetically heterogeneous and there are a large number of gene loci now established. It can also be inherited as an autosomal dominant, recessive or X-linked trait. Abnormalities in the spastin gene account for a significant proportion of the 'pure' autosomal dominant families; multiple mutations have been described and testing is not yet routine. A much rarer gene mutation in paraplegin accounts for a small number of probably autosomal recessive families. If **X-linked inheritance** is a possibility, then very long-chain fatty acids should be analysed, as **adrenomyeloneuropathy** can present with this phenotype. There are at least two other genes on the X-chromosome, including abnormalities in the gene encoding a myelin protein gene – proteo-lipid protein and a cell adhesion molecule – *L1-CAM*.

MOTOR NEURONE AND PERIPHERAL NEUROPATHIES

Genetic disorders of the motor neurone

Early-onset disease tends to be most often proximal and can produce a severe motor disorder – proximal **spinal muscular atrophy (SMA)** (see p. 265). This is the result of exonic deletions in the *SMN* gene and is readily tested. This gene does not seem to be involved in the rarer distal SMA, which clinically it can resemble. The gene(s) responsible for the much rarer distal SMA are unknown, but recently some loci have been identified.

Familial amyotrophic lateral sclerosis is a disease of much later onset, which, apart from being autosomal dominant, resembles the much more common amyotrophic lateral sclerosis (ALS) or motor neurone disease, with progressive upper motor neurone and lower motor neurone signs leading to severe disability and death, often within 2–3 years. Mutations in the gene encoding **superoxide dismutase** have been demonstrated in a number of families from around the world (see p. 267). It appears that this accounts for approximately 3–5% of all cases of ALS (familial or sporadic) and is certainly worth testing if a genetic explanation is suspected. Mutations in neurofilament genes have also been postulated to cause a similar motor syndrome.

X-linked bulbar spinal neuronopathy (Kennedy's disease, XLBSN) produces a much slower progressive lower motor neurone syndrome, with additional anti-androgenic features, including testicular atrophy and gynaecomastia. Like Huntington's disease and many ataxia genes the mutation is a **CAG repeat** in the coding region. The androgen receptor is disrupted by this repeat but the exact mechanism of cell dysfunction and death is obscure.

Hereditary motor sensory neuropathies – Charcot–Marie–Tooth (CMT) disease

Classically these hereditary motor sensory neuropathies are divided into two broad groups, type 1 or demyelinating disease (see p. 170) defined by a conduction velocity of less than 38 m/s, and type 2 the axonal form (see p. 171). Both are now known to be genetically heterogeneous. Type 1 is commoner than type 2, and in both groups autosomal dominant is commoner than autosomal recessive inheritance and one genetic form predominates. This is caused by a duplication on chromosome 17p of a 1.5 Mb segment of DNA. This is readily testable and widely available. Interestingly if the 1.5 Mb segment is deleted, the person has a **hereditary liability to pressure palsies**. Rarer, but still seen commonly enough to be worth testing for, are mutations in the following genes. *Connexin 32* causes X-linked CMT and can resemble type 1 or type 2 and is X-linked dominant and therefore females can be affected. Numerous mutations are reported and so direct sequencing is required to find mutations. Mutations in a gene encoding protein zero (*P0*) are also known to cause demyelinating CMT.

Type 2 CMT is caused by a variety of genes and at present widespread testing is not available. This situation will undoubtedly change and it is worthwhile enquiring of the local genetic services. All of the genes/mutations reported to date are rare, and dissecting out the underlying gene in this group (and probably the remainder of type 1) will be a laborious process.

Hereditary sensory and autonomic neuropathies

Hereditary sensory and autonomic neuropathies comprise a range of disorders from the pure autonomic at one end (e.g. the Riley–Day syndrome), to the pure sensory neuropathy at the other. In between there are a number of disorders with a combination of sensory and autonomic features. A clinical clue to distinguishing this group as opposed to CMT is the presence of marked sensory features, often with positive sensory symptomatology. There has been very recent progress in this area and a number of genes are now known. At the time of writing these are not in clinical service but are likely to be in specialized laboratories in the near future.

Familial amyloid polyneuropathies

Familial amyloid polyneuropathies are rare disorders (see p. 171) that are due primarily to mutations in one of two genes. Transthyretin is the commonest and numerous mutations have been described. However, the search for mutations is aided by knowledge of the population from whence the patient came, as some mutations are population specific.

In the laboratory at The National Hospital for Neurology and Neurosurgery, London, UK, three 'common' mutations are screened for. Sequencing of the whole gene only follows if there is supplementary evidence of a transthyretin in the amyloid deposit, that is, a tissue diagnosis. This is an important group to diagnose, as early liver transplantation can help protect from further deterioration.

Mutations in the apolipoprotein gene can also lead to amyloid polyneuropathy. This appears to be much rarer.

MUSCLE DISEASE

The study of genetics has contributed to all areas of neurology but nowhere is this more impressive than in the strides made towards understanding of muscle disease. Table 5.1 lists the major single gene muscle diseases. In all areas substantial progress has been made and **all specialist muscle clinic services should involve a neurogenetic component**. Although the clinical phenotype is often distinctive there is sufficient overlap between some disease groups for the full evaluation of the patient to use clinical, pathological (including immunohistochemistry) and genetic studies to define and refine the diagnosis.

The dystrophies

The commonest of the dystrophies is the **X-linked Duchenne/Becker** grouping and these result from defects within the same gene encoding the muscle membrane protein, **dystrophin**. Becker muscular dystrophy can usually be distinguished from Duchenne on clinical grounds, as it is later in onset and less severe (see p. 136). There is an associated cardiomyopathy. An electromyograph is myopathic but non-specific. Muscle histology reveals degeneration and regeneration. **Immunocytochemistry** should be performed using three antibodies, which react with the carboxy, middle and N-terminal regions of the dystrophin molecule. This technique demonstrates an absence of staining for dystrophin on the sarcolemma. A secondary reduction in the sarcoglycans is also quite common. The dystrophin gene is births and a prevalence of 2:100 000 total male population.

Both of these disorders are recessive traits. Thus males carrying the gene are affected, while heterozygous females are carriers but often unaffected. Carrier females will pass on the condition to 50% of their sons and 50% of their daughters will be carriers, that is a 25% chance that a carrier will have an affected son. Although asymptomatic carriers can be identified through minor clinical changes, such as limited weakness or occasionally bulky calves, some may have elevated CK levels and mild EMG changes. A separate group known as manifesting carriers are the result of incomplete lyonization of the maternal X chromosome.

Approximately 65% of patients with DMD have no family history and therefore appear as sporadic cases. The mutation may have arisen in the mothers or in the affected individuals. However, new techniques to identify carrier status suggest that a significant proportion of apparently sporadic cases are in fact the offspring of previously unrecognized carriers.

Becker muscular dystrophy is much milder than DMD and affected males often have families. In this case all daughters will be carriers but all sons will be normal.

Clinical and molecular features of dystrophin deficiency

The weakness of DMD usually becomes apparent at any early stage with **delayed motor milestones.** Often the child is not able to walk until the age of 2 or 3 years. There is **bilateral symmetrical proximal limb weakness, usually more profound in the pelvic girdle.** The child may exhibit Gower's sign (see p. 133). The gait is waddling and the child has difficulty rising from sitting, crouching or lying. Most patients have pseudohypertrophy of the calves as a result of accumulation of fat and connective tissue (Figure 6.1). Progression of the disease leads to marked wasting of the limb girdles with accompanying progressive weakness. Tendon reflexes are lost with the exception of the ankle jerks. Paraspinal weakness may result in kyphoscoliosis, particularly once the patient is confined to a wheelchair. This, together with weakness of the intercostal and other

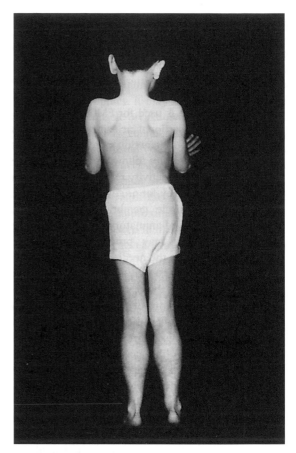

Figure 6.1 Prominent calves, wasted thighs and thinning of scapulohumeral muscles in Duchenne dystrophy.

respiratory muscles, may result in respiratory failure, although because of relative preservation of diaphragmatic function, this becomes severe only relatively late in the course of the disease.

The CK is usually very high, often scoring in the thousands, the EMG is abnormal and muscle biopsy shows a dystrophic pattern with a wide variation in fibre size, central nuclei muscle necrosis and increased connective tissue and fat (Figure 6.2). **Immunostaining with dystrophin antibodies** may show absence of expression of the protein at the sarcolemmal membrane.

Cardiac involvement is common in DMD and may result in arrhythmias, impaired contractility and, occasionally, progressive cardiac failure. Abnormalities on ECG are common and include conduction defects and tall R waves and deep Q waves. One intriguing aspect of DMD is that approximately

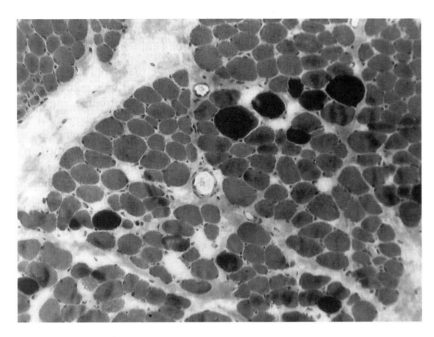

Figure 6.2 Duchenne muscular dystrophy (H & E frozen section × 120) shows large 'waxy' strongly eosinophilic (black) fibres together with great variation in fibre size. The large areas without muscle fibres are fat replacement and fibrosis as a result of progressive fibre loss.

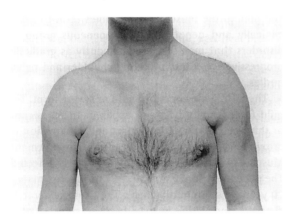

Figure 6.3 Asymmetric wasting of pectoral muscles in a man aged 40 years with Becker dystrophy.

one-third of patients have associated mental retardation. This particularly seems to affect verbal abilities. Cranial scans may show mild cerebral atrophy.

The onset and rate of progression of BMD are usually slower than in DMD. Patients with BMD present later, usually in early adolescence, although there is often a history of delayed motor milestones and difficulty keeping up with their peers at school. The pattern of muscle weakness is similar to that of DMD (Figure 6.3) and muscle hypertrophy is often a prominent feature, particularly affecting the calves. Spinal contractures are uncommon in BMD. Most patients are able to continue walking until they are aged into their 20s or 30s and whereas patients with DMD often die before the age of 20 years, those with BMD may survive much longer. **The heart may be involved in BMD** patients although usually this is less severe than in DMD. Abnormalities of ECG are seen in about half the cases of BMD. Intellect is not affected in BMD. Pathological features are similar to those seen in DMD but are usually much less severe. The expression of dystrophin in BMD is related to clinical involvement, that is the more protein expressed, the less severe the muscle weakness.

Diagnosis

The specific diagnosis of DMD or BMD rests upon demonstrating complete or partial dystrophin deficiency in the muscle biopsy. Molecular genetic diagnosis can be made by demonstrating a deletion in the dystrophin gene at the Xp21 region and this may be used in prenatal diagnosis.

The $Xp21.1$ gene is the largest known – 2.4 million base pairs. At least seven protein isoforms are encoded by this gene and these are found in skeletal

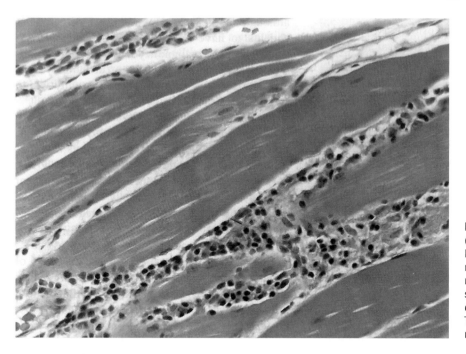

Figure 6.6 Polymyositis (paraffin section, H & E × 300): portion of three necrotic fibres with many large nuclei and macrophages and slightly more numerous round dark nuclei of lymphocytes. The intervening fibres are microscopically normal.

recovered incompletely and the remainder returned virtually to normal. The average duration of disease activity was 6 months for children who recovered and 40 months for those with sequelae. The prognosis is more favourable in adults without an underlying malignancy. Eighty per cent of patients survive 5 years.

Inclusion body myositis

Inclusion body myositis (IBM) exists in two forms, sporadic and familial. The age of onset of sporadic IBM ranges from 61 to 81 years; about 50% of patients are between the ages of 50 and 70 years. There is a 3:1 male:female preponderance. Inclusion body myositis is considered to be the most common late-onset muscular degenerative disease.

Clinically there is muscle weakness of insidious onset and slow progression

The weakness may be generalized or localized, symmetrical or asymmetrical, proximal or distal. Facial muscles are involved in 20% of patients but bulbar weakness is rare. Extraocular muscle

---

involvement is rare. Respiratory and abdominal muscles may be affected in about 10% of patients. Cardiac involvement occurs in 15–20% of cases.

Wasting is often seen and is proportionate to the weakness. Tendon reflexes may be retained until late in the disease. Dysphagia occurs in 25% of patients. There is an association of IBM with diabetes mellitus but there is no association with underlying malignancy.

The ESR and CK are usually normal or only mildly elevated; EMG shows motor unit potentials of short duration and a high proportion of polyphasic units. There are frequent fibrillation potentials and positive sharp waves. Muscle biopsy shows a variable degree of inflammatory infiltration and muscle fibre necrosis. The most typical abnormality is of rimmed vacuoles within muscle fibres. Immunohistochemistry shows that these contain a variety of proteins including ubiquitin and prion protein. Mitochondrial changes can also be seen with ragged red fibres and occasional cytochrome oxidase negative fibres. Inflammatory infiltration is predominantly with CD8+ T cells. These are sited mainly endomysially. An additional feature on light microscopy is of several small, often angulated, fibres suggesting some neurogenic component. Electron microscopy shows abnormal accumulations of filaments within the nucleus and the cytoplasm.

Familial IBM appears to be of variable inheritance patterns. Onset of weakness is usually earlier than in the sporadic form and weakness in some families appears to spare the quadriceps and affect distal muscles more. However, this pattern may vary between families. Muscle biopsy shows little in the way of inflammatory infiltration but again shows the presence of rimmed vacuoles.

Treatment of IBM is unsatisfactory. Many patients are treated with steroids or intravenous immunoglobulin but response is usually poor. Nevertheless, those with evidence of a significant inflammatory infiltrate on biopsy should be given a trial of immunosuppression.

DEFECTS OF THE NEURO-MUSCULAR JUNCTION

Myasthenia gravis

Myasthenia gravis (MG) is an autoimmune disorder caused by the production of antibodies against the acetylcholine receptor at the neuromuscular junction.

The aetiology underlying the generation of these antibodies is unknown but there is a clear association with other autoimmune disorders, particularly thyroid disease, and with abnormalities of the thymus gland, that is thymic hyperplasia or thymoma.

The typical clinical feature of MG is weakness and fatigue of voluntary muscles. Patients often present with episodic diplopia and ptosis. There may be **facial weakness** (Figure 6.7), slurring of **speech, dysphagia, dyspnoea** as a result of respiratory muscle involvement and **limb weakness which is usually proximal. Neck weakness** is a particular feature of muscle disease and is often seen in MG. There is often a clear diurnal variation in that patients may start the morning feeling normal but gradually fatigue through the day. Examination may reveal ptosis and ophthalmoplegia, which are the presenting features in 50% of patients and eventually develop in 90%.

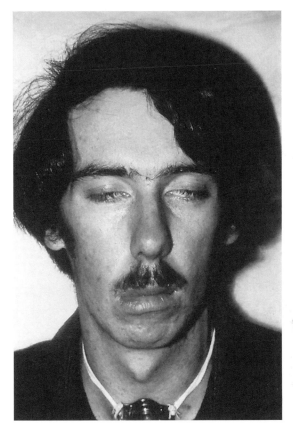

Figure 6.7 Bilateral ptosis and facial weakness in myasthenia gravis.

Diplopia is demonstrated by standard techniques. Fatigue of *levator palpebrae superioris* may be demonstrated by Cogan's lid twitch (see p. 123). Limb strength must by tested by a repetitive forced movement in order to demonstrate fatigue. Wasting of muscles is unusual, although it may develop in advanced cases. Tendon reflexes may be normal or brisk. Sensory features are absent.

Myasthenic symptoms	
Ocular	Ptosis
	Diplopia
	Weak eye closure
Bulbar	
Respiratory	
Proximal muscle weakness	
FATIGUE	VARIABLE

Table 6.3 Investigation of myasthenia gravis

Blood
  Full blood count, ESR
  Creatine kinase
  TSH, T4
  Acetylcholine receptor antibodies (+ve in some
  85% generalized myasthenia)
Muscle-specific kinase antibodies (found in c.70%
  of sero-negative myasthenics)
Striated muscle antibodies (+ve with thymoma)
Voltage-gated calcium channel antibodies
  (Lambert–Eaton)
Imaging
  Chest X-ray, CT scan chest (thymoma)
Electrodiagnosis
  Before and after exercise
  Repetitive stimulation (proximal muscle)
  Single fibre EMG – 'jitter'
Pharmacological
  Edrophonium test

ESR, erythrocyte sedimentation rate; TSH, thyroid stimulating
hormone; CT, computerized tomography; EMG, electromyography.

The investigation of MG (Table 6.3) involves the demonstration of **acetylcholine receptor antibodies**, although these may be absent in a small proportion of patients (some 15%). Those with only an ophthalmoplegia have a lower incidence of antibodies (some 50% +ve). About 85% of patients with generalized myasthenia have acetylcholine receptor antibodies (sero-positive). More recently some 70% of patients who are sero-negative have been found to have antibodies to muscle-specific kinase (about 15% of myasthenics). Other autoimmune disorders must be excluded. **Electrophysiological studies** may show decrement on repetitive stimulation and the presence of jitter and block on single fibre studies. The **edrophonium test** is an important part of the diagnosis and should be undertaken in a double-blind fashion in a hospital with appropriate resuscitation facilities to hand. A useful parameter to judge the effectiveness of edrophonium is ptosis or diplopia but proximal limb fatigue may also be used. The patient is usually given a covering dose of atropine and then 2–4 mg of edrophonium intravenously. If this produces no effect, then the remaining dose, up to 10 mg, is given. A positive effect is usually

seen within a few seconds and lasts for a few minutes. **CT scan of the thorax** is undertaken to help exclude a **thymoma** and the presence of this may be associated with **antistriatal muscle antibodies**.

The natural history of myasthenia gravis
The natural history of myasthenia gravis is that the disease remains purely ocular in less than 20% of patients; 80% of patients develop generalized myasthenia gravis within 12 months of onset.

Treatment of myasthenia gravis may be symptomatic in the form of anti-acetylcholine esterase drugs, for example pyridostigmine or neostigmine.

Pyridostigmine acts within 60 minutes and lasts from 3 to 6 hours. Typical dosages may be 30–90 mg every 6 hours but doses in excess of this may be used. Plasmapheresis may be useful in exacerbations of myasthenia gravis. In this respect, it is important to distinguish these episodes from neuromuscular blockade caused by excessive anti-acetylcholine esterases. An edrophonium test is useful in this, in that it will improve an exacerbation of myasthenia gravis but have no benefit or even worsen blockade due to drugs. The latter is treated by withdrawal of anticholinesterases and supportive therapy including ventilation if necessary.

Specific treatments include **thymectomy**, which may induce a remission rate of approximately 50% 7–10 years later. Young women with high antibody titres and a hyperplastic thymus gland respond more rapidly than men but there is no specific age or sex indication, and at 10 years no difference between male and female groups. Thymectomy is usually undertaken through a mediastinal approach as a transcervical approach may not remove all thymic tissue. The presence of a thymoma is an absolute indication for thymectomy.

Immunosuppressive therapy with alternate-day corticosteroids will induce improvement and may be used in combination with daily immunosuppressants such as azathioprine, cyclophosphamide or ciclosporin. When used initially steroids should be started at a low dose and gradually increased. Caution is necessary when starting steroid treatment as there may be an initial deterioration. Complete remission in response to steroid and other immunosuppressant therapy has been reported in 40–70% of patients. Significant clinical improvement is often not seen for about 5–6 months after initiation of therapy. Certain drugs (Table 6.4) may aggravate myasthenia gravis.

Table 6.4 Drugs that aggravate myasthenia gravis

Type of medication	Drug name
Neuromuscular block	Succinylcholine, vercuronium, *d*-tubocurarine
Cardiac drugs	Procainamide, quinidine, quinine
Calcium channel blockers	Verapamil, diltiazem
Beta blockers	Atenolol, metoprolol, propranolol, timolol eye drops
Aminoglycoside antibiotics	Gentamicin, streptomycin – rarely, ampicillin, tetracycline, ciprofloxacin
Miscellaneous	Chloroquine, ketoprofen, lithium, phenytoin
D-penicillamine*	May induce* or aggravate

Lambert–Eaton myasthenic syndrome

Lambert–Eaton myasthenic syndrome is an autoimmune disorder caused by antibodies against the voltage-sensitive calcium channel of the motor nerve terminal.

The male:female ratio is approximately 5:1 and 75% of males and 25% of females have an underlying malignancy, although this is uncommon under the age of 40 years. The majority of malignancies are small cell carcinomas of the lung.

Patients present with weakness and fatigability, particularly of the limb muscles. Seventy per cent of patients have mild ocular symptoms, such as ptosis or diplopia, there may be autonomic nervous system abnormalities including decreased salivation, lacrimation and sweating, and postural hypotension and impotence. There may be weakness, particularly in the lower limbs, at rest but isometric muscle contraction improves strength, although power may subsequently fatigue. Tendon reflexes are usually absent but may be restored by exercise.

Acetylcholine receptor antibodies are negative and edrophonium tests usually produce no response. EMG shows increased jitter and block with single fibre studies. Repetitive stimulation at 10 Hz or higher produces a gradual increase in the compound muscle action potential.

Treatment of Lambert–Eaton myasthenic syndrome includes management of any underlying malignancy. Specific treatment may include 3'4-diaminopyridine. This prolongs the duration of the presynaptic action potential and increases calcium entry into the nerve terminal. Plasmapheresis is occasionally helpful.

REFERENCES AND FURTHER READING

Hart PE, De Vivo DC, Schapira AHV (2002) *Clinical Features of the Mitochondrial Encephalomyopathies.* In: Schapira AHV, DiMauro S (eds) *Mitochondrial Disorders in Neurology,* 2nd edn. London, UK: Butterworth Heinemann, pp. 35–68.

Karpati G, Hilton Jones D, Griggs RC (eds) (2001) *Disorders of Voluntary Muscle,* 7th edn. Cambridge, UK: Cambridge University Press.

Katirji B, Kaminski H, Preston D, Ruff R, Shapiro B (eds) (2002) *Neuromuscular Disorders in Clinical Practice.* London: Butterworth Heinemann.

Rahman S, Schapira AHV (1999) *Mitochondrial Myopathies Clinical Features, Molecular Genetics, Investigation and Management.* In: Schapira AHV, Griggs RC (eds) *Muscle Diseases.* London, UK: Butterworth Heinemann, pp. 177–223.

Schapira AHV (2002) The 'new' mitochondrial disorders. *Journal of Neurology, Neurosurgery & Psychiatry,* **72**:144–149.

CHAPTER 7

PERIPHERAL NEUROPATHIES

J.G. Llewelyn

INTRODUCTION

Accurate diagnosis of a peripheral neuropathy can be difficult. This is mainly a result of the fact that the clinical features of various neuropathies seem to be very similar despite the varied aetiologies. Indeed, it is recognized that in some 30% or more of patients with an established neuropathy the cause remains unknown. The challenge therefore is to develop a sleuth-like approach to each patient, teasing out the clues in the clinical history before adding the findings of clinical examination, and then embarking on a channelled approach to investigation, which will lead to a diagnosis and from there the development of a treatment plan.

Neuropathies can be symmetric or multifocal, and can be predominantly motor or sensory or, most often, a mixture (sensorimotor). The aetiology of neuropathies is diverse and is outlined in Table 7.1. The tempo and pattern of the evolution of the neuropathy may provide a clue to the underlying cause. Inflammatory, vasculitic, diabetic, paraneoplastic and toxic neuropathies can develop over weeks to months.

Inherited conditions are often evident in childhood, and if suspected you might ask: 'Was there a delay in walking? Could you run as fast as your school friends? Were you good at sports or did you avoid sports?'

SYMPTOMS AND SIGNS

The common symmetric polyneuropathics show a pattern of sensory and motor deficit that begins distally in the limbs, slowly spreading proximally. The lower limbs are usually affected before the upper limbs.

It is useful to recognize that there are negative and positive symptoms related to neuropathies (Table 7.2). Numbness is the commonest sensory symptom, with associated loss of all sensory modalities. Sometimes the sensory loss is confined to pain and temperature sensations with preservation of light touch, vibration and joint position sense and this pattern would

Table 7.1 Causes of neuropathies

(i) Causes of sensory polyneuropathy
Diabetes, uraemia, hypothyroidism
Amyloidosis
Paraneoplastic, paraproteinaemic
Thallium, isoniazid, vincristine, cisplatin, metronidazole
Sjögren's syndrome
Leprosy
HIV, Lyme disease
Hereditary sensory and autonomic neuropathies
Fabry's disease
Vitamin B12 deficiency

(ii) Causes of sensorimotor polyneuropathy
Charcot–Marie–Tooth disease
Alcohol
Guillain–Barré syndrome (GBS); chronic inflammatory demyelinating polyneuropathy (CIDP)
Vasculitis
Paraneoplastic, paraproteinaemic
Diabetes, uraemia, hypothyroidism, acromegaly
Sarcoidosis

(iii) Causes of motor neuropathy
GBS/CIDP
Porphyria, diphtheria, lead
Hereditary motor neuropathies (HMN)

(iv) Causes of focal and multifocal neuropathies
Entrapment/compression syndromes
Polyarteritis nodosa
Connective tissue disorders
Non-systemic (tissue specific) vasculitis
Wegner's granulomatosis
Infiltration of nerve by lymphoma or carcinoma
Neurofibromatosis
Tuberculoid leprosy, herpes zoster, human immunodeficiency virus, Lyme disease
Sarcoidosis
Hereditary neuropathy with liability to pressure palsies
Multifocal motor neuropathy with conduction block

Table 7.2 Symptoms of peripheral neuropathy

Sensory symptoms

Negative	Numbness
Positive	Paraesthesiae (tingling, pins and needles)
	Pain (burning, shooting, stabbing, 'like walking on pebbles', 'like walking on hot sand', may be induced by non-painful stimuli, allodynia, hyperalgesia)

Motor symptoms

Negative	Weakness and wasting
Positive	Fasciculations
	Myokymia
	Cramps
	Restless legs
	Tremor

developing neuropathic ulcers and neuropathic joints (Charcot joints). Such neuropathies are also likely to be associated **with autonomic symptoms and signs** such as light-headedness aggravated by standing, impotence, constipation, loss of bladder control, abnormal sweating and occasionally blurring of vision. It is therefore important to check for postural hypotension and pupillary reactions in every patient with a neuropathy.

In addition to the lower motor neurone weakness and stocking sensory loss, the other cardinal sign of neuropathy is loss of or depressed reflexes (Table 7.3). When a neuropathy develops during the early growth period, skeletal deformities may be seen (clawed toes, pes cavus and kyphoscoliosis). Sometimes a clue to the cause of a neuropathy may come from palpating peripheral nerves (e.g. radial nerve at the wrist, ulnar nerve at the elbow, common peroneal nerve at the knee and the superficial peroneal nerve on the dorsum of the foot).

Conditions that cause nerve thickening are:
- Leprosy
- Hereditary motor and sensory neuropathy (HMSN) type I and II
- Acromegaly
- Amyloidosis
- Neurofibromatosis
- Refsum's disease.

indicate a predominant loss of small fibres – **a small fibre neuropathy** (e.g. diabetes, amyloidosis). The loss of pain and temperature predisposes the patient to a greater risk of painless injuries and therefore of

Table 7.3 Signs of peripheral neuropathy

Skeletal abnormalities	Pes cavus
	Clawing of toes
	Scoliosis/kyphoscoliosis
Change in skin, nails and hair	Foot ulcers
	Loss of hair to mid-calf region
	Thin dry skin
	Hypopigmentation of the skin
Motor	Normal tone with distal wasting and weakness
Reflexes	Absent or depressed
Sensory	'Stocking ± glove' loss of sensation
Gait	High stepping, foot drop
	May be unsteady

Table 7.4 Investigation of a neuropathy

Blood	**FBC, ESR, U&E, LFT**
	Glucose (+GTT if borderline)
	Serum protein electrophoresis
	Autoantibodies, TSH
	Vitamin B12, folate
	Genetic testing – e.g. PMP22, Po for CMT Type 1
Urine	**Glucose, protein**, Bence Jones protein, porphyrins
CSF	
Nerve conduction studies	Slowing of motor and sensory conduction velocities (moderate in axonal neuropathy; severe in demyelinating neuropathy).
Sensory threshold test	Reduced sensory action potential amplitude (axonal) only in suspected small fibre neuropathy when nerve conduction studies may be normal
Autonomic function tests	
Imaging	Skeletal survey for myeloma
	Chest X-ray for suspected carcinoma or sarcoidosis
Nerve biopsy	Only indicated when the cause of a progressive neuropathy has not been revealed by other investigations. It is useful to confirm the presence of a vasculitis or other inflammatory infiltration. Only sensory nerves are biopsied (sural, superficial peroneal or superficial radial)

Initial screen is in **bold type**. If this is negative, proceed to nerve conduction studies.
FBC, full blood count; ESR, erythrocyte sedimentation rate; GTT, glucose tolerance test; TSH, thyroid stimulating hormone; CMT, Charcot–Marie–Tooth disease; CSF, cerebrospinal fluid.

INVESTIGATIONS

It has to be realized that no 'battery' of laboratory tests is going to make up for a haphazard history and examination. Investigations should help towards a better understanding of the neuropathy by patients answering specific questions and hopefully establish the cause and type of neuropathy (Table 7.4). Blood tests and urinalysis are straightforward. Some are only rarely requested (e.g. anti-neuronal antibodies in suspected paraneoplastic neuropathy) and genetic tests will require the patient's consent and genetic counselling before the blood is taken.

Nerve conduction studies (NCS) will be of value if the initial clinical assessment, urinalysis and blood screen fail to suggest a diagnosis. These studies are a true extension of the clinical examination and crucial in distinguishing between an **axonal and a demyelinating process. In the latter the conduction velocities are very low (less than 35 m/s and often in the range 20–30 m/s)**. The causes of chronic demyelinating neuropathies are shown in Table 7.5.

Thermal threshold tests can be helpful when the clinical picture suggests a small fibre neuropathy and the nerve conduction tests are normal. Thermal threshold tests should only be performed in a laboratory used to interpreting these measurements as they are prone to wide variability. **Cerebrospinal fluid (CSF)** analysis is helpful again only in specific situations – when there is no clear answer from blood tests and NCS and the neuropathy is progressing rapidly. The same criteria apply to **nerve biopsy** – only consider this invasive investigation as a final test; for example, if there is suspicion of a vasculitis or where the NCS only partially suggests a chronic inflammatory demyelinating polyneuropathy (CIDP) as both are potentially treatable. Careful planning

Table 7.5 Chronic demyelinating neuropathies

Inflammatory
    CIDP and MMN

Paraproteinaemic
    Benign paraprotein (IgM, G or A)
    Myeloma (IgM,G or A)
    Waldenström's macroglobulinaemia (IgM)
    POEMS syndrome (IgG or A)

Hereditary
    CMT disease (Type 1, Dejerine-Sottas,
        X-linked CMT)
    HNPP
    Refsum's disease
    Metachromatic leukodystrophy
    Globoid cell leukodystrophy

Toxic
    Amiodarone, perhexiline, suramin
    Diphtheria

CIDP, chronic inflammatory demyelinating polyneuropathy;
MMN, multifocal motor neuropathy; Ig, immunoglobulin (M, G, A);
POEMS, polyneuropathy, organomegaly, endocrinopathy,
monoclonal protein and skin changes; CMT, Charcot-Marie-Tooth
disease; HNPP, hereditary neuropathy with liability to pressure
palsies.

is needed in selection of which nerve to biopsy (the commonest is the sural nerve) and where the biopsy is going to be processed for light and electron microscopy and who is going to report on the pathology. A nerve biopsy sent to a routine pathology laboratory without experience in dealing with peripheral nerve tissue is unlikely to yield a diagnosis.

In 25–30% of patients, no cause will be found after detailed investigation (chronic idiopathic axonal neuropathy).

TREATMENT AND GENERAL MANAGEMENT

If an underlying cause is identified, it should, where possible, be treated; for example, blood glucose control, vitamin B12 injections, immunotherapy. In

terms of overall management it is important to emphasize:

- Foot care
- Physiotherapy advice regarding use of walking aids or ankle-foot orthoses
- Occupational therapy advice regarding utensils, for example
- Input from a social worker regarding home adaptations (with community occupational therapist and physiotherapist)
- Pain control – painful neuropathy is uncommon but very difficult to treat. Symptoms can be helped with drugs such as gabapentin, carbamazepine, amitriptyline and tramadol (see p. 523).

INFLAMMATORY NEUROPATHIES

Guillain–Barré syndrome (GBS)

Guillain–Barré syndrome (GBS) is the commonest subacute neuropathy, with an incidence of 1.5–2.0: 100 000 population per year. About 4% of cases will have a further episode. Clinically it usually reaches its peak within 4 weeks of the onset of symptoms. When there is ongoing progression for between 4 and 8 weeks this is termed 'intermediate GBS' to distinguish it from CIDP, where, by definition, there is neurological progression beyond 8 weeks from the onset of the illness. **The predominant symptom is weakness, which first appears in the legs, producing often a symmetric distal pattern that ascends to involve the arms.** Only in 10% of cases does weakness start in the arms. Clinical variants of GBS have been described (Table 7.6) including some with weakness, mainly of the pharyngeal, neck and arms (cervico-pharyngeal-brachial variant), predominant leg weakness (paraparetic variant) and Miller–Fisher variant (see below). **Facial weakness** is often asymmetric and found in just over 50% of cases. Significant ophthalmoparesis occurs in 15% of patients with typical GBS.

In patients with cranial nerve involvement, including **bulbar weakness**, and associated neck

Table 7.6 Guillain-Barré syndrome (GBS) and variants

Acute inflammatory demyelinating polyradiculoneuropathy (AIDP)
  60% will have antecedent illness
  Progression is over days up to 4 weeks
  Recovery usually starts at 4 weeks
  20% will have significant neurological disability
  Mortality rate is about 5%

Acute motor and sensory axonal neuropathy
  Diarrhoeal illness is common trigger
    (*Campylobacter jejuni*)
  Acute onset of weakness, rapid progression
  Often there are early respiratory difficulties
  Longer recovery and more severe residual
    disability than AIDP
  Mortality rate is 10–15%

Acute motor neuropathy
  Diarrhoeal illness (*Campylobacter jejuni*) is usual
    trigger
  Rare in Western world
  Most commonly affects children in northern
    China and is seasonal
  Recovery and mortality rates are similar to AIDP

Miller–Fisher syndrome
  Accounts for 5% of all GBS cases
  Begins with diplopia, followed 3–4 days later by
    gait ataxia
  Evolves to complete ophthalmoplegia with
    areflexia
  Sometimes mild limb weakness is present
  >95% have IgG antibodies to ganglioside GQ1b
  Monophasic course with excellent recovery
  Intravenous immunoglobulin or plasma exchange
    is appropriate for those who cannot walk

Acute panautonomic neuropathy

Pure sensory neuropathy

and proximal arm weakness, there is a high risk of developing intercostal muscle and diaphragmatic weakness leading to potentially fatal **respiratory failure**.

Tingling, shooting pains and numbness in the feet and hands are the first symptoms of GBS and are quickly followed by **weakness**. Almost 90% of patients will complain of deep muscle pains during the course of the illness.

All reflexes are depressed or absent from an early stage.

Autonomic function may be abnormal in two-thirds of patients. Sinus tachycardia is common but rarely needs treating. Bradycardias, heart block, paroxysmal atrial tachycardia and periods of sinus arrest and asystole are life threatening and require urgent cardiological assessment and treatment. Labile blood pressure may also need treatment. Urinary retention occurs in 10–15% of cases, but frank urinary incontinence is rare. Constipation is far more common than diarrhoea.

A slow but steady recovery over weeks and up to 6 months is seen in 80% of GBS cases. A more aggressive course is seen in 10–15% of patients, who have a prolonged stay on the intensive therapy unit and a recovery period extending up to 2 years (usually acute motor and sensory axonal neuropathy variant). Sadly, even these days, about 5% of patients with GBS will die.

Poor prognostic factors in GBS are:
- Older age
- Rapid onset (<7 days)
- Requiring ventilatory support
- Small distal compound muscle action potentials
- Previous diarrhoeal illness (*Campylobacter jejuni*)
- No treatment [intravenous immunoglobulin (IVIg) or plasma exchange].

Confirmation of the clinical diagnosis comes from nerve conduction studies and from examination of the **CSF**. Both may be normal early on in the illness,

but later the CSF shows a raised protein but with a normal white cell count.

A mild lymphocytosis (10–30 cells/mm^3) is not unusual in GBS, but a higher cell count raises the possibility of human immunodeficiency virus (HIV) infection.

Table 7.7 Blood tests in Guillain–Barré syndrome (GBS)

Full blood count	White blood count may be raised Lymphoma and CLL linked with GBS
Electrolytes	Sodium may be low due to SIADH
T4/TSH	Hypothyroidism linked to GBS
ANA	Collagen vascular disease linked with GBS
Porphyrin screen	AIP may mimic GBS
HIV test (when indicated)	
Anti-GQ1b	For Miller–Fisher variant
Infection screen	*Campylobacter* serology (and stool culture), CMV, EBV, hepatitis A and C, Mycoplasma

CLL, chronic lymphatic leukaemia; SIADH, syndrome of inappropriate antidiuretic hormone; TSH, thyroid stimulating hormone; ANA, anti-nuclear antibody; AIP, acute intermittent porphyria; HIV, human immunodeficiency virus; CMV, cytomegalovirus; EBV, Epstein–Barr virus.

Nerve conduction studies show slowing of conduction velocities with patchy conduction block in the common acute inflammatory demyelinating polyradiculoneuropathy variant. Important blood tests are outlined in Table 7.7.

Management and treatment (Table 7.8)

> It is vital that the patient is monitored on a suitably staffed and equipped ward. Accurate **monitoring of respiratory and cardiac function** is vital.

If measurement of vital capacity and cardiac monitoring cannot be undertaken on the general medical ward, the patient must be transferred either to a high dependency unit or to a regional neurology unit.

Dangers of peak flow measurements

Peak expiratory flow rate (PEFR) measurements are not just unhelpful, but are misleading and dangerous as PEFR may be reasonable when the vital capacity is critically low.

Supportive care is still undoubtedly the most important component of treatment and the patient needs to be monitored carefully until the illness

Table 7.8 Management of Guillain–Barré syndrome

Early
  4-hourly recording of VC and oxygen saturation
  Continuous electrocardiogram
  Heparin 5000 units s.c. 12-hourly or tinzaparin s.c. once daily
  Regular chest physiotherapy, turning and oral toilet
  Nasogastric tube if there are swallowing problems
  Intravenous immunoglobulin (0.4 g/kg body weight per day for 5 days) or
  Plasma exchange – 5 exchanges of 50 ml/kg over 5–10 days
  Pain control – opiate analgesia may be required

Late
  Ventilatory assistance if VC is falling rapidly or is below 24 ml/kg
  Tracheostomy – if ventilation is needed for more than 10 days
  Cardiac pacemaker – for bradyarrhythmias or episodes of asystole
  Gastrostomy (PEG) – if it seems that a prolonged delay recovery of bulbar function is likely
  Continued physiotherapy, occupational therapy and speech therapy input
  Monitor pain control

VC, vital capacity; s.c., subcutaneously; PEG, percutaneous endoscopic gastrostomy.

has stabilized for at least 3 weeks. **Intravenous immunoglobulin** is the first line immunomodulating treatment, and although there are no strict guidelines as to when to start treatment, it is reasonable to consider IVIg (0.4 g/kg body weight per day for 5 days) if the patient has difficulty with walking. It is recommended that the patient or next of kin be fully informed of the 10–20% risk of relapse after IVIg, and of the small but theoretically possible risks of transmission of hepatitis A, B and C viruses and HIV and of transmission of prion proteins; a consent form should be completed before treatment is started.

There are no clinical trial data to give guidance on what to do if the patient continues to deteriorate after IVIg treatment. If it appears that the patient has relapsed after IVIg, a second treatment should be given. If on the other hand there has been no improvement after 2 weeks but a steady progression, either further IVIg or **plasma exchange** should be considered.

With early diagnosis and treatment, appropriate measures to prevent **thromboembolism, aspiration and pressure sores**, most patients with GBS recover satisfactorily. The GBS Support Group provides information and important contact with other patients who have had GBS who can reassure the patient more convincingly than any medical professional that recovery is likely to occur.

Chronic inflammatory demyelinating polyradiculoneuropathy

In some respects, CIDP is separated from GBS only by having a different time course. The former condition evolves over 12 weeks or longer (up to many months and years), and may persist for years with often incomplete recovery.

It is predominantly a symmetric polyradiculoneuropathy with symptoms of weakness, sensory loss and paraesthesiae. Proximal and distal muscles can be affected early on in the illness, and although the weakness can be severe, muscle wasting is not a major feature as a result of the fact that the problem is one of demyelination with areas of conduction block rather than marked loss of axons. Neck weakness is common, but facial weakness is rare (<15%) and is usually mild. Respiratory muscle weakness does not occur. There is hyporeflexia or areflexia and sensory loss in a stocking-and-glove distribution. Autonomic problems are uncommon.

The clinical course may be **slowly progressive** or **stepwise progressive (66%)** or **relapsing (33%)**. The CSF protein is elevated with normal microscopy. **Nerve conduction studies show demyelination, which is patchy, and regions of conduction block.** With the clinical features, detailed neurophysiology and CSF examination, there is usually no need for a nerve biopsy. A nerve biopsy is of value in those cases where either the neurophysiology is not diagnostic or where the clinical picture suggests that vasculitis is a possibility.

Table 7.9 Treatment of chronic inflammatory demyelinating polyneuropathy

Oral prednisolone	1.0–1.5 mg/kg per day until improvement is noted Dose can then be changed to alternate-day regimen Dose then slowly titrated downwards after a period of maintained maximal improvement (usually at 6–12 months) Vitamin D/calcium or a third-generation bisphosphonate to be added to prevent osteoporosis
Cyclophosphamide	No good clinical trial data. Azathioprine can be used as a steroid-sparing agent
Ciclosporin Azathioprine Intravenous immunoglobulin	Standard 0.4 g/kg per day for 5 days
Plasma exchange	3 exchanges (20 ml/kg) per week for 3 weeks followed by 2 per week for the next 3 weeks

Remember to check the patient's thiopurine methyl transferase activity to see whether it is safe to give azathioprine.

Treatment of CIDP varies with the severity of the clinical picture and three **immunomodulating therapies have been shown to be effective** – oral prednisolone, IVIg and plasma exchange (Table 7.9). The first line treatment has until recently been IVIg. With the risk of prion protein contamination, the fact that at this time IVIg does not have a licence for use in CIDP and the increasing costs of IVIg, there has been a move back to using prednisolone as first treatment, and reserving IVIg for treatment of more severely affected patients. Azathioprine is used as a steroid-sparing agent but patients on long-term steroids will need calcium and vitamin D supplements or bisphosphonate to prevent osteoporosis. Before starting azathioprine, the patient's thiopurine methyltransferase activity should be checked. Thiopurine methyltransferase metabolises azathioprine and, if activity is low, there is a high risk of myelosuppression. For patients resistant to the three main treatments, options include cyclophosphamide, azathioprine and ciclosporin but there are no clear guidelines on dosage or duration of treatment.

Although 90% of patients will show some improvement with any of the three mainline treatments, the best results are seen in those where the duration of the illness is less than 1 year, and the severity of the weakness is only mild or moderate. The relapse rate is high (>50%). A small number are resistant to all therapies and another small group show only improvement with IVIg and require this treatment on a regular (2- to 6-weekly) basis.

Multifocal motor neuropathy with conduction block

Multifocal motor neuropathy

Multifocal motor neuropathy (MMN) is an uncommon disorder but an important one to recognize because it may clinically resemble the lower motor neurone variant of motor neurone disease, and, unlike motor neurone disease, MMN is potentially treatable with immunotherapy. The other differential diagnosis is CIDP.

Clinically multifocal motor neuropathy (MMN) is characterized by **progressive and asymmetric weakness without sensory involvement**. Muscle wasting is not evident early on despite the profound weakness (like CIDP, the problem is caused by conduction block and not axonal loss). Progressive unilateral grip weakness, wrist drop or foot drop are common presenting features. Cranial nerve and respiratory involvement are rare. Cramps and fasciculations are common and the reflexes are asymmetrically depressed.

The electrophysiological hallmark is the presence of **persistent multifocal conduction block** in areas where the nerve is unlikely to be susceptible to entrapment. Evidence of peripheral demyelination is also often found. Unlike CIDP, the CSF protein is usually normal. Elevated anti-GM1 ganglioside antibody titres are of no diagnostic nor prognostic value.

Treatment with IVIg may be very effective, but the benefit is short lived (2–4 weeks), and patients require regular maintenance doses. On a long-term basis only cyclophosphamide (100–150 mg/day) has shown any consistent benefit (in 50–60% of cases), and the addition of this drug may increase the time between IVIg infusions. Unlike CIDP, steroids and plasma exchange are of no benefit.

DIABETIC NEUROPATHIES

Peripheral neuropathy occurs as a complication of both insulin-dependent and non-insulin-dependent diabetes. **The commonest form is the distal sensorimotor neuropathy.** There is evidence of a neuropathy in 7% of patients at the time of diagnosis of their diabetes, increasing to 50% after 25 years of diabetes. Occasionally the neuropathy appears before the diabetes becomes evident. Multifocal neuropathies are also common in diabetes and often coexist with the distal symmetric neuropathy.

Diabetic neuropathies

Progressive:
- distal symmetric sensory and sensorimotor neuropathies
- autonomic neuropathy

Reversible:
- acute painful neuropathy
- cranial neuropathy (IIIrd nerve palsy)
- thoraco-abdominal neuropathy
- proximal diabetic neuropathy (diabetic amyotrophy).

Distal sensory and sensorimotor polyneuropathy

For most diabetic patients the symptoms are mild, with numbness and minor tingling. In only a few cases is pain a troublesome problem (10%

of diabetics), but when present it can be debilitating and described as aching, burning, stabbing or shooting.

Tactile hypersensitivity is often present in these patients, and despite the severity of the symptoms the clinical signs may be quite trivial. **There may be mild distal weakness with loss of ankle reflexes. The sensory loss affects all modalities and begins at the toes** and evolves into a stocking distribution. It follows a length-related pattern, so that as the numbness extends up to thigh level it also begins to affect the fingers. If there is evidence of more severe distal weakness with wasting or additional proximal weakness, then the coexistence of another neuropathy, such as CIDP, vasculitis or paraproteinaemic neuropathy, has to be considered.

The **autonomic neuropathy** is also length related, with loss of sweating in the feet being an early feature. Autonomic involvement is important to recognize as it may be related to an increased mortality rate. Treatment of autonomic problems is outlined in Table 7.10.

These **progressive neuropathies** are associated with **diabetic retinopathy** and **nephropathy**, and seem to be more likely to occur the longer the patient has been suffering from diabetes, if the patient is male and tall. The cause is unknown. A multifactorial aetiology seems most likely – metabolic and vascular factors being implicated (Table 7.11). Despite all the proposed mechanisms, the only treatment to show benefit is strict maintenance of normal blood glucose levels.

Acute painful neuropathy of diabetes

Acute painful neuropathy of diabetes appears to be a distinct entity, with the onset of **severe pain distally in the legs** associated with **progressive weight loss**. The burning pains and contact hyperaesthesiae are very troublesome at night, causing insomnia and depression. With continued good diabetic control and adequate pain relief, improvement does occur but sometimes takes several months. Regaining body weight is an early indicator of improvement. This

Table 7.10 Diabetic autonomic neuropathy

Cardinal symptoms	Treatment
Impotence	Counselling. Viagra. Penile papaverine injection. Mechanical prosthesis
Postural hypotension (>30 mmHg drop)	Fludrocortisone ± indometacin
Abnormal sweating	
Gastroparesis	Metoclopramide, domperidone, erythromycin
Diarrhoea	Tetracycline with loperamide/codeine
Decreased awareness of hypoglycaemia	

Table 7.11 Possible mechanisms in the pathogenesis of diabetic neuropathy

Metabolic hypothesis
- Polyol accumulation, myo-inositol depletion, reduced Na^+K^+-ATPase
- Advanced glycosylation end-product formation
- Altered neurotrophic factors
- Oxidative stress
- Altered fatty acid metabolism

Vascular hypothesis
Altered protein synthesis and axonal transport
Immunological mechanisms

syndrome can be triggered following the institution of tight glucose control with either insulin or oral hypoglycaemic drugs. The cause is not known.

Cranial neuropathies

There is an increased incidence of **3rd and 6th cranial nerve palsies** in diabetic patients. The 3rd cranial nerve palsy is the commonest. There is intense pain around the affected eye in half of the cases and the pupil is not involved (in contrast to 3rd nerve palsy resulting from a posterior communicating aneurysm where the pupil is dilated). It is believed to be caused by ischaemia of the central core of the

3rd nerve. The prognosis is excellent, with recovery within 3–4 months.

Thoraco-abdominal neuropathy

In thoraco-abdominal neuropathy there is an acute onset of pain in a localized area over the anterior chest or abdominal wall. The patterns of sensory loss or hyperpathia produced are consistent with lesions of the spinal nerves or its branches. The pain resolves within a few days and the numbness recovers over 4–6 weeks. On the abdominal wall, muscle weakness may present as a hernia. The cause is not known.

Proximal diabetic neuropathy (lumbosacral radioplexus neuropathy)

Previously termed **diabetic amyotrophy**, this condition occurs in more elderly type 2 diabetics, affecting males more often than females. There is an **asymmetric onset of lower limb weakness and wasting which is most striking proximally** but which may be global. There is lumbar or thigh pain from the outset. The knee jerk is depressed or absent on the affected side, and often both ankle jerks are absent because of the presence of a distal symmetric sensorimotor neuropathy. There is often marked weight loss. Recovery occurs slowly over many months or years, but a number of patients have residual neurological problems. Recent studies have found either microvasculitis or non-vasculitic epineurial and endoneurial inflammatory infiltration in about one-third of cases. Whether such patients would fare better with immunotherapy is not known. Treatment is therefore based on achieving good glucose control, paying close attention to pain relief and input from physiotherapists.

TOXIC NEUROPATHIES

Nerve damage caused by drugs has always to be considered when assessing a patient with symptoms of a neuropathy. Some of the toxic drugs are highly lipophilic agents, such as amiodarone, perhexiline and chloroquine; others are chemotherapy agents – vincristine, vinblastine and cisplatin. Nucleoside analogues (ddC (zalcitabine) and ddI (didanosine)), isoniazid , metronidazole and phenytoin are other drugs that can produce a neuropathy. In all (except phenytoin), there are painful paraesthesiae with distal sensory loss but variable degrees of distal lower limb weakness.

The neuropathy caused by **alcohol** is in part a result of its toxic effect, but is also caused by an associated thiamine deficiency. There is distal sensory loss, with painful, aching feet. Distal leg weakness is uncommon unless the neuropathy has been present for a number of years. Very occasionally the neuropathy can be more acute in onset. Nerve conduction studies show an axonal process and the CSF is usually normal. Treatment is by stopping all alcohol consumption and giving generous vitamin supplements (often parenterally) including thiamine.

Neuropathy as a result of metal toxicity (thallium, mercury, arsenic and lead) is very uncommon and unless there is a specific risk that prolonged exposure has occurred a 'routine metal screen' should not be requested.

NEUROPATHIES ASSOCIATED WITH ORGAN FAILURE

While it is very unlikely that a neuropathy will be the first manifestation of an underlying metabolic disorder other than for diabetes. Patients with advanced kidney or liver disease, for example, may well develop a neuropathy. This may be because of a common cause such as vasculitis, which is potentially treatable, but most often it is attributable directly to the metabolic abnormality. Patients with such neuropathies should be appropriately investigated with detailed neurophysiology so as not to miss a potentially treatable CIDP.

Uraemic polyneuropathy occurs in over 70% of patients with chronic renal disease and is commoner in males than females.

> It is a distal symmetric sensorimotor axonal neuropathy, with prominent sensory symptoms of pain and paraesthesiae. A 'restless legs syndrome' is a common feature.

It is unusual for the upper limbs to be affected but an additional autonomic neuropathy is found in about 25% of patients with chronic renal failure. The neuropathy may improve with dialysis, but the response to renal transplantation is often dramatic. Also associated with uraemia is a focal neuropathy involving the median nerve at the wrist, ulnar nerve at the elbow and the common peroneal nerve at the fibula head. Uraemia seems to increase the susceptibility of these nerves to pressure injury, and in some cases it seems to be related to the deposition of amyloid material. These compression neuropathies should be managed as in non-uraemic patients.

Chronic liver failure rarely results in a neuropathy of any clinical significance, and likewise in patients with **chronic pulmonary disease**, the axonal sensorimotor neuropathy is mild, even though up to 75% of cases will have NCS changes consistent with an axonal process.

CRITICAL ILLNESS POLYNEUROPATHY

The neuropathy associated with critical illness becomes noticeable when a patient on an intensive therapy unit fails to be weaned off the ventilator. Most patients have a combination of adult respiratory distress syndrome, organ failure and infection. The use of neuromuscular blocking drugs also seems to be an important factor in the development of this axonal neuropathy. The degree of weakness is quite variable. There may also be an additional myopathy related to critical illness. In any patient remaining ventilator dependent, the neurophysiology becomes important in order to exclude myasthenia gravis.

Although as many as 60% of cases with septicaemia and multiple organ failure will die, for those who survive and who have a neuropathy, the prognosis for recovery of the neuropathy is surprisingly good.

PORPHYRIC NEUROPATHY

Porphyric neuropathy is rare, but an **acute axonal motor neuropathy** that is clinically similar to GBS can occur in all forms of porphyria. Features that can help distinguish this type of porphyric neuropathy from GBS include the asymmetry of the **weakness**, predominance of **proximal** rather than distal weakness that occurs in the former. Also when there is sensory involvement, this also may have a rather unusual proximal distribution ('bathing trunk' and 'breast-plate'). It can also involve respiratory, facial, ocular and bulbar muscles. There may also be autonomic involvement. It is commonly associated with abdominal pain, psychiatric disturbance and sometimes epileptic seizures.

A porphyria screen is always undertaken in cases of GBS, but a positive result is very uncommon.

Management is initially focused on withdrawing or avoiding any drugs that might exacerbate the porphyria. Adequate hydration and continuous IV glucose infusion are important. If the weakness progresses, it is worth considering IV haematin (2–5 mg/kg per day for 10–14 days depending on the clinical response), which suppresses the haem biosynthetic pathway. Recovery rate is variable.

VITAMIN DEFICIENCIES

Peripheral neuropathy is not a major feature of **vitamin B12 deficiency**, but loss of ankle reflexes confirms its presence. Sensory nerve conduction studies are abnormal. The predominant clinical features are a result of spinal cord involvement (see p. 492).

The features of **vitamin E deficiency** are gait ataxia, posterior column loss, ophthalmoplegia and a pigmentary retinopathy. There is a mild neuropathic component with loss of ankle reflexes.

Thiamine deficiency in the Western world essentially occurs in the context of chronic alcoholism where the neuropathy seen here is identical clinically to that seen in isolated thiamine deficiency. There are distal paraesthesiae and burning pains in the feet with some distal leg weakness. When there is severe nutritional deprivation, patients develop a painful sensory neuropathy, central scotomata, oral ulceration and dermatitis (Strachan syndrome). The Cuban neuropathy epidemic (1993) was probably nutritional in origin and responded to vitamin B supplementation.

INFECTIVE CAUSES

HIV

Better testing and more effective treatments with antiretroviral agents has lead to an improvement in survival for many who carry HIV or who have fully developed acquired immunodeficiency syndrome (AIDS). Heterosexual contact gives rise to 10–15% of new HIV infection cases, which has to be considered as a possible causal factor in many patients presenting with neuropathy.

HIV-related neuropathies (see p. 411)
- GBS, CIDP, sensory ataxia – at seroconversion
- Multiple mononeuropathy
- Painful distal sensorimotor neuropathy – late stage of AIDS
- Autonomic neuropathy – late stage of AIDS
- Polyradiculoneuropathy/cauda equina syndrome as a result of cytomegalovirus (CMV) infection
- Painful sensory neuropathy – related to treatment (ddC and ddI).

In the early stages of HIV infection a clinically significant neuropathy is unusual, particularly if the CD4 T-cell count is above 400/mm^3.

As patients become more immunocompromised a neuropathy will be found in up to 30% and the commonest type by far is a symmetric sensory axonal neuropathy.

The clinical presentation of HIV-related GBS or CIDP is the same as for non-HIV cases. There is usually a difference on CSF examination, where the presence of an **active lymphocytosis (20–40 cells/mm^3)**, strongly suggests the possibility of HIV infection. (In any GBS or CIDP case where the CSF shows a raised lymphocyte count, the patient should be counselled and tested for HIV.) The treatment of choice is IVIg. Plasma exchange and steroids (for CIDP) can also be used but carry greater risks in an already immunosuppressed patient. The multiple

mononeuropathy seen with HIV infection or AIDS is likely to have a varied aetiology but three factors are: CMV infection, a necrotizing vasculitis and the presence of cryoglobulins. Such patients should be screened for CMV (blood and CSF) and undergo a nerve biopsy. Anti-CMV drugs (e.g. ganciclovir) may be indicated, but if the CMV screen is negative and the biopsy confirms a vasculitis, the initial recommended treatment is IVIg, reserving steroids for those patients who fail to respond to IVIg. If cryoglobulins are found, plasma exchange can be effective.

A **distal symmetric polyneuropathy** (see p. 411) occurs in over 30% of HIV patients who are severely immunocompromised (CD4 count <150 cells/mm^3) and this incidence is increasing as a result of longer survival and improved treatment. Sensory symptoms of paraesthesiae with numbness appear first in the feet. Distal weakness is variable but usually mild. Nerve conduction studies confirm a distal axonopathy. Multiple factors are likely to be involved (nutritional state, drug therapy and other metabolic abnormalities) including the possibility of a direct neurotoxic effect of HIV itself. There is no specific treatment other than trying to control pain (e.g. gabapentin, carbamazepine), which is often resistant to therapy. Distinguishing this neuropathy from the **painful sensorimotor neuropathy caused by antiretroviral drugs** (ddC, ddI) is difficult. The neuropathy appears about 8 weeks after starting treatment and withdrawal of the drugs is the only treatment, but even then the neuropathy can worsen over the next 6 weeks (a phenomenon known as 'coasting'). Zidovudine (AZT) does not cause a neuropathy but can produce weakness as a result of a myopathy.

A **rapidly progressive cauda equina syndrome** is seen in the late stage of HIV infection. This is usually caused by CMV infection of the lumbar roots, but as CSF cultures for CMV are only positive in about 50% of cases, anti-CMV treatment should be started early if the diagnosis is suspected on clinical grounds. The syndrome begins with severe lower back pain that radiates down the legs followed by progressive leg weakness and eventually a lumbar sensory level with bladder and bowel disturbance. Usually the CSF shows an elevated white cell count with raised protein and low glucose levels. An autonomic neuropathy occurs only very late in the course of HIV infection.

Diphtheria

In the Western world, neuropathy related to diph-theria is very rare because of the success of immu-nization programmes.

> Following a throat infection, paralysis of pharyn-geal and laryngeal muscles develops, and some weeks later a generalized sensorimotor neuropathy appears with prominent paraesthesiae and often severe weakness.

This can look like CIDP. The NCS may be very slow (15–20 m/s) confirming a demyelinating process. Unless diagnosed early, when diphtheria antitoxin can be given (within 48 hours of onset), treatment is supportive.

Leprosy

Peripheral nerve damage in all forms of leprosy is caused by direct invasion of peripheral nerves by the bacillus *Mycobacterium leprae* and the immune reaction that follows. Although there are clinical and pathological differences between the various forms, the **main common feature is sensory loss**. Early on, the sensory impairment does not fit with a peripheral nerve distribution as the damage is in the intracutaneous nerves. Pinprick and temperature loss predominate with loss of sweating. Neuropathy related to leprosy is **a treatable condition**, and should be considered in the differential diagnosis of a **mono-neuropathy** or **multiple mononeuropathy** in anyone who has come from or travelled in an endemic area. If infection is suspected, the patient should be referred to a tropical disease unit where the diagnosis can be confirmed by skin or nerve biopsy. Treatment is with dapsone, rifampicin and clofazimine. A hyper-sensitivity reaction to treatment can be a potentially serious complication.

Tuberculoid leprosy causes a localized neuropathy. There may be one or two patches of cutaneous sensory loss at the site of entry of the bacillus and if it multi-plies and invades a nearby nerve trunk then a mono-neuropathy will develop. The median, ulnar, peroneal and facial nerves are most frequently affected.

In the **lepromatous** (or low resistance) form, there is a more widespread loss of sensation, beginning distally in the limbs in an asymmetric manner even-tually coalescing to produce a more symmetric pat-tern. The bacilli proliferate in cool areas, and so the ears are the first area to be affected by numbness. Haematogenous spread of bacilli in this low resistance type contributes to the eventual symmetric distribu-tion of the neuropathy, which in the later stages has a prominent motor component. The peripheral nerves become thickened but reflexes are retained, often until the neuropathy is advanced. **Borderline leprosy** shows a variable spectrum of clinical features between the tuberculoid and lepromatous types.

MALIGNANCY

> An underlying malignancy is an important consideration in the differential diagnosis of a neuropathy.

Detailed screening for malignancy should how-ever only be carried out if the neuropathy has fea-tures consistent with the syndromes outlined below. The most frequent are a **paraneoplastic sensori-motor and pure sensory neuropathy**. Direct infiltra-tion of nerve, root or plexus is well recognized but uncommon. **Chemotherapy** agents used to treat cancer can also produce a neuropathy.

The best defined paraneoplastic syndrome is the one associated with **severe sensory loss** and **result-ing sensory ataxia** with relatively normal muscle strength. It is also called a sensory neuronopathy.

> The commonest underlying tumour is a small cell lung carcinoma, but tumours of breast, ovary, prostate, testes, and stomach can be causative, as can lymphoma.

Anti-Hu antibodies may be present, but are more likely to be positive in the more complex syndrome of paraneoplastic encephalomyelitis/sensory neu-ronopathy ('anti-Hu syndrome') and some of these patients may also have an autonomic neuropathy (see p. 503).

Paraneoplastic neuropathies

- Demyelinating sensorimotor
  Acute (GBS-like) neuropathy associated with Hodgkin's disease
  Chronic form (CIDP-like), associated with non-Hodgkin's lymphoma and osteosclerotic myeloma
- Axonal sensorimotor – less well defined
- Vasculitic
  A hypersensitivity reaction related to some haematological malignancies
  Immune-complex mediated with cryoglobulin production – related to chronic lymphocytic leukaemia, lymphoma, Waldenström's macroglobulinaemia
- Sensory
  May precede finding of malignancy (small cell lung tumour) by up to 2 years Subacute in onset with pain a marked sensory ataxia
  Associated with antineuronal antibodies (anti-Hu, anti-amphiphysin)
  Females more frequently affected than males.

Treatment with IVIg has been tried without benefit. Removal of the primary tumour does not ameliorate the neuropathy.

MONOCLONAL GAMMOPATHIES

Serum protein electrophoresis should be performed on every patient with a neuropathy. A monoclonal paraprotein is associated with 10% of otherwise cryptogenic neuropathies.

Detection of a paraprotein (IgM, IgG or IgA) raises the possibility of underlying myeloma, lymphoma, macroglobulinaemia or systemic amyloidosis. If the appropriate investigations are negative, then the patient has a benign monoclonal gammopathy of unknown significance (MGUS).

Screening tests for a monoclonal gammopathy

- Full blood count, erythrocyte sedimentation rate (ESR), creatinine, calcium
- Paraprotein concentration (<3 g/dl indicates a benign paraprotein)
- Urinalysis for Bence–Jones protein
- Skeletal survey
- Bone marrow examination – ask for haematological opinion as this is often not required providing the other tests are normal.

Monoclonal gammopathy of unknown significance (MGUS)

The chance finding of a monoclonal paraprotein increases with age so that one may be detected in 1% of those aged over 50 years and 3% of those over 70 years, the vast majority of whom have no evidence of a neuropathy.

Of those with an MGUS and neuropathy, 55% will have IgM, 35% will have IgG and 10% IgA paraproteins. The light chain class is usually Kappa.

Clinical features of MGUS neuropathy

- Symmetric distal sensorimotor neuropathy; 20% pure sensory neuropathy
- Paraesthesiae a prominent early symptom
- Prominent ataxia (especially IgM-MGUS)
- Postural tremor in 49–90% of cases (especially IgM-MGUS)
- Slowly progressive over many years with evolving motor weakness
- Males more frequently affected than females
- Peak incidence 50–70 years old
- Antibody to myelin-associated glycoprotein (MAG) – in >50% of IgM-MGUS.

The NCS shows a demyelinating neuropathy in 40% of cases.

MAG is a glycoprotein that accounts for 1% of peripheral nerve myelin. Although strongly associated with IgM paraproteinaemia, and separated by some authors into an 'anti-MAG syndrome', it was at one time believed that patients with this syndrome responded better to immunotherapy than did those with the ordinary IgM-MGUS neuropathy. Recent studies reveal that IVIg does not appear to help. The role of newer immunosuppressants such as fludarabine and rituximab has yet to be studied in controlled trials.

For IgG-MGUS and IgA-MGUS neuropathies, the response to immunotherapy (prednisolone with or without cyclophosphamide, IVIg or plasma exchange) is more encouraging, and should be considered if the neuropathy is progressing at a rapid rate. Frequently, however, these neuropathies, like IgM-MGUS neuropathy, are chronic and very slowly progressive and the decision to start immunotherapy is much more difficult. Occasionally patients with MGUS neuropathy can have a clinical pattern similar to CIDP. Whether this is a distinct entity from CIDP is not known. The treatment should be as for CIDP, although the feeling is that this group (CIDP-MGUS) have a more protracted clinical course and are less responsive to therapies than ordinary CIDP.

CONNECTIVE TISSUE DISEASES AND OTHER VASCULITIDES

The peripheral neuropathy associated with connective tissue disease usually has an immune-mediated or inflammatory/vasculitic basis. Although classic teaching is that a multiple mononeuropathy is the usual clinical picture of a vasculitic process, it is in fact more common to have an overlap picture of multiple mononeuropathy together with a distal symmetric polyneuropathy.

With **rheumatoid arthritis a distal symmetric axonal sensorimotor neuropathy** occurs, which is often painful. In some but not all patients there will be an underlying vasculitis. More aggressive necrotizing vasculitis is usually associated with more chronic rheumatoid disease with evidence of digital vasculitis (e.g. nailbed infarcts) and raised ESR. The clinical picture is typically a **multiple mononeuropathy**. Nerve biopsy is needed to confirm the presence of an active vasculitis. **Entrapment neuropathies** are much more commonly found and are a result of proliferative joint and synovial fluid membrane inflammation (see p. 500).

One of four types of significant neuropathy can occur in about 10% of patients with usually **advanced systemic lupus erythematosus (SLE)** (see p. 499). The **sensorimotor type** is the commonest and as with rheumatoid arthritis, it may be vasculitic and needs nerve biopsy confirmation. A necrotizing vasculitis produces a **multiple mononeuropathy**. The third type is an **acquired demyelinating neuropathy**, which could be in the form of CIDP or GBS. Finally a **trigeminal neuropathy** can complicate SLE – it may be unilateral or bilateral and is often painful. Treatment of the trigeminal neuropathy is very difficult as it responds poorly to immunosuppression.

Peripheral nervous system complications are seen in 10–50% of patients with **primary Sjögren's syndrome** (see p. 501), and are more variable than those encountered in other connective tissue diseases. The commonest type is a **distal axonal sensorimotor neuropathy**, with the main features being pain and numbness of the feet, with only minimal weakness. Some autonomic features may also be present. This neuropathy can predate the onset of the sicca syndrome. Vasculitic changes may be seen on nerve biopsy but the response to steroids is variable, and in general treatment is only considered if this usually slowly changing neuropathy progresses more rapidly than expected. A **sensory neuronopathy** is a much rarer complication, resulting from lymphocytic infiltration of dorsal root ganglia (ganglionitis). The patient complains of paraesthesiae affecting the limbs, trunk and face, with loss mainly of large fibre function and areflexia. As the condition progresses, sensory ataxia becomes the main feature. There may be autonomic involvement. The differential diagnosis lies between a paraneoplastic and idiopathic sensory neuronopathy and as the clinical features are very similar, the diagnosis depends on the relevant antibody tests (anti-Hu or ENA (extractable nuclear antigens)) being positive or negative, a positive Schirmer test and biopsy evidence of inflammation in a salivary gland to confirm the diagnosis of Sjögren's syndrome. There is no convincing evidence supporting the role of immunosuppression. Case reports document benefit with IVIg, but it is well recognized that this neuropathy can show recovery without treatment.

Neuropathy associated with Sjögren's syndrome
- Symmetric sensorimotor (predominantly sensory) neuropathy

- Ataxic sensory neuropathy (neuronopathy)
- CIDP (as with SLE)
- Trigeminal neuropathy (as with SLE).

Systemic necrotizing vasculitis can occur in the setting of specific disorders such as **polyarteritis nodosa, Churg–Strauss syndrome** and **Wegner's granulomatosis** (see p. 501), in addition to the connective tissue disease outline above. A necrotizing vasculitis may also be tissue specific, that is, affecting only the peripheral nerve **(non-systemic vasculitis)** and this is by far the commonest type to present in the neurology clinic, and because of its restricted pathology, the prognosis is better than for a systemic vasculitis.

Whatever the type of vasculitis, the peripheral nerve manifestations are similar, and classically it presents as a **multiple mononeuropathy** affecting the common peroneal, posterior tibial, ulnar, median and radial in descending order of frequency. It has to be remembered that up to 25% of patients will present as a **symmetric sensorimotor neuropathy**, although there is often a clue in the history of an asymmetric onset to the symptoms.

Blood tests are required to assess other organ involvement and to try to identify an underlying cause (see below). Examination of the CSF rarely adds information that will change clinical management, unless the neurological picture is more complicated (i.e. CNS involvement in addition to a neuropathy).

Investigations in suspected vasculitic neuropathy

- full blood count with differential, ESR, CRP, U&E, LFT, glucose
- ANA (and anti-Ro, anti-La), RF, complement levels
- Urinalysis.

If the above are inconclusive, consider:

- ANCA, cryoglobulins, HIV, Lyme serology, hepatitis B and C
- Nerve conduction studies
- Tissue biopsy – nerve ± muscle biopsy, or a kidney biopsy if there is renal involvement.

Table 7.12 Immunosuppressive treatment for vasculitic neuropathy

Mild/moderate neuropathy
Oral prednisolone 1.5 mg/kg per day for 14 days switching to alternate day regimen thereafter. Dose to be slowly reduced
Severe neuropathy
i.v. methyl prednisolone 1 g/day for 5 days with oral cyclophosphamide 2.0–2.5 mg/kg per day (i.v. pulsed cyclophosphamide is of equal efficacy to oral treatment)
Also start on oral prednisolone 1.5 mg/kg per day

Never rely on the nerve biopsy changes alone to establish or refute a diagnosis of vasculitic neuropathy. The vasculitis is patchy and can be easily missed in the small sensory nerve biopsy. Once the diagnosis has been made, vasculitic neuropathy requires treatment with immunosuppressants (Table 7.12). Once there is clear evidence of clinical improvement, the prednisolone dose can be gradually reduced and swapped to an alternate-day regimen. Prophylactic treatment is required to prevent osteoporosis, but routine use of H2-blockers is not indicated. The cyclophosphamide will need to be continued for 1 year (maybe longer if there is ongoing renal involvement). Alternatives to cyclophosphamide are ciclosporin or methotrexate. The role of IVIg may expand as there is case report evidence that it can be effective in the acute stages of vasculitic neuropathy.

INHERITED NEUROPATHIES

Increasingly, inherited neuropathies are characterized according to their chromosomal and gene abnormalities. The field is forever changing, with the original clinical classification being replaced by a genetic classification.

Charcot–Marie–Tooth (CMT) neuropathies

The clinical classification was HMSN and this has been replaced by the genetic-based classification of

Charcot–Marie–Tooth (CMT) neuropathies. Some of the terms are interchangeable – for example, CMT1 and HMSN I, CMT2 and HMSN II – but only to a limited degree, and as expansion of the classification in the future is going to be genetically based, the terminology here will be confined to CMT. The term Dejerine–Sottas disease is preferred to the previous term HMSN III; it is not CMT3 as the genetic abnormality is the same as for CMT1 (Table 7.13).

Charcot–Marie–Tooth type 1 (CMT1) is the most frequently encountered form of hereditary neuropathy and to date three genetic variants have been identified, with **CMT1A being the commonest (70% of patients)**. The **inheritance is autosomal dominant** with symptoms appearing by late childhood.

Because of this early onset, skeletal abnormalities such as pes cavus and clawed toes are seen and may be the first clinical feature. There is distal wasting and weakness in the legs and also in a majority of cases involving the arms, with more severe cases having clawing of the fingers. Tendon reflexes are depressed or absent and distal sensory loss affects all modalities. About one-third of patients will have a positional upper limb tremor. Palpable thickening of peripheral nerves occurs in 50% of patients. Sensory symptoms are not a major feature, although patients may complain of musculoskeletal pain.

As a general rule, if there are prominent sensory symptoms one should think of another neuropathy other than CMT. The NCS show uniform slowing of motor and sensory velocities ($<30\,\text{m/s}$ in the legs).

The molecules identified so far as being involved in the pathogenesis of CMT1 are:

1 **Peripheral myelin protein (PMP-22)**, a glycoprotein of 22 kDa found in the compact region of peripheral myelin. Its exact function is not known, but it is believed to have a role as a growth arrest protein in Schwann cells and as an adhesive for the myelin sheath. In CMT1, there is duplication of the PMP22 gene. It appears that the neuropathic phenotype does

Table 7.13 Charcot-Marie-Tooth neuropathies

	Chromosome locus	Gene	Mechanism
CMT Type 1			
CMT1A	17p11.2	PMP22	Duplication
CMT1B	1q22	PO	Point mutation
CMT1C	Not known		
CMT1D	10q21.1	EGR2	Point mutation
CMT Type 2			
CMT2A	1p36	Not known	
CMT2B	3q13	Not known	
CMT2C	Not known		
CMT2D	7p14		
CMT2E	1q22	PO	
Dejerine-Sottas disease			
DSDA	17p11.2	PMP22	Point mutation
DSDB	1q22	PO	Point mutation
CMT Type 4			
CMT4A	8q13	Not known	
CMT4B	11q23	Not known	
CMT4C	5q23	Not known	
CMT4L	8q24	Not known	
X-linked dominant CMT			
(CMTX)	Xq13.1	Connexin 32	Point mutation

PMP, peripheral myelin protein; PO, protein zero; EGR, early growth response.

depend on a dosage effect, that is, whether PMP22 is either overexpressed (as in duplication) or underexpressed (as in point mutations).

2 **Protein zero (PO)** accounts for 50–60% of peripheral nerve protein and plays a vital role in myelin compaction.

3 **Early growth response gene 2 (EGR2)** is expressed by myelinating Schwann cells and plays a role in peripheral myelination. The result of alterations in these genes is a disruption in the stability of the myelin sheath. The mechanisms for these gene changes are unknown.

Charcot–Marie–Tooth type 2 (CMT2) is clinically very similar to CMT1 but much less common. In CMT2A the onset is a little later (sometimes late teens), upper limb involvement is not as prominent and nerve thickening does not occur when compared to CMT1. The neurophysiology does separate CMT2 from CMT1 in that in the former the changes are those of an axonal neuropathy. Of the CMT2 variants, CMT2B is associated with foot ulcers, CMT2C with stridor and vocal cord paralysis and CMT2D is associated with early onset of hand weakness and wasting.

The majority of cases of **Dejerine–Sottas disease** are now thought to be sporadic (rather than recessively inherited). It is now considered to be a severe variant of CMT1 as the gene defects are similar. The onset is at birth or early childhood with generalized limb and truncal weakness and often severe kyphoscoliosis, pes cavus and clawed toes. The MCVs (motor conduction velocities) are usually below 12 m/s.

Autosomal recessive CMT cases are rare, and now come under the umbrella of **CMT4**. The most recent addition is CMT4L (CMT-Lom, after the Bulgarian town where the original cases were described), which occurred in a gypsy population and is characterized by a severe sensorimotor neuropathy, deafness and skeletal abnormalities.

X-linked dominant CMT (CMTX) may account for a many as 10–15% of CMT cases. The clinical findings are similar to those of CMT1, but the clue comes from the absence of male-to-male transmission, and the fact that females who carry the gene are usually asymptomatic or very mildly affected. In affected males, NCS are similar to those in CMT1, but recent studies show that these individuals have delayed brainstem auditory evoked potentials. A number of mutations have been documented in the gene for connexin 32, a gap junction protein that allows the transfer of small molecules and ions through the compacted myelin sheath.

Hereditary neuropathy with liability to pressure palsies

Hereditary neuropathy with liability to pressure palsies (HNPP) is dominantly inherited and is usually caused by a deletion at chromosome 17p11.2 (HNPPA); those few families not linked to 17p11.2 are labelled HNPPB. It is now therefore grouped with CMT neuropathies.

> Typically the onset of symptoms is in the group aged 20–40 years, with awareness of a susceptibility to nerve palsies, usually after minor compression or trauma.

There is usually good recovery from the mononeuropathy but sometimes surgical decompression is helpful. The most frequently affected areas are the ulnar nerve at the elbow and the common peroneal nerve at the fibula head. There may be an associated mild sensorimotor neuropathy with pes cavus. Another uncommon manifestation is a painless brachial plexopathy.

Familial amyloid polyneuropathies

The majority of the dominantly inherited familial amyloid polyneuropathies are caused by mutations in the **transthyretin (TTR) gene on chromosome 18 (transthyretin amyloidoses)**. What is now clear is that with the increasing number of missense mutations being discovered, the clinical picture can be extremely variable. Onset can be from the age of 30 to 60 years, but a predominantly small fibre neuropathy with autonomic involvement should raise suspicion of a TTR amyloidosis.

> The classical clinical features are of a painful sensorimotor neuropathy with autonomic failure and an increased incidence of carpal tunnel syndrome. There is often vitreous opacification, nephropathy and cardiomyopathy, and the latter is the commonest cause of death.

As most TTR is produced in the liver, liver transplantation has been clearly shown to halt the progression of the neuropathy and even to improve the neuropathy. This however is not curative as cardiac dysfunction continues to deteriorate.

Other familial amyloid polyneuropathies are caused by mutations in the apolipoprotein A1 gene on chromosome 11, and the gelsolin gene on chromosome 9. They are clinically distinct from TTR amyloidosis, but are very rare.

The cornerstone for diagnosis for amyloid neuropathy, familial or acquired, is finding **amyloid deposition in tissue biopsy** (rectum, kidney, skin and sural nerve). Antibody kits can identify TTR. Because of patchy deposition, a negative biopsy does not exclude the diagnosis. The advent of DNA testing has not made securing the diagnosis that much easier, as most routine laboratories will only offer screening of the commonest mutations (usually methionine-30).

Hereditary sensory and autonomic neuropathies

The hereditary sensory and autonomic neuropathies (HSAN) are rare neuropathies with recent evidence linking pathogenesis to abnormalities of the nerve growth factor family of neurotrophins. The classification at present is outlined below. In addition to the groupings I to IV, many cases exist that do not fit the established clinical criteria and some have been proposed as HSAN V and HSAN VI.

Hereditary sensory and autonomic neuropathies
- HSAN I (autosomal dominant)
- HSAN II (autosomal recessive)
- HSAN III (autosomal recessive in Ashkenazi Jews)
- HSAN IV (autosomal recessive, congenital insensitivity to pain with anhidrosis).

Of the various types, HSAN I (gene locus on chromosome 9q22.1 but exact gene not identified) is the commonest, and the hallmarks of clinical presentation are spontaneous pains in the feet or painless foot ulcers. Sweating abnormalities occur but other autonomic features are not found in this type. Foot deformity as a result of repeated painless stress fractures and neuropathic arthropathy may be the presenting feature. Symptoms can start at any time between the ages of 10 and 50 years and the clinical course is slowly progressive. HSAN II starts in early childhood with painless injuries to the hands and feet, marked distal deformities and later more prominent autonomic problems. HSAN III is virtually confined to Ashkenazi Jews and has been mapped to chromosome 9q31. Onset is in infancy with bulbar problems and unexplained intermittent fevers.

REFERENCES AND FURTHER READING

Dyck PJ, Thomas PK (eds) (1993) *Peripheral neuropathy*, 3rd edn. Philadelphia: WB Saunders.

Dyck PJ, Windebank AJ (2002) Diabetic and non-diabetic lumbosacral radioplexus neuropathies: new insights into pathophysiology and treatment. *Muscle Nerve*, 25:477–491 (review).

Hughes RAC (2002) Regular review: peripheral neuropathy. *British Medical Journal*, 324:466–469.

Latov N, Wokke JHJ, Kelly JJ (eds) (1998) *Immunological and Infectious Diseases of the Peripheral Nerves.* Cambridge, UK: Cambridge University Press.

Mendell JR, Kissel JT, Cornblath DR (eds) (2001) *Diagnosis and Management of Peripheral Nerve Disorders.* Contemporary neurology series. Oxford, UK: Oxford University Press.

Rosenberg NR, Portegis P, de Visser M, Vermulen M (2001) Diagnostic investigation of patients with chronic polyneuropathy: evaluation of a clinical guideline. *Journal of Neurology, Neurosurgery and Psychiatry*, 71:205–209.

Sapperstein DS, Katz JS, Amato AA, Barohn RJ (2001) Clinical spectrum of chronic acquired demyelinating polyneuropathies. *Muscle Nerve*, 24:311–324.

Schenone A, Mancardi GL (1999) Molecular basis of inherited neuropathies. *Current Opinion in Neurology*, 12:603–616.

CHAPTER 8

NERVE AND ROOT LESIONS

T.J. Fowler

PRESSURE PALSIES

Compression of peripheral nerves may occur acutely or as part of a more chronic process. This may result in damage varying in severity. Mild compression is readily recognized and is experienced when sitting with the legs crossed, causing compression of the common peroneal nerve on the head of the fibula. With any duration of compression the blood supply to the nerve is compromised, **tingling develops and later numbness and weakness appear in the territory of the affected nerve**. With relief from the compression, there is usually rapid and complete recovery.

Moderate compression will produce damage to the insulating myelin sheath (segmental demyelination), producing a local conduction block or slowing of conduction with preservation of the continuity of the axon. This is called a **neurapraxia**. Usually the large, fast-conducting myelinated fibres are involved but small and unmyelinated fibres may be spared so that there is often preservation of some sensation. Repair is by remyelination and is usually complete with full recovery within a number of weeks or even months.

More severe compression will damage the myelin sheath and the axon leading to axonal degeneration (Wallerian) distal to the site of injury. There will be conduction block in the distal part of the affected nerve.

The muscles supplied by the nerve become inexcitable, later showing signs of denervation with the development of fasciculation and wasting. The nerve trunk remains in continuity. Small and unmyelinated fibres are commonly involved. This type of damage is termed an **axonotmesis**. Repair is by regeneration over many months at the rate of 1–2 mm/day and may be incomplete.

If the nerve is severed or torn apart, causing the connective tissue framework to separate and disrupting the continuity of the axons and myelin sheaths, the ends of the nerve are free: this is termed a **neurotmesis**. In this situation unless the two ends are sutured together or lie in close proximity, repair is by regeneration and is likely to be poor.

Nerve conduction studies will usually give appropriate information about the pathogenesis of such lesions and may demarcate the site of damage if there is a local conduction block. The electrical signs following axonal degeneration may take 5–7 days

Table 8.1 Entrapment neuropathies

Common entrapment neuropathies
  Median nerve in the carpal tunnel
  Ulnar nerve at the elbow
  Lateral cutaneous nerve of the thigh at the
  inguinal ligament
  Common peroneal nerve at the head of the fibula
Rare entrapment neuropathies
  Ulnar nerve at the wrist
  Radial nerve
  Posterior tibial nerve in the tarsal tunnel
  Lower cord of the brachial plexus by cervical rib
  or fibrous band

to appear in affected muscles after a severe injury. Electrodiagnostic tests performed too early, within 2–3 days of injury, may prove misleading.

Many compressive nerve lesions are a mixture of axonal degeneration and demyelination.

Acute compression may arise in an unconscious patient as a result of direct pressure of the weight of an inert limb against a sharp edge or unyielding surface. Patients with a depressed conscious level from sedative drugs, excess alcohol or a general anaesthetic are particularly at risk. The 'Saturday night paralysis' of the drunk is the classic example, where the radial nerve in the upper arm is compressed against the humerus as the arm hangs over a chair back. Such damage may be of varying severity so that pressure palsies may take weeks or even months to repair.

Chronic compression or entrapment is likely to arise at certain sites where peripheral nerves travel in fibro-osseous tunnels or over bony surfaces so the nerve may be constricted, stretched or deformed (Table 8.1). The damage may be persistent or intermittent and the term entrapment is often used for lesions where surgical release of the compression may afford relief. In chronic entrapment the affected nerve may appear thickened at the site and this may be palpable. It should be emphasized that nerves already 'sick' or damaged from some other neuropathic process are more liable to compression; that is, the two faults summate. Thus patients with a diabetic neuropathy are particularly prone to develop a carpal tunnel syndrome. A past history of other compressive neuropathic lesions always raises the possibility of

an underlying hereditary neuropathy with a liability to pressure palsies (see p. 171). Occasionally neoplastic or granulomatous infiltration of nerves may produce local compressive lesions, such as with leprosy, lymphoma.

Acute traction or stretch injuries can sometimes produce severe nerve damage, as when the brachial plexus is injured by a motor cyclist landing forcefully on the shoulder. In such injuries the nerve roots may actually be torn out of the spinal cord with complete loss of continuity. Such severe injuries will produce signs of denervation in the affected arm muscles and there may be no recovery. Imaging may be possible with magnetic resonance imaging (MRI) or with contrast-enhanced myelography to show such damage and electrodiagnostic studies may also be helpful.

Causalgia (see p. 520) describes the severe pain produced by a partial injury to a peripheral nerve. Such pain is often intense and burning, with contact sensitivity, and may prove difficult to control. There may be accompanying sudomotor, vasomotor and trophic changes. A complex regional pain syndrome (reflex sympathetic dystrophy) is a term used to describe an excessive or abnormal response of the sympathetic nervous system (see p. 520) most often following an injury to the shoulder or arm, less commonly the leg. Usually there are complaints of troublesome pain, with impaired motor function and sensation, sweating, temperature changes, swelling, often pallor or cyanosis, and later trophic changes, sometimes with osteoporosis.

In these excessively painful conditions treatment relies on the combination of centrally acting drugs, such as amitriptyline, with block of peripheral pain fibres, with regional guanethidine block, for example. This may be accompanied by physiotherapy. Treatments are explored further in Chapter 26.

CARPAL TUNNEL SYNDROME (CTS)

The median nerve may be compressed in the fibroosseous carpal tunnel at the wrist. The nerve is supplied from the C6, C7, C8 and T1 roots. Certain features increase the risks of carpal tunnel compression (Table 8.2): women have narrower tunnels; the

Table 8.2 Carpal tunnel syndrome

Carpal tunnel syndrome may be associated with:
Pregnancy
Diabetes mellitus
Myxoedema
Acromegaly
Rheumatoid arthritis
Previous wrist trauma
Myeloma
Amyloid

presence of rheumatoid arthritis; osteoarthritis or deformity from previous fractures, for example Colles', may encroach on the nerve. Diabetes mellitus, myxoedema, acromegaly, deposition of amyloid or even myeloma may compromise the nerve and there is an increased incidence in pregnancy. The symptoms are aggravated by use, particularly manual work.

Symptoms and signs

> **Symptoms of CTS**
> Symptoms include nocturnal painful tingling, usually described in the fingers and hand, spreading up the forearm but not usually above the elbow. The symptoms may awaken the patient from sleep or appear on waking, or with lifting, carrying in certain positions, or with driving. They are usually eased by hanging the hand down, moving it about or changing position.

There may be no abnormal signs, although with more severe lesions the thenar pad muscles appear wasted and weak, particularly the *abductor pollicis brevis*, and some sensory changes may appear in the tips of the thumb, index, middle and ring fingers (Figure 8.1). A tourniquet test may be positive in patients with no signs, when inflation of the cuff around the upper arm rapidly produces similar sensory symptoms in the affected fingers within minutes. Phalen's test describes how forced wrist flexion may provoke similar sensory symptoms.

Investigation

Nerve conduction studies in early compression will show diminution of the size of the sensory action potentials with delay seen first in the median palmar

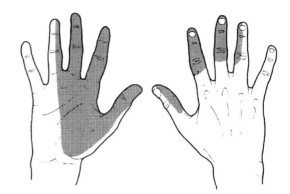

Figure 8.1 Area of sensory loss in the right median nerve lesion.

branches. Later there may be absence of the median sensory action potentials, prolonged distal motor latencies and even signs of denervation in the *abductor pollicis brevis*. These studies have some predictive value in determining the outcome from decompression. Very severe damage (absent sensory action potentials and poor motor responses) may be followed by imperfect recovery. Moderate electrical damage is usually followed by a good surgical outcome.

Treatment

Treatment depends on the severity of the lesion and whether there are any added factors, such as diabetes or pregnancy. In mildly affected patients a degree of rest and the use of a wrist splint at night may give relief. In a few patients local injection of steroids under the carpal ligament may also be of benefit, together with a reduction in the amount of manual work performed. In more severely affected patients, surgical decompression will be necessary. This will usually relieve pain and sensory upset, although severe muscle wasting (in the thenar pad) may not recover, particularly in the elderly. Occasionally surgery may not relieve symptoms, raising the possibility of an incorrect diagnosis or inadequate decompression. Further conduction studies may be useful in such instances.

ULNAR NERVE LESIONS

The ulnar nerve arises from the roots of C8 and T1. The most common ulnar nerve lesion is compression

a ganglion (which may arise from the superior tibiofibular joint) or even from the tendinous edge of *peroneus longus*.

Symptoms and signs

The presentation may be with a painless foot drop, which may become more noticeable if the patient is tired or has walked any distance. This may cause the patient to trip. There is weakness of *tibialis anterior* and often the evertors, with a preserved ankle jerk. **The sensory loss is variable** (Figure 8.4): if the deep peroneal branch is affected the area is small (Figure 8.4).

Investigation

Electromyography studies may show denervation in *tibialis anterior* and *extensor digitorum brevis*. There may be a local conduction block or slowing in the region of the head of the fibula. Usually the ascending common peroneal nerve action potential is lost. The

sural nerve action potential is preserved and tibial conduction should be unaffected, which should help to localize the lesion.

Treatment

Physiotherapy, an insert splint or foot drop appliance (orthosis), may be useful while waiting for recovery if an external compressive lesion, or acute trauma has been incriminated. In a few instances the common peroneal nerve may have to be explored to exclude a ganglion or compressive lesion.

LESS COMMON LESIONS

Radial nerve

The nerve is supplied by C7 and to a lesser extent C6 and C8. It supplies the *triceps, brachioradialis, supinator*, wrist and finger extensors and the long abductor of the thumb. Sensation may be impaired on the posterolateral aspect of the forearm or with more distal lesions over the dorsum of the web between the thumb and index finger. **An acute wrist drop is the major fault.**

Most radial palsies reflect acute compression of the nerve either in the axilla or where it winds around the humerus (Saturday night palsy) or from direct trauma. The posterior interosseous nerve may be compressed by a lipoma, ganglion or even where the nerve passes through the *extensor carpi radialis* muscle.

Sciatic nerve

The sciatic nerve is the largest peripheral nerve arising from the roots of L4–S3. It leaves the pelvis through the greater sciatic foramen and runs posteriorly down the thigh where, just above the knee, it divides into the tibial and common peroneal divisions. It lies close to the back of the hip joint and can be damaged if that joint suffers extensive trauma or following hip surgery. In its upper part, the sciatic nerve is covered by the *gluteus maximus* but in the inferior part of the buttock it is relatively superficial and so may be directly damaged by a buttock injection misplaced too medially. The sciatic nerve may also

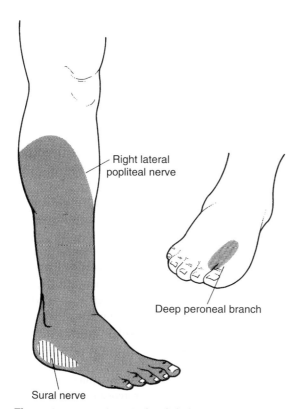

Figure 8.4 Areas of sensory loss in lesions of the right common peroneal and deep peroneal nerves.

be damaged by direct pressure in the unconscious patient: it may also be compressed by tumours on the side of the pelvis. The peroneal nerve fibres lie more laterally in the sciatic nerve and so are more prone to compression.

A high lesion of the sciatic nerve will affect the hamstrings and all the leg muscles below the knee, the calf and anterior tibial as well as the small foot muscles. **This will produce a 'flail' foot with distal wasting and weakness. There will be sensory loss involving the foot and posterolateral aspect of the lower leg** (Figure 8.3). Electrically there will be denervation of the affected muscles, with impaired conduction in the tibial and peroneal nerves and absent sural and common peroneal nerve action potentials.

Femoral nerve

The femoral nerve arises from the L2, L3 and L4 roots, passing through the *psoas* muscle and under the inguinal ligament lateral to the femoral artery, to supply the anterior thigh muscles. It may be compressed by an abscess, a haematoma (often from over anticoagulation) in the *psoas*, or be damaged acutely by fractures of the pelvis, traction during surgery, knife wounds to the groin or from thrombotic lesions of the vasa nervorum, such as in diabetes mellitus.

A femoral nerve lesion will produce weakness of the knee extensors, the quadriceps group, with muscle wasting, a depressed or absent knee jerk, and sensory loss in the anterior thigh and medial part of the knee. The terminal branch of the femoral nerve is the saphenous nerve, which supplies the medial side of the lower leg. There may be mild weakness of the hip flexors, and patients will experience difficulty walking, particularly going up stairs, and the leg may seem to buckle. On EMG there may be denervation in the *quadriceps* and a prolonged distal motor latency when the nerve is stimulated in the groin.

Tarsal tunnel

Rarely, the posterior tibial nerve may be compressed in the tarsal tunnel in the sole of the foot. Usually this will provoke tingling, pain and sometimes 'burning' in the sole and toes which may be worse at night and aggravated by inversion of the ankle. Such symptoms may be provoked by standing or walking. In severe cases there is weakness of *abductor hallucis* and sensory loss distally over the soles and toes. On EMG there may be a prolonged distal motor latency to *abductor hallucis* and in younger patients the medial plantar sensory action potential will be absent. Decompression may be effective treatment.

The long thoracic nerve (of Bell)

The long thoracic nerve (of Bell) supplies the *serratus anterior* muscle arising from C5, C6 and C7 roots. A lesion of this nerve leads to a winged scapula with inability to fix the scapula on the chest wall when the arm is being forcefully flexed, abducted or pushed forward. It may follow an injury, carrying a heavy weight on the shoulders (e.g. rucksack) or from an acute inflammation (see neuralgic amyotrophy). Most recover with time.

BRACHIAL PLEXUS LESIONS

The brachial plexus is formed from the spinal roots of C5–T1 and extends from the spinal canal to the axilla. The roots of C5 and C6 join to form the upper trunk, from C7 the middle trunk, and from C8 and T1 the lower trunk (Figure 8.5). From there they separate into anterior and posterior divisions. The three

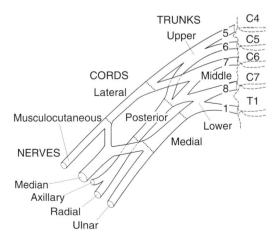

Figure 8.5 Diagram of the brachial plexus.

posterior divisions join to form the posterior cord, the anterior divisions of the upper and middle trunks join to form the lateral cord, and the anterior division of the lower trunk to form the medial cord. These cords pass through the thoracic outlet, between the first rib and clavicle.

Damage to the plexus may arise in a number of ways (Table 8.3). **Trauma** from acute stretching or traction is common and when severe may result in actual avulsion of a nerve root from the spinal cord. The upper trunk is most often affected. Penetrating injuries may also affect the plexus, for example, knife or gunshot wounds. If the lower cord is involved there is often an accompanying Horner's syndrome (Figure 8.6).

Table 8.3 Common causes of brachial plexus damage

Trauma	(a) Avulsion of root, stretch, traction (b) Penetrating injuries
Neoplastic infiltration	Local – breast or lung carcinoma, neurofibroma, sarcoma
Radiotherapy	Radiation fibrosis
Inflammatory	Neuralgic amyotrophy
Diabetic plexopathy	
Mechanical compression	Cervical rib, fibrous band

The signs and symptoms reflect the motor and sensory involvement extending over more territory than that of a single nerve root or peripheral nerve (Table 8.4).

Metastatic infiltration of the plexus most often involves the lower cord, with wasting and weakness of the thenar and hypothenar muscles and also the finger and wrist flexors. The sensory loss extends from the ulnar two fingers up the medial side of the forearm. Pain as an early symptom is common. Spread from a primary breast carcinoma or from an apical lung tumour is the most common. **Radiation fibrosis** produces patchy involvement of the plexus with early sensory symptoms and weakness, progressing slowly. It can be difficult to differentiate from metastatic infiltration.

Electromyography studies will help to confirm the anatomical localization. There is often loss of sensory action potentials, prolonged F-wave latencies, small muscle action potentials and even signs of denervation. Plain X-rays may show cervical ribs, an elongated transverse process on C7 or even an apical shadow. Modern imaging by MRI with gadolinium enhancement or computerized tomography (CT) may show the presence of tumours.

Thoracic outlet compression

The lower cord of the brachial plexus passes across the posterior triangle of the neck behind the

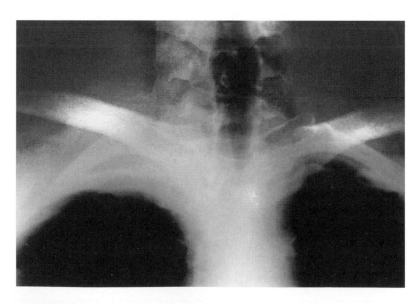

Figure 8.6 Apical chest X-ray to show shadowing at the right apex. This patient presented with wasting of the small muscles of the right hand and had a right Horner's syndrome. The shadow was caused by a lymphoma.

subclavian artery running between *scalenus anterior* and *medius*. If there is an extra cervical rib attached to the transverse process of C7 or a fibrous band attached to an elongated transverse process, either of these may compress the lower cord of the plexus. They may also compress the subclavian artery, producing **vascular symptoms**. These include Raynaud's phenomenon with complaints of coldness and colour changes in the fingers or more severe upsets from arterial or venous obstruction. The radial pulse may disappear in certain arm positions on the affected side and a bruit may be audible in the supraclavicular fossa. Rarely distal emboli may affect the fingers. **Neurological features** include aching and pain radiating down the inner forearm to the ulnar side of the hand, associated with tingling and sometimes numbness.

> Sensory loss can be demonstrated on the medial side of the forearm proximal to the wrist unlike that found in an ulnar nerve lesion. There is often wasting and weakness involving all the intrinsic muscles of the hand, the thenar and hypothenar pads and the medial forearm muscles.

Investigations

Investigations include electrophysiological studies, evoked potentials, X-rays, MRI imaging and even arteriography, if compression of the subclavian artery is suspected.

In severe symptomatic cases surgical treatment may be necessary. It is important to choose a surgeon experienced in the exploration of this region.

Neuralgic amyotrophy (Brachial Neuritis, Parsonage–Turner Syndrome)

Neuralgic amyotrophy is an acute inflammatory disturbance causing patchy damage to the brachial plexus. It is uncommon. The aetiology is unknown, although it may follow a viral infection, immunization or, on rare occasions, be linked with a hereditary liability to pressure palsies.

> The onset is with excruciating severe pain, usually in the shoulder, at the base of the neck or in the arm. Initially this is unremitting, keeping the patient awake and requiring strong analgesics.

The pain may last up to 2–3 weeks and as it remits the patient may be aware of patchy weakness of affected muscles. The most commonly affected muscles are innervated by the axillary, long thoracic and suprascapular nerves. There is associated depression or loss of reflexes and varied sensory loss, most

Table 8.4 Clinical features of disturbances of the brachial plexus

	Pain and sensory symptoms	Sensory loss	Motor loss	Reflex
Upper C5/C6	Lateral shoulder, scapula, supraclavicular fossa, arm to elbow	Deltoid and upper arm	*Deltoid, biceps brachioradialis*	BJ, SJ
Middle C7	Shoulder to hand of index, middle and ring fingers	Palmar and dorsal surfaces	*Triceps*, extensors of wrist and fingers	TJ
Lower C8/T1	Shoulder to hand	Ulnar surface of hand, forearm and arm	Long finger and wrist flexors, intrinsics	FJ
All	Neck to hand	Upper limb	Complete flaccid paralysis	

BJ, biceps jerk; TJ, triceps jerk; FJ, finger jerk.

often in the territory of the axillary nerve. The pattern of the weakness is patchy and a whole muscle may be affected, which may help to differentiate this from an acute cervical root lesion arising from a disc prolapse. **In most patients over a period of months, often 6 months, there is recovery, but in others the progress is slow, up to 18 months, suggesting repair here is by regeneration. About 90% of patients show functional recovery after 3 years.**

Electrical studies will confirm multifocal denervation in affected muscles, commonly with slowing in affected motor nerves with prolonged or absent F-waves. The cerebrospinal fluid may be normal, although a mild lymphocytic pleocytosis and protein rise have been found.

Treatment is symptomatic: analgesics and rest until the acute pain has settled. Steroids have been tried, although there is no good evidence that these are effective. Physiotherapy directed towards strengthening the affected muscles is helpful.

CERVICAL ROOT PROBLEMS

The muscles of the arm are supplied by the C5, C6, C7, C8 and T1 roots. These leave the spinal canal through the intervertebral foramina and may be irritated or compressed, causing symptoms and signs referred to that root. It should be emphasized that the pain from such a lesion is referred into the myotome, which may be different from the site of the sensory symptoms (paraesthesiae, numbness), which are referred to the dermatome (see Figure 4.19). In the cervical spine there are eight exiting nerve roots from the seven vertebrae so that the root exits above the body of the vertebra concerned; that is, the C6 root exits between C5 and C6. Below T1 the roots exit below; that is, T1 exits between T1 and T2.

Causes of cervical root damage

The most common causes of cervical root damage are:
- Compression by an acute soft disc prolapse
- Compression by a hard bony spur in degenerative spondylosis
- Compression by a neuroma, lymphoma, extradural tumour or metastasis.

Cervical root symptoms

Pain in the neck or arm is very common, affecting over 10% of the population. However, only a small number of patients have pain arising from cervical root irritation. More often pain arises from the soft tissues and joints. With cervical root disturbances the initial symptoms are usually increasing pain, often referred to the base of the neck, shoulder, scapula or upper arm. Root pain is often described as shooting, burning or like an electric shock. Later there may be weakness of affected muscles, depression or loss of appropriate reflexes, tingling and numbness.

Commonly affected roots compressed by spondylotic spurs or disc protrusions are C6 (C5/C6 disc space), C7 (C6/C7), C5 (C4/C5) and C8 (C7/T1).

In younger patients there may be an acute soft disc prolapse. If this extends laterally, it will compress the affected root. The root is initially irritated causing referred pain, but if the compression is more severe, the nerve root may infarct, leading to loss of pain but more severe weakness with signs of denervation in the affected muscles, reflex loss and sensory impairment (Table 8.5).

A large central disc protrusion in the neck will lead to compression of the spinal cord, producing a myelopathy with spastic leg weakness, sensory changes in the feet and sometimes disturbed bowel and bladder function. These will be accompanied by long tract signs, increased reflexes, clonus, extensor plantar responses and sensory loss in the feet – most often posterior column impairment.

Most patients with neck problems, particularly root irritation, show pronounced spasm of the nuchal muscles causing greatly limited neck movements. Lateral flexion is particularly affected, for most rotation occurs at the atlanto-axial joint and proximally. Sometimes a 'wry' neck may develop. Lateral flexion or rotation of the neck, which aggravates ipsilateral pain referred down the shoulder or arm, suggests root compression on that side. Neck pain that is worsened on the side contralateral to the

Table 8.5 Localizing features of cervical root disturbances

Root	Pain	Dermatome	Muscle	Reflex
C5	Neck, shoulder, lateral arm to elbow	Lateral deltoid	*Deltoid, spinati, biceps*	BJ, SJ
C6	Neck, lateral arm to thumb and index	Lateral arm, forearm, thumb and index	*Biceps, brachioradialis*	BJ, SJ
C7	Neck, lateral arm to middle finger	Lateral forearm, index, middle and ring fingers	*Triceps*, finger and wrist extensors	TJ
C8	Medial forearm and hand	Medial forearm, ring and little fingers	Finger flexors, abductor of thumb	FJ
T1	Medial arm	Medial arm	Intrinsics – all. Horner's syndrome	

BJ, biceps jerk; TJ, triceps jerk; FJ, finger jerk.

Table 8.6 Investigations of root or plexus lesions

Blood tests	Full blood count, ESR, fasting glucose, serum proteins and 'strip', calcium, phosphatases, CRP
X-rays	Spinal – for collapse, malalignment, pedicle erosion
	Chest – primary tumours, metastases
Imaging	MRI – excellent for cord and root lesions with gadolinium enhancement for neoplastic, infective/inflammatory processes
	CT – for bony lesions
	CT with contrast, intrathecal – for roots and cord lesions myelography (non-ionic contrast) if MRI not possible or not available
Electrodiagnostic	Denervation, neuropathy or myopathy, evoked potentials
Isotope scans	Bone (metastases), infective lesions (gallium)
CSF	Presence of infection/inflammation; demyelination (oligoclonal bands)

ESR, erythrocyte sedimentation rate; CRP, C-reactive protein; MRI, magnetic resonance imaging; CT, computerized tomography; CSF, cerebrospinal fluid.

lateral flexion or rotation suggests a muscular origin to that pain.

In older patients degenerative changes in the spine lead to narrowing of the intervertebral space, with bulging of the disc and hypertrophy of the surrounding ligaments causing these to thicken. The bony margins of the vertebrae become raised, producing hard osteophytic spurs, which may compress nerve roots, the spinal cord or both. The latter causes a **spondylotic radiculo–myelopathy**. Again symptoms and signs depend on the root involved and whether there is spinal cord compression. Failure to recognize spinal cord compression may lead to irreversible damage, with even a tetraplegia and lost sphincter control.

Cervical spondylosis may be aggravated by trauma, particularly if this is repeated. Occasionally patients may give a highly relevant history of trauma causing acute but transient neurological symptoms, for example, paresis in an arm or leg with sensory upset, which recover only to be followed some time later by further symptoms, which may slowly progress.

Investigations (Table 8.6 and see p. 187)

Good quality X-rays of the cervical spine with oblique views will demonstrate spondylotic degenerative changes, encroachment of the exit foramina by osteophytic spurs or malalignment. Bony collapse from unexpected malignant infiltration will also be shown. However, it should be emphasized that as patients grow older, all will show some spondylotic changes in the cervical spine so it is important to put all these in the clinical context of the patient's symptoms and signs before attributing all arm and neck pain to the blanket term 'cervical spondylosis'.

The sagittal diameter of the cervical canal is an important factor in the possible development of a myelopathy. A diameter of 10 mm or less on a true lateral film suggests the cord may be compromised.

Scanning with MRI with sagittal and axial views will show most acute root or cord compressive lesions. It will also show any intramedullary lesion.

In selected patients, CT scanning with contrast may be useful in delineating root disturbances. Myelography may still be used where MRI scanning is not available or in claustrophobic patients. However, the advent of 'open' MRI scanners has largely eliminated fears of claustrophobic patients, who have refused such imaging. Electrical studies may show denervation in appropriate root territories and help to exclude peripheral nerve entrapment or more widespread neuropathic disorders, such as motor neurone disease.

Treatment

Treatment is covered in detail in Chapter 10.

Many older patients with cervical spondylosis and a mild radiculo-myelopathy may be managed conservatively using a cervical collar and physiotherapy.

LUMBOSACRAL PLEXUS

The lumbosacral plexus is formed from the T12–S4 roots and is situated within the substance of the *psoas* muscles. It is divided into an upper part, L1–L4, and a lower part, L4–S4. Over 50% of damage arises in the lower part, about 30% in the upper part, and some 18% involves the whole plexus. Causes of damage are given in Table 8.7.

Table 8.7 Common causes of lumbosacral plexus damage

Trauma	Fracture of the pelvis
Haematoma	Psoas – anticoagulant excess, bleeding diathesis
Diabetic plexopathy	
Infection	Herpes zoster
Neoplastic infiltration	Pelvis – uterine, ovarian carcinoma
	Colonorectal carcinoma
	Lymphoma, sarcoma
Retroperitoneal fibrosis	
Mechanical compression	Traction at surgery

Note bilateral involvement suggests cauda equina/conus lesion within the spinal canal.

Retroperitoneal haematoma (often from an excess dose of anticoagulants or a bleeding diathesis) and a diabetic plexopathy (femoral amyotrophy) are common causes of upper plexus lesions. Malignant infiltration, particularly from pelvic tumours, is a common cause of a lower plexus lesion (Table 8.7).

Again, pain, weakness and sensory loss are common symptoms in one leg, extending outside the territory of a single root or peripheral nerve. **Bilateral leg symptoms suggest a lesion within the spinal canal (cauda equina or lower spinal cord).** If the pudendal nerve is damaged, there may be some impairment of bladder or bowel function. Sympathetic involvement may cause a warm dry foot. If the lymphatics or venous drainage are obstructed, the leg will swell.

A rectal and/or pelvic examination is important.

LUMBAR ROOT LESIONS

In the other mobile part of the spine, the lumbar region, nerve roots may be irritated, stretched or compressed, provoking symptoms and signs in the territory of the affected root (Table 8.8).

Table 8.8 Localizing features of lumbar and sacral root lesions

Root	Pain	Dermatome	Muscle	Reflex
L3	Front of thigh	Anterior thigh	*Quadriceps, adductors*	
L4	Front of thigh, knee and medial shin	Anteromedial shin	*Quadriceps, tib. ant. hamstrings ext. hall. longus*	KJ
L5	Back of leg, lateral lower leg, dorsum foot to great toe	Dorsum of foot to great toe evertors, hamstrings		Inner hamstring jerk
S1	Sole of foot, lateral side of foot back of thigh and leg	Sole	Plantar flexors, toe flexors, hamstrings	AJ
Lower sacral	Buttocks, saddle area	Saddle area, perianal	Anal muscles	Anal

KJ, knee jerk; AJ, ankle jerk.

Sciatica describes the pain referred down the course of the sciatic nerve from the back to the buttock, and down the back of the leg to the foot. This pain most commonly arises from compromise of the L5 and S1 roots.

Lumbar disc prolapses
In the lumbosacral region a lateral disc prolapse may compress a nerve root or sometimes more than one. A central disc prolapse will extend into the lumbar sac compressing the cauda equina and producing symptoms and signs in both legs, and more alarming disturbances of bowel and bladder control. Such symptoms of sphincter upset are a medical emergency and patients require urgent hospital admission with a view to imaging the canal and surgical decompression before irreversible damage occurs.

Over 95% of lumbar disc protrusions occur at L4/L5 and L5/S1 levels affecting the L5 and S1 roots, less often the L4 roots. In the lumbar region, roots can be involved at a higher level (Figure 8.7) so imaging is essential before deciding on surgery; for example, an L4/L5 disc protrusion can involve the L5 or L4 root. Many patients have a preceding history of low back pain and intermittent sciatica, which in the past has responded to rest or physiotherapy. Small disc protrusions will settle with rest but a large extruded fragment is likely to give continuing trouble.

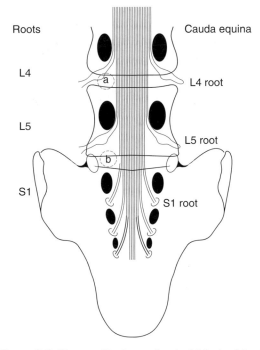

Figure 8.7 Diagram of lumbosacral roots. (a) Posterolateral disc protrusion; (b) medial disc protrusion.

Other causes of root pain need consideration, although these are less common. **Diabetic infarction** of nerve roots, the plexus or femoral nerve, may present with acute pain in the thigh and be accompanied by wasting, impaired reflexes and sensory loss (see p. 163). **Neoplastic involvement** of nerve roots may arise in the spinal canal, often secondary to

Table 8.9 Clinical features of disturbances of the lumbosacral plexus

	Pain	Sensory loss	Weakness	Reflex
Upper	Groin, anterior thigh, lateral thigh, hip	Medial and lateral thigh, anterior thigh, medial leg	*Psoas, quadriceps, adductors*	KJ
Lower	Posterior thigh, leg and foot	Foot, lateral ankle lateral and posterior leg	Hamstrings evertors, invertors, flexors toes and ankle	AJ

KJ, knee jerk; AJ, ankle jerk.

bony metastases with collapse of the vertebrae, most often from primary growths of bronchus, breast, prostate, kidney, gastrointestinal tract or lymphomas. The lumbosacral plexus on the side wall of the pelvis may be involved with gynaecological or colonorectal malignancies. Such tumours cause severe pain, which is often not relieved by rest, unlike the pain from a disc. In time the lymphatic pathways and even the iliac veins may be obstructed, leading to swelling of the leg.

Root symptoms

Root symptoms are shown in Table 8.8.

S1

S1 root lesions produce pain down the back of the buttock, thigh and leg to the heel. There will be tingling and numbness in the sole of the foot and weakness of plantar flexion (inability to stand on tiptoe), and to a lesser extent the hamstrings and glutei. The ankle jerk will be depressed or absent and there will be sensory loss on the sole and lateral border of the foot.

L5

L5 root lesions produce pain down the posterolateral side of the leg to the ankle with sensory upset on the dorsum of the foot including the great toe. Weakness involves the dorsiflexors of the great toe (*extensor hallucis longus*, which has an exclusive L5 innervation) and, to a lesser extent, the dorsiflexors of the ankle, evertors and hamstrings. The patient may show difficulty walking on their heels. The ankle jerk is usually preserved, the inner hamstring jerk depressed and there is sensory impairment over the dorsum of the foot, extending onto the lateral side of the lower leg.

L4

L4 root lesions produce pain radiating down the front of the thigh, over the knee, shin and medial side of the calf. There may be tingling and numbness on the medial side of the calf, weakness of the ankle dorsiflexors (*tibialis anterior)* and the *quadriceps*. The knee jerk is usually reduced or absent.

Root tension signs are commonly associated with L4, L5 and S1 root lesions. These include the inability to flex the fully straightened leg to a right angle at the hip. In older patients, there may be local hip joint disease, which may prevent this. If nerve roots are stretched by a disc protrusion, then straight leg raising is commonly limited on the affected side with pain referred in a sciatic radiation. Such pain may be aggravated by dorsiflexion of the foot. It should be noted that in patients exaggerating their symptoms with the suspicion of a functional component, straight leg raising may be grossly restricted lying on the couch, yet if the patient is asked to sit up to demonstrate the site of their back pain, they may be able to do this with the legs flexed at the hip to 90 degrees and the knees fully extended. Spinal movements are often restricted with lumbosacral root lesions, particularly trunk flexion. There may sometimes be a scoliosis or pelvic tilt.

Upper plexus or lumbar root lesions are uncommon but produce weakness in the hip flexors, adductors and *quadriceps*. Such patients have difficulty rising from a low chair, bath or climbing stairs. If the upper lumbar roots are stretched (L2, L3) the presence of root tension signs may be detected by the femoral stretch test. Here the patient lies prone with the knee flexed to a right angle, and the thigh is then extended at the hip. A positive test will produce pain in the front of the thigh.

All patients with lumbosacral root symptoms should be specifically questioned about their bowel and bladder function, and in the male about potency. A rectal examination, or pelvic examination, where appropriate, should be undertaken to exclude any palpable mass. At the same time this will enable sensation to be checked in the lower sacral dermatomes, the tone of the anal sphincter assessed and the anal reflex elicited. The last is tested by pricking or scratching the pigmented perianal skin and eliciting a local contraction of the muscle, which can be seen.

A cauda equina lesion usually affects both legs with lower motor neurone pattern weakness affecting distal muscles more than proximal ones, although this can be asymmetric. The weakness is usually accompanied by sensory changes, reflex loss and sphincter dysfunction.

Investigations (Table 8.6)

Blood should be taken for a full blood count, erythrocyte sedimentation rate, fasting blood glucose, and, where appropriate, estimation of the acid phosphatase and prostatic-specific antigen (PSA), serum proteins and electrophoresis. Plain X-rays of the spine may show degenerative changes, a narrowed disc space, or occasionally point to other pathology by the appearance of vertebral collapse, loss of a pedicle or abnormal density. However, MRI scanning will cover these aspects. A chest X-ray is appropriate in adults.

If there is progressive or persistent neurological deficit, continuing pain, or diagnostic doubt, imaging should be undertaken to visualize the spinal cord and roots. **This is best achieved by MRI scanning with gadolinium enhancement if there is any suggestion of an infective/inflammatory or neoplastic process.**

Spinal CT scans, best with intrathecal contrast, may also be helpful in selected patients. Where MRI is not available, myelography may be necessary using the newer non-ionic contrast media. The CSF obtained at the same time should be examined in the usual way but should also be sent for cytology to look for malignant cells, and to measure any oligoclonal bands. Isotope bone scans may be useful in showing bony lesions, particularly the presence of widespread spinal metastases. Electrodiagnostic studies may be useful in confirming the presence of denervation, pointing to more central conduction delays, or indicating the presence of an underlying neuropathy.

'Red flags'

'Red flags' indicating the need for further investigation in patients with a history of back pain include:

- Age – <20 and >55 years
- A history of trauma
- A constant progressive non-mechanical pattern of pain
- A past history of serious illness (cancer), IV drug abuse or steroid therapy
- Features of systemic illness, such as weight loss, malaise
- Fever
- Widespread neurological signs affecting more than one root territory
- Structural deformity
- Difficulty in bladder emptying, the presence of faecal soiling, loss of anal sphincter tone, or saddle anaesthesia (requires urgent referral and investigation).

Treatment

Treatment will depend on the cause, but most acute disc lesions respond to analgesics (non-steroidal anti-inflammatory drugs) and muscle relaxants. Early mobilization with greater emphasis on exercise and return to normal activities is now being promoted, although acute pain with severe muscle spasm usually results in rest. Traction has its advocates but evidence-based medicine does not support the efficacy of traction, specific exercises, bed rest or acupuncture in the relief of acute low back pain. In more chronic low back pain, exercises, multidisciplinary treatment and even behavioural therapy have been shown to help. Surgery may prove necessary where medical treatment has failed, where there is progressive or persistent neurological deficit and where a large disc is demonstrated, or there is persistent unremitting root pain. This is discussed further (see p. 221).

> **Surgical referral**
>
> Indications for **surgical referral** include:
> - Cauda equina symptoms and signs (bowel and bladder disturbance) – urgent
> - Progressive or severe neurological deficit
> - Persistent neurological deficit after 4–6 weeks
> - Persistent sciatica accompanied by root signs after 6 weeks.

SUMMARY

Common sites of peripheral nerve entrapment include the median nerve in the carpal tunnel and the ulnar nerve at the elbow.

At the more mobile parts of the spine, the neck and lumbar regions, nerve roots may be irritated or compressed. The signs and symptoms from these include:

- Pain
- Loss of use
- Sensory impairment
- Reflex changes.

Pain and sensory symptoms may be referred into the appropriate root sclerotome or dermatome. These sites are not always identical.

A working knowledge of the anatomy of such nerve and root lesions allows their recognition.

REFERENCES AND FURTHER READING

Biller J (2002) *Practical Neurology*, 2nd edn. Philadelphia, PA: Lippincott-Raven.

Brazis PW, Masdeu JC, Biller J (2001) *Localisation in Clinical Neurology*, 4th edn. Boston, MA: Lippincott, Williams & Wilkins.

Mumenthaler M (1992) *Neurologic Differential Diagnosis*, 2nd edn. Stuttgart: Georg Thieme.

Nachemson AL, Jonsson E (2000) *Neck and Back Pain*. Philadelphia, PA: Lippincott, Williams & Wilkins

Seddon H (1972) *Surgical Disorders of the Peripheral Nerves*. Edinburgh: Churchill Livingstone.

Seimon LP (1995) *Low Back Pain – Clinical Diagnosis and Management*, 2nd edn. New York, NY: Demos Vermande.

Staal A, van Gijn J, Spaans F (1999) *Mononeuropathies – Examination, Diagnosis and Treatment*. London, UK: WB Saunders.

CHAPTER 9

CRANIAL NERVE SYNDROMES

T.J. Fowler and J.W. Scadding

CRANIAL NERVE I

Anosmia

The olfactory nerve arises from nerve fibres in the nasal mucosa at the top of the nose, which pass through the cribriform plate forming the olfactory tract lying on the orbital surface of the frontal lobe. In most instances the sense of smell relies on the inhalation of very small particles (airborne chemicals) of the substance under test. **Although many patients refer to the taste of foods, in nearly all instances this involves smell, as taste only differentiates sweet, salt, bitter and sour (acid).**

Smell may be lost (anosmia), diminished (hyposmia), perverted (parosmia), distorted (dysosmia) or unpleasant (cacosmia). Olfactory hallucinations may arise, often as part of the aura of complex partial seizures. These are usually unpleasant, very brief and may arise in the uncinate lobe. Olfactory hallucinations may also occur in psychiatric disorders.

Causes of anosmia are given in Table 9.1. Temporary anosmia is found very frequently with the common cold. Head injuries may cause anosmia, most often with shearing of the delicate olfactory fibres. Such loss is often permanent: it is commonly associated with fractures of the floor of the anterior fossa. Anosmia may also arise from subfrontal tumours.

Table 9.1 Causes of anosmia

Local nasal disease	Infections, e.g. common cold, allergic rhinitis, nasal polyps
Trauma	Head injuries
Tumours	Subfrontal, e.g. meningioma, frontal glioma, pituitary
Degenerative	Alzheimer's disease, Huntington's chorea, Parkinson's disease
Endocrine	Addison's disease, diabetes mellitus

These may present with dementia or altered behaviour and the most important localizing sign may be anosmia. If the tumour is very large, it may cause papilloedema or even optic nerve damage leading to optic atrophy.

CRANIAL NERVE II

Optic disc swelling

Papilloedema
This describes swelling with elevation of the optic disc. By definition this is a pathological swelling caused by raised intracranial pressure

(ICP). As the disc swells, the veins become engorged and venous pulsation is lost (venous pulsation is best seen with the patient sitting or standing). The margins of the disc become indistinct and then radial streak haemorrhages may appear around the edges (Plates Ic,d).

Causes are shown in Table 9.2.

Optic disc swelling may be asymptomatic but usually there are symptoms related to the cause – from raised ICP or the site of a mass lesion. The visual acuity is usually unchanged and there is only slight enlargement of the blind spots. With persistent raised pressure there may eventually be a drop in acuity and some concentric constriction of the visual fields. Occasionally with very high ICP, there may be transient visual obscurations with complete loss of vision lasting a few seconds, provoked by bending, coughing or straining – measures that produce a transient rise in ICP. Causes of monocular visual loss are given in Table 9.3.

Papilloedema may develop very rapidly, for example, with a cerebral haemorrhage, but more commonly arises slowly over days or weeks, as with a tumour. It should be emphasized that only some 50% of cerebral tumours cause papilloedema.

Optic neuritis

Optic neuritis is an acute inflammation of the optic nerve causing acute visual loss, usually in one eye. If the nerve head, the papilla, is involved causing it to swell this is called a papillitis.

Papillitis
A papillitis describes local swelling of the nerve head with involvement of the optic nerve and is characterized by a fall in visual acuity and a central scotoma.

If the inflammation lies behind the nerve head, the disc may appear normal – a retrobulbar neuritis. Commonly optic neuritis affects younger patients, aged 15–40 years. In children both eyes may be affected and this may follow an acute viral infection.

Table 9.2 Causes of papilloedema

Raised intracranial pressure
Mass lesions – tumours, abscesses, haematomas
Cerebral oedema – trauma, infarcts
Infections – meningitis, encephalitis
Obstructive hydrocephalus
Venous sinus thrombosis – cavernous, sagittal
Idiopathic intracranial hypertension
Medical disorders
Severe anaemia, including B12 deficiency
Polycythaemia rubra vera
Accelerated hypertension
Lead poisoning
Carbon dioxide retention
Drugs – tetracycline, excess vitamin A, lithium, isoretinoin, ibuprofen, steroids (withdrawal)

Table 9.3 Causes of monocular visual loss (usually acute)

Optic neuritis	MS
	Viral (childhood)
	Epstein–Barr virus
	Post-infectious
	Sphenoid sinusitis
	Unknown
Ischaemic optic neuritis	GCA, atheroma (may be sequential)
Orbital tumour	
Chiasmal compression*	Usually slower
Leber's optic atrophy*	
Retinal vascular occlusion	Arterial (GCA), embolic, venous (dysproteinaemia)
Elevated ICP*	Late
Toxic*	Methyl alcohol

MS, multiple sclerosis; GCA, giant cell arteritis; ICP, intracranial pressure.
*May be bilateral.

Most patients with optic neuritis describe acute visual loss with a fall in acuity varying from mild (6/9–6/12) to severe with almost complete loss [to hand movements (HM) or perception of light (PL)]. The process may progress over hours or days, usually reaching its worst within 1 week. There may be tenderness of the globe with pain on movement in the affected eye. Most often there is a central or paracentral scotoma, sometimes very large. Colour vision is impaired and there is an afferent pupillary defect. Later pallor, indicating atrophy, may follow both optic neuritis (papillitis) or retrobulbar neuritis.

> Acute demyelination of the optic nerve may be the initial symptom of multiple sclerosis (MS) in about 25% of patients. However, if patients with an optic neuritis are followed up, some 50–70% may develop MS. An abnormal magnetic resonance imaging brain scan increases the risks of developing MS.

In most instances recovery of vision occurs over a number of weeks, often 6–8, and about 90% of patients recover acuity to 6/9 or better. In many there may be a residual afferent pupillary defect, impaired colour vision and disc pallor. A few patients are left with severe visual loss. Recurrent attacks in the same eye occur in 20–30% of patients. Visual evoked potentials will show a prolonged latency and this will persist. Magnetic resonance imaging with special sequences may show abnormal signals in the affected optic nerve.

Steroid treatment may shorten the course, relieving pain and allowing more rapid recovery of acuity. Pulsed steroids may be used: intravenous (IV) methylprednisolone 1000 mg daily for 3 days followed by oral prednisolone 1 mg/kg per day for 11 days with a 4-day taper (20 mg on day 1, 10 mg on days 2 and 4) is one regimen. It has been suggested that the use of oral steroids alone may predispose patients to more frequent bouts of optic neuritis.

The American optic neuritis trial (ONTT)
This found that the clinical diagnosis of optic neuritis was sufficient without the need for special investigations. The outcome in terms of recovery of visual acuity was not altered whether steroids were used or not. However, there was a more rapid return of acuity in patients treated with IV (pulsed) steroids.

Those patients treated with IV (pulse) steroids showed a reduced risk of relapse at 2 years when compared with those treated with placebo or oral steroids, although by 4 years the figures were not significantly different.

There was the suggestion that patients treated with IV (pulse) steroids showed a reduced rate of the development of MS during the first 2 years of follow-up in those who had shown abnormal magnetic resonance imaging (MRI) brain scans (more than two white matter lesions) at the time of the optic neuritis. An MRI brain scan showing >3 white matter lesions of >3 mm size predicted an increased risk of the development of MS. By 3 years some 43% of those presenting with an optic neuritis had developed MS.

Because IV (pulse) steroids have often required hospital admission for their administration, high dose oral methylprednisolone has also been used. This too has hastened visual recovery when compared with placebo and it appears this may not be associated with an increase in the rate of recurrence after 1 year. The more long-term results are not available.

> The most common clinical practice now is to use high dose IV (pulse) steroids in patients with:
>
> - Bilateral involvement
> - Poor vision in the fellow eye and in whom the good eye has been affected
> - Severe loss of acuity and marked pain.

The recent CHAMPS (Controlled High Risk Subjects Avonex Multiple Sclerosis Prevention Study) study suggested that the use of beta interferon Ia in a patient presenting with an acute optic neuritis and abnormal MRI brain scan reduces the risk of developing clinically definite MS over a 3-year period.

Ischaemic optic neuritis

Vascular optic nerve damage
In older patients, infarction of the optic nerve may arise from vascular damage. This may follow a giant cell arteritis (GCA) or be part of atherosclerotic arterial disease. If the posterior ciliary arteries or peripapillary choroidal vessels occlude, the anterior part of the optic nerve and its head may infarct.

Table 9.5 Causes of ocular motor palsies

	Cranial nerve		
	III	IV	VI
Trauma	13	28	11
Vascular	17	15	9
Neoplasm	18	10	31
Aneurysm	18		3
Undetermined	20	34	22
Other	14	13	24

(Figures as percentages).

one eye is obviously higher (above) the other, this is termed hypertropia, or below the other, hypotropia. A latent squint may be demonstrated by asking the patient to fix on an object and then covering each eye in turn. If the uncovered eye moves to fix on the target, a latent squint has been elicited.

The cover test will also distinguish between a concomitant squint (where the affected eye will show a full range of movement when its fellow is covered) and a true paralytic squint. The testing for diplopia has been described in Chapter 4.

Oculomotor palsy

Oculomotor palsy

In a complete oculomotor palsy the eyelid droops to cover the eye and the globe is turned down and out as a result of the unopposed actions of the unparalysed lateral rectus and superior oblique muscles (see Figure 4.11). The pupil may be enlarged and unreactive if the pupillomotor fibres that lie around the periphery of the nerve are compressed.

Thus a 'surgical' lesion such as an aneurysm (Figure 9.1) or tumour compressing the oculomotor nerve, may result in a large unreactive pupil. There will also be paralysis of the superior and inferior rectus, the medial rectus and inferior oblique muscles. Vascular lesions, which may infarct the nerve,

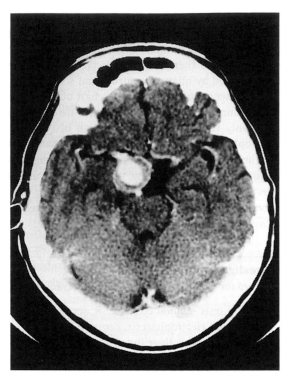

Figure 9.1 Computerized tomography brain scan with enhancement showing a large aneurysm at the termination of the internal carotid artery. The patient presented with a painful partial oculomotor palsy with pupillary involvement.

for example as a result of diabetes mellitus or an arteritis, may produce a complete oculomotor palsy with pupillary sparing. Such lesions recover spontaneously over 3–4 months. Because of the anatomical arrangement of the various divisions of the oculomotor nuclei in the midbrain tegmentum, a nuclear lesion will cause bilateral ptosis and loss of upgaze in both eyes, with ipsilateral involvement of the medial and inferior rectus and inferior oblique muscles.

Trochlear palsy

The superior oblique depresses the adducted eye and intorts the abducted eye. This will cause **diplopia on downgaze with vertical separation of images**. There is often an associated **head tilt** to the opposite shoulder. Trauma is a common cause.

Abducens palsy

The lateral rectus muscle abducts the eye, causing diplopia with horizontal separation of images maximal on gaze to the affected side. The sixth nerve has a relatively long course across the base of the skull, through the cavernous sinus and into the orbit via the superior orbital fissure. On this course it may be affected by trauma, compression from masses, or inflamed or damaged as an effect of raised intracranial pressure.

Ocular motor palsies (Table 9.5) may arise centrally within the pons and midbrain from strokes, neoplasms, plaques of multiple sclerosis and even thiamine deficiency. Usually such lesions produce other signs, particularly involvement of other cranial nerves, a Horner's syndrome, cerebellar signs and sometimes long tract signs in the limbs. At the base of the brain, nerves may be damaged by meningitis or from basal neoplasms, for example nasopharyngeal carcinoma, chordoma.

Cavernous sinus lesions

Cavernous sinus lesions cause involvement of the IIIrd, IVth and VIth cranial nerves and impaired sensation, most commonly in the territory of the ophthalmic division of the Vth (very occasionally the maxillary division if the lesion is inferior and posterior see Figure 9.2). Sometimes the optic nerve may be involved. Most often the pathology is from an aneurysm, caroticocavernous fistula or thrombosis (often secondary to infection), a tumour (pituitary, meningioma, nasopharyngeal carcinoma, metastasis) or from a granuloma (sarcoid, Tolosa–Hunt syndrome, Wegener's). More anteriorly, at the back of the orbit, mass lesions and granulomas may displace the globe producing diplopia and an axial proptosis.

Dysthyroid eye disease

An overactive thyroid (hyperthyroidism) may produce abnormal eye signs. **These include exophthalmos, a lid lag, conjunctival suffusion and diplopia.** The last

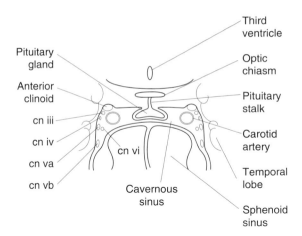

Figure 9.2 Diagram of coronal section in the parasellar region to include the cavernous sinus. cn iii, oculomotor nerve; cn iv, trochlear nerve; cn va, ophthalmic division of trigeminal nerve; cn vb, maxillary division of trigeminal nerve; cn vi, abducens nerve.

is most often diplopia with vertical separation of images from restriction of upgaze, or less commonly from limitation of abduction. Dysthyroid eye disease is a restrictive ophthalmopathy where direct infiltration of the ocular muscles causes thickening and fibrosis, which results in tethering and restricted movements, most often found in the inferior and medial rectus muscles. This leads to impaired upgaze and abduction. The affected muscles appear swollen on orbital views of a CT or MRI scan. The restricted range of eye movements can be confirmed by a forced duction test. Blood tests will usually confirm the presence of thyrotoxicosis, but sometimes the evidence for thyroid disease is subtle and requires more specialized endocrine investigation.

Myasthenia gravis (see p. 151)

In any patient with variable diplopia, the diagnosis of myasthenia gravis should be considered. This is commonly associated with weakness of eye closure, ptosis and involvement of the facial and bulbar muscles. Proximal limb muscles may also be affected. The diagnosis may be confirmed if there is a raised titre of acetylcholine receptor antibodies, or by electrodiagnostic tests. An edrophonium test may be helpful (see p. 152).

Table 9.6 Causes of facial numbness

Inflammation	MS, connective tissue diseases
Infection	Herpes zoster, leprosy
Neoplastic	Trigeminal neuroma, meningioma, cerebellopontine angle tumours, gliomas, carcinomatous infiltration, metastases, nasopharyngeal carcinoma
Toxic	Trichlorethylene, cocaine abuse, allopurinol
Vascular	Pontine and medullary infarction, basilar aneurysms, AVMs, sickle-cell disease
Granuloma	Sarcoidosis
Trauma	Head injury, dental (extractions, anaesthesia)

MS, multiple sclerosis; AVMs, arteriovenous malformations.

Table 9.7 Causes of facial palsy

Idiopathic	Bell's
Infective	Viral – zoster, mumps, EBV, Borrelia*, herpes
Vascular	Hypertension, diabetes, pontine infarction, vasculitis (collagen vascular disease)
Inflammatory	Guillain-Barré*, MS (pontine plaque), otitis media
Tumour	Cerebellopontine angle tumour, cholesteatoma, meningeal carcinomatosis, pontine glioma, parotid
Trauma	Temporal or basal skull fractures
Granuloma	Sarcoidosis*

Muscular dystrophies and myasthenia may affect the facial muscles.
*May often be bilateral.
EBV, Epstein–Barr virus; MS, multiple sclerosis.

The pathology for these may start in the pons, skull base or in the sinuses or face. Meningiomas, basal tumours, aneurysms or infiltration from a nasopharyngeal carcinoma or lymphoma are the most common symptomatic causes. Usually such pathology involves the lower cranial nerves and sometimes the long tracts as well. In MS facial numbness is common. Toxic damage may arise from substances such as trichlorethylene.

Investigations

With the trigeminal neuropathy investigations should be negative. Brain scanning with MRI and CT scanning of the skull base are combined useful measures to exclude other pathology. A CSF examination may help to confirm the presence of a malignant or infective meningitis, or MS. An ear, nose and throat (ENT) examination is important to look for sinus or nasopharyngeal lesions.

Numb chin syndrome

A small localised patchy of sensory loss may be found on the chin in some patients where the mental nerve has been involved by malignancy in the mandible. Such patients may have palpable submental lymph glands.

CRANIAL NERVE VII

Bell's palsy

Bell's palsy is a common condition that presents with an acute onset of a lower motor neurone facial weakness affecting the muscles on one side of the face.

It has an annual incidence of 23 per 100 000 and all ages may be affected, including children, although the highest incidence is in patients aged 30–50 years. The exact cause is uncertain. Certain conditions are known to be responsible (Table 9.7), but in many cases no definite answer is found.

Pathogenesis

Electrophysiological studies suggest that there is segmental demyelination resulting in a local conduction block proximally. This allows a relatively rapid and complete recovery in about 85% of cases. In others, axonal degeneration occurs, which will produce a severe paralysis. Often this is then followed by incomplete recovery associated with aberrant re-innervation, that is, fibres from the periocular muscles may regenerate and supply the mouth, and vice versa. Such faulty re-innervation may lead to 'jaw-winking', and hemifacial spasm. Where axonal degeneration has occurred, electromyography of the facial muscles will show fibrillation and features of denervation, although these changes may not appear until some 10 days after the onset. In some instances the pathogenesis is a mixture of axonal degeneration and demyelination.

Symptoms and signs

Patients may present with pain in or behind the ear preceding or appearing with the development of facial weakness. There is inability to close the eye or move the lower face and mouth.

The lack of blinking leads to tears spilling out of the eye, which waters to cause complaints of blurred vision. The cheek is flaccid and saliva and fluids may escape from the corner of the mouth. The weakness commonly progresses over 24–72 hours to reach a maximum. In many patients there are complaints of numbness in the affected side of the face, although trigeminal sensation is spared and there should be no weakness of jaw movement (supplied by the motor root of the trigeminal nerve).

About 40–50% of patients are aware of disturbed taste on the ipsilateral anterior part of the tongue. This points to a lesion in the distal part of the facial nerve below the geniculate ganglion, but above the origin of the chorda tympani. Many patients also notice hyperacusis because the stapedius muscle is supplied by a branch of the facial nerve, which leaves the nerve in the facial canal proximal to the chorda tympani. **If a zoster infection is responsible, there will be herpetic vesicles on the pinna or in the external auditory canal on the affected side.** Ramsay Hunt described a herpetic infection of the geniculate ganglion with the development of an acute facial palsy (Hunt's syndrome). In some of these patients the eighth cranial nerve may also be infected, producing acute vertigo, deafness and tinnitus. A few patients may show a bilateral facial palsy of lower motor neurone pattern; this may appear as part of a Guillain–Barré syndrome, from Lyme disease, from sarcoidosis or even carcinomatous meningitis.

Prognosis

About 85% of patients show signs of improvement within some 3 weeks of the onset. About 70% of patients recover normal function in the face but some 16% are left with asymmetry, signs of aberrant re-innervation and some weakness. An incomplete palsy at the onset or signs of recovery starting within 3–4 weeks usually are good prognostic features for recovery. This is mirrored in the electrophysiological findings. In the more severely affected, where axonal degeneration has taken place, recovery is slower and often incomplete. Recurrent facial palsies require more intensive investigation to exclude any compressive lesion in the middle ear or skull base, and to look for any systemic upset such as sarcoidosis, hypertension, diabetes.

Investigations

Blood tests – full blood count, ESR, fasting glucose, tests for Borrelia

Imaging – in selected patients MRI and/or computerized tomography scanning. Chest X-ray

EMG studies – these may assess the severity of damage and help in prognosis; they may also indicate a more widespread neuropathy

ENT examination

CSF examination – in selected patients.

Treatment

There appears to be little difference in outcome between patients treated with steroids and those who are not. Many doctors believe that a short intensive course of steroids given within 5–7 days of the onset of the palsy may reduce the swelling of the facial nerve and so prevent axonal degeneration. Prednisolone 40 mg daily for 5 days and then tapered off over the next week is a typical regimen. It has been suggested that such a course should be given to all patients seen acutely with a complete palsy at the time of consultation or with impaired taste.

Because of the possible infective causation by the herpes virus, acyclovir has also been used in the treatment of an acute facial palsy. This certainly should be given if a zoster infection (Hunt's syndrome) is suspected. The combination of acyclovir with steroids in those patients with complete facial

Table 9.8 Causes of polyneuritis cranialis

Infective	Tuberculosis, listeria, borrelia, EBV, fungal
Granuloma	Sarcoidosis, Wegener's
Neoplastic	Carcinomatous meningitis – breast, bronchus
	Lymphoma, leukaemia
	Local spread – nasopharyngeal carcinoma. chordoma
Trauma	Basal skull fracture
Vascular	Vasculitis – PAN, collagen vascular disease
Inflammatory	Guillain–Barré, Miller Fisher
Always exclude	**Myasthenia gravis – ocular, facial and bulbar involvement**

EBV, Epstein–Barr virus; PAN, polyarteritis nodosa

important. The cytology may allow identification of malignant cells and in neoplastic meningitis the CSF glucose is often very low. Staining and culture of the CSF may identify infective causes.

Treatment is that of the underlying cause. Intrathecal cytotoxic drugs, for example methotrexate, may be tried in malignant meningitis, although often with only limited benefit.

REFERENCES AND FURTHER READING

Acheson J, Riordan-Eva P (1999) *Neuro-ophthalmology: Fundamentals of Clinical Ophthalmology*. London, UK: BMJ Books.

Balcer LJ (2001) Optic neuritis. *Current Treatment Options in Neurology*, 3:389–398.

Epley JM (1992) The canalith repositioning procedure: for treatment of benign paroxysmal positional vertigo. *Otolaryngological Head and Neck Surgery*, 107:399–404.

Furman JM, Cass SP (2003) *Vestibulae Disorders. A Case Study Approach*, 2nd edn. New York: Oxford University Press.

Goebel JA (2001) *Practical Management of the Dizzy Patient*. Philadelphia, PA: Lippincott, Williams & Wilkins.

Harris W (1926) *Neuritis and Neuralgia*. Oxford, UK: Oxford Medical Publications.

Hickman SJ et al. (2002) Management of acute optic neuritis. *Lancet*, 360: 1953–1961.

Janetta P (1980) Arterial compression of the trigeminal nerve at the pons in patients with trigeminal neuralgia. *Journal of Neurosurgery*, 52:381–386.

Trobe JD (1993) *Physicians Guide to Eye Care*. San Francisco, CA: American Academy of Ophthalmology.

CHAPTER 10

SPINAL DISEASES

M. Powell, D. Peterson and J.W. Scadding

INTRODUCTION

The neurosurgical aspects of diagnosis, investigation and treatment of diseases and congenital malformations of the spinal cord, spinal nerves and the vertebral column are discussed in this chapter. It is intended that the salient diagnostic features are emphasized so that these disorders may be recognized, investigated and referred as appropriate. Spinal cord injury is not discussed.

In the past few years, there has been little change in the range and frequency of neurological diseases involving the spine. Perhaps there has been a subtle increase in the return of tuberculosis, reflecting the increasing prevalence of this disease among the urban poor.

Where there has been a difference is in the perceptions of management. It has always been a predominantly surgical disease, in that surgeons are involved in much of the management. Whereas in the recent past neurosurgeons had a broad view of spinal disease, there is a growing group of neurosurgical spinal specialists.

Along with this change in neurosurgery is a similar one in orthopaedics. From the collaboration between the two groups has developed a number of systems for spinal instrumentation, which has allowed surgeons to tackle previously impossible procedures because of the threat of instability.

Recognizing and facilitating this, manufacturers have pushed increasingly complex and expensive systems onto the market, allowing many more parts of the spine to be removed and fused to other parts. Where this form of surgery clearly has a place in the management of some diseases, the escalating costs of spinal instrumentation [always in expensive magnetic resonance imaging (MRI)-compatible titanium] strains healthcare budgets.

ANATOMICAL AND PATHOLOGICAL CONSIDERATIONS

Diseases of the spine cause neurological dysfunction either by primary pathology of nervous tissue or its blood supply, or by compression of the spinal cord, nerves or blood vessels within the spinal canal and the nerve root exit foramina. Compression of the nervous system is a frequent pathological process in neurosurgical practice, as a cause of both intracranial and spinal pathology. In the spine, compression most frequently arises from the supporting spinal elements, which form the boundaries of the spinal canal, in particular the anterior margin formed by the vertebral bodies and their principal joint, the vertebral disc. The spinal canal is inexpansible, and there is little free space outside the cord and the nerve roots. Consequently, masses or stenoses reducing the canal size lead to early compression of its contents.

Although the cord and the brain have similar nerve cells, glial cells and blood vessel constituents, within the spinal cord there is little that may be considered functionally redundant. Thus, small lesions anywhere within the cord lead to major consequences. Furthermore, despite duplication of arterial supply in most areas of the cord, derived from the segmental root arteries, there are critical areas in the thoracic cord where the arterial supply is tenuous and may depend on a single root artery, the artery of Adamkiewicz. The radial arteries that penetrate the cord substance are also end arteries. Many of the disease entities to be discussed, such as spinal canal stenosis, disc protrusion or spinal dural arteriovenous malformation (AVM), will lead to spinal cord dysfunction through ischaemia.

The vertebral column is split anatomically and functionally into five sections: (i) the craniocervical junction; (ii) cervical; (iii) thoracic; (iv) lumbar; and (v) sacral spine. Although there are similarities in the way in which a disease may affect each section, the frequency of disease occurrence and manifestations are different at the various sites.

SYMPTOMS AND SIGNS OF SPINAL DISEASE

Pain

Pain from lesions of the vertebral column is felt in the midline posteriorly in the region of the affected part. The pain may radiate up and down through a number of segments. When the spinal nerves are involved, pain is referred to the appropriate sclerotome. Associated painful muscle spasm may be present.

> Acute inflammatory disease is characterized by severe pain with marked associated muscle spasm causing spinal rigidity.

There is local tenderness, elicitable by pressure on the relevant spinous process, and an associated systemic disturbance. This symptom complex is

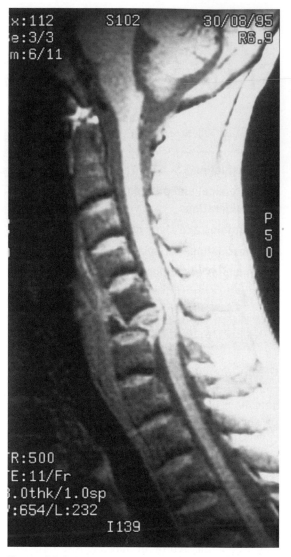

Figure 10.1 Magnetic resonance imaging cervical spine, sagittal view, showing Pott's disease with soft tissue swelling anterior to the cervical spine with deformity. This patient had severe pain but few abnormal neurological signs.

typically seen in bacterial infection of the intervertebral disc, discitis. Generally there is a recognizable source of infection present or evidence of one in the short history.

> Chronic infection, such as tuberculous or chronic staphylococcal, produces pain of more insidious onset with features similar to neoplasia (Figure 10.1).

The pain is less disabling, especially in the earlier stages, although as the disease process advances it can become very severe with marked muscle spasm and local tenderness. Clinical evidence of systemic illness may be absent. Chronic pyogenic infection is almost always seen in those debilitated by age, immune disorder or diabetes mellitus.

> Pain produced by tumours varies greatly both in its duration and severity. It depends on the particular pathology, the tissue in which it arises and the site. In general, pain as a result of tumour has a gradual and insidious onset.

When the tumour is slow growing, as in the case of spinal meningioma, minor back pain is often dismissed and even when weakness of the lower limbs develops, back pain may not be mentioned spontaneously by the patient. **Pain radiating around the trunk in a dermatomal distribution**, may give a clue to the underlying neurological problem in cases of undiagnosed abdominal or loin pain. Tumours arising within the spinal cord itself, such as an astrocytoma, do not produce pain until the cord is enlarged to occupy the vertebral canal, by which time there is usually ample evidence of cord dysfunction. Extradural tumours however, arising in the epidural space or in the bone of the vertebral column produce local spinal pain with a radicular radiation as nerve roots become involved. **Local pain and tenderness are a good guide to the site of the compression, especially if deformity (usually kyphotic) and a corresponding sensory level are present.** This contrasts with primary tumours of the spinal cord, which rarely produce a clear sensory level and local pain.

Tumours within the dura and involving the cauda equina, such as a neurofibroma in a young adult, may produce very severe pain in the legs with a virtual absence of signs in the early stages. Such patients may find it more comfortable to sleep in a chair rather than retiring to bed. Night pain is a frequent feature of intradural tumours. Decubitus pain is a common, but often disregarded, feature of significant pathology.

Spinal pain following injury must always be taken very seriously. The history of the circumstances of injury will provide some indication of the biomechanical forces that may have acted on the spine, and therefore the likely degree of disruption and instability. Spinal injuries are often missed when there is clouding of consciousness and are very easily overlooked in the comatose patient.

The slow degenerative process of ageing is generally painless, even when radiological examination of the spine shows extensive changes to be present. When pain occurs, the symptoms remit and relapse, are relieved by rest and increased by activities that increase the mechanical stresses on the spine. In a healthy individual, a clear relationship to mechanical factors, with remissions and a long history, characterizes pain as a result of wear and tear.

Clinical features of nerve root involvement

Anatomically the anterior and posterior roots emerging from the cord join before leaving the spinal canal through the intervertebral foramen. Thus in clinical practice nerve root compression, so frequently present in the vicinity of the exit foramen, will result in both motor and sensory disturbance in the myotome and dermatome. While pain may be felt over a large area, the extent of objective sensory loss is usually small. Weakness is of the lower motor neurone type with signs of wasting, sometimes fasciculation, reduced tone, and loss of tendon reflexes.

Spinal cord compression (Table 10.1)

> It is imperative that reversible causes of cord compression are recognized as quickly as possible.

However, the speed with which the clinician must act depends on the nature of the underlying pathology. Most benign tumours present with long histories and urgent neurosurgery is not required. Alternatively, compression from pyogenic infection, giant disc prolapse or metastatic deposits are emergencies requiring the immediate attention of a neurosurgeon, so that urgent diagnostic and therapeutic measures can be undertaken to preserve as much function as possible. **Failure to relieve spinal cord**

Table 10.1 Causes of spinal cord compression

Tumours
    Extradural
        Secondary carcinoma
        Reticuloses including myeloma
        Neurofibroma
        Chordoma
        Primary sarcoma
    Intradural
        Intradural extramedullary
            Neurofibroma
            Meningioma
        Intradural intramedullary
            Ependymoma
            Astrocytoma
            Angioma
    Mixed lipoma and dermoids
Infection
Extradural staphylococcal infection and tuberculosis
Intervertebral disc lesions and sequestra
Haematoma – usually extradural with defects in
    blood coagulation
Trauma

compression may condemn the patient to a permanent paraplegia and loss of sphincter control.

Spinal cord lesions

Lesions of the spinal cord above the level of the conus medullaris produce a progressive loss of all cord functions at and below the level of compression. There will be a spastic weakness of the limbs with exaggerated reflexes and extensor plantar responses, signs that characterize an upper motor neurone lesion. Sphincter disturbance is characterized by precipitancy culminating in urinary retention. If paraplegia is complete, automatic bladder emptying will be possible if the sacral segments are preserved.

Cauda equina compression

Cauda equina lesions

The cauda equina commences at the termination of the spinal cord usually at the level of L1/2.

The pattern of motor disturbance is that of a lower motor neurone lesion, weakness with flaccidity, loss of tendon reflexes and perhaps some fasciculation. The exact pattern will depend in part on the vertebral level. Sphincter disturbance is characterized by retention with overflow. In the event of permanent paraplegia automatic bladder emptying is not possible. Lesions of the conus produce a mixture of signs, some characterizing an upper motor neurone lesion and others a lower motor neurone lesion.

Intradural pathology

In the early stages, intradural but extramedullary tumours, which grow in the subdural space displacing cerebrospinal fluid (CSF) are often clinically silent. As the tumour enlarges, ultimately the spinal cord is compressed to produce symptoms which, to some extent, reflect the part of the cord receiving the greatest pressure from the tumour. A tumour growing within the substance of the cord produces loss of function, partly through infiltration and partly by distortion.

Medical causes of cord dysfunction should not be forgotten. These include infective, inflammatory (demyelination), vascular, haematological and degenerative diseases (Tables 10.2 and 10.3).

INVESTIGATIONS FOR SPINAL DISEASE

Blood tests may be specific indicators of disease in spinal cord dysfunction, such as in vitamin B12 deficiency or elevated prostatic-specific antigen in the presence of vertebral body metastases. Indirect evidence of a suspected infective discitis may be indicated by a raised peripheral white count and erythrocyte sedimentation rate. Inflammatory, metabolic and vasculitic processes will require specific screening blood tests. Patients aged over 50 years or with a history of smoking should have a **chest X-ray**.

Examination of the **CSF** is of limited value and may cause deterioration in patients with complete obstruction of the spinal canal. Infective and inflammatory disorders may cause appropriate CSF changes.

Table 10.2 Causes of acute or subacute paraparesis/quadriparesis

Trauma	
Vertebral disease	Metastatic cancer
	Acute disc prolapse
	Spondylosis
	Atlanto-axial subluxation
	Pott's disease
Infection	Pyogenic epidural abscess
	TB abscess
	Acute discitis
	HIV infection
	Syphilitic myelitis
Tumours	Extradural tumours
	Intradural tumours (Table 10.1)
	Leukaemia
	Lymphoma
Vascular	Anterior spinal artery occlusion
	Infarction due to: hypotension or aortic dissection
	Infarction or haemorrhage due to: angioma or arteriovenous malformation
	Cavernoma
	Vasculitis
Haematological	Epidural/intramedullary haemorrhage due to: thrombocytopenia; other clotting disorders including **anticoagulant treatment**
	Vitamin B12 deficiency
Inflammatory	Acute myelitis
	Multiple sclerosis
	SLE
	Sarcoidosis

SLE, systemic lupus erythematosus.

Table 10.3 Causes of chronic progressive paraparesis/quadriparesis

Vertebral disease	Cervical spondylosis
	Dorsal disc prolapse
	Pott's disease
	Ankylosing spondylitis
	Atlanto-axial subluxation
	Paget's disease
	Spinal deformity
Tumours	Meningioma
	Neurofibroma
	Ependymoma
	Chordoma
	Lipoma
	Dermoid
Infection	TSP – HTLV1 infection
	Syphilitic myelitis
Haematological	Vitamin B12 deficiency
Syringomyelia	With Chiari malformation
	Secondary to tumour
	Late effect of trauma
Vascular	Arteriovenous malformation
	Angioma
	Cavernoma
Inflammatory	Multiple sclerosis
	Sarcoidosis
	Radiation myelopathy
	Arachnoiditis
Degenerative	Motor neurone disease
Hereditary	Hereditary spastic paraparesis

TSP, tropical spastic paraparesis; HTLV1, human T-cell lymphotropic virus 1.

Plain spinal radiography is often a useful first-line investigation where bony pathology is suspected. Dynamic views taken in flexion and extension may reveal instability or abnormal movement, which may not be apparent on standard scanning protocols (Table 10.4).

Isotope scanning is particularly useful for detecting or excluding widespread metastatic deposits.

Myelography was for many years the established method of investigation of spinal root and cord compression (Figure 10.2). It has now been superseded by MRI, although myelography may still be required in complex cases where ferromagnetic (steel) implants degrade the image available on MRI or where MR is contraindicated by pacemaker or prosthetic heart valve.

Computerized tomography (CT) remains a useful tool in the investigation of bony pathology, which is less well visualized on MRI (Figures 10.3 and 10.4).

Spinal angiography may be required in cases of vascular pathology such as arteriovenous malformation. The vascular lesion may be identified with its feeding vessels and information gained concerning the cord blood supply at the relevant

Table 10.4 Spinal diseases that may be diagnosed on plain radiography

Disease	Effect
Vertebral metastasis	Bone destruction
Chordoma	Bone destruction
Neurofibroma	Foraminal widening
Intradural tumour	Scalloping of vertebral bodies
Infection	Bone destruction involving the disc space
Intervertebral disc lesions	Disc space narrowing
Deformity	
Congenital	
Acquired	Kyphoscoliosis
Degenerative disease	Spondylolisthesis
	Spondylosis
	Osteophyte formation
	Periarticular sclerosis
	Spinal instability
Rheumatoid disease	Spinal instability
	Odontoid process destruction
	Atlanto-axial subluxation
Paget's disease	Sclerotic changes

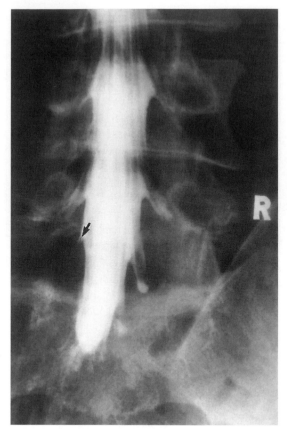

Figure 10.2 A lumbar radiculogram showing loss of contrast filling of the left S1 nerve root sleeve (arrowed) as a result of compressing disc prolapse at L5/S1.

level. Therapeutic intervention, such as embolization, may be performed at the time of diagnostic imaging.

MRI produces unrivalled imaging of the spinal cord. The range of investigations available is steadily increasing; for example, dynamic studies may yield information on CSF flow in the investigation of syringomyelia (Figure 10.5). Multiplanar imaging is readily obtained.

PRINCIPLES OF SURGICAL TREATMENT

In general, surgery may lead to a complete cure, where there is a single well circumscribed lesion, benign pathology and a patient in reasonable general health able to withstand the operation.

Other factors mitigate against success. Multiple lesions, as in metastatic cancer, make a total surgical solution impossible. Surgical exploration may be justified to provide an accurate histological diagnosis where it will affect further management and where CT-guided vertebral biopsy has failed or is contraindicated. In chronic diffuse disorders, such as osteoarthritis the search for a clear correlation between the 'surgical' abnormality and the patient's complaint is the vital part of the assessment. If the relationship between demonstrated pathology, clinical complaints and physical signs is not clear, then the outcome from operation will be poor. A clear understanding of the pathology and the mechanism producing a patient's symptoms is an essential prerequisite for the planning of successful treatment.

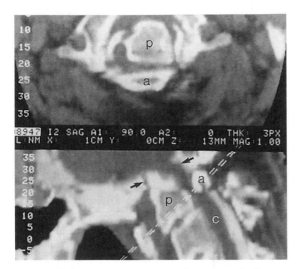

Figure 10.3 Images obtained from CT myelography. The upper image is an axial view through the C1/C2 junction, indicated by the dashed line on the lower image. The lower image is obtained by a sagittal reformat of the axial scan data. The scan demonstrates extreme pathological changes at the craniocervical junction into the foramen magnum (arrowed). There is anterior subluxation of the atlanto-axial joint causing severe cord compression between the odontoid peg (p) and the posterior arch of the atlas (a) and exclusion of contrast at this level. The contrast column and spinal cord (c) is not compressed in the subaxial spine.

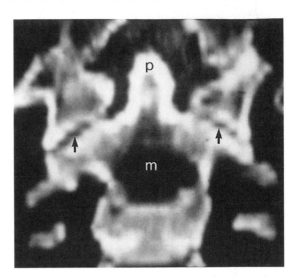

Figure 10.4 A reconstructed CT in the coronal plane obtained from axial scan data. The C2 vertebra is demonstrated with the odontoid peg (p) and atlanto-axial lateral mass joint spaces (arrows). Within the body is a lucent area secondary to a metastatic deposit (m) from a primary breast carcinoma.

The operations

The contents of the vertebral canal may be approached from a number of directions (Figure 10.6). Each section of the spine may be reached from the front, from the side and from behind, however, the optimal approach is determined by the spinal level, the type of pathology and the relationship of the pathology to the neural elements.

Laminectomy is a posterior approach and the one most commonly used, particularly in the lumbar spine. A lateral approach, **costotransversectomy**, is used primarily for the removal of thoracic disc and other high thoracic anterior lesions. **Anterior approaches** are most commonly used in the cervical spine, which is easily approached between the carotid sheath and the pharynx. Most of the thoracic and upper lumbar spine can also be approached antero-laterally, either through the chest or retroperitoneally, giving access for the treatment of thoracic disc

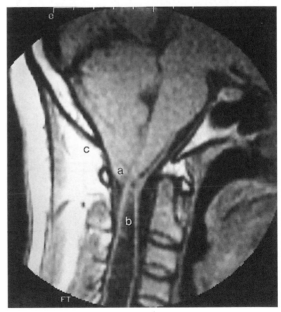

Figure 10.5 A T1-weighted sagittal MRI of the craniocervical junction demonstrating a Chiari malformation with descent of the cerebellar tonsils: (a) to the level of the C1 arch, an associated syrinx cavity; (b) and crowding at the level of the foramen magnum; (c) with loss of CSF space around the cervicomedullary junction.

lesions, osteomyelitis and fractures (Figure 10.6). Such procedures permit decompression of the contents of the vertebral canal, the removal and biopsy of tumours, evacuation of pus and the excision of disc sequestra.

Less invasive procedures are directed at specific small lesions; for example, **microdiscectomy** for cervical and lumbar disc prolapse, and **foraminotomy** for the decompression of nerve roots in the cervical and lumbar regions. In the cervical spine the merits of anterior or posterior surgery are subject to ongoing surgical debate. The anterior approach allows anterior compressive pathology to be removed directly. Single or multiple level fusion may be carried out at the same time. Posteriorly, cervical laminectomy is technically simpler than multilevel anterior procedures, but may compromise spinal stability.

When there is destruction of the vertebral body, surgical exploration must generally be accompanied by procedures to stabilize the spine, either by bone grafting, supportive metalwork, or both.

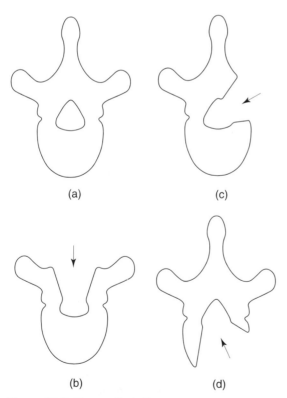

Figure 10.6 Diagram illustrating common surgical approaches to the thoracic spinal canal. The extent of bone resection is shown for each approach: (a) complete vertebra; (b) laminectomy; (c) costotransversectomy; (d) transthoracic vertebrectomy.

COMMON CAUSES OF COMPRESSION OF THE CONTENTS OF THE VERTEBRAL CANAL

The causes of compression of the contents of the spinal canal are conveniently classified according to the pathology and site (Table 10.1).

Malignant extradural tumours

Malignant extradural tumours are the commonest spinal neoplasms encountered in clinical practice. They can arise in the extradural tissue and/or bone. In many patients involvement of the spine and cord compression are the presenting features of the malignant disease (Figure 10.7).

The primary tumour, which usually has its origin in lung, breast, prostate, kidney or thyroid may defy detection. Myeloma can also present with a single spinal deposit.

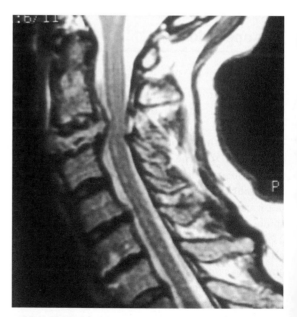

Figure 10.7 MRI scan cervical spine (T2-weighted), sagittal view, showing collapse of C3 with cord compression as a result of a metastasis from a primary breast tumour.

It needs to be emphasized that while the course of the illness may be influenced by surgery, radiotherapy, chemotherapy and endocrine manipulations, the nature of the tumour determines prognosis. Involvement of the spine often has two important consequences, namely irreversible neurological damage and spinal instability, which may represent a terminal event in an incurable disease.

Secondary carcinoma usually develops in the marrow space of the body or pedicles of the vertebrae. Local pain is an early feature and it indicates involvement of the periosteum, either directly or through stresses arising in it from loss of mechanical strength. The signs of cord compression usually herald vertebral collapse and irreversible paraplegia. Complete paraplegia may follow an anterior spinal artery thrombosis caused by the compression and will be irreversible.

It is possible that early treatment may prevent death through paraplegia even though cure of the underlying condition is not possible. The surgical issues are complex. While most deposits arise with a particular relationship to the cord, at operation they seem to surround the dural envelope. If the vertebral body has been destroyed, laminectomy may remove the only sound bone at that vertebral level and the increased instability may make an incomplete paraplegia complete. Laminectomy should be combined with a stabilization procedure, or an anterior approach should be considered. Unfortunately, anterior approaches to the thoracic and lumbar spines are major surgical undertakings in patients who are often elderly and debilitated by their disease. Treatment that decompresses the neural elements, that maintains the stability of the spine and halts the progress of the tumour can prevent paraplegia (Figure 10.8), however each case must be individually assessed to determine the treatment goals, whether palliative or curative, and the benefit/risk analysis for each. Radiotherapy or chemotherapy are essential adjuvants for the successful management of malignant spinal disease.

Extramedullary intradural spinal tumours

Neurofibromas occur at any level, but meningiomas are commonly located in the mid-dorsal region of middle-aged and elderly women (Figure 10.9). They are both usually benign tumours.

Pain at the level of the lesion is a usual but not invariable feature. These tumours may present with partial cord syndromes depending on the relationship to the spinal cord.

In tumours located between the foramen magnum and fifth cervical level, diagnosis may be difficult. Postural and discriminatory sensory loss in the hand in excess of other signs of cord compression should suggest the diagnosis. Meningiomas situated at the foramen magnum were often difficult to

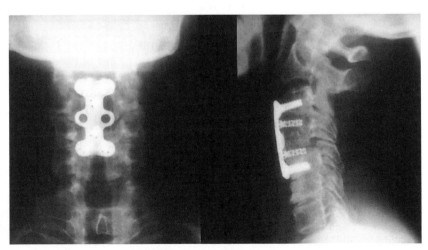

Figure 10.8 Postoperative anteroposterior and lateral radiographs of the cervical spine. The patient has undergone an excision of the C4 vertebral body with decompression of the C4 and C5 nerve root foramina for myelopathic and radiculopathic symptoms. The spine has been reconstructed using an iliac crest bone graft to replace C4 and has been stabilized with a titanium locking plate. The implant is MRI-compatible.

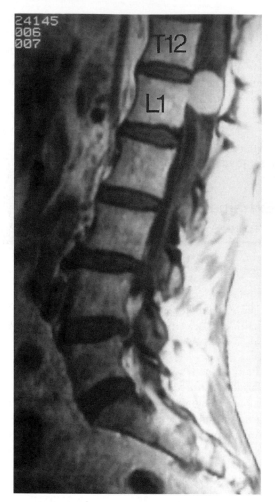

Figure 10.9 A contrast-enhanced T1-weighted sagittal MRI scan of the lumbar spine and thoracolumbar junction. At T12/L1 an enhancing mass occupies the spinal canal, compressing the conus medullaris. Histology of the excised tissue confirmed this was a meningioma.

demonstrate until the advent of MRI. Neurofibromas arise from the sensory nerve roots and may extend into the intervertebral foramen and beyond as 'dumb-bell' tumours with characteristic changes on the plain X-ray. **Most neurofibromas and meningiomas are effectively cured by removal** through a laminectomy exposure. The sacrifice of the sensory nerve root on which a neurofibroma arises rarely causes significant disability unless a major limb plexus root is involved. The neurofibromas associated with neurofibromatosis type 1 present difficult and often insoluble problems, as they may be multiple and extensive, requiring frequent operations.

Intramedullary intradural spinal tumours

The commonest intramedullary tumours are ependymomas and the astrocytomas, in approximately equal proportion and varying degrees of malignancy.

Ependymomas are generally well circumscribed, are associated with cysts and do not infiltrate the neural elements to any great extent. Slow-growing tumours often enlarge the vertebral canal, which is evident on plain film radiology. It is often possible to carry out an effective surgical removal by making an incision in the posterior aspect of the cord, and separating the dorsal columns to expose the tumour. A common site for these tumours is at the conus, where they become intimately involved with the cauda equina and are therefore difficult to remove in total.

By contrast, **astrocytomas** are frequently not well demarcated and excision is not possible without the risk of damaging functioning tissue. The mainstay of treatment is radiotherapy.

Spinal **haemangioblastomas** are less common, and may occur in any part of the spinal cord, but are usually located in the cervical region where they produce a progressive tetraparesis.

Other tumours involving the spine are rare. These include bone sarcomas, chordoma, dermoids, lipomas and dissemination of primary intracranial tumours such as medulloblastoma.

Vascular diseases affecting the spinal cord

Angiomas most frequently present with a progressive myelopathy. In the event of a haemorrhage, a sudden deterioration in function may occur if the bleed is intramedullary. Subarachnoid haemorrhage may occasionally have a spinal origin, suggested by a history of more neck pain than headache at presentation. The diagnosis should be considered where conventional four-vessel cerebral angiography is negative. Magnetic resonance imaging may demonstrate multiple signal voids suggestive of an angioma (Figure 10.10), but spinal angiography is the definitive test. Angiography is not without risk for it requires catheterization of the feeding vessels. True

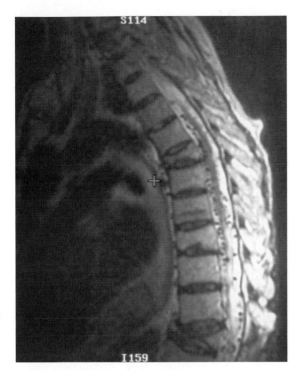

Figure 10.10 MRI scan of thoracic spine, T2-weighted, sagittal view, showing numerous small blood vessels from a dural fistula.

arteriovenous malformations are rare, more common are arteriovenous fistulae at dural level, which cause cord dysfunction through venous hypertension. Successful surgical or endovascular treatment depends on the excision or obliteration of the fistula without inflicting damage to the cord or its blood supply. The assessment is complex and requires close collaboration between neurosurgeon and interventional neuroradiologist.

Spinal infection

The clinical effects and natural history of spinal infections depend on the structures primarily involved, the organism and the host's response, modified by any treatment the patient may have received. Infection may reach the spine by contiguous spread, via the bloodstream or directly through a penetrating injury or a dermal sinus. The dura usually forms an effective barrier to local spread unless it is breached, for example by lumbar puncture.

The neurological deficit is produced by a mixture of compression and vasculitis. Those patients whose immunity is compromised through age, debility or disease present with atypical pictures, usually of chronic character when organisms of low virulence take hold.

Intradural infection

Abscess, solitary or multiple, within the dura is very rare and may be located within the spinal cord, in the subdural space or among the roots of the cauda equina, when it is usually associated with a dermal sinus. These infections are distinguished from meningitis by the fact that they are localized. Patients have a short history, often with clear evidence of the source of infection, are systemically ill, and have a bad prognosis with high mortality. Those with chronic infection present like an intramedullary tumour and respond better to surgical drainage of the pus and antibiotic treatment.

Extradural infection

Infection usually reaches the epidural space through the bloodstream from an identifiable source, commonly a staphylococcal skin infection.

Extradural infection

Characteristically the illness is acute with intense spinal and root pain, with a rapidly advancing loss of neurological function at and below the lesion. Generally, there is clear evidence of a systemic disturbance, local tenderness and muscle spasm, complemented by varying degrees of spinal cord or cauda equina dysfunction. This is an acute surgical emergency.

Once neurological deficits are well established recovery is unusual and it is probable that ischaemic damage has occurred.

Plain X-rays of the spine are usually normal. Lumbar puncture is usually safe below the level of the lesion, but it is customary to aspirate on reaching the epidural space to exclude pus before entering the subarachnoid space. Magnetic resonance imaging will provide the information necessary to plan treatment. Surgical decompression, usually by laminectomy, is essential to drain pus and provides the opportunity to identify the infecting organism and rationalize antibiotic treatment.

Infection of bone and cartilage

Osteomyelitis is uncommon in healthy individuals, but must be considered in the immune compromised, diabetics, the debilitated elderly and those with rheumatoid arthritis, who present with local spinal and root pain of short duration. The onset is insidious but progress depends on the organism and the host's response. There is local tenderness, particularly to percussion of the spines at the level of infection, muscle spasm, and, if vertebral collapse has occurred, a kyphus. While systemic disturbance is usual in children, it may well be absent in the elderly. **Tuberculosis of the spine is the most common form of infection** (Figure 10.1).

In the early stages of vertebral osteomyelitis, cord compression is unusual because infection is largely prevented from spreading to the epidural space by the strength and rigidity of the posterior longitudinal ligament. In the event of vertebral collapse, extrusion of pus and granulation tissue into the vertebral canal usually produces cord compression, with rapid loss of all functions below the level of the lesion. As in the case of early carcinoma, there are often no changes demonstrable on plain film radiology. Over a period of 4–12 weeks demineralization and the loss of the bony trabeculae become sufficient to be visible on a plain X-ray.

> Unlike carcinoma, which leaves the disc space intact, infection characteristically destroys the disc space and the two adjacent vertebrae (Figure 10.11).

Investigation by CT scan will show early bone destruction and evidence of a paravertebral abscess, and will be more informative than a plain X-ray. Needle biopsy is required to obtain pus for culture and to look for tuberculous infection. When the spinal canal is not compromised, treatment consists of immobilization and the appropriate antibiotic. Patients with extensive bone destruction and a

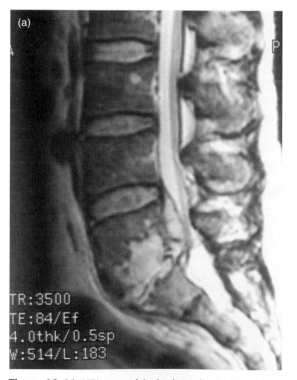
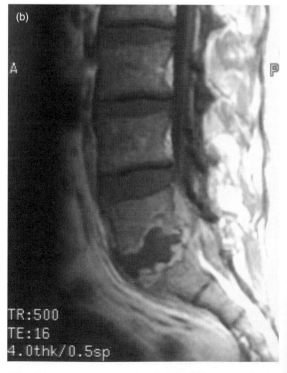

Figure 10.11 MRI scans of the lumbar spine (a) T2-weighted and (b) T1-weighted, sagittal views, showing staphylococcal infection of the L5/S1 disc. Note the infection has destroyed the disc.

compromised vertebral canal will require debridement and bone grafting. Most patients will obtain a solid fusion in 6–12 months. **For pyogenic and tuberculous infection antibiotics will be required for at least 6 months.** Where vertebral collapse is present and laminectomy is indicated for the treatment of an associated epidural abscess, an additional stabilization procedure may be necessary.

Degenerative spinal disease

Mechanical derangements and degenerative disorders are the most common disorders of the spine, and also present the clinician with some of the most difficult problems in management.

Two factors, trauma and the degenerative process of ageing, influenced by lifestyle or occupation, operate on the spine to varying degree. Sciatica as a result of a ruptured lumbar disc precipitated by a sudden strain in a young adult, contrasts with the process of attrition of diffuse degenerative spondylosis in the elderly, yet the presenting constellation of symptoms has many features in common.

Acute disc rupture may be the result of a sudden major event, but more commonly it is the end-result of repeated minor stresses, which predispose to rupture of the annulus and sequestration of disc material. Stresses of this kind predominantly affect the weight-bearing lumbar spine. The cervical section is the most mobile segment of the spine and degenerative change is a normal part of the ageing process. **Eighty percent of the population over 55 years of age has degenerative changes identifiable on plain X-ray.** These are found at C5/C6 and C6/C7 and are often clinically silent. Acute disc rupture with sequestration is rare, but narrowing of the intervertebral foramina and the reduction in the size of the vertebral canal, which occurs as a result of the degenerative process, is responsible for most myelopathy and nerve root symptoms.

The clinical syndromes of disc disease, at either single or multiple levels, fall into three categories: root, cord or cauda equina compression. There may be a combination of two types. Acute disc rupture, lumbar or cervical, often follows a history of recurrent bouts of back or neck pain, respectively. The pain is exacerbated by mechanical factors and

relieved by rest. Eventually a further episode of spinal pain is accompanied, or quickly followed by radicular pain. Sequestration of the extruded disc fragment usually takes place laterally into the vertebral canal, because the posterior longitudinal ligament is strongest in the midline.

Occasionally sequestration of the content of the disc enters the central part of the vertebral canal and may compress the spinal cord or cauda equina.

Central disc prolapse
Acute central disc prolapse with neurological involvement constitutes a neurosurgical emergency.

Radicular syndromes often respond to conservative methods, but the persistence of severe radicular pain or increasing neurological signs are indications for operation.

CONSIDERATION OF DISEASE BY SPINAL SECTION

Cervical spine

Cervical spondylosis is almost a normal part of the ageing process. Characteristically there is loss of disc space height, and reactive/osteoarthritic changes at the edges of the vertebral bodies and around the facet joints. Osteophytes around the disc margin, thickening of the soft tissues, hypertrophy of the facet joints, and the loss of disc height, which leads to a buckling of the ligamentum flavum, all contribute to a narrowing of the normally capacious vertebral canal. In some patients this results in pressure on the cord itself and/or on adjacent nerve roots.

Acute exacerbations of neck pain may be relieved by prescribing non-steroidal anti-inflammatory medication or simple analgesics. Immobilization of the neck in a collar may offer pain relief, however the collar should be worn for a limited duration, usually a maximum of 2 weeks, as prolonged passive cervical support may lead to problems with rehabilitation. Once the acute phase has settled, the spine should be remobilized by exercise or passive manipulation/stretching. This is best achieved by a specialist spinal physiotherapist.

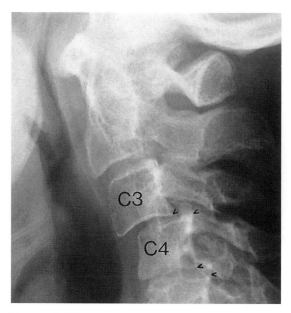

Figure 10.12 Lateral radiograph of the upper cervical spine taken in flexion. There is failure of the spinal elements to maintain their normal relationship (instability) with anterior listhesis at C3/C4 and C4/C5 indicated by the relative positions of the superior and inferior borders of the posterior vertebral bodies (arrowheads).

Where the degenerative process is also accompanied by myelopathy, a decompressive procedure may be indicated to arrest the myelopathic process. If the compressive lesion is over several segments, then a posterior decompression (laminectomy) is generally favoured. Preoperative plain X-rays in flexion and extension should be taken to exclude instability before laminectomy is considered (Figure 10.12). The anterior route, excising the degenerate disc with or without fusion best tackles localized lesions at one or two levels. **Acute disc prolapse in the cervical spine with brachalgia usually resolves with conservative treatment within 3 months.** Unremitting pain with neurological signs is an indication for investigation and consideration of discectomy.

Thoracic spine

The thoracic spine is the least mobile part of the spinal column as it is braced by the thoracic cage and symptomatic degenerative disease is rare. Symptomatic thoracic disc protrusion is exceedingly uncommon and is usually diagnosed when some other condition

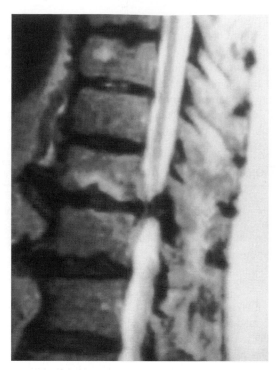

Figure 10.13 A sagittal T2-weighted MRI demonstrating extreme spinal cord compression at T10/T11. The compression is caused anteriorly by a thoracic disc prolapse in addition to ligamental hypertrophy.

is suspected. Incidental thoracic disc protrusions are not an uncommon finding on thoracic MRI.

Compressive thoracic disc lesions lie anterior to the spinal cord where the vertebral canal is narrow (Figure 10.13). Removal by a posterior approach requires caution. Careful neurosurgical evaluation is required, but generally these discs may be safely removed either by a lateral approach, costotransversectomy or anteriorly through the chest (Figure 10.6). Pain in a thoracic root distribution may present as chest pain and may even be misdiagnosed as pleurisy. It can often be reproduced by rotation of the thoracic spine. As with cervical spondylosis, the pain often settles spontaneously over a few days or weeks. Simple analgesics and reassurance may be all that are required.

Lumbar spine

Acute low back pain, the result of a sudden or repeated mechanical stress, is probably one of the most common afflictions of mankind.

Fortunately most episodes resolve with rest and simple analgesics. Occasionally, despite all kinds of conservative measures, pain persists. Plain X-rays are usually uninformative, but are carried out to exclude spondylolisthesis and more sinister pathology, such as vertebral metastases. Scanning with MRI may reveal disc disease and it may be tempting to remove the abnormal disc or fuse the spine at that level. **Decision making in surgery of the lumbar spine requires careful consideration of the patient, and correlation of the symptoms and signs with the imaging in order to achieve a successful outcome. Failure to perform this analysis will lead to inappropriate surgery, which can only worsen the clinical situation.**

Sciatica that follows a history of mechanical back pain is likely to be the result of a lumbar disc disorder, and in a young adult a soft disc protrusion with or without sequestration is the most likely explanation. **The majority of acute disc protrusions occur at the fourth and fifth lumbar intervals.** Acute rupture with sequestration is rare at higher levels. Loss of spinal movement, muscle spasm and limitation of straight leg raising and root signs are cardinal. **Similar symptoms in patients aged in their 50s or 60s are more likely to be the result of hypertrophy of a facet joint.** When a disc protrusion is present, this is often small but causes severe symptoms, as there is less available space for the nerve root as a result of the hypertrophied facet joint. Before the annulus ruptures there is often a stage when a bulging deformity is present. This may be sufficient to produce physical signs of nerve root irritation or unremitting back pain. Complete rest at this stage will generally relieve sciatica. The process is speeded up by a steroid epidural injection, which acts directly on the inflammatory process around the acutely prolapsed disc. Neurological signs often regress even if the disc material has sequestrated into the vertebral canal or exit foramen symptoms. The diagnosis will be confirmed by MRI (Figure 10.14). If signs and symptoms do not settle and an operation becomes necessary, the use of the operating microscope and improved instruments have made it possible to remove sequestrated discs with relatively little disturbance to the normal structures.

Bilateral sciatica

Bilateral sciatica, especially if accompanied by sacral root signs (loss of ankle jerks, foot drop and particularly perianal sensory loss), suggests a

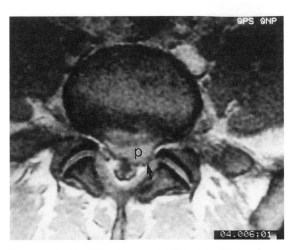

Figure 10.14 A T1-weighted axial MRI at the L5/S1 disc level. An acute anterolateral prolapse (p) of the L5/S1 disc is demonstrated. The left S1 nerve root (arrowed) is compressed concordant with the patient's symptoms of left-sided sciatica.

central disc prolapse with cauda equina compression. Any suggestion of sphincter disturbance or perianal sensory loss is reason for immediate surgical referral.

Lumbar spondylosis is almost an inevitable consequence of ageing. As in the cervical spine, the osteophytes around the disc margins, the hypertrophy of the facet joints and loss of disc height with kinking of the ligamentum flavum, narrow the lumbar canal (Figure 10.15). In most people the process remains symptomless but, in some, the nerve roots or the cauda equina become compromised.

Characteristically these patients complain of weakness and bilateral sciatica-like discomfort or pain brought on by exercise (claudication). Signs are often minimal, the diagnosis being made on the history and imaging, in addition to absent ankle jerks.

When there is a clear correlation between the history and the signs and the radiographic findings, relief of symptoms may be anticipated from a decompressive laminectomy, with decompression of the lateral recesses of the spinal canal deep to the facet joints (Figures 10.15 and 10.16). However, the duration of relief depends in part on the extent of the disease and its rate of progress.

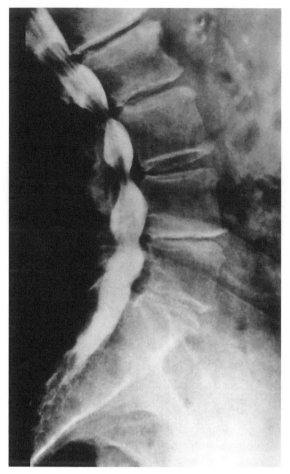

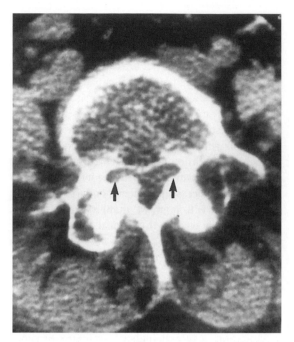

Figure 10.16 Plain lumbar axial CT through the L4 vertebral body. The spinal canal is stenosed and has a trefoil shape as a result of degenerative facet joint hypertrophy narrowing the lateral recesses (arrows) of the spinal canal.

Figure 10.15 Lateral radiculogram demonstrates extreme stenosis of the lumbar spinal canal. The lumbar theca is pinched at several levels by anterior and posterior compressive elements. The roots of the cauda equina are seen as longitudinal filling defects within the contrast column.

Syringomyelia

> Syringomyelia describes cystic cavitation in the spinal cord. The commonest cause is brainstem herniation where the cerebellar tonsils become impacted in the foramen magnum. This is the type 1 Chiari malformation (see p. 431).

A process of CSF pressure imbalance between the spine and skull leads to the development of the cavity, which can be shown to occur even in the first decade of life. The process generally begins in the cervical cord but, as the cavity expands, the brainstem and distal cord may also become involved. **Patients may present with the symptoms of brainstem compression and many have pain in the neck.** As the cavity itself expands, numbness and weakness in the hands and trunk appear, along with stiffness and weakness of the legs. **At the level of the syrinx, the grey matter of the anterior horn cells is lost, producing weakness and atrophy of the muscles with loss of tendon reflexes in the upper limb, signs of a lower motor neurone lesion. The syrinx interrupts the central decussating fibres of the spinothalamic tracts, producing dissociated loss of thermal sensibility and pain sensation, sparing the posterior columns.** As the condition advances, the loss of spinothalamic function is associated with the development of neuropathic arthropathies and other trophic changes. The symptoms and signs are seldom symmetrical. **Below the level of the syrinx there are signs of a spastic paraparesis. Sphincter function is usually preserved.**

Cavitation of the cord can occur in other circumstances, such as in association with **arachnoiditis** around the foramen magnum (another type of obstruction to the CSF pathway). Rarely, a syrinx

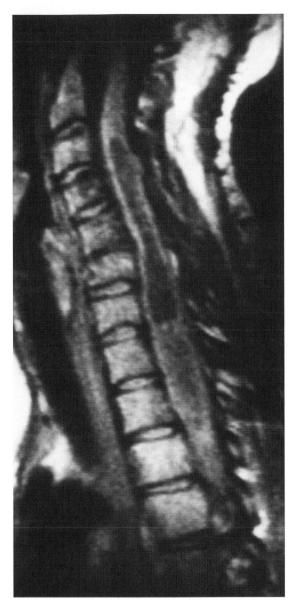

Figure 10.17 MRI scan of cervical spine, T1-weighted, sagittal view, in a patient with neurofibromatosis type 2. The spinal cord is expanded and contains a syrinx above a solid intramedullary mass.

extensions of the tumour, and not CSF-filled syrinx cavities.

Magnetic resonance imaging is the definitive investigation, which provides a clear and unequivocal picture of the syrinx, any craniocervical anomaly or other hindbrain anomaly. Management must depend in part on the aetiology and, therefore, each group should be considered separately. As a general principle, treatment must be directed at the primary cause and sometimes at the syrinx itself. Where there is an association between a Chiari malformation and a syrinx, the aim is to relieve the pressure by removing the lower central part of the occipital bone and the spines and arches of the atlas and axis at the craniocervical junction, to restore normal CSF dynamics, and prevent further extension of the syrinx. The dura may be opened leaving the arachnoid layer intact. Headache, neck and arm pain, and signs of recent and progressive character are most likely to be relieved by operation. Surgical decompression of the structures at and adjacent to the foramen magnum seems to give some benefit in about two-thirds of cases, and may prevent further deterioration. However, the extent of the improvement of the symptoms relating to development of the cavity itself may be disappointing, as the symptoms and signs reflect cord destruction.

Drainage of the syrinx into the subarachnoid space or into the pleural or peritoneal cavities may give some relief and, in particular, prevent further deterioration.

Spinal dysraphism

Most spinal dysraphism syndromes present in childhood (see p. 429). Rarely they may present in adult life with a progressive cauda equina syndrome. They may be associated with a dermoid or lipoma and sometimes with a visible tuft of hair.

develops as a late sequel to **spinal injury** and should be suspected when a patient with a traumatic paraparesis or paraplegia develops a painful ascending myelopathy. Syringomyelia-like syndromes may occur in association with **intramedullary spinal tumours** (Figure 10.17); but the cavities are cystic

REFERENCES AND FURTHER READING

Devo RA, Weinstein DO (2001) Low back pain. *New England Journal of Medicine*, **344**:363–370.

Ehni G, Clark K, Wilson CB *et al.* (1969) Significance of the small lumbar spinal canal: cauda equina compression syndrome due to spondylosis. *Neurosurgery*, **31**:490–519.

Findlay GFG (1984) Adverse effects of the management of malignant spinal cord compression. *Journal of Neurology, Neurosurgery & Psychiatry*, **47**:761–768.

Frizzell RT, Hadley MN (1993) Lumbar microdiscectomy with medial facetectomy. Techniques and analysis of results. *Neurosurgery Clinics of North America*, **4**:109–115.

Junge A, Dvorak J, Ahrens S (1995) Predictors of good and bad outcome of lumbar disc surgery. A prospective clinical study with recommendations for screening to avoid bad outcomes. *Spine*, **20**:460–468.

Nussbaum ES, Rigamonti D, Standiford H *et al.* (1992) Spinal epidural abscess: a report of 40 cases and review. *Journal of Neurosurgery*, **38**:225–231.

Rogers M, Crockard HA (1994) Surgical treatment of the symptomatic herniated thoracic disc. *Clinical Orthopaedics*, **300**:70–78.

Seppala MT, Haltia MJ, Sankila RJ *et al.* (1995) Long term outcome after removal of spinal neurofibroma. *Journal of Neurosurgery*, **82**:572–577.

Souweidane MM, Benjamin V (1994) Spinal cord meningiomas. *Neurosurgery Clinics of North America*, **5**:283–291.

Wilkinson M (1960) The morbid anatomy of cervical spondylosis and myelopathy. *Brain*, **83**: 589–616.

Williams B (1978) A Critical appraisal of posterior fossa surgery for communicating syringomyelia. *Brain*, **101**:223–250.

Young S, O'Laorie S (1987) Cervical disc prolapse in the elderly: an easily overlooked, reversible cause of spinal cord compression. *British Journal of Neurosurgery*, **1**:93–98.

CHAPTER 11

MOVEMENT DISORDERS

N.P. Quinn

INTRODUCTION

Movement disorders comprise two main categories:

1 Akinetic-rigid syndromes and
2 Dyskinesias.

AKINETIC-RIGID SYNDROMES

Akinetic-rigid syndromes are characterized by slowness of voluntary movement and muscular rigidity, often called the parkinsonian syndrome. The most important cause of an akinetic-rigid syndrome is Parkinson's disease (PD). Other causes are given in Table 11.1.

Parkinson's disease

Parkinson's disease

Parkinson's disease is a slowly progressive, degenerative disease of the basal ganglia, producing an akinetic-rigid syndrome, usually with rest tremor, and accompanied by many other motor disturbances, including a flexed posture, a shuffling gait and, later in the disease, defective balance.

Epidemiology

Parkinson's disease is a common illness of advancing years. The prevalence rate in the UK is about 170 per 100 000 of the overall population, but much higher in older subjects. There are about 100 000 patients with PD in the UK. Most series show a slight male preponderance, and the illness occurs in all races. While there are no striking differences among most populations of the world, the incidence may be somewhat less in Africa and China. Average age at disease onset is about 60 years. Survival is only modestly reduced.

Pathology

The main pathological finding in PD is loss of the pigmented neurones in the brainstem, particularly those in the substantia nigra, with the presence in some of the surviving neurones of intracytoplasmic eosinophilic inclusions known as Lewy bodies.

The substantia nigra pars compacta projects to the striatum (the caudate nucleus and putamen) via the nigrostriatal pathway, which utilizes dopamine as its neurotransmitter. Parkinson's disease is associated with a considerable loss of striatal dopamine content, 80% or more, proportional to the loss of substantia nigra neurones. **Striatal dopamine deficiency is thus the cardinal biochemical feature of PD.** This discovery led to the introduction of treatment with levodopa, the amino acid precursor for dopamine

Table 11.1 Causes of an akinetic-rigid syndrome

Idiopathic sporadic Parkinson's disease
Genetically determined 'Parkinson's diseases'
  Dominant, e.g. α-synuclein mutations on
  chromosome 4
  Recessive, e.g. parkin mutations on chromosome 6
Reversible drug-induced as a result of dopamine
  receptor blocking or dopamine depleting
  medications
Vascular 'pseudoparkinsonism'
Toxic as a result of MPTP/carbon monoxide/
  methanol/manganese
Post-encephalitic as a result of encephalitis
  lethargica or Japanese B encephalitis
Post-traumatic from repeated head trauma
  ('punch-drunk syndrome'); hydrocephalus or
  tumour
Other neurodegenerative diseases:
  Classically sporadic
    Multiple system atrophy (MSA)
    Progressive supranuclear palsy (PSP)
    Corticobasal degeneration (CBD)
  Genetic
  Dominant
    Huntington's disease
    Spinocerebellar ataxias 2 + 3
  Recessive
    Wilson's disease
    Hallervorden–Spatz disease
  Uncertain
    Parkinsonism – dementia – ALS complex of
    Guam
    PSP-like atypical parkinsonism of Guadeloupe

MPTP, 1-methyl-4-phenyl-1,2,3,6-tetrahydropyridine;
ALS, amyotrophic lateral sclerosis.

synthesis in the brain. However, the dopamine concept of PD is an oversimplification, for other brain regions and neurotransmitters also are affected.

Other dopaminergic neuronal systems degenerate, including those projecting to the cerebral cortex from the ventral tegmental area adjacent to the substantia nigra, and those in the hypothalamus.

Degeneration of the locus coeruleus leads to the loss of noradrenergic pathways to the cerebral cortex and other brain regions. There is also degeneration of cells in the raphe complex, which leads to deficiency of serotonin neurotransmission, and of cells in the substantia innominata, or nucleus basalis of Meynert, which project acetylcholine-containing pathways to the cerebral cortex. Other structures affected include cerebral cortex, dorsal motor nucleus of vagus, sympathetic ganglia, and Meissner's and Auerbach's plexuses.

Aetiology

The cause of PD is not known. In the 1920s, a pandemic of **encephalitis lethargica** was followed by many cases of post-encephalitic parkinsonism. This led to the suggestion that PD itself might be caused by a virus, but none has been found, and the microscopic pathology of post-encephalitic parkinsonism (characterized by the presence of straight neurofibrillary tangles and the absence of Lewy bodies) is quite different from that of PD.

A sizeable number of patients, perhaps 10–15%, give a history that another family member was affected by PD. Is this due to chance co-occurrence of a common disease, or does it indicate that the illness might be **inherited**? Initial clinical studies of twin pairs, one of whom had PD, showed that the risk of the second identical twin developing the illness was no different from that of non-identical twins, and no different from that among the general population. However, subsequent studies in which both twins were subjected to 18_F-fluorodopa positron emission tomography (PET) scans revealed abnormalities in clinically normal co-twins, which, if considered as evidence of subclinical disease, considerably increased concordance. A more recent large study of US World War II veteran twin pairs showed significant heritability among the population of twin pairs with onset below, but not among those with onset above, 50 years of age. In addition, rare families with multiple cases of PD have been identified, with linkage in some, and discovery of new genes responsible for parkinsonism in others. The first of these was the Contursi American–Italian–Greek kindred who presented clearly autosomal dominant inheritance of clinically fairly typical PD, apart from young age at onset (average 43 years) and shorter survival (average 9 years), and in which two autopsies revealed typical Lewy body pathology. The condition in the family is the result of a mutation in the α-synuclein gene on chromosome 4, and another German family with a different mutation in the same gene also has familial PD. Interestingly, the Lewy bodies of all other PD patients, familial or sporadic, and also the characteristic inclusions in multiple system atrophy (MSA) brains (see later), stain heavily with anti-α-synuclein antibodies, yet no mutations are present in their α-synuclein gene. More numerous are families affected by autosomal recessive early-onset 'PD'. The first of the genes responsible, the 'Parkin' mutation on chromosome 6, was discovered in Japanese families with early-onset parkinsonism, frequently consanguineous and containing affected siblings. Since then, it has been found all over the world, often in sporadic cases, without consanguinity, and subsequently at least a further two recessive loci for 'PD' have been identified on chromosome 1p. Importantly, the Parkin brains typically do not contain Lewy bodies. Thus what was previously considered as one disease, PD, is in fact a number of diseases, some genetic, others perhaps not, some with, and some without Lewy bodies.

In the majority of patients in whom heredity appears to play little or no role, might some **environmental agent** be responsible? In the early 1980s, a small outbreak of an illness clinically indistinguishable from PD, but without Lewy bodies, occurred among drug addicts on the West Coast of America. The cause was a contaminant, MPTP (1-methyl-4-phenyl-1,2,3,6-tetrahydropyridine) produced during the synthesis of a designer drug. MPTP is not the active toxin, but is converted in the brain, by monoamine-oxidase B in glia, into the toxic form MPP (1-methyl-4-phenylpyendinium), which is then taken up into dopaminergic neurones, by the normal dopamine reuptake mechanism, where it is trapped by binding to neuromelanin. MPP$^+$ poisons mitochondria to cause death of pigmented dopaminergic neurones in the brain. This, albeit imperfect, model of PD shows that environmental toxins can cause selective nigral cell death, but none has been definitely identified in the causation of PD. MPTP is one of a number of toxic species, and there have been suggestions that the incidence of PD may be higher in populations exposed to cumulative poisoning with pesticides or contaminated well water. Alternatively, exposure early in life could be followed by the effects of natural ageing in dopaminergic systems in the brain, the combination of the two leading to the appearance of the illness with increasing frequency in old age.

Main clinical features

There is no laboratory test for PD, so the diagnosis depends on clinical signs of akinesia, rigidity, tremor and postural abnormalities. The illness usually commences on one side of the body, typically in an arm, less frequently in a leg – and remains asymmetric, even when the opposite side becomes affected.

Akinesia is the most important disabling feature of PD for the patient. Akinesia means an inability to move, while bradykinesia refers to slowness of movement, and hypokinesia means reduced amplitude of movement. Typically, there is a slowness of initiation and execution of all movement, and a general poverty of spontaneous and automatic or associated movements. Alternating movements (e.g. finger-taps) show progressive fatiguing of rate and decrement in amplitude, often ultimately grinding to a halt.

Akinesia accounts for many characteristic features of PD – the masked expressionless face, reduced blinking, absence of arm-swing when walking, small cramped handwriting, soft monotonous speech, and difficulties with walking.

Rigidity of muscles is detected clinically by resistance to passive manipulation of the limbs and neck. The examiner encounters uniform resistance throughout the range of passive movement, fairly equal in agonists and antagonists (hence the terms 'plasticity' or 'lead-pipe rigidity'). When tremor is also present, rigidity is broken up ('cog-wheel' rigidity).

Tremor is the initial complaint in about two-thirds of subjects with PD, and occurs eventually in many of the remaining one-third. **The characteristic tremor is present at rest** at a frequency of 3–6 Hz; it is most common in the arms, where it can produce the typical 'pill-rolling' movement. The jaw and legs may shake as well. The tremor is intensified by mental or emotional stress but disappears during deep sleep. Many patients also, or instead, exhibit a tremor of the hands with maintained posture, at a faster frequency of 6–8 Hz.

Postural abnormalities are typical of PD. Rigidity contributes to the characteristic flexed posture.

Table 11.7 Causes of dystonia

Primary dystonia
    Generalized and segmental dystonia
        DYT1 Chromosome 9 (autosomal dominant – 40% of cases)
        Others, either genetic or sporadic
    Focal adult-onset dystonia
        Blepharospasm
        Cranial dystonia/Meige's syndrome/Breughel's syndrome
        Oromandibular dystonia
        Spasmodic torticollis
        Spasmodic dysphonia/laryngeal dystonia
        Axial dystonia
        Writer's (and other occupational) cramps
    Usually sporadic. Genetic component remains undetermined in most cases.
Dystonia plus syndromes
    Dopa-responsive dystonia (autosomal dominant – chromosome 14)
    Myoclonus dystonia (autosomal dominant – most cases chromosome 7)
Symptomatic dystonia
    Athetoid cerebral palsy
    Post-anoxic
    Post-encephalitic
    Drug-induced
        Neuroleptics (acute dystonic reactions and tardive dystonia)
        Levodopa
    Manganese poisoning/other toxins
    Hemidystonia (usually as a result of structural lesion in contralateral basal ganglia)
        Stroke/tumour/arteriovenous malformation/trauma/encephalitis
        Post-thalamotomy
    Psychogenic (rare)
Hereditodegenerative dystonias
    Various lipid storage diseases and leukodystrophies
    Acidosis (organic acidurias)
    Ataxia telangiectasia
    Mitochondrial encephalopathies/Leigh's disease
    Wilson's disease
    Huntington's disease (especially juvenile)
    Hallervorden–Spatz disease
    Neuroacanthocytosis
    PD/PSP/MSA/CBD
    Autosomal dominant spinocerebellar ataxias (especially 2 and 3)
Paroxysmal dyskinesias
    Paroxysmal kinesigenic choreo-athetosis
    Paroxysmal dystonic choreo-athetosis
    Paroxysmal exercise-induced dystonia
    Tonic spasms in multiple sclerosis

PD, Parkinson's disease; PSP, progressive supranuclear palsy; MSA, multiple system atrophy; CBD, corticobasal degeneration.

is worsened by anxiety. There is usually no tremor at rest, but a rhythmic vertical oscillation develops when the patient holds the arms outstretched. On movement, as in finger–nose testing, the tremor may worsen terminally, but does not progressively worsen throughout the movement. Tremor of the head (titubation) or legs may also be present, but is less severe than that in the hands.

There are no signs of parkinsonism, although cog-wheeling (without rigidity) may be present. A small or moderate dose of alcohol often suppresses the tremor.

Generally the illness is only slowly progressive in most patients, causing predominantly a social disability, but individuals dependent upon manual skills may be severely disabled by the tremor.

Treatment

About one-half of patients show some useful response to a **beta–adrenergic receptor antagonist** such as propranolol. **Primidone** helps some patients. Antiparkinsonian drugs have no effect. Unilateral or bilateral **thalamic DBS** can be very effective.

Chorea

Sydenham's chorea

Rheumatic fever, the cause of Sydenham's chorea (St Vitus' dance), is now a rare disease. However, chorea and other movement disorders, sometimes associated with psychiatric disturbance, but without rheumatic fever, continue to be seen in some children after group A streptococcal infection, and may be associated with anti-basal-ganglia antibodies.

Huntington's disease

Huntington's disease (HD) is a rare, dominantly inherited, relentlessly progressive illness, usually starting in middle life, characterized by a movement disorder, usually including chorea, and behavioural and cognitive changes.

It occurs worldwide and in all ethnic groups, with a prevalence in the UK of between 5 and 10 per 100 000. **The mutation, caused by a trinucleotide CAG repeat expansion (see p. 128) on the short arm of chromosome 4**, is fully penetrant, so that the children of an affected parent have a 50% risk of developing the disease. About 6% of cases start before the age of 21 years (juvenile HD) with an akinetic-rigid syndrome (the Westphal variant), caused by long trinucleotide repeats inherited, with anticipation, in 90% of cases from an affected father. About 28% of cases start after the age of 50 years (late-onset HD). 'Senile chorea' is simply chorea in an older person – once other causes are excluded, the majority of such cases turn out to have HD.

Pathogenesis

The brain is generally atrophic with conspicuous damage to the cerebral cortex and the striatum (caudate nucleus and putamen), which shows extensive loss of medium-sized spiny neurones.

Clinical features

The onset is insidious, usually between the ages of 30 and 50 years. The initial symptoms frequently are those of a change in personality and behaviour, but chorea may be the first sign of the illness.

The family may begin to notice a blunting of drive and depth of feeling, irritability and truculence, or a tendency to uncontrolled aggressive or sexual behaviour. As the disease progresses, frontal lobe deficits become more pronounced and the chorea more severe and grotesque. Akinesia, rigidity and dystonia may appear and begin to dominate the picture. Finally, the patient becomes bedridden and emaciated. Death occurs on average about 17 years after onset.

Diagnosis is not difficult if the presentation is characteristic and a positive family history is available. However, often the family history is not known, or is hidden, or chorea may be absent or a relatively minor part of the patient's motor disorder. A simple DNA test will confirm the diagnosis.

Treatment

There is no cure for the disease. The chorea may be reduced by dopamine receptor blocking or dopamine-depleting drugs, but these drugs commonly cause disabling side-effects, and the reduction in chorea may be only cosmetic, whilst the rest of the clinical state is aggravated. The mental complications of the illness often pose particular problems for the family, and eventually chronic nursing care may be required.

Genetic counselling should be made available to other family members. Presymptomatic (predictive) and prenatal testing are available in specialized centres.

Hemiballism

Hemiballism refers to wild flinging or throwing movements of one arm and leg. They are like those of chorea but predominantly involve the large proximal muscles of the shoulder and pelvic girdle. Hemiballism is rare. It is usually seen in elderly, hypertensive or diabetic patients as a result of a stroke affecting the **contralateral subthalamic nucleus or its connections**, in which case the onset is abrupt. More recently toxoplasma abscess secondary to human immunodeficiency virus infection has emerged as a cause of hemiballism in younger subjects. The intensity of the movements varies from mild to severe enough to cause injury. If a result of a stroke, hemiballism usually gradually remits spontaneously over a period of 3–6 months. In the interim, treatment with a neuroleptic or tetrabenazine may be required to damp down the movements.

Myoclonus

Generalized myoclonus

Generalized or multifocal myoclonus occurs in a wide variety of primary diseases of the nervous system, or as a manifestation of metabolic or toxic encephalopathy. In many of these conditions, myoclonus arises from spontaneous or reflex-triggered discharges in the cerebral cortex. Such cortical myoclonus is closely related to epilepsy.

Epileptic myoclonus can be a feature of primary generalized epilepsy, or may be symptomatic of progressive brain disease as in the **progressive myoclonic epilepsies**. These conditions are discussed further in Chapter 15.

Myoclonus may dominate the clinical picture in a number of cerebral diseases. In these conditions, myoclonus may occur spontaneously, on movement (action myoclonus), or in response to visual, auditory

or somatosensory stimuli (reflex myoclonus). Severe myoclonus may be the major residual deficit after cerebral anoxia **(post-anoxic action myoclonus)**, whatever the cause. Myoclonus may be the characteristic feature of a number of degenerative dementing illnesses, such as **Alzheimer's disease**, and is characteristic of **Creutzfeldt–Jakob disease**. Myoclonus, with occasional seizures, may occur in conjunction with a cerebellar syndrome in **progressive myoclonic ataxia** (the Ramsay Hunt syndrome). Myoclonus may also follow a variety of viral illnesses (post-infectious myoclonus). In all these conditions there are likely to be other signs of damage to the central nervous system.

Myoclonus–dystonia is a familial disease, inherited as an autosomal dominant trait, in which myoclonus or dystonia are the only physical abnormalities. Many patients report that alcohol helps their jerks. Most such cases have a mutation in the epsilon-sarcoglycan gene on chromosome 7.

Focal myoclonus

There are a number of conditions in which myoclonic jerking is restricted to one part of the body. Such focal myoclonus may be a result of discharges occurring anywhere from the cerebral cortex **(epilepsy partialis continua)**, the brainstem **(palatal myoclonus or tremor)**, the spinal cord **(spinal myoclonus)**, or even peripheral nerves and roots **(hemifacial spasm)**.

Such focal myoclonus is often repetitive and rhythmic; for example, in the rare occurrence of **palatal tremor** there are rhythmic contractions of the soft palate at about 2 Hz, often persisting throughout the day and night. Sometimes this rhythmic myoclonus spreads to involve the pharynx and larynx, the intercostal muscles and diaphragm, and even the external ocular muscles. Often this condition is 'idiopathic', but in secondary cases the commonest identifiable cause is an infarct involving the brainstem, in particular in the region of the olive, dentate nucleus and red nucleus (Mollaret's triangle). Much commoner is **hemifacial spasm**, in which intermittent rapid twitchy movements start at the lateral border of orbicularis oculi and spread to synchronously involve orbicularis oris on the same side (see p. 200). In addition, the affected side of the face may be drawn up by more prolonged spasms, and often there is mild facial weakness on the same side. The cause is usually irritation of the facial nerve entry zone by a pulsatile aberrant blood vessel. Most patients are helped by botulinum toxin injections. A more invasive, but usually permanently effective, alternative is facial nerve decompression via a posterior craniotomy.

Drug treatment of myoclonus

Myoclonus often responds best to a combination of drugs. **Clonazepam, sodium valproate, primidone, piracetam** and **levetiracetam** can be used in varying combinations.

Tics

Tics and Gilles de la Tourette syndrome

Many children exhibit simple tics transiently during development. Typically these consist of eye blinks, grimaces, a sniff, or a hand gesture. Often these transient tics of childhood disappear, but sometimes they persist into adult life as chronic simple tics.

In a proportion of patients, these chronic tics are accompanied by vocalizations, when the condition is known as **Gilles de la Tourette syndrome**.

This illness begins before the age of 18 years with the tics affecting particularly the upper part of the body, especially the face, neck and shoulders. Their severity and distribution tend to wax and wane with time, and one tic may be replaced by another. Sooner or later, such patients begin to make involuntary noises, such as grunting, squealing, yelping, throat-clearing, sniffing, coughing or barking. In about 15% of cases these noises become transformed into swear words (coprolalia). Many Tourette patients also exhibit features of obsessive-compulsive disorder, and many affected children also display attention-deficit hyperactivity disorder.

The illness tends to be lifelong, although its severity usually decreases in adulthood. The condition appears to be inherited possibly as an autosomal dominant trait with variable penetrance.

The tics and vocalizations may cause considerable distress to the child or adolescent. **Anti-dopamine drugs** such as haloperidol, pimozide, or tetrabenazine or sulpiride **may control the involuntary movements and noises**, although finding the appropriate dose requires careful and gradual titration in each patient. Many patients find the side-effects (extrapyramidal, drowsiness, depression) from these medications unacceptable, and instead prefer to live with their tics. **Obsessive-compulsive disorder-like symptoms may be helped by selective serotonin reuptake inhibitors or clomipramine and attention-deficit hyperactivity disorder by methylphenidate**.

Dystonia

Dystonia may affect the whole body (generalized dystonia or dystonia musculorum deformans), in which case onset is typically in childhood. Alternatively, it may affect only one part of the body (focal dystonia), typically with onset in adult life. Cases of segmental dystonia, involving two or more contiguous body parts, are intermediate between the generalized and focal types.

In **primary** or **idiopathic** dystonia, dystonia may be the only manifestation. Many patients with primary generalized or segmental dystonia give a family history, most commonly suggesting inheritance as an autosomal dominant trait. No consistent pathology has been identified in those with primary torsion dystonia.

Secondary or **symptomatic dystonia** is the result of some identifiable brain disease, in which case there are likely to be other signs and symptoms of damage to the nervous system.

Dystonia plus syndromes include dopa-responsive dystonia and myoclonus dystonia (the latter described above under myoclonus).

Various **heredito-degenerative diseases** can include dystonia as one feature.

Primary dystonia

Generalized or segmental primary dystonia

The commonest type of primary dystonia is the result of a deletion in the *DYT1* gene on chromosome 9.

Inheritance is dominant with 30–40% penetrance, so that a family history, although often evident, is not always present. *DYT1*-associated dystonia accounts for most cases of Ashkenazi Jewish patients with primary dystonia (which is common in this population as a result of a founder effect), and most cases of young-onset generalized dystonia in non-Jewish populations. This illness, with onset in childhood, usually commences with dystonic spasms of the legs

Table 12.1 Classification of cerebellar disorders

Age of onset	Conditions	Inheritance
Congenital	Congenital ataxias	Autosomal recessive (50%)
	('Ataxic cerebral palsy') with or without	Autosomal dominant
	additional features	X-linked
		Non-genetic
Early onset	Friedreich's ataxia	Autosomal recessive
(usually less than 25 years)	Other early onset hereditary ataxias	Autosomal recessive
	Metabolic ataxias	X-linked
	Vitamin E deficiency	Autosomal recessive
	DNA repair defects	Autosomal recessive
	Periodic ataxia	Autosomal recessive
		Autosomal dominant
Late onset	Late onset hereditary cerebellar ataxias	Autosomal dominant
(usually after 25 years)	Idiopathic sporadic cerebellar degenerations	Non-genetic
	Paraneoplastic	Non-genetic
	Drugs, toxins and physical agents	Non-genetic
	Infections	Non-genetic
	Hypothyroidism	Non-genetic
	Vitamin deficiency (B_1, B_{12})	Non-genetic
	Prion diseases	Non-genetic
		Autosomal dominant
	Tumours	Non-genetic
Variable	Ramsay Hunt syndrome	Non-genetic
	(Progressive myoclonic ataxia)	Autosomal recessive
		Mitochondrial
	Dentatorubropallidoluysian atrophy	Autosomal dominant

Pathologically, many cases show features of ponto-neocerebellar or granule cell hypoplasia. In early infancy, an ataxic disorder may not be obvious but eventually nystagmus, cerebellar tremor and ataxia of the trunk and limbs become apparent. Some patients have only a mild cerebellar ataxia with or without a minor degree of learning disability. This may hardly progress or even improve with age. Other patients are severely ataxic with disabling spasticity and mental retardation. In the past, such patients were often diagnosed as cases of 'ataxic cerebral palsy' but **about 50% have an autosomal recessive condition so that the recurrence risk in subsequent siblings is approximately 1 in 8.** In some families there is an autosomal dominant or X-linked pattern of inheritance and many cases are idiopathic.

Autosomal recessive congenital ataxias include:

1 **Gillespie syndrome** (congenital ataxia, aniridia, mental retardation)
2 **Marinesco Sjögren syndrome** (mental retardation, cataracts)
3 **Joubert syndrome** (retinopathy, respiratory abnormalities)
4 **Disequilibrium syndrome** (gross truncal ataxia and motor delay, autism and mental retardation)
5 **Paine syndrome** (congenital ataxia, seizures, developmental delay, myoclonus, optic atrophy)
6 **COACH syndrome** (cerebellar hypoplasia, oligophrenia, ataxia, coloboma and hepatic fibrosis) is lethal in childhood.

EARLY ONSET HEREDITARY ATAXIAS

Friedreich's ataxia

Friedreich's ataxia is the most common early onset hereditary ataxia with a frequency in the UK of approximately 1–2 per 100 000. Inheritance is autosomal recessive and the gene locus is on chromosome 9q13. The mutation is a GAA trinucleotide repeat expansion in exon 1 of a gene encoding a 210 amino acid protein (frataxin). Frataxin appears to be involved in mitochondrial iron regulation. A normal repeat of 7–22 expands to 700–800 in Friedreich's ataxia patients. Affected individuals have two expanded alleles but a few are compound heterozygotes with one expanded gene and a corresponding allele containing a point mutation.

Pathology

The principal neuropathological changes are in the spinal cord (Figure 12.1), affecting the cervical dorsal columns and lumbar pyramidal tracts with additional involvement of the spinocerebellar tracts. Brainstem and cerebellar changes are minor. The peripheral nerves show a loss of large myelinated axons.

Clinical features

The onset is typically before the age of 15 years with the majority of cases starting by the age of 20 years. The presenting feature is almost always progressive ataxia; occasional patients present with scoliosis or cardiac disease. Cerebellar dysarthria, pyramidal weakness and areflexia of the legs, extensor plantar responses and impaired vibration and joint position sense usually develop within the first few years and Romberg's test is positive. A cardiomyopathy occurs in about 75% of cases but is often mild. Many patients develop scoliosis and pes cavus as the condition progresses and distal wasting is seen in about half of cases. Diabetes, deafness, nystagmus and optic atrophy are less common features (Table 12.2)

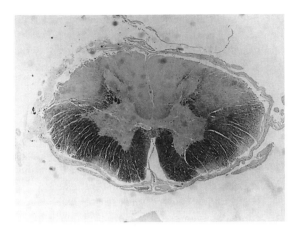

Figure 12.1 Transverse section of the spinal cord in Friedreich's ataxia (myelin stain) showing selective involvement of the dorsal columns. (Courtesy of Dr J. Broome.)

Table 12.2 Clinical features of Friedreich's ataxia

Clinical feature	Frequency (%)
Ataxia	100
Lower limb areflexia	99
Dysarthria	96
Extensor plantar responses	89
Pyramidal weakness	88
Impaired vibration sense	84
Impaired proprioception	78
Scoliosis	80
Pes cavus	55
Distal wasting	49
Optic atrophy	30
Nystagmus	20
Diabetes	10
Deafness	8
Investigation results	
Abnormal ECG	75
Absent sensory action potentials	92

ECG, electrocardiogram.
Figures in the table base on Harding (1981).

and cognitive function is not impaired. The progression of the disease is usually relentless, with patients losing the ability to walk after a mean of 15 years and nearly always by 45 years of age. Death often occurs in the fourth decade but some patients survive much longer.

Clinical variants have long been recognized but their relationship to Friedreich's ataxia was questionable prior to the very recent demonstration of the Friedreich's ataxia mutation in such cases. The most important variants are:

1 **Late onset Friedreich's ataxia** may develop after the age of 25 years, often in the fourth decade and occasionally as late as 51 years of age. There is slower progression, less skeletal deformity and lower GAA repeat numbers in the mutation.
2 **Early onset ataxia with retained reflexes**. The retention of lower limb reflexes has been regarded as incompatible with a diagnosis of Friedreich's ataxia but some of these patients have a cardiomyopathy. In some families the condition has been mapped to chromosome 9q13, and some have a Friedreich's ataxia trinucleotide expansion. It is likely that early onset ataxia with retained reflexes is heterogeneous however and that not all such patients have Friedreich's ataxia.
3 An **Acadian variant** has been described, particularly in Italy, among French Canadians and among the Acadian population of Louisiana. Onset is between the ages of 21 and 30 years but cases with onset as late as 36 years of age have been described. Progression is slower, with less frequent scoliosis and pes cavus and survival is prolonged.
4 Occasional **atypical cases** have presented with chorea or scoliosis.

Investigations

The electrocardiogram is invaluable as almost no other form of early onset ataxia is associated with cardiac disease. Widespread T wave inversion and left ventricular hypertrophy are the most common abnormalities. Cardiac arrhythmias and echocardiographic abnormalities are less common.

Most patients have reduced or absent peripheral nerve sensory action potentials as a result of degeneration of dorsal root ganglion neurones. Motor nerve conduction velocities are normal, in contrast to hereditary motor and sensory neuropathy type I, which can also present in childhood with ataxia and areflexia but in which motor conduction velocities are slowed. Visual-evoked potentials are of reduced

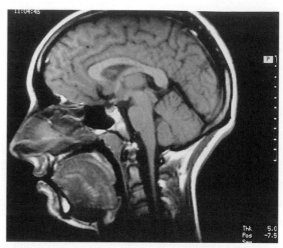

Figure 12.2 Magnetic resonance imaging scan showing cervical cord atrophy in a patient with Friedreich's ataxia.

amplitude in many patients and somatosensory and brainstem auditory evoked potentials are frequently abnormal.

Magnetic resonance imaging (MRI) reveals atrophy of the cervical cord but the appearance of the cerebellum is normal (Figure 12.2).

Vitamin E levels are normal but should always be checked, as the spinocerebellar ataxia associated with vitamin E deficiency is indistinguishable on clinical grounds and is potentially treatable.

Diagnostic confirmation by DNA testing to detect the gene mutation directly is now possible.

Management

No treatment has been shown to improve the neurological deficit. Cardiac disease is treated symptomatically and may improve with correction of scoliosis, and diabetes usually requires insulin therapy. Prevention of postural deformities by appropriate seating and physiotherapy is essential and orthopaedic correction of lower limb deformity or scoliosis is helpful in selected cases. Some patients will require hearing aids or low visual aids. The management of hypostatic oedema can be particularly difficult but elevation is often more effective than diuretics. Depression is a common and easily overlooked treatable cause of additional morbidity.

Genetic counselling is vital but many parents have completed their families by the time a child is affected; the risk to siblings is 1 in 4. Affected patients survive into adult life and have children. Pregnancy does not exacerbate the disorder but the practical difficulties of caring for children are obvious. The recurrence risk in children is very low, approximately 1 in 220, based on the risk of a partner being a heterozygote gene carrier of 1 in 110. DNA testing of patients requires specialized expertise and should follow nationally agreed guidelines.

Early onset ataxia with retained reflexes

Early onset ataxia with retained reflexes is distinguished from Friedreich's ataxia by normal or increased upper limb and knee reflexes (the ankle jerks may be absent); the plantar responses are extensor. The onset is before the age of 20 years but progression is slower than in Friedreich's ataxia. Severe skeletal deformity, optic atrophy and diabetes do not occur. Cerebellar atrophy is revealed by brain MRI.

Inheritance is autosomal recessive. In some families the gene locus has been mapped to the Friedreich's ataxia region on chromosome 9q13 and some of these patients have had a cardiomyopathy. Recently, the Friedreich's ataxia mutation has been detected in some patients and it is now clear that this condition is sometimes a manifestation of Friedreich's ataxia.

X-linked ataxia

X-linked ataxia causes cerebellar ataxia with lower limb spasticity and hyper-reflexia. Skeletal and cardiac abnormalities are absent and progression is variable. In contrast to early onset ataxia with retained reflexes, motor conduction velocities are reduced. X-linked ataxia should be considered during genetic counselling of affected males. Adrenoleukodystrophy and Pelizaeus Merzbacher disease (see below) must be considered.

Other early onset hereditary ataxias

A detailed discussion of other rare early onset hereditary ataxias is outside the scope of this chapter but the clinical features seen in addition to ataxia include optic atrophy and spasticity (**Behr syndrome**), hypogonadism (**Holmes' ataxia**), deafness, extrapyramidal features and retinopathy. The syndrome of cerebellar ataxia with myoclonus (**Ramsay Hunt syndrome**) is discussed later in this chapter.

EARLY ONSET METABOLIC ATAXIAS

The intermittent metabolic ataxias of childhood are rare. Affected children have a fluctuating cerebellar ataxia which tends to appear for a few weeks and then remit. Seizures, episodes of coma and mental retardation are often associated. Attacks may arise spontaneously or in association with infections or dietary changes. Females with X-linked **ornithine transcarbamylase deficiency** may be only mildly affected in between attacks of encephalopathy and cerebral oedema. A photosensitive rash is characteristic of **Hartnup disease**. The most likely metabolic derangements are:

- **Hyperammonaemias** (several autosomal recessive forms and X-linked ornithine transcarbamylase deficiency)
- **Aminoacidurias** (Hartnup disease, maple syrup urine disease and isovaleric acidaemia)
- **Congenital lactic acidosis** (various inborn errors of metabolism including pyruvate dehydrogenase deficiency and pyruvate carboxylase deficiency).

Vitamin E deficiency is discussed in Chapter 7 and will be mentioned only briefly here. **Autosomal recessive ataxia with vitamin E deficiency (AVED) causes a spinocerebellar degeneration indistinguishable from Friedreich's ataxia**. Cardiomyopathy can occur but retinopathy is extremely rare. The cause of AVED is mutations of the alpha tocopherol transfer protein (aTPP) gene on chromosome 8q13. The genetic defect causes a selective intestinal malabsorbtion of vitamin E.

Vitamin E deficiency is also associated with abetalipoproteinaemia (autosomal recessive, caused by mutations of the microsomal triglyceride transfer protein gene) and hypobetalipoproteinaemia (autosomal dominant, resulting from mutations of the apolipoprotein β-100 gene). In addition to the lipoprotein abnormalities, such patients have small stature, fat malabsorbtion with deficiencies of other fat-soluble vitamins (A, D and K). The neurological disorder is similar to Friedreich's ataxia and AVED but a retinopathy is also seen, probably as a result of vitamin A deficiency. A similar neurological disorder may occur with intestinal malabsorbtion resulting from biliary or intestinal disease. **Vitamin E deficiency is treatable** with oral or intramuscular vitamin E supplements to prevent further neurological deterioration.

Mitochondrial diseases are characterized by defective mitochondrial respiration as a result of abnormal mitochondrial or nuclear genes. Neurological manifestations occur alone or in association with fatigable muscle weakness (see p. 147). Ataxia is a prominent feature, often with shortness of stature, deafness, neuropathy, dementia, retinopathy, optic atrophy, ophthalmoplegia or myoclonus. Mitochondrial disease must be considered in the differential diagnosis of the Ramsay Hunt syndrome (see below). Features suggestive of mitochondrial diseases are shown in Table 12.3.

The diagnosis may be confirmed by DNA testing or muscle biopsy, which often shows 'ragged red fibres'. Blood and especially cerebrospinal fluid (CSF) lactate levels may be elevated. Many cases are single but some affected families show maternal or occasionally autosomal dominant inheritance. Recurrence risks to siblings or children are generally low. No treatment is available.

Hexosaminidase A deficiency (GM2 gangliosidosis) is an autosomal recessive disorder, which usually causes a fatal cerebromacular degeneration of infancy (Tay–Sachs disease). However, rare patients have a later onset ataxia associated with eye movement abnormalities, facial grimacing, anterior horn cell disease or neuropathy. The diagnosis is established by measurements of hexosaminidase A.

Cholestanolosis (cerebrotendinous xanthomatosis) presents as a childhood-onset cerebellar ataxia with spasticity, epilepsy, cognitive impairment, cataracts, neuropathy and xanthomas on tendons. The level of CSF protein is elevated and cholestanol levels are also increased as a result of an abnormality of bile salt synthesis; early treatment with chenodeoxycholic acid is partly effective. The condition is caused by mutations of the sterol 27-hydroxylase (*CYP27*) gene.

Niemann–Pick disease type C (juvenile dystonic lipidosis) is characterized by ataxia, dystonia, loss of vertical eye movement (the key clinical clue) and cognitive impairment (dementia or psychosis); cataplexy can be prominent, along with dysarthria and dysphagia. A multiple sclerosis-like presentation (on the MRI scan) with dementia has been described. Abnormal 'sea-blue histiocytes' may be seen in bone marrow biopsies but filipin staining of cultured skin fibroblasts is more reliable. Various mutations of the *NPC1* gene on chromosome 18q have been associated with this condition.

Leukodystrophies (see Chapter 22, p. 443) usually present in infancy or childhood but later onset variants may occur. Cerebellar ataxia is accompanied by other neurological features such as cognitive impairment, spasticity and visual loss but is sometimes the main presenting feature. The diagnosis is suggested by an associated peripheral neuropathy, characteristic appearances in the white matter on brain MRI and the results of white cell enzyme studies.

Table 12.3 Clinical features of mitochondrial disorders

Fatigable proximal myopathy (especially in combination with CNS disease)
Ptosis, progressive ophthalmoplegia or pigmentary retinopathy, optic atrophy
Short stature
Deafness (sensorineural)
Myoclonus, seizures
Diabetes mellitus, hypoparathyroidism
Cardiomyopathy, cardiac conduction defects
Lipomas
Unexplained stroke before 40 years of age
Migraine
Lactic acidosis
Raised CSF protein/lactate
Muscle biopsy (ragged red fibres, COX negative fibres)

CNS, central nervous system; CSF, cerebrospinal fluid; CO, cytochrome oxidase.

Partial hypoxanthine guanine phosphoribosyl transferase (HGPRT) deficiency arises from point mutations of the *HGPRT* gene on chromosome Xq26. Hyperuricaemia is associated with gouty arthritis and renal stones but about 20% of affected boys have a spinocerebellar ataxia. Allopurinol is effective treatment for arthritis and nephrolithiasis but does not help the neurological features.

DNA REPAIR DEFECTS

Ataxia telangiectasia

Ataxia telangiectasia (AT) is an autosomal recessive disorder, with an incidence of 1 in 100 000 births.

A progressive ataxia develops as the child starts to walk but sometimes later. Subsequently, dysarthria and a marked eye movement disorder appear along with other signs, including chorea, dystonia, myoclonus, areflexia and eventually some cognitive impairment. Telangiectasia of the conjunctivae appear at 4–6 years of age and may develop on the face, ears, neck and limbs; occasionally they are absent. Frequent infections are common as a result of impaired immunity, and malignancies, often lymphoma or leukaemia, develop in 10% of patients.

Characteristic laboratory findings are an elevation of alpha fetoprotein and deficiency of IgA or other immunoglobulins. The AT gene (*ATM*) is on chromosome 11q23 and a variety of mutations have been detected in AT patients. Recurrence risk to siblings is 1 in 4.

Xeroderma pigmentosum and Cockayne syndrome

Xeroderma pigmentosum and Cockayne syndrome are very rare autosomal recessive neurocutaneous disorders, which are caused by various mutations in the same family of DNA repair genes.

- Xeroderma pigmentosum causes a severe photosensitive rash, skin carcinomas and malignant melanoma. Neurological features appear in some patients and include ataxia, areflexia, dementia, spasticity and movement disorders; some patients have only a peripheral neuropathy.
- Cockayne syndrome produces a characteristic dwarfism with microcephaly, ataxia, spasticity, retinopathy, deafness and neuropathy. There may be a photosensitive rash and neuroimaging shows basal ganglia calcification.

PERIODIC ATAXIA

There are several forms of autosomal dominant ataxia in which ataxia occurs in intermittent attacks.

1 In **episodic ataxia with myokymia (EAM/EA type 1)** the attacks start in early childhood and last seconds to minutes with myokymia (rippling of muscles) evident between attacks. Persistent ataxia does not develop. Mutation analysis of the voltage gated K^+ channel gene, *KCNA1*, on chromosome 12p has identified different mis-sense point mutations. The attacks may respond to acetazolamide or carbamazepine.

2 In **episodic ataxia with nystagmus (EAN/EA type 2)**, the attacks develop in later childhood or adolescence, last hours or days and may be relieved by acetazolamide. There is no myokymia. In between the episodes there may be nystagmus and mild gait ataxia; some patients do not experience any acute attacks. Cerebellar atrophy is seen on brain MRI. Similar neurological signs are seen in some patients with autosomal dominant familial hemiplegic migraine. Familial hemiplegic migraine and periodic ataxia without myokymia are allelic disorders on chromosome 19p13 caused by point mutations of the alpha 1A calcium channel gene (*CACNL1A4*). Trinucleotide CAG expansions within the same gene cause a mild autosomal dominant adult-onset cerebellar ataxia (SCA6 – see below).

3 In **episodic ataxia type 3** there is episodic acetazolamide-responsive ataxia. Epilepsy may also occur. Episodic ataxia type 3 is the result of mutations of the calcium channel beta 4 subunit (*CACNB4*) gene on chromosome 2q.

4 Another form of episodic ataxia, **periodic vestibulocerebellar ataxia**, can also

be associated with a mild persistent ataxia; it is not linked to episodic ataxia type 1,2 or 3.

LATE ONSET HEREDITARY CEREBELLAR ATAXIAS

The autosomal dominant cerebellar ataxias (ADCA) are clinically, pathologically and genetically heterogeneous and their classification is controversial. Pathologically there is degeneration of the cerebellum, brainstem and other regions, including the optic nerves, basal ganglia, cerebral cortex, spinal cord and peripheral nerves. It is not possible to classify or define these conditions in terms of neuropathological features because these are so inconsistent, even within the same genetic type of ADCA.

Advances in molecular genetics have led to a new genetic reclassification and DNA diagnosis is now possible for some forms of ADCA. At present there are 19 known genes underlying the autosomal dominant ataxias. There are 15 'spinocerebellar ataxia – SCA genes' (an unfortunate terminology as it ignores the many earlier onset recessive genes which also cause 'spinocerebellar ataxia'), the gene for dentatorubropallidoluysian atrophy (DRPLA, see below) and the three episodic ataxia genes. These are summarized in Table 12.4.

Harding proposed a clinical classification (ADCA types I–IV) in 1984 which has required revision but is still useful in the clinic. Types III and IV are probably obsolete but the ADCA types I–III are recognizable. It must be emphasized that there is a very poor correlation between the phenotype of a dominant ataxia and the genotype underlying it. The main phenotypes (ADCA types I, II and III along with Biemond's ataxia (ADCA with severe sensory peripheral neuropathy) and the episodic ataxias are

Table 12.4 Autosomal dominant cerebellar ataxia genes

Gene	Locus	Mutation type	Gene product (approximate)	Trinucleotide repeats
SCA1	6p23	CAG expansion	Ataxin 1	38–68 (normal = 7–34)
SCA2	12q24	CAG expansion	Ataxin 2	35–59 (normal = 14–31)
SCA3	14q32	CAG expansion	Ataxin 3	65–84 (normal = 13–44)
SCA4	16q22	Unknown	Ataxin 4	–
SCA5	11cen	Unknown	Ataxin 5	–
SCA6*	19p13	CAG expansion	α-1A calcium channel	21–27 (normal = 4–16)
SCA7	3p12	CAG expansion	Ataxin 7	38–130 (normal = 7–17)
SCA8	13q21	CTG expansion	Ataxin 8	107–127 (normal = 16–37)
SCA10	22q13	Unknown	Ataxin 10	
SCA11	15q14-21	Unknown	Ataxin 11	
SCA12	5q31	CAG expansion	Ataxin 12	66–78 (normal = 9–28)
SCA13	19q	Unknown		
SCA14	19q	Unknown		
SCA15	?	Unknown		
SCA16	8q	Unknown		
DRPLA	12p13	CAG expansion	Atrophin 1	49–85 (normal = 5–35)
EA-1	12p13	Point mutations	KCNA1 potassium channel	–
EA-2*	19p13	Point mutations	α-1A calcium channel	–
EA-3	2q22-23	Point mutation	CACNB4 calcium channel	–

SCA, spinocerebellar ataxia; EA, episodic ataxia; DRPLA, dentatorubropallidoluysian atrophy.
*SCA6 and EA-2 are allelic, resulting from different mutations of the alpha 1A calcium channel (CACNL1A4) gene.
Note: SCA9 is currently not utilized.

summarized in Table 12.5 with the genes associated with each clinical type.

Autosomal dominant cerebellar ataxia type I

The age of onset for ADCA type I is nearly always after the age of 20 years, usually in the fourth decade, but can be as late as 65–70 years of age. Progressive ataxia with cerebellar dysarthria are the salient features.

Supranuclear eye movement disorders, eyelid retraction, nystagmus and optic atrophy are common, along with parkinsonism, chorea and dystonia. Some patients have fasciculation of the face and tongue and occasionally the limbs. The tendon reflexes can be brisk, normal or absent and often decline over time in the same patient. Sensory loss and pyramidal leg weakness may be seen and mild dementia occurs in about 40% of cases. Retinopathy is not seen in ADCA type I and any optic atrophy is associated with mild visual loss.

No treatment is available for ADCA, which is progressive. Patients require physiotherapy, occupational therapy and speech therapy in some cases. Genetic counselling of patients and their families is important. In those with marked parkinsonian features, levodopa may be partly effective.

Cerebellar and brainstem atrophy is apparent on MRI or computerized tomography (CT) scans, abnormal visual, brainstem auditory or somatosensory evoked potentials are common and there may be abnormal nerve conduction studies if a peripheral neuropathy is present.

Inheritance is autosomal dominant and the risk to children is 50%. Eight genes causing ADCA type I have been discovered (Table 12.5) but **the clinical features are not a reliable guide to the molecular diagnosis**.

- *SCA1* is reported in 15–35% of ADCA I families. Larger repeat numbers are associated with earlier age of onset and increased severity.

Table 12.5 Clinical and genetic classification of autosomal dominant cerebellar ataxias

Clinical classification	Additional features	Associated genes identified
ADCA type I	Variable combinations of abnormal eye movements, optic atrophy, spasticity, extrapyramidal signs, fasciculation, neuropathy, dementia	*SCA1*; *SCA2*; *SCA3*; *SCA8*; *SCA12*; *SCA13**; ?*SCA15*; ?*SCA16*; others *SCA7*; ? other loci
ADCA type II	Retinopathy	*SCA3*; *SCA5*; *SCA6*;
ADCA type III	None but nystagmus, or pyramidal signs in some	*SCA10**; *SCA11*; *SCA14***; others
Ataxia with sensory neuropathy (Biemond's ataxia)	Severe sensory neuropathy	*SCA4*
DRPLA	Myoclonus, seizures, chorea, dementia	*DRPLA* gene (atrophin 1)
Episodic ataxia type 1 (with myokymia)		*KCNA1*
Episodic ataxia type 2 (without myokymia)		*SCA6/CACNL1A4*
Episodic ataxia type 3 (without myokymia)		*CACNB4*

SCA10 is associated with epilepsy.
**SCA13* develops in early infancy and is more correctly a hereditary congenital ataxia.
***SCA14* can cause earlier onset ataxia with myoclonus.

The gene product, ataxin 1, is an 8 kDa protein of unknown function. Clinically, the eye movements are affected late and reflexes are commonly brisk. A bulbar palsy often appears, along with cognitive decline. Optic atrophy, facial fasciculation and parkinsonism are less common.

- *SCA2* was first described in Cuba but subsequently elsewhere. The clinical features are similar to *SCA1* but slow eye movements and hyporeflexia are more common. This mutation has been reported in 20–40% of ADCA I cases.
- *SCA3* accounts for 15–40% of ADCA I cases and has also been described as Machado–Joseph disease and Azorean disease of the nervous system. Prominent dystonia or parkinsonism, facial and tongue fasciculation, a staring expression (as a result of eyelid retraction) and distal wasting are common but are also seen in *SCA1*. Some patients have a parkinsonian syndrome with peripheral neuropathy but no ataxia, while others have only a spastic paraparesis.
- *SCA8* is a rare cause of ADCA type I. This mutation has also been reported as a normal polymorphism and its status as an ADCA (*SCA*) gene is controversial.
- *SCA12* has been associated with an ADCA type I phenotype with prominent tremor and cognitive decline.
- *SCA13* produces an ADCA I phenotype but in some cases onset is in infancy. This gene may more correctly be placed among the congenital ataxias. Only one family has been described.
- *SCA15* and *SCA16* are very rare.

Some ADCA I families have none of these genes. The proportion is uncertain with different frequencies of the various *SCA* mutations in different case series.

Autosomal dominant cerebellar ataxia type II

In ADCA type II, there is progressive ataxia with visual failure as a result of a retinopathy.

The age of onset is highly variable, ranging from infancy to the seventh decade. Sometimes parents develop symptoms after their affected children. There are also abnormalities of eye movement and pyramidal signs in the limbs. Some affected children have a severe lethal cerebromacular degeneration. In this condition, the *SCA7* mutation (Table 12.5) is usually the cause. ADCA II is the exception to the generally useful rule concerning age of onset and dominant and recessive transmission (Table 12.1); all ages are affected. The visual loss may be inconspicuous and electroretinography may be needed in doubtful cases. Some ADCA II families do not have the *SCA7* gene.

Autosomal dominant cerebellar ataxia type III

In ADCA type III there is a pure cerebellar ataxia with nystagmus and pyramidal signs in some cases. Onset is late, usually after the age of 50 years and progression is slow. Similar families have been found to have a gene locus on the centromeric region of chromosome 11 (*SCA5*). Some patients with *SCA3* have this phenotype and the *SCA6* mutation is typically associated with a mild, pure cerebellar ADCA III phenotype. Note that point mutations of the same gene (*CACNL1A4*) can cause familial hemiplegic migraine or episodic ataxia type 2 (see above). Other *SCA* genes (listed in Table 12.5) associated with this type of ataxia are extremely rare.

SPORADIC DEGENERATIVE CEREBELLAR ATAXIA

Two out of three cases of adult-onset degenerative cerebellar ataxia are non-genetic and of unknown cause.

Pathologically these patients have **olivoponto-cerebellar atrophy** or **cortical cerebellar atrophy**. However, the term olivopontocerebellar atrophy should be reserved for the cerebellar presentation of multiple system atrophy (see below). Age-of-onset tends to be a bit later than in ADCA, optic atrophy and retinopathy are absent and ophthalmoplegia is uncommon.

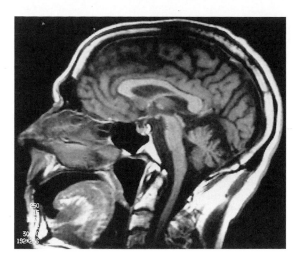

Figure 12.3 Magnetic resonance scan showing severe cerebellar and brainstem atrophy in a patient with idiopathic late onset ataxia. (Courtesy of Dr T.P. Enevoldson.)

It is essential in late onset ataxia, where there is no family history, to exclude a posterior fossa structural lesion (such as a tumour or Chiari malformation), hydrocephalus, vitamin B_{12} deficiency (and vitamin E where there is any doubt), thyroid function tests and, where indicated (see below), a systemic malignancy. In most patients these tests are all normal and a sporadic cerebellar degeneration is left as a diagnosis of exclusion. Within this group, four phenotypes are recognized:

1 **Dejerine–Thomas type:** The onset is typically between 35 and 55 years of age. There is cerebellar ataxia, and varying combinations of dementia, parkinsonism, supranuclear eye movement abnormalities and areflexia. Optic atrophy or retinopathy are rare (Figure 12.3).

2 **Multiple system atrophy (MSA)** (see Chapter 11) may take the form of **a late onset degenerative cerebellar ataxia as well as atypical parkinsonism or primary autonomic failure. A cerebellar syndrome is associated with parkinsonism, pyramidal signs and sometimes autonomic features such as postural hypotension, bladder dysfunction and impotence.** The parkinsonism rarely responds well to levodopa. Nystagmus may occur but not severe gaze palsies, optic atrophy or retinopathy; dementia is not a feature of MSA. There is cerebellar and brainstem atrophy on MRI scans, which may also show

abnormal signal in the putamen. Denervation of the external urethral sphincter detected by electromyography is characteristic. Pathologically there is degeneration of the cerebellum, brainstem (including substantia nigra), basal ganglia and sometimes the intermediolateral columns of the spinal cord with characteristic glial and neuronal cytoplasmic inclusions in these areas. Severe and early autonomic failure or bladder dysfunction is suggestive of MSA. Perhaps a quarter of those with the Dejerine–Thomas type of sporadic ataxia actually have MSA.

3 **Marie-Foix – Alajouanine type**. These patients develop ataxia later, often after 55 years of age. There is unsteadiness of gait but less limb ataxia, corresponding to a degeneration of the cerebellar vermis.

4 **Dyssynergia cerebellaris progressiva**. The onset of ataxia is between 40 and 60 years of age and is followed by increasingly severe tremor of the limbs (intention tremor with resting and postural elements).

THE RAMSAY HUNT SYNDROME (PROGRESSIVE MYOCLONIC ATAXIA)

> **Progressive myoclonic ataxia (Ramsay Hunt syndrome)**
> Progressive myoclonic ataxia (Ramsay Hunt syndrome) is a syndrome of progressive cerebellar ataxia, myoclonus and sometimes seizures. None of the disorders leading to the syndrome is treatable but myoclonus may respond to valproate, clonazepam or primidone.

Causes of progressive myoclonic ataxia include:

1 **Unverricht–Lundborg disease** (Baltic or Mediterranean myoclonus) is an autosomal recessive early onset spinocerebellar degeneration (see above). The onset is in childhood with seizures and myoclonus, ataxia and mild cognitive impairment appear later. The condition is caused by mutations of the cystatin B gene on chromosome 21q22.3.

2 **Lafora body disease** is also an autosomal recessive disorder with onset in adolescence and severe epilepsy and dementia with milder myoclonus. A milder later onset form exists. Characteristic periodic acid Schiff-positive inclusions are seen in skin, muscle, brain and liver. Various mutations of the *EPM2A* gene on chromosome 6q24 have been identified; the function of the gene product, laforin, is unknown.

3 **Neuronal ceroid lipofuscinosis** can occur at various ages, with combinations of epilepsy, myoclonus, visual failure and ataxia. Characteristic inclusions are seen in neurones (detectable in rectal or skin biopsies). Inheritance can be autosomal recessive or dominant. An axillary skin biopsy can detect ceroid lipofuscinosis or Lafora bodies.

4 **Sialidosis** is inherited as an autosomal recessive disorder, caused by α-N-acetylneuraminidase (sialidase) deficiency. The onset is in adolescence or early adult life with epilepsy, myoclonus, visual failure (with cherry red maculae) and ataxia. Various mutations of the sialidase gene on chromosome 6p21 have been detected.

5 **Mitochondrial disease** takes many forms including the MERRF syndrome (myoclonic epilepsy with ragged red fibres). The ragged red fibres are a muscle biopsy feature caused by an accumulation of abnormal mitochondria. In addition to myoclonic ataxia, there is often smallness of stature, deafness, dementia and sometimes subcutaneous lipomas. The majority of MERRF cases are caused by a point mutation of the mitochondrial lysine transfer RNA gene (at position 8344). A few cases have been associated with other mutations of mitochondrial DNA (at positions 8356 and 3243) and, in some, the molecular basis has not been determined.

6 **Dentatorubropallidoluysian atrophy (DRPLA)** is described below. A Ramsay-Hunt phenotype may occur.

7 **Coeliac disease** (see p. 493) may be associated with a cerebellar ataxia with myoclonus or other neurological complications including cerebral calcification, seizures, peripheral neuropathy or a Friedreich's ataxia-like illness. Diagnosis is by antibodies (to gliadin or endomysial) or small bowel biopsy. The neurological disorder does not respond to a gluten-free diet.

8 **Whipple's disease** (see p. 493) is associated with several neurological complications, including focal brain lesions, ataxia (with myoclonus), supranuclear eye movement abnormalities and dementia. Myoclonus may affect the eyes and face (oculomasticatory myorhythmia). Biopsy of the small bowel or detection of the organism *Tropheryma whippelii* in bowel or CSF may allow the diagnosis. Treatment is with antibiotics.

9 **Creutzfeldt–Jacob disease** (see p. 285) classically presents with rapidly progressive cerebellar ataxia and myoclonus, as well as dementia and sometimes cortical visual disturbances.

DENTATORUBROPALLIDO-LUYSIAN ATROPHY

The inheritance of DRPLA is autosomal dominant and the gene is located on chromosome 12p12-ter (ter = telomere); the mutation is a CAG trinucleotide repeat expansion. Larger repeat numbers are associated with earlier age of onset and greater severity. Onset for DRPLA is extremely variable in terms of age and clinical features, even within the same family. Childhood onset is often associated with rapidly progressive myoclonic epilepsy and dementia. Adult onset is characterized by chorea, ataxia and dementia. **The condition may closely resemble Huntington's disease.** Affected families commonly contain individuals with each phenotype. Brain MRI scans show cerebral and cerebellar atrophy and abnormal lesions in the cerebral white matter and basal ganglia. **DNA testing for DRPLA is useful in the investigation of families with features of Huntington's disease but in whom the Huntington's disease mutation cannot be detected.**

MISCELLANEOUS CEREBELLAR SYNDROMES

In addition to the hereditary and degenerative ataxias, the cerebellum may be affected by a wide range of pathologies (Table 12.1). Some of these, such as vascular disease, are covered in other chapters.

Paraneoplastic cerebellar degeneration

> **Paraneoplastic cerebellar degeneration**
>
> Paraneoplastic cerebellar degeneration is a rare disorder most commonly seen in association with small cell lung cancer, ovarian or uterine cancer or lymphoma and may precede the appearance of the tumour. Severe ataxia develops rapidly, over weeks or months, along with dysarthria, vertigo, oscillopsia and nystagmus. The condition then stabilizes but the patients are severely disabled. **It is the severe subacute onset and rapid deterioration that is characteristic of paraneoplastic ataxia**.

CT or MRI brain scans are normal initially but cerebellar atrophy can appear later. The CSF usually contains a mild lymphocytic pleocytosis with elevated protein level and positive oligoclonal bands. Serum markers such as cancer antigen 125 and carcinoembryonic antigen may be positive. In about 50–75% of cases, antineuronal antibodies are detected. These react with cerebellar Purkinje cells (anti-Yo or anti-PCA1) or occasionally a wider range of neurones (anti-Hu). Passive transfer of anti-Yo antibodies has failed to produce cerebellar degeneration in animal studies and the role of these antibodies is unclear. Some patients have anti VGCC (voltage gated calcium channel) or anti-Ri antibodies.

Treatment is usually unsuccessful but improvement after treatment of the underlying tumour, plasma exchange, immunoglobulin therapy, steroids or cytotoxic drugs has been reported occasionally. Symptomatic improvement may be seen with clonazepam.

Drugs

1 **Anticonvulsants** particularly phenytoin, carbamazepine and phenobarbitone lead to reversible ataxia, nystagmus and dysarthria if serum levels are elevated. Permanent cerebellar damage can follow phenytoin intoxication.
2 **Lithium** toxicity can produce cerebellar ataxia, even with normal serum levels. Occasionally a combination of ataxia with myoclonus can occur with a clinical picture very similar to Creutzfeldt–Jacob disease.
3 **Cytotoxic drugs and immunosuppressants**, such as 5-flurouracil, vincristine, cytosine arabinoside and ciclosporin are associated with a reversible cerebellar syndrome.
4 **Other causes** include benzodiazepines, piperazine and amiodarone.

Toxins and physical agents

1 **Alcohol abuse** is associated with a characteristic cerebellar syndrome with similarities to that seen in Wernicke's encephalopathy. The relative roles of thiamine deficiency and direct toxicity are unclear (see below).
2 **Organic solvents** are highly lipid soluble and so are potent neurotoxins. Prominent cerebellar features may occur but a diffuse encephalopathy is more common.
3 **Organic mercury** causes a cerebellar syndrome with optic neuropathy and cognitive changes.
4 Acute **thallium** poisoning can lead to an encephalopathy with prominent cerebellar features.
5 **Acrylamide** causes a toxic peripheral neuropathy with additional cerebellar features.
6 **Heatstroke** may be followed by permanent cerebellar damage.

Infections

1 **Acute cerebellar ataxia** is seen mainly in children and rarely in adults. There is myoclonus and a prominent eye movement disorder (opsoclonus) in some patients.

> This gives rise to a striking clinical picture with irregular multidirectional saccadic eye movements, jerking of the limbs and ataxia (**'dancing eyes**

Table 12.6 Spastic paraplegia (*SPG*) genes

Gene	Locus	Inheritance
SPG1	Xq28 (L1CAM)	X-linked
SPG2	Xp21 (PLP)	X-linked
SPG3	14q11	Autosomal dominant
SPG4	2p22 (Spastin)	Autosomal dominant
SPG5	8p12-q13	Autosomal recessive
SPG6	15q11	Autosomal dominant
SPG7	16q24 (Paraplegin)	Autosomal recessive
SPG8	8q23-24	Autosomal dominant
SPG9	10q23-24	Autosomal dominant
SPG10	12q13	Autosomal dominant
SPG11	15q13-15	Autosomal recessive
SPG12	19q13	Autosomal dominant
SPG14	3q27-28	Autosomal recessive
SPG16	Xq11	X-linked
SPG17	11q12	X-linked

1 **Autosomal dominant HSP** shows high
penetrance but variable expression within
families. Severely affected children can have
affected but asymptomatic parents. Dominant
pure HSP appears to be heterogeneous with
infantile, early (before 35 years of age) and later
onset (after 35 years of age) variants. The early
onset type is more common and typically starts
between 12 and 35 years of age.

A number of genes may cause autosomal
dominant HSP (Table 12.6); the most common
(*SPG4*) is that associated with mutations of the
spastin gene on chromosome 2p22.

Pathologically there is degeneration of
the corticospinal tracts with less prominent
involvement of the dorsal columns and
spinocerebellar tracts, motor cortex and
anterior horn cells.

> HSP presents as a spinal cord disease with pro-
> gressive spasticity of the legs. Tendon reflexes
> are increased and plantar responses extensor.
> The abdominal reflexes are often preserved. In
> advanced later onset cases there may be upper
> limb involvement, impairment of vibration
> sense in the feet, ankle areflexia, distal muscle

> wasting, and bladder dysfunction. The rate of
> deterioration is variable. Progression in the later
> onset type is more rapid, with greater disability.

Diagnosis of HSP must be made with caution.
In many cases the family history is incomplete
or unreliable, in which case it is vital to examine
both parents if possible. In doubtful cases,
treatable conditions such as spinal cord
compression, vitamin B_{12} deficiency, multiple
sclerosis, dopa-responsive dystonia (which may
resemble HSP closely; see Chapter 11) must
always be excluded by a therapeutic trial of
levodopa.

Investigations are unhelpful and serve only
to exclude other disorders but somatosensory
evoked potentials may be abnormal indicating
subclinical involvement of peripheral and
central sensory pathways.

Treatment of HSP is limited to symptomatic
management of spasticity with baclofen and
physiotherapy together with management of
bladder symptoms if present. Genetic counselling
is essential; the recurrence risk in siblings or
children of affected patients is 50% and the
severity is difficult to predict.

2 **Autosomal recessive pure HSP** families are
rare. The distinction from the early onset
form of dominant HSP is very difficult,
making examination of the parents essential
before diagnosing recessive HSP. The *SPG7*
type on chromosome 16q24 is caused by
homozygous mutations of the paraplegin
gene; the paraplegin protein is a mitochondrial
ATPase.

3 **X-linked pure HSP** is genetically heterogeneous.
Clinically it is similar to early onset autosomal
dominant HSP but carrier females are normal.
In *some* families there has been genetic linkage
to the proteolipid protein (PLP) gene on
chromosome Xq22 (also referred to as *SPG2*).
Mutations of the same gene can cause a
complex HSP phenotype (see below) and
X-linked sudanophilic leukodystrophy
(Pelizaeus–Merzbacher disease) indicating that
these conditions and some cases of pure
X-linked HSP are allelic disorders. It is

important to check very long chain fatty acid levels as **adrenoleukodystrophy** may present with a pure spastic paraparesis without clinical or MRI evidence of cerebral involvement and with normal adrenal function in both affected males **and in heterozygous carrier females**.

Complex hereditary spastic paraplegias

In the complex HSP syndromes, additional neurological features are seen with the spastic paraplegia, such as mental retardation, optic atrophy, retinopathy, deafness, ataxia (especially of the upper limbs), extrapyramidal features, muscle wasting, peripheral sensory neuropathy and skin changes. The key to the diagnosis is the predominant spastic paraplegia that forms the 'core' of the syndrome.

Selected complex autosomal HSPs include:

- **Sjögren–Larsson syndrome** (autosomal recessive) presents at birth with icthyosis. Spastic paraplegia, mental retardation and retinopathy appear subsequently. Patients have mutations of the fatty aldehyde dehydrogenase (FALDH) gene on chromosome 17p11.2.
- **Behr syndrome** (autosomal recessive) is characterized by optic atrophy and HSP. A similar dominant form exists.
- **Kjellin syndrome** causes childhood mental retardation and retinal degeneration; spasticity appears later in adult life. Inheritance is autosomal recessive.
- **Complex HSP with severe sensory neuropathy** causes severe small fibre sensory loss and mutilating lower limb acropathy. This may be autosomal recessive or dominant. There is a dominant form with mild large-fibre neuropathy.
- **Complex HSP with distal muscle wasting** may be inherited as an autosomal dominant or recessive trait.

- **Complex HSP with cerebellar ataxia** usually develops in adult life with lower limb spasticity and cerebellar signs in the arms. There may be cerebellar eye movement abnormalities and dysarthria. This may be autosomal dominant or recessive.

X-linked complex hereditary spastic paraplegias

A rapidly progressive spastic paraplegia of childhood with optic atrophy is caused by a gene on chromosome Xq21. This condition, some cases of pure X-linked HSP and Pelizaeus–Merzbacher disease are all caused by mutations of the PLP gene (see above). Different PLP gene mutations are associated with different phenotypes. The PLP gene encodes two proteins required for myelin synthesis, PLP and an isoform, DM-20.

Allan–Herndon syndrome comprises variable mental retardation, hypotonia, gross motor delay, ataxia and spastic paraplegia. The gene for this disorder is also on chromosome Xq21, close to the PLP gene and possibly allelic.

MASA syndrome leads to mental retardation, aphasia, shuffling gait and adducted thumbs. A spastic paraplegia develops later. A distinct form of X-linked complex HSP also maps to this locus as do X-linked hydrocephalus and X-linked corpus callosum agenesis. All are caused by mutations of the *L1* gene, which encodes the L1 neural cell adhesion molecule (L1CAM). This gene is also referred to as *SPG1*.

REFERENCES AND FURTHER READING

Burk K, Abele M, Fetter M *et al.* (1996) Autosomal dominant cerebellar ataxia type I clinical features and MRI in families with SCA1, SCA2 and SCA3. *Brain*, 119:1497–1505.

Durr A, Cossee M, Agid Y *et al.* (1996) Clinical and genetic abnormalities in patients with Friedreich's ataxia [see comments]. *New England Journal of Medicine*, 335:1169–1175.

Fletcher NA (2001) Tremor, ataxia and cerebellar disorders. In: Donaghy M. (ed.) *Brain's Diseases of the Nervous System*, 11th edition. Oxford, UK: Oxford University Press, pp. 973–1014.

Harding AE (1981) Friedreich's ataxia: a clinical and genetic study of 90 families with an analysis of early diagnostic criteria and intrafamilial clustering of clinical features. *Brain*, **104**:589–620.

Marsden CD, Obeso JA (1989) The Ramsay Hunt syndrome is a useful clinical entity. *Movement Disorders*, **4**:6–12.

CHAPTER 13

MOTOR NEURONE DISEASE AND SPINAL MUSCULAR ATROPHIES

C.E. Shaw

INTRODUCTION

The first section will include an account of the typical clinical presentation and diagnostic work-up of a patient with motor neurone disease (MND) and a brief description of the conditions that cause or mimic motor neurone degeneration. The second section will cover the pathological features of MND and what is understood of its pathogenesis from molecular genetic and cell biology research. Therapies designed to alter the course of the disease and symptom management will be discussed.

WHAT DO WE MEAN BY MOTOR NEURONE DISEASE?

The term 'motor neurone disorders' covers a range of conditions in which the motor neurone bears the brunt of the disease process. Clinical, pathological and, more recently, molecular genetic studies have helped distinguish many of these from typical MND. The principal features of the group of motor neurone disorders are summarized in Table 13.1 and those mimicking MND in Table 13.2.

The clinical definition of motor neurone disease

Motor neurone disease (MND) is known as **amyotrophic lateral sclerosis (ALS)** in most parts of the world other than the UK, and Lou Gherig's disease in the USA. It was originally thought to be a degenerative muscle disorder until Charcot in 1869 published clinicopathological studies that emphasized the involvement of both upper motor neurones (UMN) and lower motor neurones (LMN) and sparing of the sensory and autonomic pathways. He used the words amyotrophic (muscle wasting), lateral (corticospinal

Table 13.1 Clinical classification of motor neurone syndromes

	UMN signs	LMN signs	Other features	Diagnostic tests
MND/ALS	+	+	Emotional lability Rapid progression	Clinical signs, supported by EMG and MRI
SBMA/Kennedy's	–	–	Arm tremor Slow progression	Androgen receptor gene expansion
SMA	–	+	Young onset, distal and bulbar muscle sparing	Survival motor neurone gene deletion

UMN, upper motor neurone; LMN, lower motor neurone; MND, motor neurone disease; ALS, amyotrophic lateral sclerosis; EMG, electromyography; MRI, magnetic resonance imaging; SBMA, spinobulbar muscular atrophy; SMA, spinal muscular atrophy.

Table 13.2 Conditions mimicking motor neurone disease

Condition	Diagnostic screening tests
Spinal disease causing myeloradiculopathy	MRI spine
Multifocal motor neuropathy	Antiganglioside antibodies: EMG: NCS
Other autoimmune neuropathies	Autoreactive antibodies
Paraproteinaemias	Protein electrophoresis
Thyrotoxicosis	Thyroid and stimulating hormone assays
Hyperparathyroidism	Calcium, phosphate
Diabetic amyotrophy	EMG: glucose, glycosylated haemoglobin
GM2 gangliosidoses	Hexosaminidase A and B levels
Myopathies (e.g. inclusion body myositis)	Muscle biopsy: EMG
Myasthenia gravis (bulbar weakness)	Autoantibodies: EMG

MRI, magnetic resonance imaging; EMG, electromyography; NCS, nerve conduction studies.

tracts) and sclerosis (scarring) to describe the cardinal features, and it is from these that the term ALS is derived. The features that distinguish this disorder from others affecting the motor system are a combination of UMN and LMN signs. Lower motor neurones reside in the anterior horn of the spinal cord or motor nuclei of the brainstem and project in peripheral nerves to make direct contact with muscle fibres. When LMNs degenerate, the muscles they activate become weak, wasted and fasciculate (small twitches). Upper motor neurones reside in the pre-central gyrus of the cerebral cortex and project to the LMNs. When UMNs degenerate, muscles become spastic, tendon reflexes are exaggerated and plantar responses are extensor. **Neurones of the sensory and autonomic pathways are usually spared** as are motor neurones controlling eye movements and bladder and bowel sphincters. Most MND patients have a mixture of UMN and LMN signs. There is no definitive diagnostic test and essentially the diagnosis of MND is clinical, supported by investigations that exclude other conditions.

The clinical course of typical motor neurone disease

In the majority of patients, MND begins in one arm – causing weakness of grip, or one leg – causing foot drop. Affected muscles become wasted and weak as LMNs in the spinal cord degenerate and die. Sometimes muscle cramps or spasms precede wasting and weakness, reflecting early UMN involvement. Usually symptoms progress in that limb before becoming more generalized.

Sensation remains normal throughout the illness.

In 25% of patients, symptoms begin in the tongue or throat with dysarthria and dysphagia. Bulbar symptoms arise when motor neurones in the brainstem (previously known as the bulb) degenerate and cause wasting and weakness of the tongue and pharyngeal muscles. This is often combined with poor elevation of the soft palate on vocalizing and an exaggerated gag reflex or jaw jerk. The disorder has been named **'progressive bulbar palsy'** but is essentially a variant of MND. Over 90% of patients will eventually develop bulbar symptoms at some stage. Motor neurone disease causes significant disability at an early stage and progresses relentlessly so that most patients ultimately lose the ability to speak, swallow, walk, feed and toilet themselves. A particular cruelty is that intellectual function is often spared so that people with MND are fully aware of their circumstances but are trapped in bodies that no longer work and are isolated by an inability to touch or communicate verbally. Death is most commonly the result of respiratory failure and the mean survival from symptom onset is 3 years and only 10% of patients are alive at 10 years. Those patients who are elderly, female, or who have a bulbar onset of symptoms have a worse prognosis.

Diagnosis of motor neurone disease

Making the diagnosis can be difficult. While the symptoms and signs on examination may be suggestive of MND, there is no specific diagnostic test for MND. Furthermore, as the implications are so grim, clinicians may delay discussing the possibility of MND until they are absolutely certain of the diagnosis.

Investigations
The **investigations** that are most useful are those that exclude other conditions that mimic MND (Table 13.2).

- The most important investigation is **magnetic resonance imaging (MRI) of the spine and/or head** to exclude an extrinsic or intrinsic lesion
- **Nerve conduction studies** are essential to exclude a generalized or multifocal neuropathy and to search for nerve entrapment and conduction block
- **Electromyography** is necessary to confirm evidence of widespread LMN loss, particularly in regions not symptomatically affected and to exclude myopathy. Typical electromyography features of MND are spontaneous fibrillations and slow frequency fasciculations (0.3 Hz), with unstable and complex motor unit potentials on voluntary activation
- **Blood tests** – serum creatine kinase levels may show a mild rise. If the value is very high, an inflammatory myopathy should be considered
- Thyroid function tests help to exclude **thyrotoxicosis** as a reversible cause of bulbar palsy or proximal weakness
- Acetylcholine receptor antibodies will be found in **generalized myasthenia gravis** presenting with bulbar weakness
- Muscle biopsy or lumbar puncture are not routinely required unless the presentation is atypical and an alternative diagnosis is suspected.

SPINAL MUSCULAR ATROPHY AND KENNEDY'S DISEASE

Disorders of the motor neurone that may be mistaken for MND/ALS include **spinal muscular atrophy (SMA)** and **Kennedy's disease or spinobulbar muscular atrophy (SBMA)** (clinical features are summarized in Table 13.1). Proximal SMA usually develops in infancy or childhood and was originally classified according to the age at onset, mobility achieved and survival. SMA type 1 (Werdnig–Hoffmann disease) has an onset within the first 6 months, few children learn to sit and death usually occurs by the age of 2–3 years. SMA type 2 (intermediate form) has an onset before 3 years but these children never walk and may survive up to 10 years of age. SMA type 3 (Kugelberg–Welander disease) has an onset between

3–18 years; these children walk and many survive well into adulthood. Patients with all three of these clinical phenotypes have a pure lower motor neurone syndrome charcterized by proximal muscle weakness, absent reflexes and sparing of distal limb muscles, speech and swallowing. Although SMA types 1, 2 and 3 were thought to be distinct disease entities, most patients were found to be recessive and linked to Chromosome 5q13, and the survival motor neurone gene (*SMN1*) is found to be deleted or disrupted in >95–99% of cases. The severity of the disease course (type 1 or 3) is largely due to deletion of an almost identical gene (*SMN2*); those with no copies of *SMN2* have a worse prognosis.

Kennedy's disease (SBMA) is another purely LMN syndrome that presents in adult life and is characterized by very slowly progressive wasting of both proximal and distal muscles in the limbs with prominent involvement of the tongue and facial musculature. Inheritance is X-linked recessive and female carriers are asymptomatic. The gene defect is an expanded CAG nucleotide repeat sequence in the androgen receptor gene. Clinical pointers to SBMA include a fine, rapid tremor of the outstretched hands, gynaecomastia and testicular atrophy. Nerve conduction studies commonly show a sensory neuropathy, even though there may be no clinical accompaniment.

CONDITIONS THAT MIMIC MOTOR NEURONE DISEASE

Signs suggestive of motor neurone degeneration are seen in a variety of other degenerative, inflammatory, metabolic and multisystem neurodegenerative diseases that need to be considered in the differential diagnosis (Table 13.2).

The most common mimic of MND is spinal cord and/or nerve root compression as a result of **degenerative spinal column disease**. This can present with painless muscle wasting, weakness and fasciculation in one or more limbs, and sensory loss may be difficult to detect in the early stages. Magnetic resonance imaging of the spinal cord is essential to exclude this, and MRI may also reveal rarer intrinsic cord lesions, such as a

tumour or syringomyelia (see p. 222) **Multifocal motor neuropathy (MMN)** is another important condition to exclude. This autoimmune condition usually presents as an asymmetrical weakness of the upper limbs, which can progress to cause significant wasting and disability without generalized fasciculation (see p. 161). Often, but not invariably, MMN is associated with conduction block demonstrated by careful neurophysiological studies and/or the presence of anti-GM1 ganglioside antibodies in the serum. This mimic of MND is not lethal and can improve following immunoglobulin or cyclophosphamide treatment. **Post–polio syndrome** (see p. 397) may appear as a slowly progressive muscular atrophy.

EPIDEMIOLOGY OF MOTOR NEURONE DISEASE

Motor neurone disease is most commonly a disease of middle age with a mean age at onset of 60 years and a range of 20–90 years. Males develop MND more frequently than females, with a ratio of 1.7:1, and often at a younger age. The annual incidence of MND is approximately 1.4 per 100 000 per year, which is roughly half that of multiple sclerosis. Because of a relatively short survival, the prevalence rate is only approximately 4 per 100 000, a figure that is fairly consistent throughout the world apart from in Guam and the Kii Peninsular in Japan, where a clustering of ALS cases occurred in the 1950–70s; here it was seen alone or in combination with frontotemporal dementia or parkinsonism. Case-control studies have usually failed to identify an environmental event, toxin or infection that might be a risk factor for MND, but a history of previous musculoskeletal injury and exposure to electric shock appear mildly to increase disease risk.

PATHOGENESIS OF MOTOR NEURONE DISEASE

Although the brain and spinal cord usually look normal at post mortem, the microscopic changes may be dramatic. Motor neurone loss from the anterior spinal cord and motor cortex is usually severe and associated with proliferation and hypertrophy of neighbouring astrocytes. Pathological staining techniques often reveal neurofilament and other protein aggregates in the cell body of motor neurones. The binding of **ubiquitin** to a protein targets it for degradation and is the cell's way of putting damaged or unwanted proteins in a molecular rubbish bag. Thread-like and globular protein aggregates containing ubiquitin are an early pathological feature in MND. It seems likely that damaged proteins build up and may be toxic to neurones, although there is no proof yet of a causal link between aggregates and motor neurone cell death.

MECHANISM OF DEGENERATION: CLUES FROM MOLECULAR GENETICS

The most important clues to the pathogenesis of MND have come from **molecular genetics.** Although the majority of MND occurs sporadically, in approximately 10% of cases other members of the family are affected. Most commonly familial MND is an autosomal dominant disorder, being passed down through the generations. Linkage to a region on chromosome 21 was reported in 1991 and 2 years later mutations in the **copper/zinc superoxide dismutase (*SOD1*)** gene were discovered (see p. 124). To date more than 100 different mutations have been described. Most cause only a single amino acid to be substituted but that is sufficient to make the mutant SOD1 protein toxic to motor neurones. Mutations in *SOD1* are found in approximately 20% of familial and 3% of apparently sporadic MND cases but the pathology of patients with or without *SOD1* mutations is not substantially different. Transgenic mice have been developed that express mutant human *SOD1* and prove that motor neurone degeneration is the result of a toxic 'gain-of-function', not a loss of normal anti-oxidant function as was originally predicted. The exact mechanism by which mutant *SOD1* has a toxic effect and why motor neurones are particularly vulnerable is still not known.

Several studies point to **oxidative injury** as a result of the increased production of superoxide

(O^-), hydroxyl (OH^-) and peroxynitrite $(ONOO^-)$ – **free radicals**, which may damage many cellular components. An alternative hypothesis suggests that copper-mediated catalysis is irrelevant and that mutations in *SOD1* cause the protein to unfold and aggregate, which may be toxic to neurones or may block the ubiquitin protein degradation pathway. Aggregates of SOD1 protein however are rarely visible and many other proteins may be implicated in a common final pathway that results in motor neurone death and the clinical picture of MND.

OTHER HYPOTHESES

There are a number of disease mechanisms postulated to play a role in MND. Although viral infection, toxin exposure and autoimmunity have been implicated by some studies, an extensive body of research has consistently failed to support these hypotheses. Experimental evidence does implicate protein aggregation, excitotoxicity, oxidative injury and a loss of neurotrophic support. Glutamate is an important neurotransmitter in the brain but in excess it is very toxic to neurones, causing death by overexcitation. One theory is that astrocyte glutamate transporters, responsible for mopping up excess glutamate, are defective in MND. Another is that the composition of glutamate receptors expressed on the surface of motor neurones makes them prone to excitotoxicity, but the role of glutamate in the pathogenesis of MND is still controversial. Neurones are not replaced and so must continue to function for many years. Their metabolic activity generates free radicals capable of causing oxidative damage to protein, lipid and nucleic acids, which need to be repaired or replaced. This continuous oxidative stress is likely to be most severe in cells with a high metabolic demand, such as motor neurones. Signs of free radical injury can be found at post mortem in degenerating motor neurones in MND and mutant *SOD1* transgenic mice, but the evidence is still circumstantial and does not prove that oxidative injury has a primary role in causing MND.

Developing neurones require a variety of trophic factors for survival and growth. One hypothesis is that motor neurones lose this support over time and degenerate as a result. Although benefit from neurotrophins has been demonstrated in some animal models of neurodegeneration, trials in MND patients have been disappointing so far.

PRACTICAL MANAGEMENT ISSUES IN MOTOR NEURONE DISEASE

Giving the diagnosis to someone with symptoms and signs of MND can be a difficult task and should be done in a private space with a relative or friend present to provide support. In the absence of a diagnostic test, some explanation is required as to how the diagnosis of MND has been reached (i.e. excluding all other possible explanations). While it is important to be honest about the seriousness of this illness, a precise account of the disease course and prediction of survival is unhelpful at the outset. The shock of receiving the diagnosis often means that relatively little additional information will be taken in, so it is important to give the patient information to take home, such as pamphlets about MND and contact details of support groups, and to see the patient again soon to answer their questions. It is important to take a positive approach to treatment and tackle practical problems early and so diminish feelings of hopelessness and helplessness. Anxiety and depression are common after diagnosis and in response to the very substantial disabilities that develop. Psychological counselling and antidepressant medication should be used judiciously to support patients and carers through the most difficult periods.

DRUGS THAT ALTER THE COURSE OF DISEASE OR PROVIDE SYMPTOMATIC RELIEF

A large number of drugs have been tested in MND but only the glutamate-release inhibitor, **riluzole**, has been shown to have a significant effect, with a 3 month increase in survival over an 18 month trial period. The result is modest but has been reproduced in other studies and the early administration of riluzole after diagnosis may be more effective. Although side-effects from riluzole are uncommon, monitoring with regular blood tests for evidence of toxicity is essential, with particular attention being paid to any increase in liver enzymes.

Symptomatic relief

Many patients' experience **lower limb spasticity**, including painful tonic spasms. These can be diminished by careful titration of anti-spasticity agents such as baclofen, tizanidine or, occasionally, dantrolene. **Dysphagia** accompanied by dribbling may respond to low-dose amitriptyline, glycopyrrolate tablets, 1% atropine drops or hyoscine patches. In severe cases irradiation or botulinum toxin injection of the salivary glands may be beneficial but it is difficult to judge the dose. Excessive dryness of the mouth may be irreversible after irradiation.

THE MULTI-PROFESSIONAL APPROACH TO CARE

Until a cure is discovered, the major focus of therapy is on symptom management. Relentless disease progression and an escalating level of disability means that it is vital to anticipate problems and respond early so that the impact of the disease is ameliorated. The physician involved is likely to play an important role and may have expertise in neurology, rehabilitation, palliative care or general practice, but they are only one part of a team of professionals who are essential to maintain and improve a patient's quality of life.

Increasingly patients are managed in dedicated MND clinics in neurological centres with out-reach support from various agencies, including the MND association.

Physiotherapists can advise on and provide aids to improve mobility and posture. Self-care exercises, splints and orthoses can help avoid contractures and reduce pain. Occupational therapists can advise on mechanical aids and modifications to the home and workplace that will maximize patient independence and the assistance of carers.

Early referral to speech and language therapists when bulbar symptoms develop will help in the assessment of swallowing difficulties and advise on safe swallowing techniques. They will also provide advice on enhancing speech and eventually the use of computers to generate speech. Loss of the ability to communicate easily is one of the most frustrating aspects of MND. Dietary assessment and advice is increasingly recognized as important for maintaining quality of life and survival. Malnutrition is common in MND, even in patients without major bulbar symptoms, and early gastrostomy is advised before respiratory complications develop. This can be achieved by **percutaneous endoscopic gastrostomy** or radiologically inserted gastrostomy if the patient has insufficient respiratory reserve safely to tolerate sedation and being lain flat.

When patients become symptomatic from breathlessness, usually when the vital capacity is <60% of that predicted for age, sex and height, they may develop carbon dioxide retention, particularly overnight. This causes frequent nocturnal wakening, morning headache, daytime sleepiness, anorexia and even mental confusion. The use of a **non-invasive positive pressure ventilation** mask overnight can dramatically reduce these symptoms and prolong survival. As the disease progresses, however, the time spent on ventilation tends to increase and daytime use may be required for symptom control. Some patients elect to have endotracheal intubation and long-term mechanical ventilation. However, the quality of life for patient and carers is often poor and long-term ventilation is uncommon in the UK.

There are many parallels in MND care with the management of cancer patients and **early referral to a local hospice can be helpful to provide advice and practical support at home, in day centres and on in-patient respite care** to support the patient and their carers. If breathlessness at rest becomes distressing, anxiolytics, such as benzodiazepines and opiates, can be very useful in the terminal stages of the illness and most patients have a peaceful death.

REFERENCES AND FURTHER READING

Al-Chalabi A, Leigh PN (2000) Recent advances in amyotrophic lateral sclerosis. *Current Opinions in Neurology*, 13:397–405.

Gendron NH, Mackenzie AE (1999) Spinal muscular atrophy: molecular pathophysiology. *Current Opinions in Neurology*, 12:137–142.

Kuncl RW (ed.) (2002) *Motor Neurone Disease*. London, UK: WB Saunders.

Morrison K (2002) Molecular characterisation of motor neurone disorders. *Advances in Clinical Neuroscience and Rehabilitation*, 2:10–12.

Shaw CE, Al-Chalabi A, Leigh PN (2001) Progress in pathogenesis of amyotrophic lateral sclerosis. *Current Neurology and Neuroscience Reports*, 1:69–76.

Table 14.5 Investigations in dementia

---

1 Essential investigations to exclude remedial conditions in all patients
- Blood tests
  Blood count, ESR, CRP
  B12 and folate levels
  TSH, serology for treponemal infections
  Biochemical – renal and liver function, calcium
- Chest X-ray
- Imaging – CT or better MRI (may not be necessary in all cases)

2 Investigations often indicated, but dependent on age of presentation and specific clinical features
- Blood tests – autoantibody studies, angiotensin converting enzyme (ACE), HIV serology, serum copper and caeruloplasmin
- Urine – urinary copper
- EEG
- CSF examination – cells, protein, 14-3-3 protein, oligoclonal bands

3 Investigations occasionally indicated
- Blood tests
  Measurement of white cell enzymes, e.g. metachromatic leukodystrophy, hexosaminidase deficiency.
  DNA testing – screening for specific mutations e.g. Huntington's disease, familial prion disorders, familial Alzheimer's disease
- CSF examination – for JC virus and antibodies in suspected progressive multifocal leukoencephalopathy
- Biopsy of peripheral tissues, e.g. temporal artery, muscle, peripheral nerve, liver in dementia with systemic disease as in arteritis; rectal biopsy in storage disorders; small bowel biopsy in coeliac disease and in Whipple's disease; tonsillar biopsy in new variant CJD
- Functional imaging – single photon emission tomography; positron emission tomography
- Brain biopsy – usually a last resort in younger patients in whom all other tests have been negative, or when tests indicate that a histological diagnosis may determine a specific therapy: e.g. suspected chronic meningeal inflammation

---

structural lesions has been superseded by CT and MRI. In certain circumstances the EEG can be revealing, as in subclinical epilepsy (which may be severe enough to cause intellectual failure) and CJD, in which periodic sharp wave complexes against a slow background are typical in the later stages. Loss of normal rhythms with diffuse slowing usually indicates a widespread or metabolic disorder, while in unusual dementias, such as those associated with cerebral lymphomas, focal slow and sharp waves may precede structural changes.

Imaging techniques

Scanning with CT and MRI both provide a detailed picture of intracranial neuroanatomy. Cerebral atrophy can be convincingly dis-played (Figures 14.1 and 14.2) but does not correlate with intellectual function, and cannot be used by itself as evidence of primary cortical degeneration.

Both methods are more diagnostically useful in the assessment of structural disturbance such as tumours (Figure 14.3), or the development of hydrocephalus (Figure 14.4). In dementia as a result of cerebrovascular disease multiple infarcts may be seen (Figure 14.5), although lacunar strokes may not be visible even on high resolution CT scans. Scanning with MRI may show diffuse white matter abnormalities ('leukoaraiosis' – see Figure 3.7). These are often non-specific, do not correlate well with cognitive changes, and can be caused by many different types of pathology, including mixed Alzheimer's disease and MID. Recent evidence indicates that increased signal intensity in the basal ganglia and thalamus on T2-weighted MRI scans is a characteristic feature of variant CJD (vCJD), and can also be seen in other forms of CJD (Figure 14.6).

The measurement of cerebral blood flow by single photon emission computerized tomography (SPECT) (Figure 14.7) or positron emission tomography (PET), has only a limited role in investigation of dementia, but can reveal focal changes in regional cerebral blood flow before structural changes are evident on MRI. Such perfusion changes correlate well with cognitive abnormalities. The advantage of SPECT over PET as a clinical tool is that it is widely available and cheaper with comparable resolution.

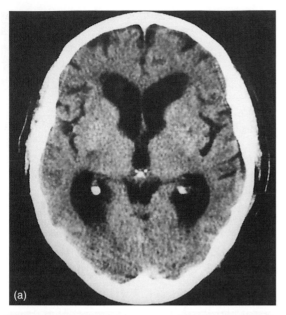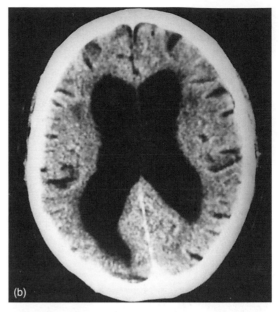

Figure 14.1 (a, b) CT brain scan showing cerebral atrophy. The ventricles are enlarged, the cisterns and surface sulci are widened.

TYPES OF DEMENTIA

The cortical degenerative dementias

Alzheimer's disease

Since its description in 1907, Alzheimer's disease has become recognized as the commonest of the primary degenerative dementias. In clinical research, the diagnosis of Alzheimer's disease is currently made in patients who meet specific criteria for dementia [DSM IV, and NINCDS/ADRDA (National Institutes of Neurological and Communicable Diseases and Stroke/Alzheimer's Disease and Related Disorders Association)].

> **Pathology of Alzheimer's disease**
> The pathological hallmarks of Alzheimer's disease comprise senile plaques, composed of β-amyloid and dystrophic dendrites, and neurofibrillary tangles, composed mainly of hyperphosphorylated microtubule-associated tau protein. Tangles are found within cortical pyramidal neurones.

There is widespread cortical neuronal loss in areas of plaque and tangle formation, and in addition there is subcortical neurone loss (and tangle formation) particularly in the nucleus basalis of Meynert and locus coeruleus. Other intraneuronal changes include granulo-vacuolar degeneration and Hirano bodies. Earliest manifestations of pathology probably occur in the hippocampus and medial temporal cortex. Plaques and tangles are most abundant in the frontotemporal, temporo-parietal and temporo-occipital regions. The pathological process tends to spare the primary motor and sensory cortex, and the primary visual and auditory cortex.

Clinical features

The evolution of symptoms can be divided into three stages, although there is no precise demarcation between these stages. The **first phase, lasting between 1 and 3 years,** is marked by progressive loss of memory and topographical sense with relative preservation of speech, minor personality changes and normal locomotor function. Household tasks become more difficult and are exacerbated by the increasing difficulty in spatial orientation, so that the patient becomes lost in unfamiliar, then familiar surroundings and exhibits impairment of constructional skills. The ability to concentrate is impaired. Vocabulary is restricted but language is otherwise normal early on.

As the disease progresses the features of the second stage become more apparent. Memory

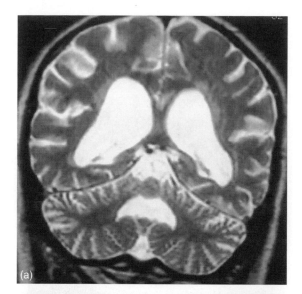

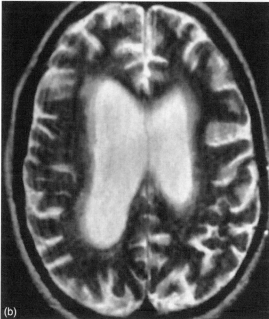

Figure 14.2 T2-weighted MRI brain scan: (a) coronal view; (b) axial view. Note the enlarged ventricles, surface sulci and basal cisterns in a patient with Alzheimer's disease.

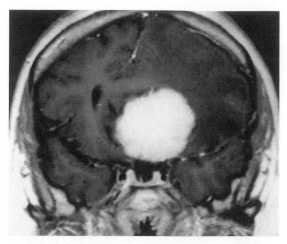

Figure 14.3 Gadolinium-enhanced coronal view MRI brain scan to show a large subfrontal meningioma presenting with dementia and apathy

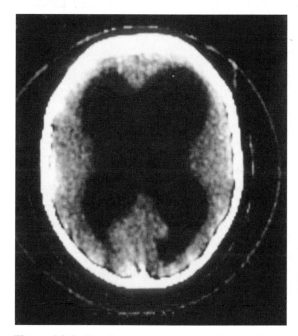

Figure 14.4 CT brain scan to show gross hydrocephalus. This was the result of an obstruction of the aqueduct.

impairment increases with severe disorientation so that the patient is lost in time and space. Speech becomes empty of coherent meaning and although elementary motor skills and coordination are preserved, even simple constructional skills decline. Insight is lost, being replaced by indifference and irritability. Although in younger patients the final phase may be reached within 3 or 4 years of onset, up to double this is more usual. This **final stage** is marked by almost complete loss of intellectual function, with incontinence and emergence of primitive reflexes and severe motor disabilities, with spasticity developing terminally.

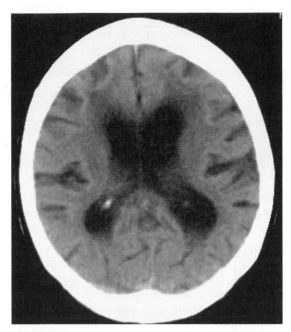

Figure 14.5 CT brain scan showing multi-infarct damage. Note the scattered low density patches and the enlarged ventricles.

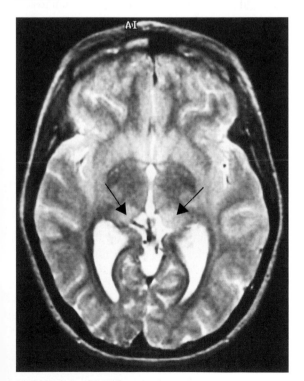

Figure 14.6 T2-weighted MRI brain scan, axial view, to show increased signal in the pulvinar (posterior nuclei of the thalamus) in a patient with vCJD.

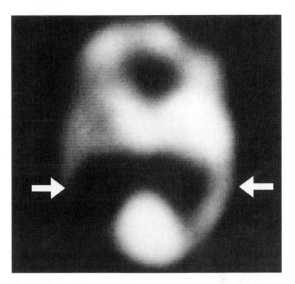

Figure 14.7 The single photon emission computerized tomography (SPECT) scan is obtained by injecting a radio-isotope tracer, which delineates cerebral perfusion. The marked decrease in concentration in the parietal regions, especially on the left (arrowed) is characteristic of Alzheimer's disease. (Picture courtesy of Dr Testa, Manchester Royal Infirmary.)

There is no clear clinical cut-off between the early and late presentation of Alzheimer's disease. The late onset form is more common, and has a female preponderance with longer life span, while speech disorders and early spatial disorientation are less marked than in younger patients.

Summary

In summary, the clinical diagnosis of (probable) Alzheimer's disease is based upon the recognition of:

- Dementia, documented by a validated scale such as the Mini-Mental Examination and confirmed by appropriate neuropsychological tests
- The presence of deficits in two or more areas of cognition
- Progressive deterioration in memory and other cognitive functions
- No disturbance of consciousness
- Onset between the ages of 40 and 90 years, usually after 65 years of age
- Absence of other conditions that could account for the progressive deficits in memory and other cognitive functions.

The above represents a part of the diagnostic criteria developed by the NINCDS/ADRDA. There are many research diagnostic schemes, which attempt to refine the accuracy of diagnosis in life, but proof is only possible through neuropathological examination.

In the early stages, when increasing forgetfulness is often the only complaint by the patient or relatives, it is important to differentiate memory problems from those of normal ageing. Alzheimer's disease pathology occurs in varying degrees in the brains of many (but not all) very elderly people, without being associated with significant cognitive abnormalities. Such changes are common in the medial temporal regions, including the hippocampus, and probably represent a stage in the evolution of more widespread pathology.

There is debate about the nature of age-associated memory impairment or benign forgetfulness of old age. Subtle changes in language functions or spatial disorientation may suggest evolving Alzheimer's disease, but often follow-up with neuropsychological testing is required to document the presence or absence of progressive deficits. It is especially important to consider depression and anxiety as triggers to complaints of memory loss or impaired concentration. The concept of mild cognitive impairment has been introduced to indicate these mild cognitive changes. Some of these individuals will progress to AD, but this is not inevitable, and mild cognitive impairment should not be uncritically regarded as an early manifestation of Alzheimer's disease. Longitudinal MRI with measurement of hippocampal volume and PET or SPECT scanning may prove to be helpful in distinguishing truly 'benign' memory loss of old age from the early stages of Alzheimer's disease.

There is overlap between Alzheimer's disease and Lewy body disease, as discussed below.

Familial Alzheimer's disease

Of patients with Alzheimer's disease, 5–10% have a family history suggestive of an autosomal dominant mode of inheritance. Genetic factors contribute to the risk of developing Alzheimer's disease in cases without a family history. Clinically, presentation at a younger age (sometimes in the third or fourth decades), myoclonic jerks, seizures, and depression

are more common than in non-familial Alzheimer's disease, although families differ in these features.

Molecular genetics and pathogenesis

Senile plaques contain beta amyloid. Identification of this protein led to the cloning of the amyloid precursor protein (APP) gene on chromosome 21q.

When linkage to this locus was found in familial Alzheimer's disease, APP was an obvious candidate gene and indeed point (missense) mutations of the APP gene were identified in a few families, perhaps 4% in all. These mutations are thought to be causative in these families. Mutations of the APP gene can also cause a rare familial disorder known as **hereditary cerebral haemorrhage with amyloidosis (Dutch type)**. Amyloid precursor protein is a membrane-spanning protein that is widely expressed. It is cleaved by enzymes known as β- and γ-secretase to produce several fragments, the longer of which (the 42 amino acid fragment, $A\beta_{42}$) is abnormally amyloidogenic, and which forms the major component of β-amyloid. Current research into methods of inhibiting the production of harmful $A\beta_{42}$ peptide involves searching for clinically useful inhibitors of β-secretase (β-site APP cleaving enzyme). So far, transgenic mice overexpressing mutant APP and presenilin proteins do not entirely reproduce the pathological features of human Alzheimer's disease.

In addition, mutations have been identified in other Alzheimer's disease families in two other genes (presenilin 1 and presenilin 2). The presenilin gene mutations account for the majority of early onset familial Alzheimer's disease cases.

The presenilin proteins are transmembrane proteins implicated in interneuronal signalling and the intracellular processing of proteins, and it is now apparent that presenilins regulate the activity of one of the enzymes (γ-secretase) that cleaves APP. In addition to APP and the presenilin genes as causative factors in familial Alzheimer's disease, an association exists between a locus on chromosome 19 and late onset Alzheimer's disease. The gene on chromosome 19 codes for a glycoprotein known as apolipoprotein E (ApoE) that exists in three allelic variants $\varepsilon2$, $\varepsilon3$ and $\varepsilon4$.

The frequency of the $\varepsilon4$ allele is increased in late onset Alzheimer's disease, and possession of the $\varepsilon4$ allele is associated with earlier age of onset in sporadic Alzheimer's disease and, in some families, with Alzheimer's disease. It is clear that multiple genetic factors influence the risk of developing Alzheimer's disease, perhaps interacting with environmental factors such as aluminium exposure, previous head trauma, viral infections or exposure to toxins.

Neurochemistry

> The neurochemical hallmark of Alzheimer's disease is loss of presynaptic cholinergic markers (choline acetyl transferase, acetyl choline, acetylcholinesterase) in the cerebral cortex, particularly the medial temporal cortex and hippocampus.

Loss of cholinergic input to the cortex is thought to follow degeneration of the nucleus basalis of Meynert. There is also loss of presynaptic and postsynaptic 5-hydroxytryptamine and noradrenaline markers, reflecting degeneration of the dorsal raphe nucleus and locus coeruleus, respectively. Loss of these enzymes is more pronounced in early onset cases. Identification of the cholinergic deficit has prompted attempts at symptomatic treatment. Acetylcholinesterase inhibitors may improve memory function in a subgroup of patients. Some of these are now being used to treat patients, usually with disease of mild to moderate severity.

Lewy body dementia

As noted above, in some pathological surveys the second most common diagnosis after Alzheimer's disease is **Lewy body dementia**. Other terms for this clinicopathological complex are dementia of Lewy body type, diffuse Lewy body disease, cortical Lewy body disease and the Lewy body variant of Alzheimer's disease.

Lewy body disease

Lewy bodies are intraneuronal inclusions, most commonly found in pigmented neurones of the substantia nigra in idiopathic Parkinson's disease, for which they are the pathological hallmark. Lewy bodies contain many proteins, but of particular interest are ubiquitin (a protein implicated in the breakdown of abnormal proteins) and α-synuclein. Mutations of the α-synuclein gene have been identified in a small number of families with autosomal dominant familial Parkinson's disease, but antibodies against α-synuclein strongly label Lewy bodies in sporadic disease, including Lewy body dementia. It was long known that Lewy bodies could be found in many other locations in the central and autonomic nervous system, but more recently they have been identified in the cerebral cortex, particularly in the medial temporal and limbic areas, in Parkinson's disease. However, although dementia is more common in patients with Parkinson's disease, rising to about 65% by the age of 85 years, the relationship between cortical Lewy bodies and the dementia of Parkinson's disease is not clear. In most cases of Parkinson's disease with mild and slowly progressive dementia in the late stages of the disease, cortical Lewy bodies are scanty and there is little by way of Alzheimer's disease pathology.

> **Lewy body dementia**
> Widespread and abundant cortical Lewy bodies associated with senile plaques and, to a lesser extent, neurofibrillary tangles have been linked to a syndrome of rapidly progressive dementia characterized by marked fluctuations in cognitive impairments, visual (and sometimes auditory) hallucinations, paranoid delusions, mild extrapyramidal features or sensitivity to neuroleptics, and unexplained falls or variations in consciousness.

The syndrome of Lewy body dementia

> The syndrome may be mistaken for delirium or MID. Cognitive impairments include memory loss, language difficulties, apraxia and spatial disorientation.

> Patients with Lewy body dementia seldom present with Parkinsonism, but treatment with neuroleptics may result in profound rigidity and akinesia.

The relationship between Lewy body dementia and Alzheimer's disease is debated. In Lewy body dementia, abundant cortical Lewy bodies are associated with Lewy bodies in the substantia nigra and varying degrees of nigral degeneration. Such changes are either absent or less marked in typical Alzheimer's disease. It appears that the two types of pathology have an additive effect, but may represent two distinct pathological processes. Some patients have been treated with the cholinesterase inhibitor rivastigmine.

Frontotemporal dementia, frontal lobe dementia, Pick's disease

Frontotemporal dementia accounts for about 20% of primary cerebral atrophy in the presenium (age less than 65 years) and 5–10% of dementia overall in pathological series. It is distinct from Alzheimer's disease clinically and pathologically. Pick described aphasia with frontotemporal atrophy but did not describe Pick bodies, the characteristic neuronal inclusions found (by Alzheimer) in a subgroup of patients with the syndrome of frontotemporal dementia. **It is probably best to avoid the term Pick's disease** and to use the generic term of frontotemporal dementia to denote these clinical syndromes.

Pathology
Cortical atrophy is usually confined to the frontal and temporal lobes and may be striking. Histologically there is cortical cell loss with superficial laminar spongy change (not identical to the spongiform changes seen in CJD) and astrocytosis in grey and white matter. Only about one-third of such cases show argyrophilic tau-positive and ubiquitin-positive Pick bodies and swollen neurones known as Pick cells. Occasionally frontotemporal dementia coexists with motor neurone disease (MND). In such patients, ubiquitin-positive but tau-negative inclusions are often present in frontal and temporal cortical neurones and in dentate granule cells of the hippocampus. Patients with tau pathology can be classified to some extent by the type of tau abnormality detected immunochemically. There are six isoforms of tau protein in the human brain, and these express either three or four microtubule binding domains [3-repeat or 4-repeat tau (3R and 4R tau)]. Frontotemporal dementia with Pick bodies has predominantly 3R tau, whereas progressive supranuclear palsy and corticobasal degeneration are associated with 4R tau, and in Alzheimer's disease both 3R and 4R tau are detected.

Frontotemporal dementia
Two main syndromes are associated with frontotemporal dementia, although there is overlap between the extremes. In one form, disinhibition, distractibility and overactivity predominate. In the other, affected individuals show mainly apathy, inertia and withdrawal.

Clinical features
Patients with **overactivity** tend to become more **withdrawn and apathetic** as the disease progresses. Subtle changes in social and personal behaviour, depression or atypical psychotic illness may precede progressive deterioration in mental function. Sometimes an episode such as a minor sexual misdemeanour, quite out of character, brings the individual to psychiatric attention or to court. An early feature is **loss of concern for others** and a lack of empathy. As the disease **progresses, motor perseveration, stereotyped movements, and ritualistic behaviour may emerge**.

Behavioural changes may be sufficiently pronounced to resemble the Kluver–Bucy syndrome (loss of emotional response, altered sexual activity, bulimia and apparent visual and sensory agnosia). Memory, mathematical abilities and parietal function are otherwise relatively preserved, but **speech deteriorates**, with circumlocution, vocabulary restriction and other features of empty speech, progressing to mutism with widespread pyramidal signs. As in the other cortical dementias laboratory investigations are non-contributory.

A **family history** is forthcoming in about 40% of cases, and often suggests an autosomal dominant mode of transmission. Linkage to chromosome 3 has been found in one large kindred and linkage to chromosome 17q in others. The latter have mutations of the gene coding for the microtubule-associated protein tau. Individuals with tau gene mutations usually present with symptoms typical of frontotemporal dementia but may present with extrapyramidal features and a few develop a form of MND.

In some patients with **frontotemporal dementia associated with MND**, the pathology consists of ubiquitin-immunoreactive inclusions that are not labelled by antibodies against tau. In these cases, dementia may precede or follow the evolution of MND. Parkinsonism may also manifest as part of the frontotemporal dementia syndrome but is not associated with Lewy body disease. The spinal cord pathology is essentially the same as that seen in MND without dementia. Many cases of MND with dementia are familial, and in some such families linkage has been identified to a locus on chromosome 9q.

Finally, some patients who present with **progressive aphasia have lobar atrophy** with the pathological changes seen in frontotemporal dementia. Thus frontotemporal dementia presents a spectrum of clinical syndromes that may be associated with at least two types of non-Alzheimer's disease pathology.

Dementia from cerebrovascular disease (see p. 460)

Cerebrovascular disease is well recognized as a cause of intellectual failure, usually by causing neuronal loss from infarction. This may arise from **embolic or thrombo-occlusive events**, but although dementia may complicate most disease states characterized by cerebrovascular involvement, the major causes are **cerebral atheroma and hypertension**. However derived, the effects of infarction depend on size, location and number. **Cerebral infarcts over 100 ml in size may be associated with dementia**, and although smaller single lesions do not cause widespread cognitive deficits, a strategically placed lesion affecting the dominant angular gyrus may simulate Alzheimer's disease, demonstrating the importance of location. Likewise, **focal infarction in the medial diencephalon** (particularly the anterior and dorsomedial thalamus) can produce dementia with **profound memory loss** and marked **apathy**. Occlusion of both anterior cerebral arteries

can result in profound neuropsychological changes amounting to a frontal lobe dementia, with apathy, inertia, loss of insight and loss of social inhibitions.

> Intellectual function is susceptible to multiple minor vascular insults causing MID.

The type of dementia depends on the location of the damage. Multiple cortical infarcts cause defects of cortical function but, unlike Alzheimer's disease, the motor strip and visual pathways are vulnerable with resulting **long tract signs and visual field loss**. Such changes can be seen on CT or MRI scans, but are rare in comparison with subcortical infarcts known as **lacunes**. These are usually associated with hypertension. Lacunes range from 2 to 15 mm in diameter, and may be undetectable by CT, although MRI is more sensitive in identifying small lesions and also identifies white matter changes (leukoaraiosis), which are often attributed to MID but which can also occur in primary degenerative disorders (Figure 14.8 – and see Figure 23.11).

> The term **Binswanger's disease** or progressive arteriosclerotic encephalopathy, refers to a syndrome of progressive neurological dysfunction, usually with focal signs such as hemiparesis, associated with hypertension, systemic vascular disease and stroke. The pathology is that of lacunar infarction with widespread white matter degeneration, that is, leukoaraiosis. Patients with this syndrome often develop dementia of a subcortical type.

Lacunar infarcts show predilection for the basal ganglia and upper pons resulting in a subcortical picture with **slowing, dysarthria, clumsiness, gait disturbance (marche à petits pas) and extrapyramidal features**. In most cases, however, features of cortical and subcortical involvement are apparent and both types are characterized by abrupt onset, stepwise deterioration and fluctuating course. These features form the basis of the Hachinski ischaemic score, which can be used to identify a vascular origin in some cases of dementia.

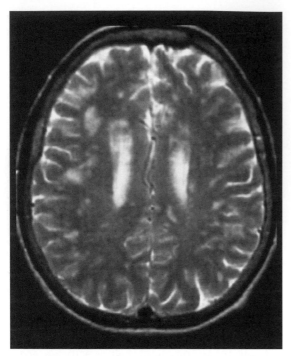

Figure 14.8 MRI brain scan T2-weighted, axial view, showing multiple small patches of high signal in the periventricular white matter, particularly in the right hemisphere. The patient had high blood pressure and these patches were thought to reflect vascular damage.

Such identification is valuable because the control of blood pressure and other treatable risk factors for cerebrovascular disease may be helpful in preventing further deterioration, although this is not proven.

Ischaemic score (after Hachinski et al., 1975)

All score 2 each

Abrupt onset
Fluctuating course
History of strokes
Focal neurological symptoms
Focal neurological signs

All score 1 each

Stepwise deterioration
Nocturnal confusion
Relative preservation of personality
Somatic complaints
Emotional lability

Depression
History of hypertension
Evidence of associated atherosclerosis
Scores of 7 and above are likely to be associated with multi-infarct vascular damage, while values of <5 are not.

Dementia from trauma and structural lesions

Head injury

Cognitive dysfunction following **trauma**, while not uncommon, is often neglected as a cause of dementia. It is a frequent cause of severe intellectual impairment with a UK incidence of 1600 cases per annum, usually resulting from road traffic accidents. Most commonly a non-penetrating injury causes multiple contusions and shearing lesions of the white matter; the frontal and temporal poles are particularly at risk.

> The length of retrograde amnesia, the extinction of memories prior to injury and post-traumatic amnesia, the inability to lay down new information subsequently, indicates its extent.

The vulnerability of the frontal lobes is reflected in the frequency of personality change as a result of the development of the **frontal lobe syndrome**.

This is marked by increased rigidity in thinking, reduction in powers of concentration, abstraction, planning and problem solving with loss of fluency, and an inability to change rapidly from one task to another. This is associated with emotional blunting, loss of insight and facile or apathetic mood. Such disturbance may be difficult to quantify, particularly in previous 'high flyers', and may not be easy to separate from secondary affective responses caused by insight into the consequences of the injury.

Although dementia usually results from a single episode, **recurrent trauma, as in boxing, results in a characteristic picture (dementia pugilistica)** of progressive ataxia, dementia, extrapyramidal features, dysarthria and personality impairment.

Structural causes

> Between 5 and 10% of patients with dementia have intracranial neoplasms.

Impairment of cognition may result from focal compression or infiltration, oedema or impairment of CSF circulation causing hydrocephalus (Figure 14.4). Development may be very slow as with a subfrontal meningioma, but is usually less than 12 months in duration. Tumours causing lateralizing deficits are normally easy to identify, but those in unusual sites such as the corpus callosum may present with mental change only.

> Subdural haematomas have such varied presentations that they may mimic other causes of dementia, even causing a metabolic encephalopathy as a result of inappropriate ADH secretion.

Subdural haematomas are most commonly seen in the elderly and investigation is sometimes misleading. Suspicion of a subdural haematoma should always be aroused by fluctuations in cognitive and neurological findings (see p. 356).

Dementia from transmissible, infectious and inflammatory causes

Transmissible spongiform encephalopathies

Transmissible spongiform encephalopathies affect humans and a variety of animals, including sheep (scrapie) and, notoriously, cattle (bovine spongiform encephalopathy – BSE). **Spongiform encephalopathy** was first recognized as a cause of dementia by Creutzfeldt in 1920 and Jakob in 1921. The disorder is rare, with about 50 new cases each year in the UK, an incidence of around one per million. Until about 1990, there had been no obvious increase in the annual incidence over the previous two decades. Recently, however, there has been great public concern over the recognition of a new form of CJD in young people. This clinically, pathologically and biochemically distinct syndrome is known as variant CJD (vCJD).

Pathology

The characteristic changes comprise spongiform degeneration with neuronal loss in the cerebral cortex. The spongiform change consists of vacuole formation within cortical (and subcortical) neurones. Amyloid plaques are found in some forms of the disease (such as Kuru, and vCJD) and there is widespread gliosis.

> **Creutzfeldt–Jakob disease**
> In Creutzfeldt–Jakob disease there is a rapid evolution of dementia from a stage of nonspecific confusion or behavioural change to the development of frank widespread neurological abnormalities terminating in a vegetative state. Creutzfeldt–Jakob disease is normally fatal within 12 months and in some patients more rapid progression over a number of weeks may occur.

Clinical features

In typical late onset sporadic CJD, although there may be a variety of extrapyramidal and long tract signs, diagnostically the presence of **startle myoclonus** is the most useful sign, while typical EEG findings occur ultimately in 75% of patients (Figure 14.9). Myoclonus may, however, appear late in the evolution of the disease. Some patients develop muscle wasting and evidence of anterior horn cell degeneration; others may exhibit **ataxia** (see p. 259).

> Five to ten per cent of patients with this disorder have a family history of a similar dementing illness, usually with autosomal dominant mode of inheritance, associated with mutations of the prion gene.

Several familial variants of the disease occur, including **Gerstmann–Sträussler syndrome** with slowly progressive ataxia and late dementia (as in kuru), and **fatal familial insomnia**, in which progressive insomnia occurs with autonomic and motor dysfunction and severe degeneration of the

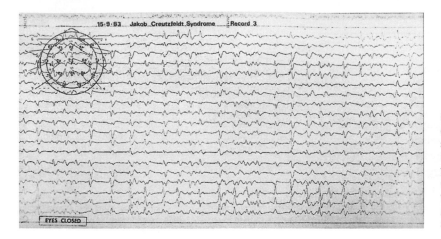

Figure 14.9 The characteristic changes of periodic synchronous sharp waves superimposed on an isoelectric background are seen in this tracing from a patient with Creutzfeldt–Jakob disease. A few weeks earlier the electroencephalogram only showed non-specific slowing.

anterior and dorsal thalamic nuclei. Some patients with familial Creutzfeldt–Jakob disease have slowly progressive dementia, leading to confusion with Alzheimer's disease.

Pathogenesis

Transmission was first demonstrated in 1966 by Gajdusek and colleagues who inoculated brain from a patient with kuru into chimpanzees. Kuru was an unusual form of spongiform encephalopathy that occurred in the Fore people of Papua New Guinea, and is thought to have been transmitted by **ritual cannibalism**. Clinically, it was characterized by emotional lability, behavioural changes and progressive ataxia, with dementia as a late feature. Cultural changes have led to its disappearance. Evidence for the transmissible nature of the disease in humans also derives from patients who have developed Creutzfeldt–Jakob disease following **neurosurgical procedures**, including dural grafts or after **corneal grafts** or dental intervention, and in people who received **cadaveric pituitary hormones** for endocrine disturbances in childhood.

throughout the body, but in the disease form it is altered in a way that makes it resistant to protease digestion. The prion protein is coded by the prion gene in which a number of different mutations have been found in the familial spongiform encephalopathies.

Thus spongiform encephalopathies in humans can be **sporadic or inherited**, but both forms share **transmissibility**. Disease transmitted from one person to another, as by injection of pituitary hormone extracts, tends to produce symptoms after 10–20 years incubation and a syndrome reminiscent of kuru, with behavioural change and ataxia as initial features. The recognition of similar cases in young people without exposure to pituitary hormones or other known sources of infective prions has led to concern that BSE may be transmissible to humans, although definite proof is lacking. How the altered prion protein causes progressive neuronal damage is not known.

There is no treatment that will alter the course of these disorders.

Prion transmissible agent

The transmissible agent originally thought to be an atypical or 'slow' virus , is now thought to be a protein, termed prion protein. This 253 amino acid protein (whose normal function is unknown) is highly conserved and widely expressed

---

HIV dementia

Human immunodeficiency virus (HIV) can result in dementia (see p. 410) through a variety of mechanisms. Dementia is common in acquired immunodeficiency syndrome (AIDS) (greater than 65%) and may precede other manifestations. It is referred to as the AIDS-dementia complex, or HIV-1-associated motor/cognitive complex. The AIDS-dementia complex is the most common form of dementia in young people.

Pathological changes are most marked in the white matter and deep grey matter, with relative sparing of the cortex. White matter loss reflects axonal damage and demyelination. Perivascular and parenchymal collections of inflammatory cells are seen, and multinucleated cells of macrophage or microglial origin in the white matter are characteristic. The virus can be detected in such cells but not usually in neurones. Cortical neuronal loss has been reported but is not usually striking. Clinically, the picture is typical of **'subcortical dementia'**.

Early symptoms comprise poor concentration, lapses of recent memory, and slowness completing or coping with complex tasks. There may be apathy and loss of initiative with mood changes. Impaired coordination with mild extrapyramidal features, including tremor, may be evident. As the disease progresses, speech is affected and motor abnormalities become more marked. Frontal release signs such as a pout response and grasp reflexes may appear and eventually it progresses to tetraplegia, mutism and death. In one-fifth of patients it may be rapidly progressive (see p. 410).

Azidothymidine (AZT; zidovudine) has been shown to stabilize or improve cognitive impairments in AIDS-dementia complex and in the early stages the symptoms are potentially reversible. In the differential diagnosis, opportunistic infections including tuberculosis and cryptococcal disease must be considered (see p. 405).

Other infections

Generally, infections cause relatively few cases of dementia but are important because some cases are responsive to treatment. The brain may be affected in a number of ways. Dementia may arise from the development of a **chronic meningitis** with secondary damage to the brain often associated with impaired immunity. *Cryptococcus neoformans* is the most common infection, but *Candida*, *Aspergillus*, toxoplasmosis and *Plasmodium falciparum* malaria have all been implicated. Some causative agents cause a more extensive meningovascular response such as **tuberculous meningitis**, while others additionally involve the brain parenchyma; for example, Whipple's disease, which causes a chronic meningo-encephalitis. These conditions evoke an inflammatory response, which may also cause cerebral infarction or hydrocephalus from thickened basal meninges. **Syphilis** may cause dementia through any of these mechanisms as well as, rarely, from the mass effect of a gumma (see p. 400).

In contrast, in **subacute sclerosing panencephalitis** the parenchyma of the brain is damaged by a chronic reaction to the measles virus in children. The progress from behavioural changes through intellectual deterioration and widespread neurological changes with prominent myoclonus to death, may occur within months. Direct destruction of the grey and white matter without an inflammatory response may also cause dementia.

Progressive multifocal leukoencephalopathy (see p. 407) is caused by viral infection of the brain. The causative agent is a papovavirus which, in the presence of chronic disturbed immunity, causes widespread progressive cerebral demyelination resulting in focal neurological signs and cognitive abnormalities. It is now most commonly seen in AIDS, but may complicate lymphoma, sarcoidosis, or long-term immunosuppression. Antiviral treatment is unhelpful and, although death can be expected within 1–2 years, the condition occasionally stabilizes and, rarely, may improve.

Inflammatory and granulomatous conditions without an infective cause may also result in dementia. **Mood disturbance is common in multiple sclerosis**: depression is more common than euphoria, but the latter is often associated with **cognitive impairment** with widespread frontal demyelination, the extent of the cognitive impairment reflecting the underlying severity of the disease.

Rarely, malignancies, particularly oat-cell carcinoma of the lung, may be associated with a paraneoplastic inflammatory process **(limbic encephalitis)** without obvious cause. Vascular disorders such as

Behçet's disease and systemic lupus erythematosus cause neuronal damage secondary to microcirculatory impairment, while granulomatous disorders, notably sarcoid, can affect cerebral function through the development of basal meningitis or strategically placed granulomas, especially in the hypothalamus.

Metabolic, nutritional and toxic causes

Chronic disturbance of electrolyte balance, particularly **hyponatraemia** from any cause, may disturb brain activity through the development of cerebral oedema, while cognitive function is sensitive to the accumulation of toxic metabolites in **chronic renal failure and portosystemic encephalopathy**. These conditions are marked not only by neuropsychiatric disturbance, but also by a variety **of movement disorders** such as myoclonus and asterixis. Constructional apraxia is said to be specifically disturbed in hepatic failure but probably reflects overall cortical deterioration, rather than a specific parietal dysfunction. Uraemic encephalopathy should be distinguished from dialysis dementia, which occasionally occurs after several years treatment of any form of renal failure with haemodialysis (see p. 489). It causes a distinctive picture of personality disturbance and prominent alteration of articulation and language formation, myoclonus, epilepsy, incoordination and a characteristic EEG. The cause is unknown, although aluminium deposition has been suggested and improvement only rarely follows transplantation.

Endocrine dysfunction

Thyrotoxicosis may cause behavioural disturbance resembling an anxiety state but may present in the elderly as an apathetic form with widespread psychomotor slowing, while 5% of **hypothyroid** patients also have non-specific slowing of cognition and lethargy. Similar patterns of dysfunction may complicate **Cushing's disease**, and **hypopituitarism** from any cause. The means is unknown but probably reflects electrolyte disturbance. Hypercalcaemia

may result in reversible neuropsychiatric disturbance, while **hypocalcaemia**, when associated with basal ganglia calcification in hypoparathyroidism, is sometimes associated with subcortical dementia having extrapyramidal features.

Vitamin deficiencies

Thiamine deficiency causes a specific type of amnesia rather than dementia (Korsakoff's psychosis). While neuropsychiatric disturbance may follow B_{12} **deficiency**, this is very much rarer than subacute combined degeneration of the cord. The dementia of **pellagra** (niacin deficiency) is more conspicuous, with pathological changes in the Betz cells and brainstem nuclei giving rise to extrapyramidal rigidity and primitive reflexes as well as cognitive dysfunction.

Toxic causes

A variety of therapeutic agents have been implicated in dementia. Immunosuppressants permit the development of opportunistic central nervous system infections, while most **drugs are toxic in excess**. Some may exacerbate an underlying dementia process, particularly hypotensive drugs, tranquillizers and those used in antiparkinsonian therapy. **Anticholinergics and industrial organophosphates** may affect central nervous system neurotransmission. A number of drugs cause inappropriate ADH secretion, while some **anticonvulsants**, especially phenytoin and barbiturate, in long-term high dosage can cause intellectual impairment which may not be reversible.

   Alcohol abuse causes intellectual deterioration in several ways and is an appreciable cause of dementia, a mild to moderate frontal lobe syndrome being the commonest form of encephalopathy (see p. 495). In rare instances, alcohol may cause subacute demyelination in the corpus callosum (Marchiafava–Bignami disease). More commonly it results in dementia indirectly through dietary deficiency, cerebral trauma and increased incidence of infection. **Heavy metal poisoning**, although rare, causes intellectual deterioration. The effect of chronic inhalation of lead on intelligence in children is currently a matter of concern and 'hatter's shakes' and 'mad as a hatter' describe the

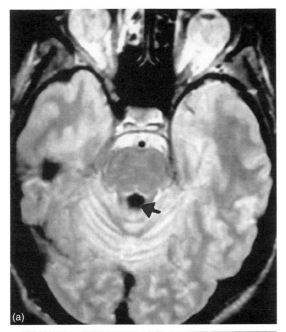

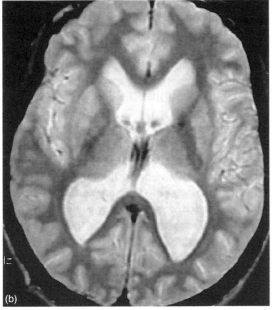

Figure 14.10 (a, b) Communicating hydrocephalus MRI brain scan, T2-weighted axial views, showing ventricular enlargement and flow void [arrowed in (a)], which has similar low signal to that seen in the basilar artery. The flow void lies in the bottom of the aqueduct.

mental disturbance, ataxia and restlessness found in workers who dressed hats with mercury. Contaminated seafood and mercury-treated seed corn have more recently been reported as sources of dementia.

Miscellaneous conditions

There are a large number of **inherited disorders**, sometimes with a demonstrable biochemical or enzyme defect, which affect the brain often as part of a multisystem disorder. For instance **porphyria** and **homocystinuria** may be associated with variable intellectual deficits, while storage diseases such as metachromatic leukodystrophy result in a progressive picture of dementia and neurological abnormality. Pathologically the white matter is particularly vulnerable to abnormal lipid deposition. Mild diffuse intellectual impairment often accompanies the **muscular dystrophies and spinocerebellar degenerations** and may be pronounced in **dystrophia myotonica**. The association of dementia with epilepsy is varied. In some conditions, such as Unverricht–Lundborg disease (progressive myoclonic epilepsy), dementia is an essential part of the syndrome, while in symptomatic epilepsies it may be an epiphenomenon. In severe chronic epilepsy, dementia may arise through repeated anoxic or traumatic insults, although the effects of long-term anticonvulsants are a far more common cause of intellectual deterioration.

Hydrocephalus

Hydrocephalus (see p. 367), whether communicating or non-communicating, can cause dementia. The typical picture of a **normal pressure hydrocephalus** is of a progressive disturbance of gait, incontinence and cognitive changes (Figure 14.10).

MANAGEMENT OF DEMENTIA

Ideally patients are best kept in familiar surroundings with support, if necessary, from attendance at day-centres or from home visits by health visitors and nurses. Further help at home may be provided by the local Social Services, such as, meals-on-wheels, home helps, incontinence laundry service. Attention to correctable deficits may give further aid; for example, providing hearing aids or correct spectacles. It is important to discuss the likely outcome with the family to help them plan the future. As the patient's condition deteriorates, along with an increasing number of others, they will be admitted to psychogeriatric wards or long-stay units.

> **Generalized seizures**
> Generalized seizures are characterized by the bilateral involvement of the cortex at the onset of the seizure. Patients experiencing generalized seizures lose consciousness at seizure onset, so that there is usually no warning.

Generalized tonic clonic seizures

Generalized tonic clonic convulsions, or convulsive seizures, previously termed **grand mal** attacks, are common. In this type of seizure, there is no warning, but the patient may experience a prodrome of general malaise. In some epilepsies, increasing frequency of another generalized seizure type, such as **myoclonic jerks** or **absences**, may herald a **tonic-clonic seizure**.

> The initial phase (tonic phase) is marked by rigidity; often the patient will cry out as air is expelled. Apnoea occurs, and the patient often becomes cyanosed. The tongue may be bitten, usually on one side, and the patient falls. Then clonic movements, usually involving all four limbs, develop. These are followed by muscle relaxation. The frequency of these movements gradually decreases and eventually the clonic movements cease altogether, marking the end of the seizure. Incontinence can occur at the end of the clonic phase. Most convulsions last less than 2 minutes. There is then a post-ictal period characterized by drowsiness and confusion lasting a variable period (sometimes as long as 20 minutes). It is not uncommon for people to fall asleep after a convulsion and this may sometimes be misinterpreted as unconsciousness.

Although patients are unaware of what has occurred, they will often be aware that they have had a seizure because of a variety of symptoms such as lethargy, generalized muscle aching, headache, bitten tongue and incontinence.

Absence seizures

> Typical **absence attacks**, previously known as **petit mal**, occur almost exclusively in **childhood** and adolescence. The child appears suddenly blank and stares: fluttering of the eyelids, swallowing, and flopping of the head may occur. The attacks last only a few seconds and often pass unrecognized.

Children may have many of these attacks a day, and not infrequently they are misdiagnosed as learning difficulties at school. **Absence attacks are associated with a characteristic electroencephalography (EEG) pattern – three per second generalized spike-and-wave discharges**. They may be precipitated by **hyperventilation**, which can be a useful diagnostic manoeuvre during EEG recordings, and sleep deprivation. There are also atypical absences, which are usually associated with more severe epilepsy syndromes, such as the Lennox–Gastaut syndrome. In these the EEG usually demonstrates less homogeneous, slower and more irregular spike/wave discharges. The onset and cessation of the seizure is not as abrupt as with typical absence seizures, and additional features such as eyelid flutter and myoclonic jerking are usually pronounced.

Myoclonic seizures

Myoclonic seizures are abrupt, very brief, involuntary movements that can involve the whole body, or just part of it such as the arms or the head. In idiopathic generalized epilepsies (see below), they occur most commonly in the morning, shortly after waking. They may sometimes cause the patient to fall, but recovery is immediate. The majority of myoclonic seizures occur in relatively **benign seizure** conditions, but sometimes they herald more severe disorders such as **the progressive myoclonic epilepsies.** These are rare, progressive conditions, which often begin in childhood. They consist of **mental deterioration** and **myoclonus** in association with other **neurological deterioration**, depending on aetiology. Not all myoclonus is the result of epilepsy: non-epileptic myoclonic jerks occur in a variety of other neurological conditions including lesions of the brainstem and spinal cord. In addition, myoclonic phenomena also occur in healthy people, particularly when they are just going off to sleep (hypnic jerk). Myoclonus is epileptic if it occurs in the context of a seizure disorder, and is cortical in origin.

Atonic and tonic seizures

Atonic and tonic seizures are very rare generalized attacks, accounting for less than 1% of epileptic attacks. They are often termed **'drop attacks'** and usually occur during the course of some forms of severe epilepsy, often starting in early childhood, such as **Lennox–Gastaut syndrome** or **myoclonic astatic epilepsy. Atonic seizures** (sometimes called akinetic attacks) involve a **sudden loss of tone in the postural muscles, and the patient falls to the ground.** There are no convulsive movements. Recovery is rapid, with no perceptible post-ictal symptomatology. During tonic seizures, there is a sudden increase in the muscle tone of the body and the patient becomes rigid, usually falling backwards onto the ground. Again, recovery is generally rapid.

The International Classification of Epilepsies (ICE), epileptic syndromes and related disorders

Epilepsy syndromes are defined by the features of the seizures, the presence of characteristic structural lesions, the age of onset of the condition, the presence of a family history, and by typical changes in the EEG. It is important to categorize epilepsies according to the syndromic classification because this may have implications both for management and prognosis. The classification scheme for epileptic syndromes proposed by the International League Against Epilepsy (ILAE) is currently the most widely used (Table 15.2). This classification does have a number of limitations, in particular it does not take into account recent progress in neuroimaging and neurogenetics; this classification is thus being revised and updated. The ILAE classification divides epileptic syndromes into four groups: localization-related (partial or focal), generalized, undetermined and special syndromes. Within these groups the syndromes are further divided into three subgroups: primary or idiopathic, secondary or symptomatic, and cryptogenic. When epileptic seizures are the only symptom of an inherited or genetic disorder, the syndrome is termed primary; when they occur as symptoms of a condition associated with structural brain lesions, the syndrome is termed secondary, and when the aetiology of the condition is unknown the term cryptogenic

is used. Below, the commoner epilepsy syndromes are divided by the age at which they occur.

Neonatal

Neonatal seizures (ICE 3.1)

Neonatal seizures are seizures occurring in the **first 4 weeks of life**: the syndrome is defined solely by age of onset, with no regard for the background aetiology or ictal manifestations. Causes of neonatal seizures include infection, anoxia, ischaemia, trauma, metabolic imbalance and nutritional disturbances. In around a quarter of cases no aetiological factor is identified. In a few babies, seizures are genetically determined.

> Seizures are often subtle and include clonic movements, eye deviation and blinking, usually of short duration; very rarely, more conventional seizure types may occur. These clinical features probably reflect the immaturity of the neonatal brain.

The EEG in the neonate is often difficult to interpret, but it may be possible to identify an epileptic focus. About 0.5% of babies have neonatal seizures. The prognosis is related to the underlying pathology, but the **overall outcome is not good**; approximately 25% die in the first year of life, and about half of those living longer either carry on having seizures into adult life or have evidence of neurological damage. Only about 25% make a full recovery. Indicators of poor prognosis include prematurity, early onset of seizures (especially within the first 2 days of life), focal cerebral lesions or malformations, intracranial bleeding and the presence of a very abnormal EEG.

Infancy

West syndrome (infantile spasms) (ICE 2.2)

West syndrome is also known as **infantile spasms, salaam spasms and hypsarrhythmia.** The onset is usually around the age of 6 months (range 3–9 months), and the child may have identifiable brain lesions (such as tuberous sclerosis, cortical dysplasias, malformations, or anoxic-ischaemic insults) prior to

Table 15.2 Summary of International League Against Epilepsy classification of epilepsies, epileptic syndromes and related seizure disorders (1989)

1 Localization-related
   1.1 Idiopathic
        Benign childhood epilepsy with centrotemporal spikes
        Childhood epilepsy with occipital paroxysms
        Primary reading epilepsy
   1.2 Symptomatic
        Chronic progressive epilepsia partialis continua of childhood
        Syndromes characterized by seizures with specific modes of precipitation
        Temporal lobe epilepsies
        Frontal lobe epilepsies
        Parietal lobe epilepsies
        Occipital lobe epilepsies
   1.3 Cryptogenic
        As 1.2, but aetiology is unidentified
2 Generalized
   2.1 Idiopathic
        Benign neonatal familial convulsions
        Benign neonatal convulsions
        Benign myoclonic epilepsy in infancy
        Childhood absence epilepsy (pyknolepsy)
        Juvenile absence epilepsy
        Juvenile myoclonic epilepsy (impulsive petit mal)
        Epilepsies with grand mal seizures on awakening
        Other generalized idiopathic epilepsies
        Epilepsies with seizures precipitated by specific modes of activation (reflex epilepsies)
   2.2 Cryptogenic or symptomatic
        West syndrome (infantile spasms)
        Lennox–Gastaut syndrome
        Epilepsy with myoclonic–astatic seizures
        Epilepsy with myoclonic absences
   2.3 Symptomatic
        2.3.1 Non-specific aetiology
               Early myoclonic encephalopathy
               Early infantile epileptic encephalopathy with suppression bursts
               Other symptomatic generalized epilepsies
        2.3.2 Specific syndromes
               Epileptic seizures may complicate many disease states
3 Undetermined epilepsies
   3.1 With both generalized and focal features
        Neonatal seizures
        Severe myoclonic epilepsy in infancy
        Epilepsy with continuous spike-waves during slow wave sleep
        Acquired epileptic aphasia (Landau–Kleffner syndrome)
        Other undetermined epilepsies
   3.2 Without unequivocal generalized or focal features
4 Special syndromes
   4.1 Situation-related seizures
        Febrile convulsions
        Isolated seizures or isolated status epilepticus
        Seizures occurring only when there is an acute or toxic event as a result of factors such as alcohol, drugs, eclampsia, non-ketotic hyperglycaemia

the onset, but in about one-third of cases no aetiology can be found. In this syndrome a **characteristic EEG pattern, termed hypsarrhythmia**, is seen. This consists of a chaotic pattern of high amplitude, irregular, slow activity intermixed with multifocal spike and sharp wave discharges.

The seizures may be flexor, extensor, or mixed, the latter being most common. Flexor spasms consist of sudden flexion of the neck, arm and legs. Sudden flexion of the trunk causes so-called 'salaam' or 'jack-knife' seizures. During extensor spasms, sudden movement of the neck, trunk and legs occurs, while in mixed spasms, there is flexion of the neck, trunk and arms, and extension of the legs. Seizures often occur in clusters, particularly soon after the child has been awoken.

The prognosis for West syndrome is poor. Overall, only about 20% of children make a complete recovery, with death occurring in a further 20% in childhood. Almost 65% of survivors have ongoing epilepsy, and up to 50% have persistent neurological handicap. The response to treatment with most anti-epileptic drugs (AEDs) is poor in West syndrome, but in some children the outcome may be improved if adrenocorticotropic hormone is given early in the condition. Vigabatrin has recently become the treatment of choice, particularly in children in whom the condition is associated with tuberous sclerosis.

Childhood

Lennox-Gastaut syndrome (ICE 2.2)

The **Lennox-Gastaut syndrome** is characterized by multiple seizure types including tonic and atonic seizures and complex absences. Tonic–clonic convulsions and myoclonic seizures may also occur.

It is a rare condition, accounting for perhaps 1% of all new cases of epilepsy, although because of its poor outcome it may represent as many as 10% of cases of severe epilepsy. Lennox–Gastaut syndrome is frequently associated with **learning difficulties** and **neuropsychiatric disturbances**. In about half of the cases no definite aetiological factor can be identified. A past history of West syndrome is the commonest identifiable cause, being present in 30–40% of children. Other causes include brain damage at birth, infections, tumour and severe head trauma. The condition typically has its onset between ages 3 and 5 years, although it may start at as early an age as 1 year or as late as 8 years of age (rarely even older). **Patients are at high risk of developing status epilepticus**, either tonic–clonic or non-convulsive. The **prognosis** of Lennox–Gastaut syndrome is **poor**, both with regard to seizure control (seizures persisting in 60–80% of patients) and mental development. Cognitive and behavioural problems are very common, and it is unusual for patients ever to lead independent lives. The EEG pattern in Lennox–Gastaut syndrome is almost invariably abnormal. The background activity is slow, and 2.0–2.5 Hz spike and wave and polyspike and wave discharges, often most marked over the anterior and posterior head regions, are characteristically seen. Such discharges may sometimes dominate the EEG for hours or days at a time. The complexes are not usually induced by hyperventilation or by photic stimulation. Rhythmic 10 Hz spikes are seen particularly during slow-wave sleep. Polypharmacy and sedation may worsen

seizures. Valproate and benzodiazepines are the drugs of choice, although the new AEDs lamotrigine, felbamate, levetiracetam and topiramate appear to be of benefit. A ketogenic diet may also be of benefit, but compliance is usually poor.

Benign childhood epilepsy with centrotemporal spikes (ICE 1.1)

Benign partial epilepsy of childhood also known as **Rolandic epilepsy or centrotemporal epilepsy** is the commonest of the idiopathic partial epilepsies. The onset of seizures is between the ages of 2 and 14 years, usually between 5 and 10 years. This syndrome accounts for about 10–15% of epilepsy in this age group. Children with this benign epilepsy usually have simple partial seizures, occasionally with progression to complex partial or to secondarily generalized seizures. Seizures tend to occur during the night or on awakening, and usually involve the face, lips and the tongue. Consciousness is usually preserved.

The **inter-ictal EEG** tracing has a **characteristic appearance** in this syndrome; it consists of frequent paroxysms of slow spike and wave discharges over the centrotemporal ('Rolandic') region, with a normal background rhythm. About 30% of the children have a family history of epilepsy. It has an **excellent prognosis** for complete seizure remission by puberty. Long-term treatment is usually not required, but if seizures are frequent then carbamazepine is the drug of choice. A variety of this syndrome is **benign occipital epilepsy**, in which the EEG disturbance is in the occipital lobe and the children may present with visual disturbances during the seizures.

Childhood absence epilepsy (ICE 2.1)

Childhood absence epilepsy is common, and occurs at the age of 3–13 years, more commonly in girls than boys. Typical **absences** lasting 5–15 seconds (no longer than 30 seconds) may be **'simple'** or **'complex'** and may occur many times a day. Up to 40% may develop tonic–clonic seizures. The EEG shows characteristic 3 Hz spike and wave. Absence seizures are usually well controlled with valproate or ethosuximide, and they usually resolve by adult life.

Febrile convulsions (ICE 4.1)

Febrile seizures are seizures occurring in the context of a **febrile illness**, often of viral aetiology, in children **between the ages of 6 months and 6 years.**

They affect as many as 3% of children in the general population and there is often a **family history** of febrile convulsions or epilepsy.

The seizures usually take the form of short, generalized tonic–clonic convulsions, without other features, with body temperatures over 38° C, particularly following a rapid rise in temperature. Acute treatment, in addition to supportive treatment, consists of diazepam, either rectally or intravenously, reducing the child's temperature and treatment of the underlying condition if appropriate. **Febrile convulsions do not usually require long-term prophylactic treatment unless complications develop.** However, parents should be counselled about the risk of recurrences and measures to avoid these. Risks for recurrence include age less than 15 months, epilepsy in first-degree relatives, febrile convulsions in first-degree relatives, and first febrile seizure with partial onset. In some children intermittent prophylaxis with a benzodiazepine is helpful. Investigation by EEG is usually not indicated. The most important differential diagnosis in this condition is with seizures that are triggered by central nervous system infections such as meningitis, encephalitis or brain abscess. If there is suspicion of a central nervous system infection, imaging, lumbar puncture (if safe) and antibiotic treatment are necessary.

In the great majority of children presenting with febrile convulsions, even if recurrent, the overall prognosis is excellent with no further seizures or other problems.

However, in a **few** children, **chronic seizures** subsequently develop, so that the risk of epilepsy occurring by the age of 25 years is about 7%.

> The risk is greatest in children with prolonged convulsions (lasting more than 20–30 minutes), those with previous signs of developmental delay, and those with partial seizures. The probability of epilepsy subsequently developing is also greater in children with a family history of afebrile seizures in a first-degree relative.

Adolescence

Juvenile absence epilepsy (ICE 2.1)

Juvenile absence epilepsy is similar to childhood absence epilepsy, but there is an equal sex incidence and later onset. Tonic–clonic seizures occur in 80%, and are *less* likely to remit.

> **Juvenile myoclonic epilepsy (ICE 2.1)**
> Juvenile myoclonic epilepsy is a common disorder that is probably underdiagnosed. It begins at the age of 8–18 years, and a family history is common. Seizures consist of bilateral or unilateral myoclonic jerks, usually affecting the upper limbs. Tonic–clonic seizures may also occur and approximately 10% of those affected have typical absences. Seizures often occur shortly after waking, and can be precipitated by sleep deprivation and alcohol. Investigation by EEG shows irregular spike and wave, and high frequency spikes. Approximately one-third have a response to photic stimulation. Spontaneous remission is rare, although the seizures respond well to valproate. Carbamazepine, vigabatrin and barbiturates may worsen the myoclonus.

Epilepsies that present in both childhood and adulthood

Epilepsies occurring in both childhood and adulthood are most commonly **cryptogenic or symptomatic partial epilepsies,** and are usually divided by the cortical origin of the seizures into temporal, frontal, parietal and occipital lobe epilepsies.

Temporal lobe epilepsy

Approximately 60–70% of localization-related seizures originate in the temporal lobes. Seizures commonly derive from the **hippocampus**, with **hippocampal sclerosis** (Figure 15.1) being the commonest aetiology. Seizures originating from temporal neocortex are similar in nature, but it is **common** to find a **structural lesion** such as glioma, angioma (Figure 15.2), neuronal migrational defects (Figure 15.3), post-traumatic change, hamartoma (Figure 15.4) or dysembryoplastic neuroepithelial tumour underlying the seizure disorder.

The seizures take the form of complex partial seizures and less commonly simple partial seizures and are described in Table 15.3.

Frontal lobe epilepsy

Frontal lobe epilepsy accounts for approximately 30% of partial epilepsy syndromes in adults

(Figure 15.5). The clinical features of frontal lobe seizures are given in Table 15.4.

Seizures originating in the motor cortex most commonly involve the face and limbs, particularly the hands. A well-known, though rather uncommon, form of simple partial motor seizure is the **'Jacksonian seizure'** (see Table 15.5). This starts as clonic jerking in one part of the body, often in a hand, which slowly spreads to contiguous muscle groups in the so-called 'Jacksonian march'. This parallels the slow progress of the epileptic discharge along the motor cortex (Figure 15.6).

Parietal and occipital lobe epilepsy

About 10% of all localization-related epilepsies originate in **the parietal and occipital lobes** (Figure 15.7).

Their clinical features are described in Table 15.6.

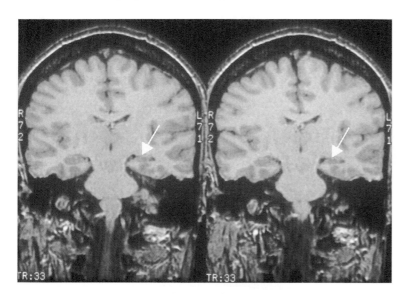

Figure 15.1 MRI brain scans, coronal views, to show hippocampal sclerosis on the left side (two contiguous cuts).

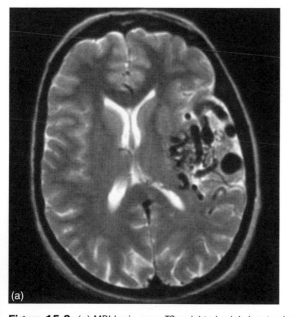

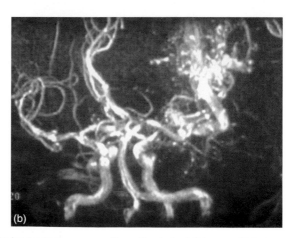

Figure 15.2 (a) MRI brain scan, T2-weighted axial view, to show large arteriovenous malformation in the left temporal lobe. (b) MRI angiogram of the same malformation.

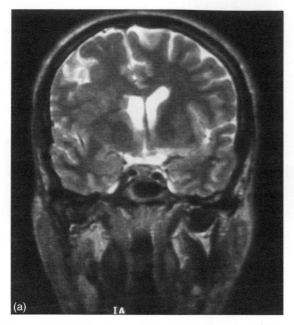

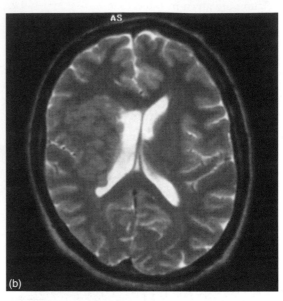

Figure 15.3 MRI brain scan, T2-weighted: (a) coronal view and (b) axial view, to show heterotopia in the right hemisphere.

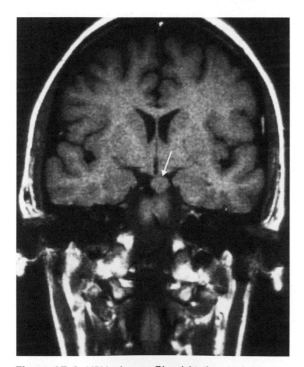

Figure 15.4 MRI brain scan, T1-weighted coronal view, to show hypothalamic hamartoma, presenting with complex partial seizures.

Table 15.3 Clinical features of temporal lobe seizures – 60–70% of partial seizures

Complex or simple partial seizures
Usual duration 2–10 minutes – slow evolution over 1–2 minutes
Aura
   Epigastric – nausea, borborygmi, belching, a rising epigastric sensation
   Olfactory, gustatory hallucinations (often unpleasant)
   Autonomic symptoms – change in heart rate, blood pressure, pallor, facial flushing, pupillary dilatation, piloerection
   Affective – fear (may be intense), anger, depression, irritability, dreamy states, depersonalization
   Dysmnestic – déjà vu, déjà entendu, recall of childhood or even former lives
Motor – arrest and absence prominent
   Automatisms – oro-alimentary (lip smacking, chewing, grimacing), gestural (fidgeting, undressing, walking)
   Vocalizations common, recognizable words suggests origin in dominant temporal lobe
May be secondary generalizations
Post-ictal confusion common

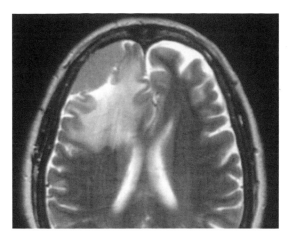

Figure 15.5 MRI brain scan, T2-weighted axial view, to show a right frontal meningioma with surrounding high signal. This patient presented with seizures suggestive of a frontal lobe origin.

Table 15.4 Partial seizures arising from the motor cortex – rare

Simple partial seizures
Duration variable – may be prolonged
Motor onset – corner of mouth, side of face, thumb, finger and hand, foot. Jacksonian march spreading proximally
Post-ictal – Todd's paresis
May have secondary generalization

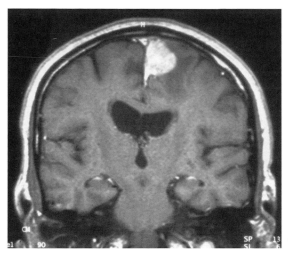

Figure 15.6 MRI brain scan, T1-weighted coronal view with enhancement, to show a meningioma. This patient presented with simple partial seizures with onset in the foot.

EPIDEMIOLOGY OF EPILEPSY

Incidence

The incidence of epilepsy in the general population has been estimated to be between 20 and 70 cases

Table 15.5 Clinical features of frontal lobe seizures – 30% of partial seizures

Complex partial	May be nocturnal
Duration very brief – c. 30 seconds	Abrupt onset
Aura	Cephalic:
	Non-specific dizziness, strange feelings in the head
	Forced thinking, ideational and emotional manifestations
Automatisms	Violent and bizarre
	Ictal posturing and tonic spasms
	Legs kick, cycle, step, dance
	Vocalization shrill loud cry, occasional speech fragments
	Version of head and eyes: version of the body causes circling
	Abduction and external rotation of the arm with flexion of the elbow in the contralateral arm with version of the eyes to the affected limb
	Autonomic symptoms may arise
	Sexual automatisms with pelvic thrusting, obscene gestures and genital manipulation
Secondary generalization common	
Post-ictal confusion brief with rapid recovery	

Table 15.10 Treatment according to seizure type

Seizure type	Drugs tried first	Other drugs that are used
Partial seizures		
Simple partial	Carbamazepine	Acetazolamide
Complex partial	Lamotrigine	Clobazam
Secondary	(Phenytoin)	Gabapentin
generalized	Valproate	Levetiracetam
		Oxcarbazepine
		Phenobarbitone
		Primidone
		Tiagabine
		Topiramate
		(Vigabatrin)
Generalized seizures		
Absences	Ethosuximide	Acetazolamide
	Lamotrigine	Clonazepam
	Valproate	Levetiracetam
		Topiramate
Atonic/tonic	Lamotrigine	Acetazolamide
	Valproate	Carbamazepine
		Clobazam
		Oxcarbazepine
		Phenobarbitone
		Phenytoin
		Primidone
		Topiramate
Tonic–clonic/	Carbamazepine	Acetazolamide
clonic	Lamotrigine	Clobazam
	(Phenytoin)	Gabapentin
	Valproate	Levetiracetam
		Oxcarbazepine
		Phenobarbitone
		Primidone
		Tiagabine
		Topiramate
		(Vigabatrin)
Myoclonic	Clonazepam	Acetazolamide
	Valproate	Piracetam

How treatment is started

If started at too great a dose, AEDs may result in side-effects and the abandonment of a potentially useful therapy. Therefore AEDs are introduced cautiously. The titration of an AED dose is usually symptom led, and if seizures are not controlled by an AED, it is then titrated slowly up to the maximum tolerated dose, regardless of serum concentrations. Possible dose-related side-effects are discussed with patients and carers and they are given instructions to reduce the dose if they occur. For most AEDs the serum concentration is linearly related to dose. The exception is phenytoin, which has saturation kinetics. Here an increase in serum concentration is not linear so a small dose increase will produce a disproportionate rise in serum concentration. Carbamazepine induces its own metabolism (autoinduction) resulting in a drop in serum concentration after 20–30 days. Occasionally the maximum tolerated dose may be higher than that recommended under the licence. With some AEDs (notably valproate) there is little benefit in exceeding the recommended dose.

If one first-line AED fails (at the maximum tolerated dose), it is substituted by another first-line therapy. The first-line therapies are then tried in combination and finally second-line AEDs are added. The aim of AED treatment is to achieve seizure control with one drug because polytherapy leads to poor compliance, drug interactions, increased teratogenicity and increased long-term toxicity.

Pharmacokinetics and drug monitoring

Therapeutic drug monitoring

The adherence to AED 'therapeutic' serum concentrations is often misconceived, and may lead to either under-treatment or over-treatment. Of patients on phenytoin monotherapy, 20–40% are well controlled with 'subtherapeutic' serum concentrations. Conversely, some patients are only controlled with phenytoin serum concentrations above the 'therapeutic' range, and yet experience no side-effects. This effect is seen with other AEDs, and in some cases (notably valproate) the serum concentration bears little relationship to either efficacy or side-effects. The titration of an AED should thus be symptom led, and if seizures are not controlled by an AED, it should then be titrated up to the maximum tolerated dose, regardless of serum concentrations. Measurement of AED serum concentrations, however, is helpful under certain circumstances: if poor seizure control occurs

Table 15.11 Commoner side-effects of anti-epileptic drugs

Drug	Idiosyncratic	Dose-related	Chronic
Acetazolamide	Rash, Stevens–Johnson syndrome, aplastic anaemia	Anorexia, lethargy, paraesthesiae, headache, thirst	Renal calculi
Benzodiazepines		Sedation, dizziness, fatigue, behavioural changes	
Carbamazepine	Rash, Stevens–Johnson syndrome, aplastic anaemia, leucopoenia, lupus-like syndrome	Nausea, headache, diplopia, dizziness, hyponatraemia	
Ethosuximide	Dyskinesia, rash, Stevens–Johnson syndrome, aplastic anaemia	Anorexia, headache, gastrointestinal disturbances	
Gabapentin		Sedation, diplopia, dizziness	Weight gain
Lamotrigine	Rash, Stevens–Johnson syndrome, aplastic anaemia, acne	Drowsiness, headache, diplopia, dizziness,	
Levetiracetam		Drowsiness, dizziness, ataxia, irritability	
Oxcarbazepine	Rash, Stevens–Johnson Syndrome, aplastic anaemia	Nausea, headache, diplopia, dizziness, hyponatraemia	
Phenobarbitone	Rash	Sedation, fatigue, confusion, cognitive impairment, impotence, paradoxical aggression and irritability	Dupuytren's contracture, osteomalacia, folate deficiency, acne
Phenytoin	Rash, Stevens–Johnson Syndrome, lupus-like syndrome	Sedation, fatigue, cognitive impairment, unsteadiness	Gum hypertrophy, coarsening of facies, acne, hirsutism, Dupuytren's contracture, osteomalacia, lymphadenopathy
Tiagabine		Dizziness, nervousness, diarrhoea, seizure worsening, emotional lability	
Topiramate		Impaired concentration, sedation, dizziness, paraesthesiae	Weight loss, renal calculi
Valproate	Pancreatitis, hepatitis (in children), thrombocytopenia, hyperammonaemia	Gastrointestinal symptoms, alopecia, tremor	Weight gain, polycystic ovarian syndrome
Vigabatrin*	Depression, psychosis	Dizziness, sedation	Weight gain, irreversible field defects (in approximately 40%)

*New patients now starting treatment with vigabatrin must be made aware of the potential for visual loss.

Table 15.12 Costs of 1 month's treatment with anti-epileptic drugs using an average dose each day (*BNF* 2003)

Anti-epileptic drug	Dose (mg/day)	Cost/month (£)
Carbamazepine	800	6.42
Clonazepam	4	3.36
Ethosuximide	750	9.00
Gabapentin	1800	89.00
Lamotrigine	200	64.37
Levetiracetam	750	44.45
Oxcarbazepine	1200	48.00
Phenobarbitone	90	2.16
Phenytoin	300	2.52
Primidone	750	1.59
Tiagabine	30	81.67
Topiramate	200	64.80
Valproate sodium	1000	8.88
Vigabatrin	1000	26.90

(serum concentrations may have fallen or very high serum concentrations occasionally may cause a paradoxical decrease in seizure control); if suspected drug toxicity occurs; if there is suspected non-compliance; if concomitant drug therapy is modified (to check for drug inter-actions); during pregnancy and illness; and during clinical trials. Lastly, in the case of phenytoin, which shows saturation kinetics, the serum concentration is a useful guide to the dosage increments that should be used.

Surgery

It has been estimated that there are approximately 750–1500 new patients per annum in the UK who could benefit from **epilepsy surgery**, and who thus require presurgical assessment (International League Against Epilepsy, 1991). The potential and the success of surgery may increase as MRI techniques improve and the cause of seizures may be identified in more patients. Epilepsy surgery is a major undertaking as it involves removing the part of the brain where the seizures begin and obviously carries some risks. In patients with a progressive underlying lesion (such as a tumour) or a lesion that carries other inherent risks (such as the risk of haemorrhage

from an arteriovenous malformation) the need for surgery is often determined by these considerations, regardless of seizure control. In other patients, the seizure disorder is the primary determinant. There is wide agreement that **epilepsy should have been shown to be intractable to medical treatment** before surgery is contemplated. Such a trial of therapy should include treatment separately with at least two first-line drugs appropriate to the type of epilepsy, and with adequate compliance. Although it is often reasonable to try several different drugs alone or together over a period of time, the chance of a patient becoming seizure-free diminishes if control is not achieved with initial first-line drugs, and evaluation for surgery is not usually delayed while every possible combination of medication is tried.

Patients considered for epilepsy surgery need to fulfil a number of criteria:

- It has to be felt that the seizures are one of the main causes of a patient's disability
- Similarly, it has to be considered that stopping the seizures would result in a significant improvement in quality of life (severe learning difficulties and psychiatric disease are relative contraindications)
- The patient must be able to understand the possible risks and benefits of the epilepsy surgery
- Seizure origin can be located (there should preferably be concordant data from psychometry, EEG and imaging)
- The risks of surgery do not outweigh the benefits (e.g. removal of dominant temporal lobe may result in unacceptable memory deficits even if seizures are halted).

Assessment for surgery thus involves a **multidisciplinary approach** including: neurologist, neurosurgeon, psychologist, psychiatrist, neurophysiologist and radiologist.

There are two main strategies for the surgical treatment of seizures. The first involves **resective surgery**, in which the aim of the surgery is the **removal of the epileptic focus** itself. Examples of this type of surgery are: anterior temporal lobectomy; selective amygdalo-hippocampectomy (in which only the mesial temporal structures are removed); or resection of a frontal lobe lesion. At the other extreme of resective surgery are patients in whom most or all of one hemisphere is abnormal, as in hemimegalencephaly or Rasmussen's encephalitis (an uncommon inflammatory condition causing seizures, progressive hemiparesis and intellectual deterioration), **hemispherectomy** may be necessary. The other strategy for surgical treatment is **to interrupt the pathways of seizure spread**, so isolating the epileptic focus from the rest of the brain. Examples of this type of surgery include section of the corpus callosum, and multiple subpial transection. **Callosotomy** is used to prevent secondary generalization of seizures, and its chief indication is in the treatment of intractable generalized seizures, particularly tonic seizures. **Multiple subpial transection** is a technique that relies upon the theory that seizure spread occurs tangentially through the cerebral cortex, while impulses controlling voluntary movement travel radially. In this operation, multiple cuts are made vertically in the cortex in an effort to isolate the epileptogenic area from the surrounding cortex. It may be helpful in the treatment of seizures arising in eloquent areas of the brain, such as the speech area or motor cortex.

Importantly, the social and medical results of surgery are better earlier on in the course of the epilepsy. The prognosis for epilepsy surgery depends upon the surgery and the underlying cause for the epilepsy, **but in patients in whom there is an identifiable lesion, approximately 70% will become seizure-free following surgery.**

Temporal lobe surgery (anterior temporal lobectomy, selective amygdalo-hippocampectomy) results in approximately 60% of patients becoming seizure-free, and 30% are improved. The overall mortality of temporal lobectomy is less than 0.5%, and the risk of permanent hemiparesis less than 1%. Memory problems and visual field defects are the other common morbidities. Extratemporal surgery is performed less frequently and the results are less impressive, with 40% becoming seizure-free and 30% improved. The morbidity is related to the site of resection. Hemispherectomy is particularly effective in controlling seizures, with approximately 80% becoming seizure-free, but this operation is reserved for patients with a profound hemiplegia.

Corpus callosotomy results in 70% of patients having a worthwhile improvement, but only 5% become seizure-free.

Other treatment modalities

Diet

It was the observation that starving patients had fewer seizures that resulted in the introduction of the ketogenic diet in the 1920s, in which 80% of calories were given as fat. The diets are usually unpalatable, cause gastrointestinal symptoms and are poorly tolerated. Nevertheless, these diets have been shown to be effective in children with severe intractable epilepsy and neurological deficits.

Vagal nerve stimulation

Stimulation of the **vagal nerve** involves surgically implanting a small **stimulator** under the skin in the neck, which intermittently stimulates the nerve. Recent data on the vagal nerve stimulator in patients with intractable partial seizures show a significant decrease in seizure frequency, with few side-effects. The efficacy was comparable to short-term results in new AED trials, but, as described above, the impact of new AEDs on the prognosis of intractable epilepsy has been modest, and it is at present difficult to see how this approach offers any advantages over the use of newer AEDs.

Drug treatment in special circumstances

Pregnancy

Conception

Frequent seizures may result in hormonal abnormalities that could contribute to infertility; however, AEDs possibly have a greater effect on fecundity. Some AEDs decrease libido and can induce impotence in men (e.g. phenobarbitone). There have been recent concerns of the association of polycystic ovarian syndrome and valproate, but the extent of this association is unclear; valproate should be prescribed cautiously in women who are obese or who have menstrual irregularities.

The metabolism of the contraceptive pill is increased with certain AEDs (e.g. phenytoin, carbamazepine). Women taking these drugs should use a higher dose pill (containing 50–100 μg ethinyloestradiol is generally recommended). Breakthrough bleeding is a sign that the contraceptive dose is not adequate.

> The **fetal malformation rate** in infants born to mothers with epilepsy is: higher than that of the general population; higher in those treated with AEDs; higher in those with high plasma AED concentrations; and higher in those on polytherapy. An attempt is thus often made to reduce therapy in women who wish to fall pregnant. In addition, women should be given folate supplements (5 mg daily) prior to conception and through the first trimester.

The most common abnormality in infants born to mothers with epilepsy is cleft lip/palate, comprising approximately 30% of the abnormalities. Specific syndromes have been described for different AEDs, the most well known being the fetal hydantoin syndrome, consisting of dysmorphic features and learning difficulties; other such syndromes have been described with other anti-epileptic drugs, in particular valproate. Also of note is the risk of spina bifida, which is most common with valproate (1–2% of births), and carbamazepine (0.5–1.0% of births). Women on these drugs require α-fetoprotein measurement and fetal ultrasound for the early detection of neural tube defects. Some new AEDs appear free from teratogenic effects in animals, but it is not certain that these data can be extrapolated to humans. Indeed, trials of new AEDs are not carried out on pregnant patients, and patients of child-bearing potential involved in drug trials have to be on adequate contraception. There are thus scarce data on the teratogenic potential of new AEDs, and caution is needed when new AEDs are used in women likely to fall pregnant.

The pharmacokinetics of AEDs may substantially change during pregnancy, requiring regular monitoring of seizures and serum drug concentrations. Furthermore, it is not uncommon for problems of compliance to occur during pregnancy, usually from maternal concern of the effects of AEDs on the developing fetus. It is essential to emphasize the importance of compliance, as frequent seizures may damage the fetus, and seizures can complicate the puerperium. Pharmacokinetic effects that occur are: a decrease in protein binding, resulting in an increase in the 'free' plasma concentrations of drugs that are predominantly protein bound (phenytoin, valproate and diazepam); an increase in hepatic metabolism and renal clearance of drugs; an increase in volume of distribution also increases during pregnancy, and a fall in total plasma concentrations of AEDs is thus not uncommon, especially in the third trimester. In the case of phenytoin, the increase in 'free' concentrations may result in toxicity despite a fall in total concentrations, and thus monitoring of 'free' phenytoin is recommended. However, as with all treatment, the absolute indication for changing drug dosages is an increase in seizures or drug toxicity.

In the last month of pregnancy women should be given oral vitamin K if they are taking enzyme-inducing drugs, and at birth the baby should receive vitamin K. **Breast feeding is not usually contraindicated**, except for women taking phenobarbitone or ethosuximide; other AEDs are present in insignificant amounts in breast milk. Breast feeding should only stop if the baby becomes drowsy or irritable following feeds.

Management of status epilepticus

> **Status epilepticus**
> Status epilepticus is defined as a condition in which a patient has a seizure or a series of seizures that last more than 30 minutes without regaining consciousness. Emergency treatment of convulsive seizures should, however, begin if the seizure has lasted more than 5 minutes or with repeated convulsions within an hour.

The term **status epilepticus** can apply to **all seizure types**, but it is convulsive status epilepticus (CSE) that is of most importance. The **mortality of CSE is approximately 20%** and relates mostly to the underlying aetiology. Approximately half the patients with CSE have chronic epilepsy, and in these **AED withdrawal** is the commonest identifiable cause. Reintroduction of a withdrawn AED often helps to terminate CSE.

> Other important causes are: cerebral trauma, cerebral tumour, cerebrovascular disease, intracranial infection, metabolic disturbances and alcoholism.

In treating CSE, there are three important considerations:

1 CSE is associated with severe physiological and metabolic compromise
2 Prolonged CSE can result in significant neuronal damage even after the clinical manifestations have halted, and there is only on-going electrographic status epilepticus
3 The longer that CSE continues, the harder it is to treat.

General measures are critical in the treatment of CSE. These are outlined in Table 15.13.

Drug treatment can be divided into stages. Although opinion varies as to which are the preferred therapeutic options, the use of a protocol for the treatment of CSE is mandatory as this simple measure results in the rapid administration of adequate doses of effective drugs and thus improves prognosis.

Early status (Table 15.13)
Intravenous lorazepam. This can be repeated after 10 minutes, or intravenous diazepam. If intravenous access is difficult, midazolam can be given buccally (between the gum and teeth), rectally or intramuscularly.

Established status (Table 15.13)
Intravenous fosphenytoin – the prodrug fosphenytoin can be used with greater speed and less risk. This is given in a dose of 20 mg/kg as PE (phenytoin equivalents – 1 mg of phenytoin being equivalent to 1.5 mg of fosphenytoin). Alternatively phenytoin (15–20 mg/kg given at 25–50 mg/minute (with EEG and blood pressure monitoring) can be used. If this has no effect, then intravenous phenobarbitone can be tried.

Refractory status (Table 15.13)
Transfer to intensive care unit. General anaesthesia is used with concomitant EEG monitoring, and continued for 12–24 hours after the last EEG/clinical seizure.

Once the patient is stable, the underlying cause needs to be identified and patients may require lumbar puncture, chest X-ray, neuroimaging and further blood tests.

To control the seizures, intravenous propofol is often used. Propofol is neuroexcitatory, as many anaesthetists recognize, so that slow withdrawal is necessary. An alternative is thiopental. Thiopental is cumulative in the body and a proportion of patients may develop hypotension. It is possible to monitor the blood level. Again a slow withdrawal of the drug is necessary.

> Seizures that do not respond to therapy should always raise the question of whether they may be non-epileptic attacks.

Non-convulsive status epilepticus

> In this condition, no convulsion is apparent. It may present with confusion, obtundation and psychiatric symptoms. Diagnosis is usually made with EEG. It usually responds well to benzodiazepines. It may be underdiagnosed in the elderly and psychiatric populations.

Furthermore 'electrical' status epilepticus (on EEG) with minimal visible signs can occur after acute hypoxic events and may be a cause of continuing coma. It is underdiagnosed and the **diagnosis should be considered in all comatose patients.** Diagnosis is by EEG.

THE PROGNOSIS OF EPILEPSY

The prognosis for full seizure control is relatively good. **Studies have shown that about 70–80% of all people developing epilepsy will eventually become seizure–free and about half will successfully withdraw their medication.** Once a substantial period of remission has been achieved, the risk of

Table 15.13 Acute management of status epilepticus

General measures

- Secure airway and resuscitate: monitor respiration, blood pressure and pulse
- Venous access
- Oxygen should be given – hypoxia is common during a convulsion
- Monitor urea, electrolytes, blood gases, pH, blood count and temperature
- Monitor neurological signs and GCS level
- ECG
- EEG (where possible)
- Intravenous glucose (25 g) and thiamine 250 mg (10 ml Pabrinex) (if poor nutrition or alcoholism suspected)
- Correct any metabolic abnormalities
- Save blood for AED levels

Medication

1 Immediate

   IV lorazepam 4 mg slowly for adults: 0.1 mg/kg for children
   or IV diazepam 10–20 mg in adults (0.25–0.5 mg/kg in children at 2–5 mg/minute as an alternative
   if difficult venous access, midazolam:

       buccally (between teeth and gum) 10 mg in adults (0.2–0.4 mg/kg)
       rectally 5–10 mg (0.15–0.3 mg/kg)
       or IM 0.15–0.3 mg/kg

2 If seizures continue after 5–10 minutes add IV fosphenytoin (as PE 20 mg/kg) given slowly c. 150 mg/minute
   (1 mg of phenytoin is equivalent to 1.5 mg of fosphenytoin) or IV phenytoin (20 mg/kg) at 50 mg/minute
   If seizures continue, try IV phenobarbitone 10 mg/kg given slowly at 100 mg/minute
   Monitor respiration and BP. **Could seizures be non-epileptic?**
   Treatment for refractory seizures – continuing after 30–40 minutes:

   - Transfer to ITU for intubation and GA
   - Continuous EEG monitoring (if possible)
   - IV propofol – loading dose 2 mg/kg – infuse 1–10 mg/kg per hour. Slow taper when all seizure activity disappeared ('burst suppression')
   - Or IV thiopental – loading dose 100–250 mg, infuse 3–5 mg/kg per hour. Cumulative drug with possible hypotension. Slow withdrawal. Can monitor blood level 40 mg/litre
   - Ensure maintenance AEDs are continued

GCS, glasgow coma score; ECG, electrocardiogram; EEG, electroencephalography; PE, phenytoin equivalents; ITU, intensive therapy unit; AEDs, anti-epileptic drugs.

further seizures is greatly reduced. A minority of patients (20–30%) will develop **chronic epilepsy**, and in such cases treatment is more difficult. Patients with symptomatic epilepsy, more than one seizure type, associated learning difficulties, or neurological or psychiatric disorders are more likely to develop a chronic seizure disorder. Five per cent of patients with intractable epilepsy will be unable to live in the community or will be dependent on others for their day-to-day needs. In a minority of patients with severe epilepsy, physical and intellectual deterioration may occur.

Stopping treatment

Because of the possible long-term side-effects of the drugs, it is common clinical practice to consider drug withdrawal after a patient has had a substantial period of remission (usually 2 years). After this period of seizure freedom, the chance of successfully coming off medication is approximately 60%. Even after being seizure-free for 2 years, there is still a chance of relapse while continuing the same medication; this chance of relapse is about half that of withdrawing medication.

The prognosis for AED withdrawal is worse in those who:

- Are 16 years or older
- Are taking more than one AED
- Have seizures after starting AEDs
- Have a history of generalized tonic–clonic seizures or of myoclonus
- Have an abnormal EEG.

The mortality of epilepsy

Epilepsy is often assumed to be a benign condition with a low mortality. Although this is usually the case, it does carry an **increased mortality**, particularly in younger patients (<40 years of age) and those with severe epilepsy (tonic–clonic seizures). Common causes of death in people with epilepsy include chest infections, neoplasia, and deaths directly related to seizures. Deaths directly related to seizures fall into several categories: status epilepticus; seizure-related death; **sudden unexpected death**; and accidents. There is extensive literature on death in status epilepticus, which is estimated to occur in about 20% of all cases of generalized tonic–clonic status. Sudden unexpected death in epilepsy is defined as a non-traumatic unwitnessed death occurring in a patient with epilepsy who had been previously relatively healthy, for which no cause is found even after a thorough post-mortem examination. Suggested explanations for the cause of death have included suffocation during a seizure, deleterious action of AEDs, autonomic seizures affecting the heart, and the release of endogenous opioids, although the pathophysiology (if indeed there is a single mechanism) is still unknown. The annual mortality rate is 1 sudden death for every 400 people with epilepsy in the community; this risk is probably doubled for those with uncontrolled seizures. Another possible cause of mortality and morbidity in people with epilepsy is as a result of accidents during seizures or as a consequence of a seizure. The precise extent of this problem is unknown. However, mortality rates for traumatic death have been shown to be increased, indicating that accidents and trauma are a more frequent cause of death in patients with epilepsy than in the general population. There is also an increased mortality from drowning among people with epilepsy. Mortality rates also indicate that patients with epilepsy are at a higher risk of committing suicide. Patients with temporal lobe epilepsy and severe epilepsy, or epilepsy with a handicap have a much greater risk of suicide: 25 times greater in the cases of temporal lobe epilepsy and five times greater for severe epilepsy.

SOCIAL IMPLICATIONS OF EPILEPSY

It is important to realize that there are many social implications of epilepsy; for instance, in regard to driving, schooling, employment and relationships. Unfortunately, there is still some unnecessary prejudice against those who have epilepsy, but there are also certain laws governing driving and employment for people with epilepsy.

Driving

Seizures while driving are still one of the commonest preventable causes of road traffic accidents. In the UK the rules laid down about driving are straightforward, and there is little excuse not to follow them.

Driving and epilepsy

It is the obligation and responsibility of every person who has any condition that may impede their driving (this includes all people with epilepsy) to inform the Driver and Vehicle Licensing Authority (DVLA). Anyone who fails to inform the DVLA and continues to drive is committing a criminal offence. Furthermore, failing to inform the DVLA may invalidate the driver's insurance.

This applies to all people with seizures, and for this purpose even the smallest epileptic event (for example, an aura or a myoclonic jerk) is counted as a seizure. Once the DVLA has been informed, the patient should stop driving and can reapply for a licence only when the following criteria have been fulfilled: either that **no epileptic attacks while awake (including aura, etc.) have occurred during** the **past year**, or that if epileptic attacks have occurred, that these were **only during sleep and that this pattern has been present for at least 3 years**. Following a single epileptic seizure, or if there is loss of consciousness of no known cause, patients are also barred from driving for 1 year.

If a patient has been seizure free, and has thus regained his driving licence, but wishes to come off medication, the advice from the DVLA is that the patient should not drive during the changes in medication and for 6 months after the withdrawal from medication.

The rules for heavy goods vehicle and passenger carrying vehicle licences are much stricter, and it is not possible to hold these licences if a person has a continuing liability to epileptic seizures. This is interpreted as meaning no epileptic seizure or anti-epileptic medication for the previous 10 years and no evidence of a continuing risk of seizures (e.g. 3 per second spike and wave on the EEG or a brain lesion).

Employment

There are a few occupations that are barred by statutory provision for people with epilepsy and these include: aircraft pilot; ambulance driver; taxi driver; train driver; merchant seaman; or working in the armed services, fire brigade or police. There are also certain jobs that involve substantial risks if a seizure should occur and thus cannot be recommended (e.g. scaffolder), and common sense should apply when considering such jobs. Furthermore there are jobs in which epilepsy is not explicitly mentioned but may be considered a bar (e.g. midwifery). For insurance purposes it is generally important that employers are aware if employees have epilepsy.

NORMAL SLEEP AND ABNORMALITIES OF SLEEP

Adults require on average 7–8 hours sleep a night. This sleep is divided into two distinct states – rapid eye movement (REM) sleep and non-REM sleep. These two sleep states cycle over approximately 90 minutes throughout the night, with the REM periods becoming progressively longer as sleep continues and accounting for about one-quarter of sleep time. During REM sleep, dreams occur; there is hypotonia or atonia of major muscles that prevents dream enactment. Rapid eye movement sleep is also associated with irregular breathing and increased variability in blood pressure and heart rate. Non-REM sleep is divided into four stages (stages I–IV) defined by specific EEG criteria. Stages I/II represent light sleep, while stages III/IV represent deep, slow-wave sleep. Dreams do occur during non-REM sleep, but these tend to be more rational and have less emotional association.

Abnormalities of sleep are divided into three main categories:

1 Dysomnias or disorders of the sleep–wake cycle;
2 Parasomnias or disordered behaviour that intrudes into sleep;
3 Sleep disorders associated with medical or psychiatric conditions.

Dysomnias

Dysomnias are divided into: intrinsic sleep disorders, such as idiopathic insomnia, idiopathic hypersomnolence (a diagnosis by exclusion) or narcolepsy; extrinsic sleep disorders, in which there is an extrinsic cause for the sleep disorder such as drugs, poor sleep hygiene or high altitude; and disorders of the circadian rhythm, which can be intrinsic (e.g. delayed sleep-phase syndrome) or extrinsic (e.g. caused by shift-work).

Insomnia

Although **insomnia** can be idiopathic, in the majority of patients there is an underlying cause. This cause can be an intrinsic sleep problem, such as **periodic limb movements, restless legs or sleep apnoea**, or an extrinsic problem, such as **high altitude, drugs** (e.g. certain AEDs, and certain antidepressants) or **poor sleep hygiene**. This last problem is usually easy to address – no caffeine or alcohol in the evening, avoidance of exercise close to bedtime, no daytime naps, regular bedtime, and so on. Other **medical conditions**, such as chronic obstructive lung disease, asthma, cardiac failure, gastro-oesophageal reflux and nocturia can all contribute to insomnia, and certain neurological conditions can also have a significant impact (see below). Among the commoner causes, however, are **depression, fibromyalgia, anxiety and old age.** The elderly tend to have more fragmented sleep patterns, with less slow wave sleep and more early morning awakenings.

The treatment of insomnia should first of all address possible underlying causes and sleep hygiene. For short-term insomnia, hypnotics can be useful, but long-term use of these drugs, especially benzodiazepines, can result in tolerance, dependence and poor sleep. Certain cases of insomnia benefit from a behavioural approach, in which the patient is retrained in normal sleep behaviour; such an approach should be considered in all with chronic insomnia.

Narcolepsy

> ### Narcolepsy
> Narcolepsy is a specific, well-defined disorder with a prevalence of approximately 1 in 2000; it is a lifelong condition usually presenting in the late teens or early 20s. Narcolepsy is a disorder of REM sleep and the main symptom is excessive daytime sleepiness. This is manifest as uncontrollable urges to sleep, not only at times of relaxation (e.g. when reading a book, watching television), but also at inappropriate times (e.g. when eating a meal or while talking). The sleep is usually refreshing. The other typical symptoms are cataplexy, sleep paralysis and hypnagogic/hypnapompic hallucinations.

These represent REM sleep phenomena such as hypotonia/atonia, and dreams occurring at inappropriate times. **Cataplexy** is a sudden decrease in voluntary muscle tone (especially jaw, neck and limbs) that occurs with sudden emotion like laughter, elation, surprise or anger. This can manifest as jaw dropping, head nods or a feeling of weakness or, in more extreme cases, as falls with 'paralysis' lasting sometimes for several minutes. Consciousness is preserved. Cataplexy is a specific symptom of narcolepsy, although narcolepsy can occur without cataplexy. **Sleep paralysis** and **hypnagogic hallucinations** are not specific and can occur in other sleep disorders and with sleep deprivation (especially in the young). Both these phenomena occur shortly after going to sleep or on waking. Sleep paralysis is a feeling of being awake, but unable to move. This can last for several minutes and is often very frightening, so can be associated with a feeling of panic. Hypnagogic/hypnapompic hallucinations are visual or auditory hallucinations occurring while dozing/falling asleep or on waking; often the hallucinations are frightening, especially if associated with sleep paralysis.

Narcolepsy in humans is rarely familial. However, the lifetime risk for developing narcolepsy is increased to 1% in first-degree relatives of narcoleptic patients.

> Approximately 90% of all narcoleptic patients with definite cataplexy have the human leukocyte antigen (HLA) allele, HLA DQB1* 0602, compared with approximately 25% of the general population. The sensitivity of this test is decreased to 70% if cataplexy is not present. The strong association with HLA type has raised the possibility that narcolepsy is an autoimmune disorder. There is probably a functional defect in hypocretin secretion (hypocretins are expressed in neurones in the hypothalamus).

Because narcolepsy is a lifelong condition with possibly addictive treatment, the diagnosis ideally should be confirmed with a **multiple sleep latency test (MSLT).** During this test, five episodes of sleep are permitted during a day; rapid onset of sleep and REM sleep within 15 minutes are suggestive of narcolepsy. A low level of cerebrospinal fluid hypocretin also has been suggested as a diagnostic test for narcolepsy.

The excessive sleepiness of narcolepsy can be treated with modafinil, methylphenidate or dexamphetamine and regulated daytime naps. The cataplexy, sleep paralysis and hypnagogic/hypnapompic hallucinations respond to antidepressants (fluoxetine or clomipramine are the most frequently prescribed). People with narcolepsy ironically often have fragmented, poor sleep at night, and good sleep hygiene can be helpful.

in those with sleep apnoea. Multisystem atrophy and some other neurodegenerative diseases are associated with central sleep apnoea. In addition, brainstem strokes can result in Ondine's curse, in which automatic respiratory control is lost, resulting in severe nocturnal apnoea. The two syndromes of RLS and PLMS can be associated with neuropathies, spinal cord lesions and Parkinson's disease.

Perhaps one of disorders that is most indicative of an underlying neurological cause is **REM sleep behaviour disorder**, which is most commonly associated with extrapyramidal syndromes such as Parkinson's disease, multisystem atrophy and cortical Lewy body disease, but is also associated with other neurodegenerative conditions, strokes and brainstem tumours. Dopaminergic agents used to treat parkinsonism are also associated with REM sleep disorders, especially nightmares.

Epilepsy has a complex association with sleep. Certain seizures are more common during sleep, such as frontal lobe seizures, which occur during non-REM sleep. Rarely, nocturnal seizures may be the only manifestation of an epileptic disorder and these can be confused with a parasomnia – this has been especially true for autosomal-dominant nocturnal frontal lobe epilepsy, the seizures of which were thought originally to represent a nocturnal paroxysmal dystonia. Activation of EEG in epilepsy commonly occurs during sleep, so that sleep recordings are much more likely to demonstrate epileptiform abnormalities. Rarely, non-convulsive status epilepticus can occur during slow wave sleep; the clinical manifestation of this is usually intellectual regression and autism. Lack of sleep can precipitate seizures, especially in the idiopathic generalized epilepsies, and sleep apnoea has been reported to worsen seizure control. Sleep disturbances also commonly occur in people with epilepsy in whom there is a higher incidence of sleep apnoea, fragmented sleep and insomnia as well as daytime somnolence (often drug related).

Specific clinical approach to patients with sleep disorders

As in most neurological conditions **the history of patients with sleep disorders is paramount**. In the history of the presenting complaint, it is often important to have **a witnessed account** and to determine at what stage of the night the sleep disturbance is occurring or under what circumstances daytime somnolence occurs. Sleepiness at times of relaxation may be as a result of sleep deficit, but sleepiness at inappropriate times is much more likely to be indicative of a condition such as narcolepsy. A history of a typical night is often helpful, as are sleep diaries and an exploration of sleep hygiene. Family history can be informative, as many sleep disorders such as insomnia, restless leg syndrome and parasomnias run in families. Alcohol and drug history are critical as many drugs can influence sleep and can contribute to or trigger sleep disorders. Specific scales have been developed to assess somnolence, and the **Epworth sleepiness scale** (Table 15.14) is one of the commonest and most frequently used.

The mainstay of sleep investigation is **polysomnography**. Full polysomnography measures EEG to sleep stage, respiration either by chest movements or nasal airflow, electrocardiography and oxygen

Table 15.14 Epworth Sleepiness Scale (ESS)

How likely are you to doze off or fall asleep during the following situations, in contrast to just feeling tired? For each of the situations listed below, give yourself a score of 0 to 3 where 0 = would never doze; 1 = slight chance; 2 = moderate chance; 3 = high chance. Work out your total score by adding up your individual scores for situations 1 to 8.

Situation	Chance of dozing
Sitting and reading	
Watching television	
Sitting inactive in a public place, e.g. theatre, meeting	
As a passenger in a car for an hour without a break	
Lying down to rest in the afternoon	
Sitting and talking to someone	
Sitting quietly after lunch (when you have had no alcohol)	
In a car while stopped in traffic	

An ESS score of greater than 10/24 or more is considered abnormally sleepy saturations. For suspected cases of sleep apnoea, an overnight measure of oxygen saturations is a cheap and effective screening process that can be carried out at home. Polysomnography is indicated for the investigation of all patients with suspected narcolepsy, sleep apnoea and REM sleep disorders. It can be used to monitor treatment in these conditions, and this is especially useful for obstructive sleep apnoea treatment with continuous positive airway pressure in order to optimize the machine settings. In addition, **multiple sleep latency tests** are used for the diagnosis of hypersomnolence. The patient is permitted to sleep for up to 15 minutes on five occasions through a day. Short latency to sleep indicates hypersomnolence; REM sleep occurring in two or more of the sleep episodes is indicative of narcolepsy. Other investigations are determined by the clinical picture.

As well as the treatment suggested above. Social aspects should be discussed, as sleep disorders can have a considerable psychosocial impact. Depression, anxiety and loss of libido can result directly from sleep disorders. In addition, driving should be discussed and patients with daytime somnolence should not drive unless their condition is being adequately treated. This is especially important for those with narcolepsy and sleep apnoea in whom naps at inappropriate times can occur.

REFERENCES AND FURTHER READING

Chokroverty S (1999) *Sleep Disorders Medicine*. London, UK: Butterworth-Heinemann Medical.

Crawford P, Appleton R, Betts T, Duncan J, Guthrie E, Morrow J (1999) Best practice guidelines for the management of women with epilepsy. The Women with Epilepsy Guidelines Development Group. *Seizure*, 8(4):201–217.

Douglas NJ (2002) *Clinicians' Guide to Sleep Medicine*. London, UK: Arnold.

Sander JW, Hart YM (1997) *Epilepsy: questions and answers*. Basingstoke, UK: Merit.

Sander JW, Shorvon SD (1996) Epidemiology of the epilepsies. *Journal of Neurology and Neurosurgery and Psychiatry*, 61:433–443.

Shorvon SD, Walker MC (2000) Tonic–clonic status epilepticus. In: Hughes RAC (ed.) *Neurological Emergencies*, 2nd edn. London, UK: British Medical Journal. pp. 143–172.

Walker MC (2001) Diagnosis and treatment of nonconvulsive status epilepticus. *CNS Drugs*, 15(12):931–939.

HEADACHE

P.J. Goadsby

Headache is the most common neurological problem. This is clearly correct in general practice, while headache dwarfs other out-patient problems for consultant neurologists. In the UK it is estimated by the Association of British Neurologists that 20% of referrals in out-patients are for headaches, with epilepsy next at 12%.

GENERAL PRINCIPLES

The International Headache Society (IHS) classification, currently being revised, is used, deviating only where it is clear that there will be a change in the second edition of the classification. There are many types of headache, and diagnosis is the key to proper management. The IHS system is explicit, in the sense that it uses features of the headache to make the diagnosis, summing features to make the diagnosis more certain. The general concept is that there are primary and secondary forms of headache (Table 16.1).

Broadly, **primary headaches** are those in which headache and its associated features are the disease in themselves, and **secondary headaches** are those where the headache is a manifestation of another disease, such as headache associated with fever. Mild secondary headache, such as that seen in association with upper respiratory tract infections is common but only rarely worrisome. The clinical dilemma remains that while life-threatening headache is relatively uncommon in Western society, it is present and requires suitable vigilance by doctors. Primary headache, in contrast, often confers considerable disability over time and, while not life-threatening, certainly robs patients of quality of life.

SECONDARY HEADACHE

It is imperative to establish in the patient presenting with any form of head pain whether there is an important secondary headache that is declaring itself. Perhaps the most crucial clinical feature to elicit is the length of the history. Patients with a short history

Table 16.1 Common causes of headache (after Olesen *et al.*, 2000)

Primary headache Type	Prevalence(%)	Secondary headache Type	Prevalence(%)
Migraine	16.0	Systemic infection	63.0
Tension-type	69.0	Head injury	4.0
Cluster headache	0.1	Sub-arachnoid haemorrhage	<1.0
Idiopathic stabbing	2.0	Vascular disorders	1.0
Exertional	1.0	Brain tumour	0.1

Table 16.2 Warning signs in head pain

- Sudden onset pain
- Fever
- Marked change in pain character or timing
- Neck stiffness
- Pain associated with higher centre complaints
- Pain associated with neurological disturbance, such as clumsiness or weakness
- Pain associated with local tenderness, such as of the temporal artery.

require prompt attention and may require quick investigation and management. Patients with a longer history generally require time and patience rather than alacrity. There are some important general features, including associated fever or sudden onset of pain (Table 16.2); these demand attention.

Patients with a history of recent onset headache or neurological signs need a positive diagnosis that it is benign or brain imaging with computerized tomography (CT) or magnetic resonance imaging (MRI) (Figures 16.1 and 16.2).

Patients with a history of recurrent headache over a period of 1 year or more, fulfilling IHS criteria for migraine (Table 16.3) and with a normal physical examination, have abnormal scans in only 0.1% of cases. In general it should be noted that brain tumour is rare relative to other causes of headache, and rarely a cause of isolated long-term histories of headache.

The **management** of secondary headache is generally self-evident: treatment of the underlying condition, such as an infection or mass lesion. An

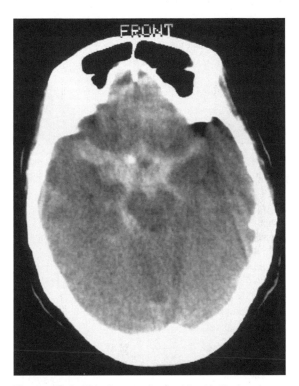

Figure 16.1 CT brain scan showing blood in the basal cisterns following an acute subarachnoid haemorrhage causing an acute onset headache – 'first and worst'.

exception is the condition of **chronic post-traumatic headache** (see p. 359) in which pain persists for long periods after head injury. This is an interesting generic problem that may be seen after central nervous system (CNS) infection, trauma, both blunt and surgical, intracranial bleeds and other precipitants. While the syndrome is generally self-limiting up to 3–5 years after the event, treatment of the headache may be required if it is disabling (see Chronic daily headache, below).

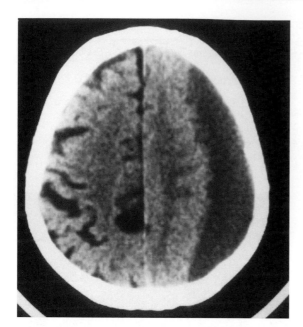

Figure 16.2 CT brain scan showing an extensive left-sided subdural collection in a patient with troublesome headaches.

Table 16.3 Simplified diagnostic criteria for migraine adapted from the International Headache Society Classification (Headache Classification Committee of The International Headache Society, 1988)

Repeated attacks of headache lasting 4–72 hours that have these features, normal physical examination and no other reasonable cause for the headache:

At least two of:	At least one of:
• Unilateral pain	• Nausea/vomiting
• Throbbing pain	• Photophobia and
• Aggravation by movement	phonophobia
• Moderate or severe intensity	

PRIMARY HEADACHE SYNDROMES

The primary headaches are a group of disorders in which headache and associated features are seen in the absence of any exogenous cause. The common syndromes (Table 16.1) are tension-type headache, migraine and cluster headache. The collection of headaches known as primary chronic daily headache form the greatest part of the neurologists burden.

Other less common syndromes will be mentioned because they are easily treated when recognized.

Anatomy and physiology of headache

The disabling primary headaches, migraine and cluster headache, have been studied extensively in recent times and they are now relatively well understood. It is the intracranial extracerebral vessels and the dura mater, and not the brain, that are responsible for, or at least perceived as, generating pain from within the head.

The key structures involved in the nociceptive process
- The large intracranial vessels and dura mater
- The peripheral terminals of the trigeminal nerve that innervate these structures
- The central terminals and second-order neurones of the caudal trigeminal nucleus and dorsal horns of C_1 and C_2 (trigeminocervical complex).

The innervation of the large intracranial vessels and dura mater by the trigeminal nerve is known as the trigeminovascular system.

The **cranial parasympathetic autonomic innervation** provides the basis for symptoms, such as lacrimation and nasal stuffiness, which are prominent in cluster headache and paroxysmal hemicrania, although they may also be seen in migraine. It is clear from human functional imaging studies that vascular changes in migraine and cluster headache are driven by these neural vasodilator systems so that these headaches should be regarded as **neurovascular**. The concept of a primary **vascular** headache is no longer tenable, because it neither explains the pathogenesis of what are complex CNS disorders, nor does it necessarily predict treatment outcomes.

Migraine is an episodic syndrome of headache with sensory sensitivity, commonly to light, sound and head movement, probably resulting from

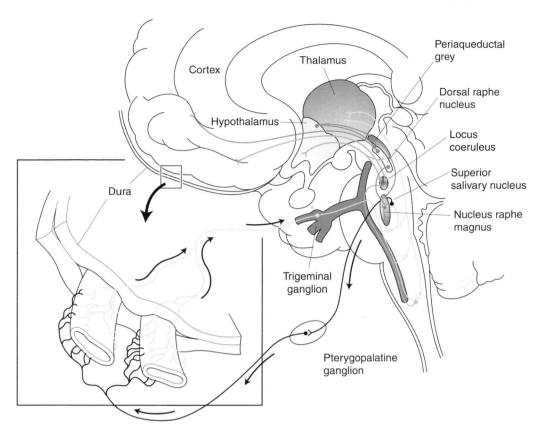

Figure 16.3 Pathophysiology of migraine. Migraine involves dysfunction of brainstem pathways that normally modulate sensory input. The key pathways for the pain are the trigeminovascular input from the meningeal vessels, which passes through the trigeminal ganglion and synapses on second-order neurones in the trigeminocervical complex. These neurones in turn project in the quinto-thalamic tract, and after decussating in the brainstem, synapse on neurones in the thalamus. There is a reflex connection with neurones in the pons in the superior salivary nucleus, which provides an efferent cranial parasympathetic outflow synapsing in the pterygopalatine, otic and carotid mini-ganglia. This trigeminal-autonomic reflex is present in normal subjects and expressed most notably in patients with trigeminal-autonomic cephalgias, such as cluster headache and paroxysmal hemicrania; it may be active in migraine. Important modulation of the trigeminovascular nociceptive input, as suggested from brain imaging studies, comes from the dorsal raphe nucleus, locus coeruleus and nucleus raphe magnus.

dysfunction of aminergic brainstem/diencephalic sensory control systems (Figure 16.3).

The first migraine genes have been identified for familial hemiplegic migraine, in which about 50% of families have mutations in the gene for the $Ca_V2.1$ (α_{1A}) subunit of the neuronal P/Q voltage-gated calcium channel and another. These findings and the clinical features of migraine suggest it might be part of the spectrum of diseases known as channelopathies, disorders involving dysfunction of voltage-gated channels. Functional neuroimaging has suggested that brainstem regions in migraine (Plate 3a,b), and the posterior hypothalamic grey matter site of the human circadian pacemaker cells

of the suprachiasmatic nucleus in cluster headache (Plate 4a,b), are good candidates for specific involvement in primary headache.

MIGRAINE

Migraine is generally an episodic headache with certain associated features, such as sensitivity to light, sound or movement, and often with nausea or vomiting accompanying the headache (Table 16.3).

None of the features is necessarily present, and indeed given that the migraine aura, visual disturbances with flashing lights or zigzag lines moving across the fields or other neurological symptoms, is reported in only about 15% of patients, a high index of suspicion is required to diagnose migraine. A headache diary can often be helpful in making the diagnosis, although in reality it usually helps more in assessing disability or recording how often patients use acute attack treatments.

> In differentiating the two main primary headache syndromes seen in clinical practice, **migraine at its simplest level is headache with associated features, and tension–type headache is headache that is featureless,** furthermore **most disabling headache presenting in primary care is probably migrainous in biology.**

If headache with associated features describes migraine attacks, then **headachy** describes the migraine sufferer over their lifetime. The migraine sufferer **inherits a tendency** to have headache that is amplified at various times by their interaction with their environment, the much-discussed triggers. The brain of the migraine sufferer seems more sensitive to sensory stimuli and to change, and this tendency is even more notably amplified in females during their menstrual cycle. The migraine sufferer does not habituate to sensory stimuli easily and so can be unfairly and often stimulated in the world in which they live and work. Migraine sufferers may have headache when they sleep in, when they are tired, when they skip meals, when under stress or when they relax. They are less tolerant to change and part of successful management is to advise them to maintain regularity in their lives. It is this biology that marks migraine and in clinical practice must override the phenotype of individual headaches.

It has been said that migraine can never occur daily, but few biological issues respect absolute rules. **Chronic migraine**, which is part of the group of headaches known as **chronic daily headache** (see below), is the most severe end of a complex biology and often requires neurological input. Only development of specific disease markers will settle issues around **daily headache** clearly. After making a diagnosis, the second step is to ascertain how much headache the patient has and, more important, what

the patient is unable to do. What is their degree of disability? One can ask the patient directly, keep a diary, or obtain a quick but accurate estimate using the migraine disability assessment scale, which is well-validated and very easy to use in practice (Figure 16.4).

Management of migraine

After diagnosis the management of migraine begins with an explanation of some aspects of the disorder to the patient.

- Migraine is an inherited tendency to headache; this is caused by the patient's genes, therefore it cannot be cured; *however*:
- Migraine can be modified and controlled by life-style adjustment and the use of medicines
- Migraine is not life-threatening nor associated with serious illness, with the exception of females who smoke and are taking oestrogenic oral contraceptives, but migraine can make life a misery
- Migraine management takes time and cooperation when, for example, a headache diary has to be collected, or inquiry made concerning the disability.

Non-pharmacological management

Non-pharmacological management of migraine is to help the patient identify things that make the problem worse and encourage them to modify these. Pamphlets from the Migraine Trust and Migraine Action Association in the UK are very helpful. However, many patients will not find any success with this approach. Patients need to know that the brain sensitivity that is migraine varies, so that the effect of triggers will vary. This fact alone will remove considerable frustration on the patient's part, will ring true to most as they have had the experience, and is biologically plausible because it is exactly what one would predict from the channelopathic

INSTRUCTIONS: Please answer the following questions about ALL your headaches you have had over the last 3 months. Write your answer in the box next to each question. Write zero if you did not do the activity in the last 3 months

1. On how many days in the last 3 months did you miss work or school because of your headaches? . . . . ☐☐ days

2. How many days in the last 3 months was your productivity at work or school reduced by half or more because of your headaches (*Do not include days you counted in question* 1 *where you missed work of school*)? . . . . ☐☐ days

3. On how many days in the last 3 months did you not do household work because of your headaches? . . . . ☐☐ days

4. How many days in the last 3 months was your productivity in household work reduced by half or more because of your headaches (*Do not include days you counted in question* 3 *where you did not do household work*)? . . . . ☐☐ days

5. On how many days in the last 3 months did you miss family, social, or leisure activities because of your headaches? . . . . ☐☐ days

A. On how many days in the last 3 months did you have a headache? (If a headache lasted more than one day, count each day) . . . . ☐☐ days

B. On a scale of 0–10, on average how painful were these headaches? (*where* 0 = *no pain at all, and* 10 = *pain as bad as it can be*) . . . . ☐☐

Figure 16.4 Migraine disability assessment scale questionnaire (MIDAS version 3.0, reproduced courtesy of Innovate Medical Research 1997.

theory of migraine pathogenesis. **The crucial life–style advice is to explain to the patient that migraine is a state of brain sensitivity to change**. This implies that the migraine sufferer needs to regulate their life: eat a healthy diet; take regular exercise; observe regular sleep patterns; avoid excess caffeine and alcohol; and, as far as practical, modify or minimize stress.

Preventive treatments for migraine

The decision to start a patient on a preventive drug requires crucial input from the migraine sufferer. The patient needs to have come to terms with the fact that they have an inherited, incurable but manageable problem, and that they have sufficient disability to wish to take a medicine to reduce the effects of the disease on their life. Only then can the doctor explain the choices available and why one might be better than another. The basis of considering preventive treatment from a medical viewpoint is a combination of acute attack frequency and attack tractability. Attacks that are unresponsive to abortive medications

are easily considered for prevention, while simply treated attacks may be less obviously candidates for prevention. If a patient's diary shows a clear trend of an increasing frequency of attacks, it is better to begin preventive treatment early rather than wait for the problem to become chronic.

A simple rule for frequency is that for 1–2 headaches a month there is usually no need to start preventive medication, for 3–4 headaches a month it may be needed but not necessarily, and for 5 or more headaches a month prevention is likely to be needed.

Options available for treatment are covered in detail in Table 16.4 and vary somewhat by country even within the European Union.

The problem with preventives is that often the doses required to reduce headache frequency produce marked and intolerable side-effects. It is not clear how preventives work, although it seems likely that they modify the brain sensitivity that underlies migraine. Another key clinical point is that generally each drug should be started at a low dose and gradually increased to a reasonable maximum if there is going to be a clinical effect.

Table 16.4 Preventive treatments in migraine[†]

Drug	Dose (mg)	Frequency	Selected side-effects
Pizotifen	0.5–2.0	Daily	Weight gain Drowsiness
β-blocker Propranolol	40–120	b.d.	Reduced energy Tiredness Postural symptoms *Contraindicated in asthma*

Tricyclics
    Amitriptyline
    Dothiepin
    Nortriptyline
	all 25–75	Nocte	Drowsiness
			Note: some patients are very sensitive
			and may only need a total dose of 10 mg,
			although generally 1.0–1.5 mg/kg body
			weight is required for a response

Anticonvulsants Valproate	400–600	b.d.	Drowsiness Weight gain Tremor Hair loss Fetal abnormalities Haematological or liver abnormalities
Gabapentin	900–3600	Daily	Dizziness Sedation
Topiramate	25–200	Daily	Confusion Paraesthesiae Weight loss
Methysergide	1–4	Daily	Drowsiness Leg cramps Hair loss Retroperitoneal fibrosis (1 month drug holiday is required every 6 months)
Flunarizine	5–10	Daily	Drowsiness Weight gain Depression Parkinsonism

No convincing controlled evidence
    Verapamil

Controlled trials to demonstrate no effect
    Nimodipine
    Clonidine
    SSRIs: fluoxetine

[†] Commonly used preventives are listed with reasonable doses and common side-effects. The local national formulary
  should be consulted for detailed information.
b.d., twice daily; nocte, at night; SSRIs, selective serotonin reuptake inhibitors.

Acute attack therapies for migraine

Acute attack treatments for migraine can be usefully divided into disease non-specific treatments – analgesics and non-steroidal anti-inflammatory drugs (NSAIDs) – and disease-specific treatments – ergot-related compounds and triptans (Table 16.5).

Most acute attack medications seem to have a propensity to aggravate headache frequency and induce a state of refractory daily or near-daily headache, **medication overuse headache** (see below). Codeine-containing compound analgesics are a particularly pernicious problem when available in over-the-counter preparations. Patients with migraine who have two headache days a week or more should be advised to avoid their regular use.

Most patients who stop taking regular analgesics will experience substantial improvement in their headache, with a reduction in frequency, although about one half will relapse, most in the subsequent 12 months.

Table 16.5 Oral acute migraine treatments

Non-specific treatments*	Specific treatments
Aspirin (900 mg)	Ergot derivatives
Paracetamol (1000 mg)	• Ergotamine (1–2 mg)
NSAIDS	Triptans
• Naproxen (500–1000 mg)	• Sumatriptan (50 or 100 mg)
• Ibuprofen (400–800 mg)	• Naratriptan (2.5 mg)
• Tolfenamic acid (200 mg)	• Rizatriptan (10 mg)
	• Zolmitriptan (2.5 or 5.0 mg)
	• Eletriptan (40 or 80 mg)
	• Almotriptan (12.5 mg)
	• Frovatriptan (2.5 mg)

* Often used with anti-emetic/prokinetics, such as domperidone (10mg) or metoclopramide (10mg)

It is crucial to emphasize to the patient that standard preventive medications will simply not work in the presence of regular analgesic use. It is generally a waste of time to start a preventive in migraine patients if they are using regular analgesics; the analgesic problem must be tackled first (see below).

Treatment strategies

The simplest approach to treatment has been described as **stepped care**. In this model all patients are treated, assuming no contraindications, with the simplest treatment, such as aspirin 900 mg or paracetamol 1000 mg with an anti-emetic. Aspirin is an effective strategy, has been proven so in double-blind controlled clinical trials, and is best used in its most soluble formulations. The alternative would be a strategy known as **stratified care**, by which the physician determines, or stratifies, treatment at the start based on likelihood of response to levels of care.

An intermediate option may be described as stratified care by attack. The latter is what many headache authorities suggest and what patients often do when they have the options. Patients use simpler options for their less severe attacks, relying on more potent options when their attacks or the circumstances demand them (Table 16.6).

Non-specific acute migraine attack treatments

Simple medications, such as **aspirin** and **paracetamol**, are cheap and can be very effective and therefore they can be employed in many patients. Dosages should be adequate and the addition of **domperidone** (10 mg p.o.) or **metoclopramide** (10 mg p.o.) can be very helpful. When tolerated, **NSAIDs** can be very useful. Their success is often limited by inappropriate dosing, and adequate doses of naproxen (500–1000 mg p.o. or p.r., with an anti-emetic), ibuprofen (400–800 mg p.o.) or tolfenamic acid (200 mg p.o.) can be extremely effective.

is male, with a 3:1 predominance, who has bouts of 1–2 attacks of relatively short duration unilateral pain every day for periods of 8–10 weeks a year. The patients are generally perfectly well between times. Patients with cluster headache tend to move about during attacks, pacing, rocking or even rubbing their head for relief. The pain is usually retro-orbital, boring and very severe. It is associated with ipsilateral symptoms of cranial (parasympathetic) autonomic activation: a red or watering eye, the nose running or blocking, or cranial sympathetic dysfunction: Horner's syndrome. Cluster headache is likely to be a disorder involving central pacemaker regions of the posterior hypothalamus (Plate 4).

The TACs, cluster headache, paroxysmal hemicrania and short-lasting unilateral neuralgiform headache attacks with conjunctival injection and tearing (SUNCT) syndrome, present a distinct group to be differentiated from short-lasting headaches that do not have prominent cranial autonomic syndromes, notably trigeminal neuralgia, idiopathic (primary) stabbing headache and hypnic headache. By determining the cycling pattern, length of attack, frequency of attack and timing of the attacks, most patients can be usefully classified.

The importance of clinical classification of this group is threefold. First, the clinical phenotype

Table 16.7 Primary headache-cluster headache, other TACs and short-lasting headaches

Trigeminal autonomic cephalgias (TACs)	Other short-lasting headaches
Cluster headache	Idiopathic stabbing headache[†]
Paroxysmal hemicrania	Trigeminal neuralgia
SUNCT syndrome	Benign cough headache
	Benign exertional headache
	Benign sex headache
	Hypnic headache

†Likely to be primary stabbing headache in the revised IHS classification.
SUNCT, short-lasting unilateral neuralgiform headache attacks with conjunctival injection and tearing.

determines the likely secondary causes that must be considered and appropriate investigations ordered (Figure 16.5). Second, the appropriate classification gives clarity to the patient with a clear diagnosis and allows the physician to comment on natural history. Third, the correct diagnosis determines therapy that can be very different in these conditions, being very good if the diagnosis is correct but probably ineffective if it is not (Table 16.9).

Management of cluster headache

Cluster headache is managed using acute attack treatments and preventive agents. Acute attack

Table 16.8 Simplified diagnostic criteria for cluster headache (after IHS with anticipated modifications) (Headache Classification Committee of The International Headache Society, 1988)

Cluster headache has two key forms
Episodic: Occurs in periods lasting 7 days for 1 year separated by pain-free periods lasting 1 month
Chronic: Attacks occur for more than 1 year without remission or with remissions lasting less than 1 month

Diagnostic criteria for attacks
A   At least five attacks fulfilling B–D.
B   Severe or very severe unilateral orbital, supraorbital and/or temporal pain lasting 15–180 minutes untreated.
C   Headache is accompanied by at least one of the following signs that have to be present on the side of the pain:
  1 Conjunctival injection
  2 Lacrimation
  3 Nasal congestion
  4 Rhinorrhoea
  5 Forehead and facial sweating
  6 Miosis
  7 Ptosis
  8 Eyelid oedema
Or
Headache is associated with a sense of restlessness or agitation.
D   Frequency of attacks: from 1 every other day to 8 per day.

treatments are usually required by all cluster headache patients at some time, while preventives are essential for the patients with chronic cluster headache and are often needed to shorten the active periods in patients with the episodic form of the disorder.

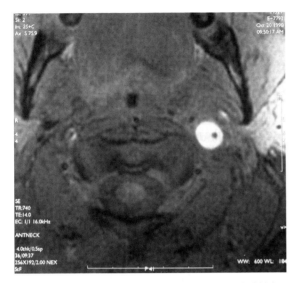

Figure 16.5 MRI brain scan, axial view, to show vivid high signal around the left carotid artery ('bull's eye') at the skull base from a dissection. The patient presented with acute headache and a right-sided Horner's syndrome.

Preventive treatments for cluster headaches

The options for preventive treatment in cluster headache depend on the bout length (Table 16.10). Patients with short bouts require medicines that act quickly but will not necessarily be taken for long periods, whereas those with long bouts or indeed those with chronic cluster headache require safe, effective medicines that can be taken for long periods. Most experts would now favour **verapamil** as the first-line preventive treatment when the bout is prolonged, or in chronic cluster headache, whereas limited courses of oral **corticosteroids** or **methysergide** can be very useful strategies when the bout is relatively short.

Verapamil has been suggested as a useful option for the last decade and compares favourably with **lithium**. What has clearly emerged from clinical practice is the need to use higher doses than had initially been considered and certainly higher than those used in cardiological indications. Although most patients will start on doses as low as 40–80 mg twice daily, doses up to 960 mg daily or more may be needed. Side-effects, such as constipation and leg swelling, can be a problem, but more difficult is the issue of cardiovascular safety. Verapamil can cause heart block by slowing conduction in the atrioventricular

Table 16.9 Differential diagnosis of short-lasting headaches

Feature	Cluster headache	Paroxysmal hemicrania	SUNCT	Idiopathic* stabbing headache	Trigeminal neuralgia	Hypnic headache
Gender	M > F 3:1	F > M 3:1	M > F	F > M	F > M	M = F
Pain						
Type	Boring	Boring	Stabbing	Stabbing	Stabbing	Throbbing
Severity	V. severe	V. severe	Moderate/severe	Severe	V. severe	Moderate
Location	Orbital	Orbital	Orbital	Any	V2/V3>V1	Generalized
Duration	15–180 min	1–45 min	15–120 sec	Secs–3 min	<5 sec	15–30 min
Frequency	1–8/day	1–40/day	1/day–30/hour	Any	Any	1–3/night
Autonomic	+	+	+	–	–	–
Alcohol	+	–	–	–	–	–
Indometacin	?	+	–	+	–	–

*Or primary stabbing headache.
SUNCT, short-lasting neuralgiform headache attacks with conjunctival injection and tearing; ?, Not formally tested.

Table 16.11 Classification of chronic daily headache

Primary		Secondary
>4 hours daily	**<4 hours daily**	

Chronic migraine[†]	Chronic cluster headache[‡]	Post-traumatic:
		  head injury
		  iatrogenic
		  post-infectious

Chronic tension-type
  headache[†]
	Chronic paroxysmal
	  hemicrania
		Inflammatory, such as:
		  giant cell arteritis
		  sarcoidosis
		  Behçet's syndrome

Hemicrania continua[†]	SUNCT	Chronic CNS infection
New daily persistent headache[†]	Hypnic headache	Substance abuse headache

[†] May be complicated by analgesic overuse. In the case of substance abuse headache, the headache is completely resolved after the substance abuse is controlled (Headache Classification Committee of The International Headache Society, 1988).
[‡] Chronic cluster headache patients may have more than 4 hours per day of headache.
SUNCT, short-lasting unilateral neuralgiform headache attacks with conjunctival injection and tearing.

patients with frequent headache, some of which fulfils standard criteria for migraine and some for tension-type headache, have a single migrainous biology is a very vexed one. Given that tension-type headache describes a phenomenology that is indistinct at best it seems unlikely that all its phenotype will have a single biological generator.

About two-thirds of daily headache patients have chronic tension-type headache and about one-third satisfy the criteria for chronic migraine (transformed migraine in the old nomenclature). The concept behind chronic migraine is that some patients who inherit a migrainous biology end up with CDH. About 90% of patients in referral headache clinics have headache of a dull, non-specific type, punctuated by more severe attacks that would often, in isolation, fulfil standard criteria for migraine. In headache speciality clinics this chronic migraine is usually associated with analgesic overuse.

The diagnosis of **chronic tension-type headache (CTTH)** is made when the patient has 15 days or more a month of entirely featureless generalized dull or pressure-like pain. When any of the attacks on some days have migrainous features, such as nausea,

photophobia, phonophobia, throbbing or aggravation with movement, then chronic migraine is a more useful diagnosis. The problem is not that both chronic migraine and CTTH do not exist, but some patients must simply have CTTH and episodic migraine, that is, two conditions; it is, however, simply impossible on clinical or other grounds to determine who they are. The approach outlined overdiagnoses chronic migraine, and underdiagnoses the coexistence of CTTH and episodic migraine. The converse would be true if one were to diagnose them all as CTTH and episodic migraine, as then chronic migraine would be missed. In clinical practice the concept of chronic migraine is helpful. Given that the lifestyle advice is identical for both TTH and migraine, and that the range of therapeutic options for preventive treatment in migraine is so much greater, the clinician loses absolutely nothing diagnosing chronic migraine, and the patient has much to gain.

Management of chronic daily headache

The management of CDH can be very rewarding. Most patients overusing analgesics respond very sensibly when the problem is explained.

The keys to managing daily headache
- Exclude treatable causes (Table 16.12)
- Obtain a clear analgesic history
- Make a diagnosis of the primary headache type involved.

Management of medication overuse – outpatients

It is essential that analgesic use be reduced and eliminated. Patients can reduce their use gradually over several weeks, or by immediate cessation.

Either approach can be facilitated by first keeping a careful diary over a month or two to be sure of the size of the problem. A small dose of an NSAID, such as naproxen 500 mg b.d. if tolerated, will help as the analgesic use is reduced. Overuse of NSAIDs does not seem to be a common issue in daily headache with once or twice daily dosing, whereas with more frequent dosing problems may develop. When the patient has reduced their analgesic use substantially a preventive should be introduced.

> It must be emphasized that **preventives simply do not work in the presence of analgesic overuse**, so the patient must reduce the analgesics or the entire use of the preventive is a wasted effort.

The most common cause of intractability to treatment is the use of a preventive when analgesics continue to be used regularly. For some patients this is very difficult and often one must be blunt that some degree of pain is inevitable in the first instance if the problem is to be controlled.

Management of medication overuse – inpatient

Some patients will require admission for detoxification, including those who fail outpatient withdrawal or who have a significant complicating medical indication, where withdrawal may be problematic

as an outpatient. When such patients are admitted, acute medications are withdrawn completely on the first day, unless there is some contraindication. **Anti-emetics**, preferably domperidone oral or suppositories, and fluids are administered as required, as well as clonidine for opiate withdrawal symptoms. For acute intolerable pain during the waking hours **aspirin** (1 g IV) is useful, and at night **chlorpromazine** by injection, ensuring adequate hydration. If the patient does not settle over 3–5 days, a course of **intravenous dihydroergotamine** can be given. Dihydroergotamine is indispensable in this setting; administered 8-hourly for 3 days, it can induce a significant remission that allows a preventive treatment to be established. Often 5-HT$_3$ antagonists, such as ondansetron or granisetron, will be required with dihydroergotamine as it is essential to minimize nausea.

Preventive treatments for chronic daily headache

Tricyclics, amitriptyline or dothiepin, at doses up to 1 mg/kg are very useful in patients with CDH. Tricyclics are started in low dose (10–25 mg) daily and are best given 12 hours prior to when the patient wishes to wake up, in order to avoid excess morning sleepiness. **Anticonvulsants**, such as valproate, gabapentin, and, more recently, topiramate, are also useful. For valproate doses up to 1500 mg daily are used, gradually increasing over several weeks. For gabapentin the dose is 1800–3600 mg daily; it is well tolerated, although probably less effective. For some patients flunarizine (where available) can be very effective, as can methysergide or phenelzine.

New daily persistent headache

New daily persistent headache (NDPH) is a clinically distinct syndrome with a range of important possible causes (Table 16.13), and the term serves both patients and clinicians by highlighting a group of conditions, some of which are curable. There can be both primary and secondary forms of NDPH

Table 16.13 Differential diagnosis of new daily persistent headache

Primary	Secondary
Migrainous-type	Sub-arachnoid haemorrhage
Featureless	Low CSF volume headache
(tension-type)	Raised CSF pressure headache
	Post-traumatic headache*
	Chronic meningitis

*Includes post-infective forms.

(Table 16.13) and neurologists will be called on to diagnose and treat these patients.

Clinical presentation of new daily persistent headache

The onset of headache is abrupt, and typically the patient will recall the exact day and circumstances. It is a female-predominant disorder with a marked continuous daily headache with some associated migrainous symptoms. In about one-third of patients the headache appeared to follow a 'flu-like illness.

The pressing issues arise from considering the differential diagnosis, particularly of the secondary headache forms. Although subarachnoid haemorrhage is listed for some logical consistency, as the headache may certainly come on from one moment to the next, it is not likely to produce diagnostic confusion in the majority of patients with NDPH. Other important causes of secondary NDPH are listed in Table 16.13.

Low cerebrospinal fluid volume headache

The syndrome of persistent low CSF volume headache is most commonly encountered **after lumbar puncture**. In that setting the headache settles rapidly with bed-rest. In the chronic situation, the patient typically presents with a history of headache from one day to the next. The pain is generally not present on waking, worsens during the day, and is relieved by lying down, usually within minutes, and recurs quickly when the patient is again upright. The patient may give a history of an index event: lumbar puncture or epidural injection, or a vigorous Valsalva manoeuvre, such as with lifting, straining, coughing, clearing the Eustachian tubes in an aeroplane or orgasm. **Soft drinks** with **caffeine** sometimes provide temporary respite. Spontaneous CSF leaks are recognized, when there is no obvious index event. As time passes from the index event the postural nature may be less obvious. The term low volume rather than low pressure is used because there is no clear evidence at which point the pressure can be called low. While low pressures, such as 0–5 cm are usually identified, pressures of up to 14 cm CSF have been recorded with a documented leak.

The investigation of choice is MRI with gadolinium, which produces a striking and typical pattern of diffuse pachymeningeal enhancement, although in about 10% of cases a leak can be documented without enhancement. It is also common to see Chiari malformations on MRI with some degree of descent of the cerebellar tonsils. This is important from the neurologist's viewpoint because surgery in such settings simply makes the headache problem worse. Alternatively the CSF pressure may be determined, or a leak sought, with ^{111}In-DPTA CSF studies, which can demonstrate the leak and any early emptying of tracer into the bladder, indicative of a leak.

Treatment is bed rest in the first instance. Intravenous **caffeine** (500 mg in 500 ml saline administered over 2 hours) is the standard and often very effective treatment. The ECG should be checked for any arrhythmia prior to administration. A reasonable practice is to carry out at least two infusions separated by 4 weeks after obtaining the suggestive clinical history and MRI with enhancement. Intravenous caffeine is safe and can be curative, by an unknown mechanism, so it spares many patients the need for further tests. If that is unsuccessful, an abdominal binder may be helpful. If a leak can be identified, either by radioisotope study, CT myelogram, or spinal T2-weighted MRI, an autologous blood patch is usually curative. In more intractable situations theophylline is a useful longer-term treatment.

Raised cerebrospinal fluid pressure headache

Brain imaging will often reveal the cause of raised CSF pressure headache. Patients with **idiopathic intracranial hypertension** (see p. 380) who present with headache without visual problems, particularly with normal fundi, are included in the spectrum of secondary NDPH. It is recognized that intractable chronic migraine can be triggered by persistently raised intracranial pressure. These patients typically give a history of generalized headache that is present on waking and improves as the day goes on. It is generally worse when lying down. Visual obscurations are frequently reported. Diagnostic difficulty should only arise in patients without papilloedema.

If raised pressure is suspected, brain imaging is mandatory, and it is simplest in the long run to obtain an MRI, and include magnetic resonance venography (MRV), if a mass lesion or hydrocephalus are to be excluded. In suspected idiopathic intracranial hypertension, following imaging, the CSF pressure should be measured by lumbar puncture, taking care to do so when the patient is symptomatic, so that both the pressure and response to removal of 20 ml of CSF can be determined. A raised pressure and improvement in headache with removal of CSF is diagnostic of the problem. The fields should be formally documented even in the absence of overt ophthalmic involvement. Initial treatment is with **acetazolamide** (250–500 mg twice daily). If this is not effective, topiramate has many actions that may be useful in this setting: carbonic anhydrase inhibition, weight loss, and neuronal membrane stabilization, probably through actions on phosphorylation pathways. A small number of patients who do not respond to medical treatment will require CSF shunting.

Post-traumatic headache

The issue of post-traumatic headache (see p. 359) is a vexed one, and the clarity of medical analysis of the condition has frequently been obscured and confused by associated medicolegal issues. The term is used here to indicate trauma in a very broad way. New daily persistent headache may be seen after a blow to the head, usually starting within 2 weeks of the injury. It may also appear after an infective episode, typically viral, or even malarial meningitis. The headache starts during that episode and is continuous and investigation reveals no current cause for it. It has been suggested, but not proven, that some patients with this syndrome have a persistent Epstein–Barr infection. A complicating factor will often be that the patient underwent a lumbar puncture during that illness, so a persistent low CSF volume headache needs to be considered. Persistent post-traumatic headache may be seen after carotid dissection (Figure 16.5), subarachnoid haemorrhage, and following intracranial surgery for a benign mass. The underlying theme seems to be that a traumatic event involving the dura mater can trigger a headache process that lasts for many years after that event.

> The treatment of this form of NDPH is empirical. **Tricyclics**, notably amitriptyline, and **anticonvulsants**, valproate, gabapentin and **phenelzine** have all been used with good effect. The headache usually runs a course of not more than 3–5 years.

Primary new daily persistent headache

In primary NDPH, migrainous features are common, with unilateral headache in about one-third and throbbing pain in about one-third. Nausea, photophobia and phonophobia are present in about half the patients. A small proportion of these patients have a previous history of migraine. Primary NDPH is perhaps the most intractable and least therapeutically rewarding form of headache. In general one can classify the dominant phenotype, migraine or tension-type headache, and treat with preventives according to that subclassification, as for patients with CDH. Primary NDPH with a tension-type headache phenotype is very unresponsive to treatment.

OTHER PRIMARY HEADACHES

Idiopathic stabbing headache

Idiopathic stabbing headache, soon to be called primary stabbing headache, is well documented in association with most types of primary headache.

> **The essential clinical features of idiopathic stabbing headache**
> - Pain confined to the head, although rarely is it facial
> - Stabbing pain lasting from 1 to many seconds and occurring as a single stab or a series of stabs
> - Recurring at irregular intervals (hours to days).

The sites of pain generally coincide with the site of the patient's habitual headache. Retro-auricular and occipital region pains are also well described and these respond promptly to indometacin. Stabbing headaches have been described in conjunction with cluster headaches, usually in the same area as the cluster pain. Idiopathic stabbing headache also occurs in chronic paroxysmal hemicrania. The response of idiopathic stabbing headache to **indometacin** (25–50 mg two to three times daily) is generally excellent.

Benign cough headache

Sharp pain in the head on coughing, sneezing, straining, laughing or stooping has long been regarded as a symptom of organic intracranial disease, commonly associated with obstruction of the CSF pathways. The presence of an Arnold–Chiari malformation or any lesion causing obstruction of CSF pathways or displacing cerebral structures must be excluded before cough headache is assumed to be benign. Cerebral aneurysm, carotid stenosis and vertebrobasilar disease may also present with cough or exertional headache as the initial symptom. The term 'benign Valsalva's-manoeuvre-related headache' covers the headaches provoked by coughing, straining or stooping, but **cough headache** is more succinct and so widely used it is unlikely to be displaced.

> **The essential clinical features of benign cough headache**
> - Bilateral headache of sudden onset, lasting minutes, precipitated by coughing
> - May be prevented by avoiding coughing
> - Diagnosed only after structural lesions, such as posterior fossa tumour, have been excluded by neuroimaging.

Comparing benign cough with benign exertional headache, the average age of patients with benign cough headache is 43 years of age – older than patients with exertional headache. **Indometacin** is the medical treatment of choice in cough headache, and it may be relieved, by an unknown mechanism, by lumbar puncture.

Benign exertional headache

The relationship of this form of headache, first described by Hippocrates, to cough headache is unclear, though they are similar.

> **The clinical features of benign exertional headache**
> - Pain specifically brought on by physical exercise
> - Bilateral and throbbing in nature at onset and may develop migrainous features in those patients susceptible to migraine
> - Lasts from 5 minutes to 24 hours
> - Prevented by avoiding excessive exertion, particularly in hot weather or at high altitude.

The acute onset of headache with straining and breath-holding, as in weightlifter's headache, may be explained by acute venous distension. The development of headache after sustained exertion, particularly on a hot day, is more difficult to understand. Anginal pain may be referred to the head, probably by central connections of vagal afferents and may present as exertional headache, so-called cardiac cephalgia. The link to exercise is the main clinical clue. Phaeochromocytoma may occasionally be responsible for exertional headache. Intracranial lesions or stenosis of the carotid arteries may have to be excluded as discussed for benign cough headache. Headache may be precipitated by any form of exercise and often has the pulsatile quality of migraine.

Management

The most obvious form of treatment is to take exercise gradually and progressively whenever possible. **Indometacin** at daily doses varying from 25 to 150 mg is generally very effective in benign exertional headache. Indometacin 50 mg, **ergotamine tartrate** 1–2 mg orally, ergotamine by inhalation, or **methysergide** 1–2 mg orally given 30–45 minutes before exercise are useful prophylactic measures.

Benign sex headache

Sex headache, formerly called coital cephalgia, may be precipitated by masturbation or coitus and usually starts as a dull bilateral ache while sexual excitement increases, suddenly becoming intense at orgasm. The term orgasmic cephalgia is not useful because not all sex headache requires orgasm. Three types of sex headache are discussed: a dull ache in the head and neck, which intensifies as sexual excitement increases; a sudden severe ('explosive') headache occurring at orgasm; and a postural headache resembling that of low CSF pressure developing after coitus. The last is simply another form of low CSF pressure headache arising from vigorous sexual activity, usually with multiple orgasms over a short period, and is more usefully considered with NDPH as a secondary CDH (Table 16.13).

> **The essential clinical features of sex headache**
> - Precipitation by sexual excitement
> - Bilateral at onset
> - Prevented or eased by ceasing sexual activity before orgasm.

Headaches developing at the time of orgasm are not always benign. Subarachnoid haemorrhage is occasionally precipitated by sexual intercourse. Sex headache affects men more often than women and may occur at any time during the years of sexual activity. It may develop on several occasions in succession and then not trouble the patent again. In patients who stop sexual activity when headache is first noticed it may subside within 5 minutes to 2 hours, and it is recognized that more frequent orgasm can aggravate established sex headache. About half the patients with sex headache have a history of exertional headaches, but there is no excess of cough headache in patients with sex headache. In about 50% of patients sex head-ache will settle within 6 months. Migraine is probably more common in patients with sex headache.

Management

Benign sex headaches are usually irregular and infrequent in recurrence, so management can often be limited to reassurance and advice about ceasing sexual activity if a milder, warning headache develops. When the condition recurs regularly or frequently, it can be prevented by the administration of **propranolol**, but the dosage required varies from 40 to 200 mg daily. An alternative is **diltiazem** 60 mg t.d.s. **Ergotamine** (1–2 mg) or **indomethacin** (25–50 mg) taken about 30–45 minutes prior to sexual activity can also be helpful.

Thunderclap headache

Sudden-onset, severe headache may occur in the absence of sexual activity. The differential diagnosis includes the sentinel bleed of an intracranial aneurysm, cervicocephalic arterial dissection and cerebral venous thrombosis. Headaches of explosive onset may also be caused by the ingestion of sympathomimetic drugs or tyramine-containing foods in a patient who is taking monoamine oxidase inhibitors, and can also be a symptom of phaeochromocytoma. Whether thunderclap headache can be the presentation of an unruptured cerebral aneurysm is unclear.

Follow-up studies of patients whose CT scans and CSF findings were negative have shown headache – thunderclap, migraine or tension type – to recur in two-thirds of patients.

> **Investigation of any sudden onset severe headache,** be it in the context of sexual excitement or isolated thunderclap headache, should be driven by the **clinical context**. The first presentation should be investigated with CT and CSF examination, preferably within 3 days, and where possible MRI/MRV/MRA.

Intra-arterial **cerebral angiography** should be reserved for when no primary diagnosis is forthcoming, and the clinical situation is particularly suggestive of intracranial aneurysm. A proportion of patients with idiopathic thunderclap headache without any demonstrable intracranial aneurysm, develop multifocal reversible cerebral vasospasm.

Hemicrania continua

The essential features of **hemicrania continua** are unilateral pain, which is moderate and continuous, but with fluctuations, and associated autonomic features when the pain is bad (tearing and redness of the eye). Analgesic overuse may aggravate the pain. There is complete resolution of the pain with **indomethacin**, given either as a diagnostic test, using 50 mg intramuscularly, or an oral trial, starting at 25 mg t.d.s., increasing slowly to 75 mg t.d.s., allowing 2 weeks for any dose to have an effect.

Hypnic headache

The syndrome of hypnic headache occurring in **elderly patients**, women more than men (4:1), aged from 67 to 84 years, comprises unilateral or bilateral headache of a moderate severity that typically **comes on a few hours after going to sleep**. The headache lasts from 15 to 30 minutes, is typically generalized, although it may be unilateral, and can be throbbing. Patients may report falling back to sleep only to be awoken by a further attack a few hours later with up to three repetitions of this pattern during the night.

Management

Patients with hypnic headache generally respond to a bedtime dose of **lithium** carbonate (200–600 mg) and in those who do not tolerate this, verapamil, methysergide, flunarizine or caffeine at bedtime are alternatives.

REFERENCES AND FURTHER READING

Goadsby PJ (2000) The pharmacology of headache. *Progress in Neurobiology*, **62**:509–525.

Goadsby PJ, Lipton RB (1997) A review of paroxysmal hemicranias, SUNCT syndrome and other short-lasting headaches with autonomic features, including new cases. *Brain*, 120:193–209.

Goadsby PJ, Lipton RB, Ferrari MD (2002) Migraine: current understanding and management. *New England Journal of Medicine*, 346:257–270.

Goadsby PJ, Silberstein SD (eds) (1997) *Headache*. Asbury A, Marsden CD (eds) Blue Books in Practical Neurology, vol 17. New York, NY: Butterworth-Heinemann.

Headache Classification Committee of The International Headache Society (1988) Classification and diagnostic criteria for headache disorders, cranial neuralgias and facial pain. *Cephalalgia*, **8(7)**:1–96.

Lance JW, Goadsby PJ (1998) *Mechanism and Management of Headache*, 6th edn. London, UK: Butterworth-Heinemann.

May A, Bahra A, Buchel C, Frackowiak RSJ, Goadsby PJ (1998) Hypothalamic activation in cluster headache attacks. *The Lancet*, **351**:275–278.

Olesen J, Goadsby PJ (1999) Cluster headache and related conditions. In: Olesen J (ed.) *Frontiers in Headache Research*, vol 9. Oxford, UK: Oxford University Press.

Olesen J, Tfelt-Hansen P, Welch KMA (2000) *The Headaches*, 2nd edn. Philadelphia, PA: Lippincott, Williams & Wilkins.

Silberstein SD, Lipton RB, Goadsby PJ (1998)
   Headache in Clinical Practice. Oxford, UK: ISIS
   Medical Media.
Tfelt-Hansen P, Saxena PR, Dahlof C *et al.*
   (2000) Ergotamine in the acute treatment of
migraine – a review and European consensus.
   Brain, 123:9–18.
Weiller C, May A, Limmroth V *et al.* (1995) Brain stem
   activation in spontaneous human migraine attacks.
   Nature Medicine, 1:658–660.

HEAD INJURY

G. Neil-Dwyer

Epidemiology

The estimated incidence of head injury is 430/100 000 of population. There are approximately 1 million patients in the UK who present to hospitals each year with head injuries. Males outnumber females by more than 2:1 and over 50% of admitted patients are younger than 20 years. Of those patients with head injuries admitted to hospital, 2.5% die there. While 85% of patients who sustain severe head injuries and 63% of adult patients who sustain moderate head injuries remain disabled 1 year after their accident, patients with minor head injuries also have difficulties. Three months after sustaining mild head injuries 79% of patients have persistent headaches, 59% have memory problems and 34% are still unemployed. In fact only 45% of patients who have sustained a minor head injury have made a good recovery 1 year after admission.

While the commonest cause of injury in developed countries is a road traffic accident, falls and assault are also frequent causes. Injuries at work, during sport and leisure are less common. There are a number of associated factors – alcohol (38%), drugs (7%) and suicide (10%).

Over the course of the past two decades measures aimed at prevention of head injury have gained more prominence. Alcohol is a well documented cause of road crashes. In the UK a level of 80 mg alcohol per dl is the upper level and in the last two decades a dramatic fall in drunk driving has been reported. Other preventive measures have been improvements in road construction, speed control, better vehicle design (seat belts, air bags, windscreens) and motorcycle and bicycle helmets.

Considerable progress has been made over the past 30 years in the understanding of the mechanisms involved in the production, progression and reduction of brain damage. In many series the mortality of patients suffering a severe head injury has been reduced from 45 to 34%, with a similar fall in morbidity. The recognition of the need to deal with hypotension, hypoxia and hypercarbia, early evacuation of mass lesions and the development of modern principles of critical care have accounted for this reduction in mortality and morbidity, as well as a reduction in the number of vegetative survivors.

There has been progress in the understanding of the pathophysiology of severe head injuries and the effect of secondary insults. **The recognition that the brain is 2% of the body mass, demands 13% of the cardiac output, and consumes 20% of the total energy expenditure highlights some of the problems.** In addition the brain has a high substrate demand, with no energy stores, no oxygen reserves and, importantly, cerebral metabolism is tightly coupled with cerebral arterial blood flow (CBF).

The study of the causes of death following head injury focuses attention on the important areas. The major cause of death is primary brain damage followed by multiple injuries, cerebral oedema and airway obstruction. These are the commonly recognized causes, the least common cause being intracranial haematomas.

PATHOPHYSIOLOGY OF BRAIN INJURY

The classical division of brain injury is into primary and secondary damage. This division is clinically useful. **Primary brain damage occurs at the time of the injury**, produces its clinical effect immediately and has proved resistant to most treatments. **Secondary brain damage**, on the other hand, occurs some time after the primary impact and is **largely preventable and treatable**. The importance of managing a head-injured patient is to recognize and document the primary brain damage and subsequently to prevent and treat secondary damage.

While traumatic brain injury results in an extraordinary cascade of neurochemical events, and there is much speculation as to its importance, most research has focused on injuries to the axon, the neurone and the glia. While axonal injury was considered to be irreversible with progressive changes in ultrastructure, the blood–brain barrier and neuronal function over time may provide some potential for treatment. While future research may yield more and provide ideas on future treatment, currently the main emphasis remains on secondary brain damage which may begin very soon after the impact, necessitating important early management decisions.

Primary brain damage

The clinical effects of primary brain damage may be greatly aggravated by secondary brain damage.

Diffuse axonal injury, contusions and lacerations of the brain will produce immediate clinical effects, varying from concussion, with mild diffuse axonal injury, to coma and death.

Focal primary damage may produce an immediate neurological deficit depending upon the site of injury. Any further increase in a neurological deficit or deepening of level of consciousness will be the result of secondary brain damage.

The nature of progressive injury has three components:

1 cytotoxic oedema, membrane damage and mitochondrial failure and inhibition of protein synthesis causing destruction of cells;
2 micro-circulatory disturbance leading to vasogenic oedema, loss of autoregulation and vasospasm;
3 ischaemia, which develops in the injured brain around areas of haematoma, oedema, contusion and with local compression around mass lesions. This leads to focal ischaemia, high intracranial pressure (ICP), diminished cerebral perfusion pressure (CPP) and global ischaemia.

Brain ischaemia is found in 88–92% of brains at post mortem. If global ischaemia as a result of raised ICP is associated for long periods with a low CPP (under 50 mmHg), then the mortality rate will be 90% or more. The three main causes of brain ischaemia are:

1 inadequacy of flow delivery;
2 inadequacy of cerebral artery content of oxygen and substrate;
3 inability of the brain to utilize oxygen, which is a cytotoxic problem.

The systemic secondary insults to be avoided are listed in Table 17.1.

Table 17.1 Effects of hypoxia and hypotension on the outcome of brain injury (after Gentleman and Jennett, 1981)

Hypoxia
Hypotension
Hypercapnia
Hypocapnia
Hyperthermia
Hyperglycaemia
Hypoglycaemia
Hyponatraemia
Hypoproteinaemia

Pressure/volume relationship

The skull is a rigid compartment within which lies the brain, cerebrospinal fluid (CSF), blood and extracellular fluid. The volume within the cranial vault is constant and any increase in volume results in an increase in ICP. The relationship between the pressure and volume is expressed in Figure 17.1. The major intracranial volumes are brain parenchyma (1200–1600 ml), blood (100–150 ml) and CSF (100–150 ml). The latter two constitute about 20% of total intracranial volume and part of each is capable of rapid extracranial displacement. The initial increase in intracranial volume is catered for by the loss of CSF from the intracranial compartment, reduction in the amount of blood in the cerebrum followed by compression of brain tissue with herniation of the brain and a decrease in CBF. **The redistribution of the CSF and venous blood have little pathological consequence but a reduction in CBF and the occurrence of brain herniation results in cerebral ischaemia and secondary cerebral damage.**

Intracranial pressure/cerebral perfusion pressure

The normal range of ICP is between 0 and 10 mmHg. Raised ICP is regarded as being 20–25 mmHg. Raised ICP in the head-injured patient is associated with

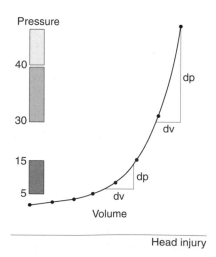

Figure 17.1 Pressure-volume curve (see text).

increased mortality. Patients whose ICP remains between 0 and 20 mmHg have a mortality rate of 23% while those whose pressures rise above 60 mmHg have a 100% mortality. It is doubtful whether raised ICP itself directly alters neuronal function but it seems likely that the level of ICP is not as important as its effect on CPP and its relationship to brain herniation. **Reduced CPP and brain herniation are principal mechanisms of secondary brain damage following severe head injury.** In support of this is the observation that a raised ICP, even over 60 mmHg, without displacement with adequate CPP may produce no neurological deficit. This is seen quite dramatically in idiopathic intracranial hypertension.

Cerebral perfusion pressure

This is equal to the mean blood pressure minus the mean ICP. Normally within a range of CPP of 60–160 mmHg cerebral blood flow remains constant. However, in brain injury this autoregulatory relationship may be altered by a number of factors.

Cerebral perfusion pressure is equivalent to the transmural pressure across the cerebral vessel walls; at the arteriolar level, CPP is the stimulus for the autoregulatory response, and at the capillary level is the driving force for fluid exchange.

There are a number of observational studies with the general consensus that maintaining the CPP at 70 mmHg may be associated with a decrease in head injury morbidity and mortality. **Evidence shows that aggressive action in the head-injured patient to maintain normal blood volume or induced systemic hypertension to maintain a CPP of 70 mmHg has no deleterious effect on ICP, morbidity or mortality.**

In managing a head-injured patient attention must be paid to both ICP and CPP.

Cerebral blood flow and head injury

Cerebral blood flow is affected by arterial PaO_2; an arterial PaO_2 of below 7 kPa produces an increase in CBF. Variations in arterial $PaCO_2$ can cause marked changes in CBF because CO_2 is a very potent vasodilator. If the P_aCO_2 is increased above 6 kPa, CBF increases, while it falls if the P_aCO_2 drops below 4 kPa. The maintenance of CBF in response to various changes has been termed autoregulation and this may be impaired by ischaemia, hypoxia or brain trauma. Cerebral blood flow is the critical factor in terms of function and survival. While a wide range in CBF values has been reported for different brain locations, in general, it is agreed that the mean hemispheric CBF is about 55 ml/100 g per minute. A CBF of below 18 ml/100 g per minute is the threshold for global ischaemia and infarction will occur if these levels are sustained for more than 1–3 hours. While CPP would have to fall to 40 mmHg in the normal brain before CBF fell, following trauma a CPP of 50 mmHg would indicate a low CBF.

Cerebral oedema

Cerebral oedema is an important but variable secondary response to trauma, the causes and consequences of which are poorly understood. Five different types have been described:

1 Vasogenic oedema
2 Cytotoxic oedema
3 Hydrostatic oedema
4 Osmotic brain oedema
5 Interstitial brain oedema.

Cerebral oedema can produce a rise in ICP either locally or generally, which then reduces CBF.

Shift and distortion

Expanding lesions in head-injured patients produce a well established sequence of events. The ventricle on the side of the expanding lesion becomes smaller and, with distortion and compression of the third ventricle, dilatation of the opposite ventricle occurs.

If the uncus of the temporal lobe is pushed through the tentorial edge, the third cranial nerve and the posterior cerebral artery are compressed causing a third nerve palsy and a homonymous hemianopia.

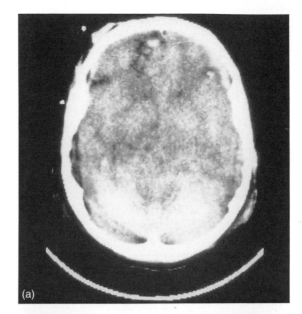
(a)

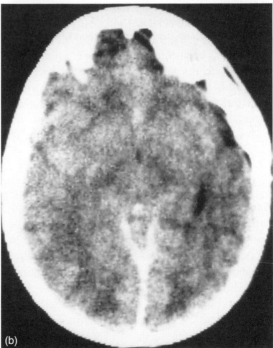
(b)

Figure 17.2 (a) and (b) CT brain scans showing raised intracranial pressure with the loss of basal cisterns.

A computerized tomography (CT) scan at the time of the clinical syndrome shows the disappearance of the subarachnoid space in the supratentorial compartment with loss of the basal cisterns (Figure 17.2a,b);

crowding of the brainstem in the tentorial hiatus occurs. Central areas of the brain are pushed in a downwards axial direction towards the foramen magnum, and coning occurs. The compression of the midbrain produces ischaemia of central areas, leading to a loss of consciousness and increasing neurological signs.

MEDICAL MANAGEMENT OF THE HEAD-INJURED PATIENT

When considering management of head-injured patients it is important to integrate clinical expertise with the best available external evidence from systematic research – to try and apply an evidence-based approach. In this arena categories of evidence are important and these are highlighted in Table 17.2. They are appropriate to the following discussion and the strength of the evidence will be identified on the basis of those categories of evidence.

There has been considerable effort to disseminate widely guidelines with regard to the modern treatment of head-injured patients. Two main sets of guidelines, which are similar, have been produced by the Brain Trauma Foundation in co-operation with the American Association of Neurological Surgeons and the European Brain Injury Consortium.

When considering treatment, the trimodal distribution of death after injury needs to be recognized. The first peak occurs within seconds or minutes of the injury, the second peak is within several hours as a result of subdural/extradural haematomas, pneumothoraces, abdominal injuries including ruptured spleen, pelvic fractures and other conditions leading to hypovolaemia and hypotension. The final peak happens several days to weeks after the injury and is caused by sepsis or multiple organ failure. The most important treatment area lies within the second peak and is termed the 'golden hour'. However, minutes count and it is now recognized that the first 20 minutes after an injury can be the most vital.

It is clear on reviewing the pathophysiological effects of head injury that the main clinical challenge

Table 17.2 Categories of evidence for consideration in management of head-injured patients

I	Randomized controlled trials
II	Prospective study and control
III	Retrospective study and controls
	Correlation/case control studies
IV	Opinion of experts/expert committees

Table 17.3

Head injury management – initial assessment/primary survey
Airway and cervical spine control
Breathing and ventilation
Circulatory control and management
Conscious level (Glasgow Coma Scale)
Limb movement and sensation
Site of pain
Extracranial injuries and fractures

in its management is the prevention and treatment of secondary damage.

During the pre-hospital phase the prime aim is to reduce any initial hypoxic/ischaemic damage using principles of resuscitation that have been set out in the advanced trauma life support system (ATLS – American College of Surgeons, 1993). This phase (primary survey) requires a major emphasis on airway maintenance, control of external bleeding and shock, immobilization and immediate transfer to the closest and most appropriate hospital. The ABC of such a resuscitation is laid out in Table 17.3.

The effects of hypotension and hypoxia need to be fully recognized. There is increased morbidity and mortality if the systolic blood pressure drops below 90 mmHg. This must be avoided and rapidly corrected if it occurs (Class II evidence). It has also been demonstrated (strong Class II evidence) that elevation of the blood pressure in a hypotensive head-injured patient improves outcome. The effects of hypoxia and hypotension on the outcome of head injury are shown in Table 17.4.

Resuscitation takes place with the airway secured and, if necessary, the patient intubated, paralysed and ventilated. The critical factors are a blood pressure >90 mmHg systolic, PaO_2 at a minimum of 9 kPa

Table 17.4 Effects of hypoxia and hypotension on the outcome of brain injury
(after Gentleman and Jennett, 1981)

	Patients (*n*)	Dead (%)	Good recovery (%)
Hypoxia and hypotension	5	100	0
Hypotension only	12	75	8
Hypoxia only	29	59	17
Neither factor	104	34	34

(90 mmHg) and a P_aCO_2 maintained between 3.5 and 4.0 kPa (35–40 mmHg). Venous access is achieved and volume replacement carried out if necessary. Electrocardiogram monitoring, pulse oximetry and blood pressure monitoring should be instituted. In addition the patient's level of consciousness needs to be recorded and this is undertaken using the Glasgow Coma Scale (see Table 4.7).

In the hospital Accident and Emergency Department the second phase of assessment (secondary survey) is undertaken. The airway is maintained with continued control of the cervical spine. Breathing and ventilation are maintained. Circulation is maintained and haemorrhage is controlled. The patient is completely undressed and the conscious level documented. **This is the most important clinical assessment with the post-resuscitation coma score recorded then subsequent measures made at regular intervals.** Severe head injuries have a Glasgow Coma Scale (GCS) score of 3–8, moderate head injury GCS 9–12, minor head injury GCS 13–15. Subsequently, assessment of the severity of a closed head injury is also possible using the duration of post-traumatic amnesia (PTA) (Table 17.5).

Criteria for hospital admission
- All patients with impaired consciousness or confusion
- Skull fracture or diastasis
- Persisting neurological symptoms or signs
- Nausea/vomiting persisting after 4 hours observation in the Accident and Emergency Department
- Difficulty in assessing (e.g. suspected drugs or alcohol; possible non-accident injury; epilepsy; attempted suicide; children who are difficult to assess; or pre-existing neurological conditions such as stroke, Parkinson's disease, Alzheimer's disease)

- Other medical conditions such as coagulation disorders (e.g. patients being treated with warfarin
- Lack of responsible adult to supervise the patient at home
- Any uncertainty in diagnosis
- There is an additional point in that transient unconsciousness or amnesia with full recovery is not necessarily an indication to admit an adult but may be so in a child.

Table 17.5 Severity of head injury assessed by the duration of post-traumatic amnesia

Duration	Severity
Less than 5 minutes	Very mild
Less than 1 hour	Mild
1–24 hours	Moderate
1–7 days	Severe
More than 7 days	Very severe
More than 4 weeks	Extremely severe

After the initial assessments, observation in hospital includes continued monitoring of respiratory function, blood pressure, conscious level and neurological signs including the pupillary reactions. The simplest method available to assess conscious level is the GCS, which is now universally acceptable.

X-Rays and imaging

Resuscitation should be completed before X-rays are taken. The indications for skull X-ray are given in Table 17.6. It is recognized that these indications will depend on whether CT scanning is immediately available. It is important to recognize that children

Table 17.6 Indications for skull X-ray

- History of loss of consciousness or amnesia
- Suspected penetrating injury, CSF or blood loss from nose or ear
- Scalp laceration, bruise or swelling
- Violent mechanism of injury (e.g. falling >60 cm)
- Persisting headache and/or vomiting
- In a child who has fallen from a significant height and/or onto a hard surface – tense fontanelle
- Suspected non-accidental injury

Table 17.7 Indications for CT brain scan in head-injured patients

- Patients with a GCS of 8 or less
- Patients with a GCS of 9–14, with or without a skull fracture
- Patients with focal neurological signs
- Patients with a depressed skull fracture or penetrating brain injury
- Patients with a skull fracture should be scanned before discharge
- Patients with epileptic seizures following injury
- Patients with a lucid interval followed by decline in conscious level or the appearance of focal signs
- All patients who are drowsy for more than 24 hours should be scanned before discharge
- Unstable systemic state precluding transfer to neurosurgery
- Diagnosis uncertain
- Tense fontanelle or suture diastasis in a child

may have a significant intracranial injury in the absence of a skull fracture. Absence of a skull fracture in itself is not a reliable criterion for deciding on whether to admit a patient. It is also recognized that children are more likely than adults to need a CT scan in certain situations.

A skull X-ray is not necessary if a CT scan is to be performed.

In patients after major trauma the initial plain X-rays should include a lateral cervical spine, chest and pelvis. Once all life-threatening injuries have been treated, further views of the cervical, thoracic and lumbar spine may be necessary. In the case of the less severely injured patient guidelines have been produced with the initial management of head-injured patients.

The indications for CT brain scanning are listed in Table 17.7.

If there are difficulties in scanning patients locally there should be a discussion with the regional neurosurgical unit (NSU) to determine whether CT should be performed locally or in the NSU. This will depend on the patient's condition (including the presence or absence of extracranial injuries) and local policies. All patients with skull fractures should be detained in hospital for observation and should undergo CT scanning prior to discharge. A patient who remains drowsy for 24 hours or more should be scanned before discharge. It is important to be aware that an early CT scan (within 6 hours) may have to be repeated to exclude a developing/enlarging haematoma in a patient failing to recover, or if there is a deteriorating level of consciousness. If the initial CT scan is performed more than 6 hours after admission, another cause for the patient failing to improve

or for deterioration should be sought before further scanning as a repeat scan is less likely to explain the patient's condition.

After a head injury the CT appearances allow classification of head injuries based on the patho-physiological disturbances described earlier. Four classifications of diffuse brain injury are distinguished from patients with an intracranial mass lesion or an evacuated intracranial mass lesion.

This classification is important because management can be structured on a pathophysiological basis. In addition, these different CT appearances have a direct relationship with the mortality rate. Patients with diffuse brain damage with no visible pathology on CT have the lowest mortality rate (10%); by contrast, patients with diffuse brain damage on a CT scan in category 4 have a mortality rate greater than 50%. Thus, in conjunction with the known outcome of patients with extradural, subdural and intracranial haematomas, the risk of intracranial hypertension and other fatal outcome can be assessed. Patients can also be targeted for specific treatment, and importantly patients with a low risk assessment on clinical grounds but who are identified on CT to have a high risk of a poor outcome, can be identified.

Diffuse brain injury on CT scanning

The four categories of brain damage are:

1 No visible pathology on CT;
2 Basal cisterns present – no lesions >25 ml in volume and/or midline shift 0–5 mm;
3 Compressed or absent cisterns, midline shift 0–5 mm and no parenchymal lesions of more than 25 ml;
4 Midline shift >5 mm and no parenchymal lesion >25 ml.

Guidelines for transfer to regional neurosurgical unit

In the UK currently only a small proportion (3–5%) of head-injured patients are transferred to an NSU, usually because of a deteriorating level of consciousness, progressive focal neurological deficits, the detection of recognized risk factors for developing intracranial haematoma or their confirmation by local CT imaging, or because of specific complications requiring neurosurgical intervention (e.g. CSF leak, depressed fracture). Patients with a GCS less than 9 persisting after resuscitation, those with a deteriorating level of consciousness and those with an open brain injury should be transferred urgently to an NSU (Table 17.8). It is often expedient for a CT scan to be performed in the NSU (Figures 17.3 and 17.4).

When a patient is to be transferred to an NSU arrangements should follow the protocol set out in recommendations for the transfer of patients with acute head injuries to NSUs.

Staff to be notified or linked to transfer

- A consultant from the referring hospital with overall responsibility
- Contact and discussion with the duty consultant neurosurgeon
- An attending transfer doctor (usually an anaesthetist)
- Transfer team – appropriately trained nurses.

Table 17.8 Indications for urgent discussion and possible transfer of a head-injured patient to a neurosurgical unit

- Coma – GCS less than 9 – persisting after resuscitation
- Deteriorating level of consciousness or progressive focal neurological deficits
- Fracture of the skull with any of the following:
    Confusion or deteriorating impairment of consciousness
    Fits or neurological symptoms or signs
- Open injury:
    Depressed compound fracture of skull vault
    Base of skull fracture or penetrating injury
- Patient fulfils criteria for CT of the head within referring hospital but this cannot be performed within a reasonable time (e.g. 2–4 hours)
- Abnormal CT scan
- After neurosurgical opinion on images transferred electronically
- A normal CT scan but unsatisfactory progress

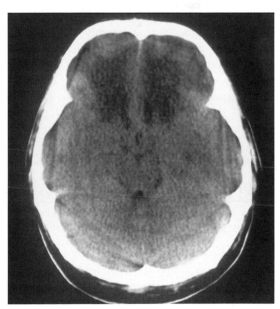

Figure 17.3 CT brain scan to show bilateral frontal low density changes in keeping with damage at these sites.

The patient must be resuscitated and stabilized before transfer. It is imperative that continued intensive care should continue during transfer. A key factor in the success of a transfer is that any previous

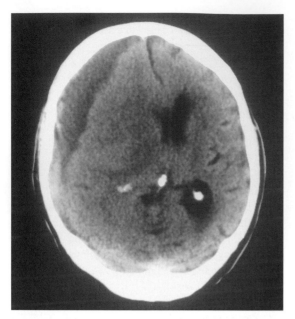

Figure 17.4 CT brain scan showing a left frontal subdural collection with considerable midline shift.

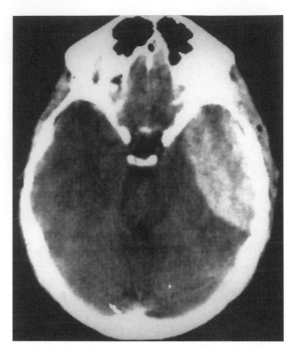

Figure 17.5 CT brain scan showing extradural haematoma.

insult (hypotension, hypoxia) is predictive of further problems. Insults before and during transfer leading to greater problems after transfer increase morbidity and mortality.

MANAGEMENT OF SPECIFIC COMPLICATIONS OF HEAD INJURY

Depressed skull fracture

Simple depressed skull fractures

Surgical elevation should be considered if the injury is cosmetically disfiguring, the depressed fragment has significant mass effect or there is an underlying haematoma. However, this approach needs to be modified if the simple depression is located over a major venous sinus.

Compound depressed or comminuted skull fractures

Surgery for patients with compound depressed or comminuted skull fractures is initially local wound closure after thorough cleaning and removal of foreign bodies. The surgical requirement is to achieve haemostasis and prevent infection. If there is no dural laceration, this may well be the definitive treatment. However, definitive surgery must be performed as soon as possible if there is a suspected dural laceration, intracranial haematoma or moderate to severe wound contamination.

Complications as a result of a depressed fracture include intracranial infection (meningitis or an intracerebral abscess) and epilepsy. Up to 30% of patients with a depressed skull fracture develop epilepsy if the dura is torn or if there is an associated cortical contusion or laceration.

Haematomas

Extradural haematoma (Figure 17.5)

Typically extradural haematoma may arise after a mild injury and more than half the patients with this complication are under the age of 20 years; it is rare after the age of 40 years. It is also rare before the age of 2 years when trauma tends to indent the more pliable skull and dura together so damage tends to occur to the brain and haematomas are subdural. In infants the large head size relative to the body means that the volume of the extradural space is large in relation to the blood volume, so that hypovolaemia may be the primary presenting feature with an infantile extradural haematoma. In an adult the blow causes the dura to become separated from the skull immediately below the point of impact and this is where the clot forms. Bleeding commonly arises from a torn middle meningeal artery but may also bevenous. It needs to be recognized that extradural haematoma is rare, with only 0.5% of head-injured patients admitted to hospital developing the condition.

Extradural haematoma

The single most important clinical feature of extradural haematoma is a deterioration in the level of consciousness, occasionally a period of increasing restlessness (not resulting from a full bladder, which may be a cause). Extradural haematomas are extracerebral lesions and there may be little or no primary brain damage so that initially consciousness may recover before further deterioration in conscious level occurs, the so called 'lucid interval'. To wait for the classic textbook description of a unilateral dilated pupil, hemiparesis, slow pulse and rise in blood pressure is to accept a high morbidity and mortality.

While a view has been expressed that extradural haematomas 'should be treated at the hospital where the condition is diagnosed as soon as it is recognized, this would require local surgical expertise. It is well recognized that for a successful outcome in this condition the haematoma must be removed within 2 hours of the first sign of deterioration, an event that will vary from one patient to another. Nevertheless in the UK there should be time for neurosurgical consultation.

The mortality rate for extradural haematoma is 10% or less.

Acute subdural haematomas

Acute subdural haematomas are relatively common (Figures 17.5 and 17.6), occurring at any age, and tending to occur following more severe impact

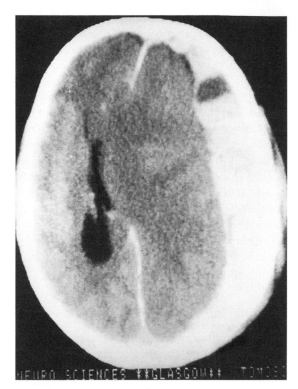

Figure 17.6 CT brain scan showing a large acute subdural haematoma with significant shift.

damage than that which occurs with extradural haematomas, so morbidity and mortality tends to be higher in this group of patients.

Acute subdural haematoma

There are two common causes of traumatic acute subdural haematomas. A haematoma may accumulate around a parenchymal laceration, usually frontal or temporal lobe with a severe underlying primary brain injury – usually unilateral so that patients with acute subdural haematomas are more likely to present in coma in contrast to extradural haematomas. There is no 'lucid interval'. The second cause is as a result of the tearing of veins bridging the extradural space during violent head motion. In this case primary brain damage is less severe and a lucid interval may occur followed by rapid deterioration.

Acute subdural haematoma may also occur in patients receiving anticoagulation therapy, usually following minor trauma.

In some 15–20% of cases the haematoma may be bilateral and about 50% are associated with a skull fracture. Brain scanning with CT establishes the diagnosis. Factors indicating the need for an operation include the size of the haematoma, the degree of midline shift (may be caused by isodense collections), obliteration of the third ventricle or basal cisterns and dilatation of the contralateral ventricle. Acute subdural haematomas often carry a poor prognosis because of delay in diagnosis and because of the severity of the underlying brain damage. The mortality rate is often over 50%, with an associated high morbidity, although there is some suggestion that patients operated on within 4 hours of receiving the injury may have a lower mortality. The treatment is urgent surgical evacuation via a craniotomy. These patients will require intensive care.

Traumatic intracerebral haemorrhage

Traumatic intracerebral haemorrhage may be related to cerebral contusions, may be part of a complex intracerebral haemorrhage or result from penetrating injuries (Figure 17.7). The haematoma may remain within the parenchyma, or burst into the ventricles or extradural spaces. Serial CT scans show that after 24–72 hours these haematomas are commonly surrounded by an area of oedema. Increasing mass effect will lead to a rise in ICP and a decrease in CPP and ultimately CBF. Much of the appearance on CT of the area around the haematoma is the result of ischaemia, and, although surgical removal of the mass will reduce ICP, it will do little to relieve the ischaemic neuronal damage. Surgical management will be to protect the patient from the harmful effects of raised ICP but is unlikely to improve neurological deficits.

Chronic subdural haematomas

Head injury is identified in less than 50% of adults who present with a chronic subdural haematoma (CSDH) and the injury is usually mild. There are a number of risk factors including cerebral atrophy, alcoholism, epilepsy, CSF shunts and coagulopathies, including patients on anticoagulant therapy and patients with a tendency to fall.

There is a tendency for CSDH to occur in **older people** around 60 years of age with a male

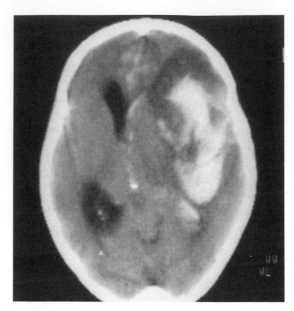

Figure 17.7 CT brain scan showing a traumatic intracerebral haematoma.

preponderance. Most CSDH are seen in the parietal region, the majority are unilateral with **20–25% of cases being bilateral**.

Chronic subdural haematoma

Patients usually present with minor symptoms of headaches, which are accompanied by a change in personality, variable drowsiness or confusion, impaired consciousness and a hemiparesis. While it is often emphasized that major fluctuations in consciousness and neurological signs are characteristic features in CSDH, these signs only occur in about one-third of patients. Impairment of upward gaze is commonly present: this should alert the doctor (it can be found in normal elderly people).

A CT scan will usually show a CSDH, although isodense lesions may be difficult to identify (Figure 17.8a,b), particularly if there are bilateral CSDH, in which case there may be no midline shift.

A CSDH is usually drained through one or two burr holes, although in a few cases, if the haematoma is clotted or multilocular, a craniotomy may be required.

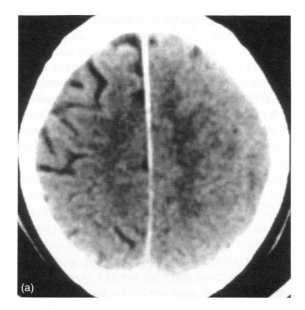

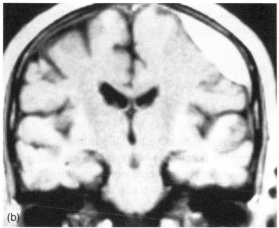

Figure 17.8 (a) CT brain scan, axial view, showing an isodense subdural haematoma: note the effacement of the surface sulci. (b) MRI brain scan, coronal view, of the same patient showing the presence of a more obvious subdural haematoma.

Cerebrospinal fluid leaks

Traumatic CSF leaks occur in adults in about 2% of closed head injuries. The risk of CSF leak is especially high in penetrating head injuries, where a frequency of 9% has been reported. Traumatic CSF leaks usually appear within the first 48 hours after injury but can develop several years later. The severity of the head injury has little, if any, correlation with the occurrence of a leak.

Cerebrospinal fluid rhinorrhoea (via the nose) is the most common type of CSF leak. The fluid can be confirmed as CSF if the glucose level is greater than 30 mg %, identified using a dipstick. β_2 transferrin is present in CSF but is absent in tears, saliva, nasal secretion and is a useful test to employ if there is doubt. Most cases of CSF rhinorrhoea (70%) stop within 1 week and the remainder usually by 6 months. The great risk is, of course, meningitis and the incidence is around 5–10% but this increases if the leak persists for more than 7 days. In a long-term study of patients who had CSF leaks that were not repaired, 80% developed meningitis over a 20 year period. Leaks of CSF should be identified and the fistula repaired if possible. The exception is CSF otorrhoea (via the ear), which usually stops spontaneously within 3 weeks. An operation is only required for persistent CSF otorrhoea.

Conscious patients are nursed head up to reduce the intracranial CSF pressure. There is no evidence supporting the use of prophylactic antibiotics.

Localization of the fistula in patients with CSF rhinorrhoea is best undertaken with CT, using 2 mm slices and bone windows in axial and coronal planes. Intrathecal contrast is only of value in patients with an active CSF leak. Careful MRI scanning using T2 sequences and coronal cuts may reveal a protrusion of the subarachnoid space through an unsuspected bony defect.

Traumatic aerocoele

Air may enter the skull after basal fractures and is usually readily visible on 'brow up' lateral skull X-rays and is always evident on CT. The air may be subarachnoid, subdural, intraventricular or intracerebral. Urgent decompression may be required if the aerocoele is responsible for a clinical deterioration, but usually a delayed dural repair is required after the patient has recovered from the acute effects of the head injury.

Craniofacial repair

Complex disruption of the craniofacial skeleton with associated cerebral and ophthalmological problems

Table 17.9 Glasgow outcome scale

> 1 Good recovery – resumption of normal life
>   despite minor deficits
> 2 Moderate disability (independent but disabled)
> 3 Severe disability (conscious but dependent)
> 4 Vegetative state – unresponsive and speechless;
>   after 2 or 3 weeks may open eyes and have
>   sleep/wake cycles.
> 5 Dead – most deaths as a result of primary head
>   injury occur within 48 hours of the injury.

rehabilitationists. This is a multidisciplinary and specialized process. There is a recognition that if it is to be successful, it needs to be started early and so minimize the development of physical and behavioural complications.

OUTCOME

The development of the Glasgow Outcome Scale has been important not only in assessing the individual patient but in allowing comparison of a variety of treatment options (Table 17.9).

There are a number of predictors of outcome after severe head injury, including the GCS after resuscitation, the pupillary responses, age, ICP and the intracranial diagnosis on CT scanning. After a severe head injury overall mortality at 6 months is 36% in patients looked after in NSUs experienced in and committed to the care of head-injured patient. In non-specialist units, head injury mortality varies from 43% less than expected to more than 52% greater than expected. These differences are largely explained by variation in outcome in patients with a low risk of death and not in the high risk group of patients. There is, therefore, a compelling argument that neurosurgical assessment and supervision are as important for the less severely injured patient as for the severely injured one. Unfortunately, limited neurosurgical facilities are available in some areas, particularly dedicated intensive care beds. Clinicians responsible for the care of head-injured patients should be experienced and have access to neurological intensive care facilities. Flexible CT and MRI

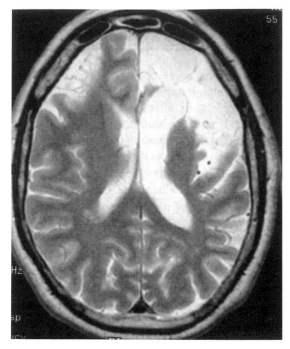

Figure 17.9 MRI brain scan, T2-weighted axial view, to show bifrontal areas of high signal, more obvious on the right side where the lateral ventricle was also enlarged. This was the result of a severe head injury.

scanning policies, the latter producing more pathological detail (Figure 17.9), are required to allow an appropriate selection of patients for treatment, coupled with adequate facilities for monitoring the effects and complications of therapy.

REFERENCES AND FURTHER READING

American College of Surgeons (1993) *Advanced Trauma Life Support Course Manual*. Washington, DC: American College of Surgeons. p.168.

Brain Trauma Foundation, American Association of Neurological Surgeons (1996) Joint Section on Neurotrauma and Critical Care. Guidelines for the management of severe head injury. *Journal of Neurotrauma*, 13:641–734.

Gentleman D, Jennett B (1981) Hazards of interhospital transfer of comatose head-injured patients. *Lancet*, ii:853.

Jennett B (1975) *Epilepsy after Non-missile Head Injuries*. London, UK: Heinemann.

Jennett B, Bond M (1975) Assessment of outcome after severe brain damage. *Lancet*, i:480–484.

Maas AI, Dearden M, Teasdale GM *et al.* (1997) EBIC guidelines for management of severe head injury in adults. European Brain Injury Consortium. *Acta Neurochirurgie (Wien)*, **139**:286–294.

Neuroanaesthesia Society of Great Britain and Ireland and the Association of Anaesthetists of Great Britain and Ireland (1996) *Recommendations for the Transfer of Patients with Acute Head Injuries to Neurosurgical Units*. London.

Teasdale GM, Nicoll JAR, Murray G, Fiddes M (1997) Association of apolipoprotein E polymorphism with outcome after head injury. *Lancet*, **350**:1069–1071.

lying flat overnight. One diagnostic pitfall is that the vomiting can occur in the absence of nausea, and even in the absence of headache. This presentation of 'pure' vomiting is most often caused by a brainstem lesion affecting the floor of the fourth ventricle; it may be a result of local stimulation of vomiting reflexes before the tumour has caused much increase in the ICP. Vomiting with a diurnal pattern, or if sudden and 'effortless' in nature, is highly suspicious of raised ICP.

If the vomiting is accompanied by headache, the patient often notices that the headache worsens as they vomit (because this further raises ICP due to straining). Each bout of vomiting increases ICP, so the patient may reach a crescendo of vomiting, often leading to presentation at an Accident and Emergency Department.

Visual symptoms and signs

Visual obscuration

Raised ICP, particularly if rapid in onset, may lead to transient loss of vision, referred to as visual obscuration or an amblyopic attack.

Papilloedema

As ICP progressively rises, fundoscopy will often reveal loss of the normal venous pulsations in the retinal veins around the optic disc. With a further increase, axonal transport in the optic nerve becomes compromised, leading to the characteristic swelling of the disc: initially progressive loss of the cup and then the more obvious 'heaped up' appearance. Severe venous obstruction can then lead to retinal haemorrhages around the disc.

> ### Presence or absence of papilloedema
> Although papilloedema is a significant sign, it is important to realize that it is frequently not present. Less than half of patients with raised ICP will demonstrate papilloedema. Thus, papilloedema is diagnostic, but lack of papilloedema should never be taken as reassurance.

Apart from its usefulness as a sign of raised ICP, papilloedema is also significant because it represents

a risk to vision. Left unresolved, papilloedema can lead to expansion of the blind spot, loss of visual acuity and eventually to blindness.

It should be noted that fundoscopy to check for papilloedema should not require a mydriatic to dilate the pupil (this is usually performed in the context of full retinal screening). Indeed, in many contexts where papilloedema is relevant, it will also be important to preserve normal pupil reactions as a part of the clinical assessment.

In some cases of hydrocephalus, or space-occupying lesions in the region of the optic chiasm, visual deterioration can occur even in the absence of papilloedema because of the direct effect of pressure on the chiasm. Thus, in some patients with obstructive hydrocephalus, visual deterioration can sometimes occur even without characteristic symptoms or papilloedema. For this reason, patients with CSF shunts should have regular visual checks as part of their ongoing surveillance; visual deterioration may sometimes be the first and only sign that their shunts are malfunctioning.

Abnormalities of eye movements

Raised ICP, particularly if a result of obstructive hydrocephalus, can lead to distortion or 'kinking' of the tectal plate region, producing a loss of up-gaze. In infants with severe hydrocephalus, this can lead to the characteristic sign of 'sunsetting', where the iris is displaced downwards and partially obscured by the lower lid, like the sun disappearing over the horizon at sunset. In the very elderly, there is sometimes a physiological loss of up-gaze and so it is a less useful sign in that age group.

Diplopia can be a symptom of raised ICP. This is sometimes caused by an abducens palsy, probably as a result of a non-specific pressure effect on the brainstem. It is thus a 'false localizing' sign, because there is usually not a lesion pressing directly on the abducens nerve, and it does not provide useful information as to the location of an intracranial lesion. On the other hand, diplopia can be caused by an oculomotor palsy from herniation of the uncus over the tentorial edge and this is a 'localizing' sign, because it occurs as a result of the direct pressure on the nerve and is usually ipsilateral with the lesion producing the mass effect.

Decreased level of consciousness

A decreased level of consciousness implies severely raised ICP. Either the homeostatic mechanisms have been exhausted and overall CBF has fallen too low to maintain brain function, or specific areas critical to maintaining arousal (reticular formation, midbrain) have been compromised by brain shift (see p. 108). In either case, the situation is serious and further rises in ICP can lead to deterioration into coma and death.

Pressure gradients, shifts and herniations

The intracranial space is divided by incomplete partitions formed from folds of dura. The tentorium separates the cerebral hemispheres from the cerebellum, medulla and pons; the falx separates the two cerebral hemispheres. The midbrain straddles the tentorial hiatus, with the medial part of the temporal lobe (uncus) adjacent on each side. This basic anatomy helps us to understand the three main patterns of brain shift: subfalcine, transtentorial (or uncal) and foramen magnum (or tonsillar). Each of these patterns is sometimes referred to as 'coning' (Figure 18.1).

Subfalcine herniation

A unilateral supratentorial lesion produces an asymmetrical mass effect and, as it increases, leads to progressive displacement of midline structures towards the contralateral side, forcing brain tissue to herniate underneath the edge of the falx. If there is decreased conscious level or an accompanying focal deficit, urgent treatment to reduce mass effect will be required. Even in an otherwise well patient, if the midline displacement is more than 5 mm, the patient is considered at significant risk of rapid deterioration. As the medial surface of the cerebral hemisphere herniates under the tentorial edge, bridging veins, draining blood from the hemisphere into the sagittal sinus, can become kinked leading to sudden worsening of swelling and rapid decompensation; for example, a small chronic subdural haematoma would require urgent burr-hole drainage if there was decreased conscious level, focal deficit or midline shift >5 mm. On the other hand, in a well patient with less than 5 mm of midline shift, a small chronic

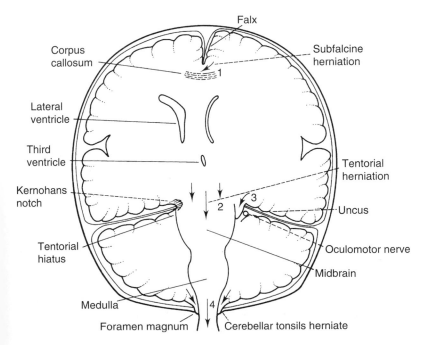

Figure 18.1 Coronal section of the brain to show the sites of possible herniation. Note: the oculomotor nerve (III) lies by the free edge of the tentorium cerebelli. (1) Subfalcine herniation; (2) transtentorial herniation; (3) uncal herniation; (4) tonsillar herniation (foramen magnum).

subdural haematoma might be considered for conservative management.

Transtentorial/uncal herniation

As supratentorial pressure increases, structures begin to herniate through the tentorial hiatus. In the case of a unilateral supratentorial mass, the first structure to herniate will be the uncus on the medial aspect of the temporal lobe. The oculomotor nerve running along the free edge of the tentorium is compressed by the herniating uncus leading to the **cardinal sign of an ipsilateral increase in pupil size. As the effect increases the pupil becomes fully dilated and unreactive.** As the uncus herniates, it also presses on midbrain structures leading to a **decrease in conscious level.** Eventually, the compressed tissue within the tentorial hiatus also compromises the contralateral oculomotor nerve, leading to bilateral fixed dilated pupils.

Kernohan's notch describes the situation whereby lateral displacement of the midbrain by a supratentorial mass leads to impingement of the opposite cerebral peduncle onto the hard tentorial edge. This produces an indentation or 'notch' in the contralateral cerebral peduncle and can produce a hemiparesis ipsilateral to the causative supratentorial mass. Thus, hemiparesis can be misleading as a localizing clinical sign. Occasionally, a posterior fossa mass can produce transtentorial herniation upwards. Thus, there is a small but definite risk of producing this complication when associated obstructive hydrocephalus is relieved in the presence of a posterior fossa mass.

Foramen magnum/tonsillar herniation

Once all the compensatory intracranial mechanisms are exhausted, the only further displacement possible is through the foramen magnum. At this stage the cerebellar tonsils are displaced downwards and, as they become crowded into the foramen magnum, they cause compression of the medulla. Because this is usually the final stage of ICP decompensation, the patient is likely to be comatose, but, **if conscious, the patient will complain of severe occipitocervical pain and neck stiffness.** Typically, the patient will find a particular head position in which the pain is minimized

(this can be flexed, extended or neutral) and will then resolutely hold their head fixed in that position.

Brainstem reflexes may become compromised, leading to cardiorespiratory irregularities (see p. 112). However, these signs are very late, usually occurring just prior to respiratory arrest, and so their absence should not be taken as reassurance.

It is important to note that performing lumbar puncture in the presence of brain shift either with a supratentorial or a posterior fossa mass can be rapidly fatal.

The sudden reduction of pressure within the spinal CSF can worsen the displacement, leading to further compression of vital structures. It is therefore critical to differentiate between possible meningitis and headache/neck stiffness caused by an intracranial mass. This will usually be suspected on clinical features, but if there is any doubt an urgent CT scan should be performed prior to any attempt at lumbar puncture.

CAUSES OF RAISED INTRACRANIAL PRESSURE

Head injury

Head injury is a common problem (see p. 346). In terms of overall numbers, it is the most significant cause of raised ICP.

Although it is an oversimplification, brain damage from head trauma is customarily divided into primary and secondary injury: primary injury is the damage at the moment impact, whereas secondary injury results from ongoing causes (see p. 347). The most potent causes of secondary injury are hypoxia and hypertension (often sustained before the patient even reaches hospital). Intracranial causes of secondary injury predominantly act by raising ICP, decreasing CBF and thus causing brain tissue metabolic failure.

Raised ICP following trauma can be the result of haematoma (extradural, subdural or intracerebral), contusion or diffuse brain swelling (see p. 353). It is particularly important not to miss the diagnosis of an intracranial haematoma, because such lesions are often eminently treatable by surgery, but such treatment needs to be instituted quickly.

Hydrocephalus

Basic principles

Cerebrospinal fluid is continuously produced by the choroid plexus, mainly in the lateral ventricles but also, to a lesser extent, in the third and fourth ventricles. An even smaller amount is produced directly by the ependymal lining of the ventricles. The daily rate of production varies very little for a particular individual. It is generally around 500 ml per day in an adult and does not change even with quite wide variations of other physiological parameters. It is very difficult to reduce CSF production, although carbonic anhydrase inhibitors such as acetazolamide can achieve minor reduction.

The CSF leaves the ventricular system through the foramina of Magendie and Luschka to enter the subarachnoid space. Some fluid will flow around the spinal cord, while some will enter the basal subarachnoid spaces (cisterns), but eventually all CSF circulates over the surface of the cerebral hemispheres to be reabsorbed through the arachnoid granulations into the intracranial venous sinuses.

The production of CSF being essentially fixed, hydrocephalus (the abnormal accumulation of CSF) is caused by impairment of flow somewhere in the pathways outlined above. If blockage occurs within the ventricular system (e.g. a tumour occluding the fourth ventricle, or aqueduct stenosis), this leads to 'obstructive' or 'non-communicating' hydrocephalus. If, however, impairment of flow is a result of scarring of the arachnoid granulations or the cisternal subarachnoid spaces (e.g. following meningitis or subarachnoid haemorrhage), the resulting hydrocephalus is said to be 'communicating'.

Clinical presentation

In children, hydrocephalus can be caused by congenital malformations (e.g. aqueduct stenosis or malformations associated with dysraphism) or can be produced by perinatal intracranial haemorrhage. Raised ICP in infants produces bulging of the fontanelles and increasing head circumference. Depending on the severity, this may be less apparent and may merely cause delayed closure of the fontanelles. In an older child, hydrocephalus can present gradually with decreased educational achievement and

subtle cognitive decline. In addition, any of the features of raised ICP discussed above can be present.

In adults, the presentation is more likely to be with the general features of raised ICP. In addition, middle aged and elderly adults can present with a disorder known as **normal pressure hydrocephalus (NPH)**. This is probably a misnomer, because it is thought to be a result of intermittently raised ICP: such patients were found to have 'normal' pressure at lumbar puncture, but subsequent studies using 24-hour ICP monitoring have shown that plateau waves of raised ICP do occur.

Patients with NPH classically present with the triad of dementia, gait ataxia and urinary incontinence (Table 18.2). It is not necessary, however, for all the features to be present. Some patients present with an akinetic-rigid Parkinsonian gait.

The diagnosis of NPH may be supported by MR imaging (see Figure 14.10 a,b) (e.g. dilatation of the temporal horns is more likely to represent a hydrocephalic process rather than atrophy or small vessel disease, both of which are also common in the elderly). Additionally, ICP monitoring may demonstrate characteristic plateau waves, and some clinicians rely on a timed walking test, before and after therapeutic lumbar puncture. However, all of the above methods of assessment have a significant false-negative rate and so, if the clinical presentation is convincing, it is worth discussing with the patient and their family whether the insertion of a CSF shunt is worthwhile, even though improvement cannot be guaranteed.

Treatment of hydrocephalus

As with other causes of raised ICP, there are two aspects of treatment of hydrocephalus: treating the causative lesion and directly reducing ICP, in this

Table 18.2 Symptoms and signs of normal pressure hydrocephalus

Impaired cognitive function
Gait disorder – short shuffling steps, unsteady, falls, 'magnetic gait', astasia-abasia
Urinary incontinence – urgency, frequency, then incontinence with lack of concern

case by draining CSF (usually by insertion of a CSF shunt, although acutely an external ventricular drain may be used). A catheter is inserted into the ventricle and linked via a subcutaneous tube to another body cavity, generally the peritoneal cavity, but sometimes the right atrium or, more rarely, the pleural cavity or the transverse venous sinus. The system will contain a valve to regulate the CSF flow, with various degrees of sophistication depending on the type of valve.

Some valves are now capable of being adjusted non-invasively after insertion, allowing a variety of pressure settings to be tried without requiring revision surgery. Such valves can be reset by strong magnetic fields and so, if a patient requires MRI, it is important to ascertain whether their shunt system is MR compatible and, if it is an adjustable valve, it will need to be checked and possibly reset immediately after the imaging. Thus, such patients should be dealt with at a centre familiar with hydrocephalus and shunt problems. Complications from the use of shunts include blockage, infection and the development of a subdural collection.

Obstructive hydrocephalus, particularly as a result of aqueduct stenosis, is increasingly treated by endoscopic third ventriculostomy, whereby the floor of the third ventricle is punctured to allow CSF to 'bypass' directly to the basal cisterns, avoiding the blockage in the aqueduct or fourth ventricle. Such operations are only indicated if the ventricular system is sufficiently dilated to allow safe introduction of the endoscope, and only achieve a 60–70% rate of independence from subsequent CSF shunting. However, if successful, the patient then generally remains shunt-independent indefinitely, and is therefore spared the many possible complications of lifelong shunting.

It has often occurred to clinicians that hydrocephalus could also be treated by reducing the production of CSF. In practice, this is of little clinical value: acetazolamide can produce a minor reduction in CSF production; endoscopic coagulation of the choroid plexus is also sometimes used in cases where other therapeutic options have been exhausted, but it has a low rate of success. However, research is currently exploring molecular approaches aimed at selectively destroying the choroid plexus and such techniques may become available in the near future.

Tumour

Glioma

Gliomas

Gliomas are the most common primary brain tumours. As the name implies, they can arise from any of the glial components of the brain: astrocytoma, oligodendroglioma and ependymoma. Gliomas are classified into one of four grades (The World Health Organization system being the most widely accepted), depending on histological characteristics such as anaplasia, presence of necrosis, vascular proliferation, and so on.

- Grade 1 correspond to a specific entity known as pilocytic astrocytoma; this occurs almost exclusively in children and has a very good prognosis
- Grade 2 gliomas are generally referred to as 'benign' and tend to be slow growing; often the history extends to many years and they may present with epilepsy rather than mass effect
- Grade 3 and 4 gliomas are referred to as 'malignant' because they are fast growing and have a worse prognosis (Figure 18.2). In this case, however, 'malignant' does not imply metastatic potential: gliomas metastasize only very rarely outside the central nervous system
- The most malignant Grade 4 gliomas are commonly known as glioblastoma multiforme, because the cells may take on multiple forms as they dedifferentiate into more primitive tumour cells (Figure 18.3).

The earliest presentation is often with **epilepsy** and this may be associated with a relatively better prognosis because the diagnosis is being made at an early stage before the onset of mass effect. Later presentation can be with **focal effects**, such as hemiparesis or dysphasia, depending on the site of the tumour, or with the more generalized features of **raised ICP**.

If the presentation is with symptoms of mass effect, **surgery** can provide a useful palliative role, particularly if the tumour is in a non-eloquent area. However, there has been little definitive evidence

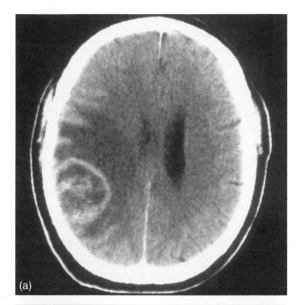

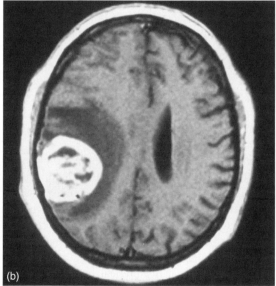

Figure 18.2 Right parietal glioma: (a) contrast-enhanced CT brain scan; (b) T1-weighted MRI brain scan with contrast enhancement.

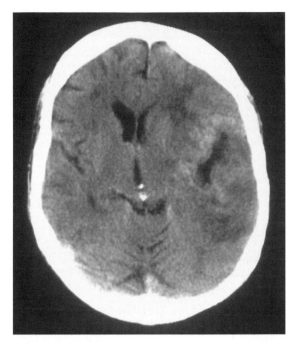

Figure 18.3 CT brain scan showing a left-sided glioblastoma multiforme with slight enhancement by contrast and considerable midline shift.

that surgery improves life expectancy (this remains controversial) and so, if symptoms are not attributable to mass effect or are easily controlled by medical means, then surgery is usually limited to biopsy to establish diagnosis.

Surgery, of whatever extent, is generally followed by **cranial radiotherapy**, which has been shown to extend survival (although overall prognosis remains poor), and sometimes by **chemotherapy**, which has also been shown to have a relatively small but positive effect. The selection of patients for radiotherapy depends on their 'performance status' by the degree of pre-existing disability; a significantly disabled patient may be more appropriate for palliative measures rather than radical radiotherapy.

Peritumoural oedema can often be dramatically relieved by **high dose steroids**, and often the terminal phases of the disease are marked by balancing the beneficial effect of steroids against their increasing side-effects, until eventual inevitable decompensation occurs.

Grade 2 gliomas generally present with much more subtle symptoms and signs, often with epilepsy alone. Usually a biopsy is performed to establish diagnosis. Thereafter, some clinicians recommend surgery to remove as much abnormal tissue as possible, but generally it is thought that such a radical approach has no effect on outcome. Instead, simple surveillance and symptomatic treatment (e.g. anticonvulsants to control epilepsy) is widely practised. In the case of oligodendroglioma, such tumours often respond well to chemotherapy. For astrocytomas, radiotherapy remains the best option but is

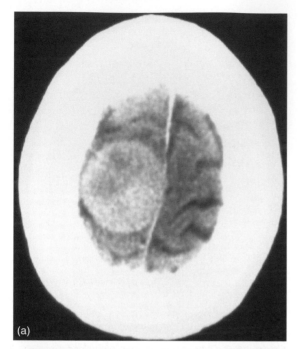

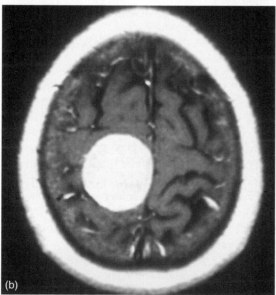

Figure 18.4 Right-sided convexity meningioma: (a) contrast-enhanced CT scan; (b) T1-weighted MRI scan with contrast.

usually reserved for tumours that have shown definite increasing size; irradiation at the time of diagnosis may have little biological effect if the tumour is 'quiescent', but then leaves no good therapeutic option if the tumour later increases its rate of growth.

Grade 1 (pilocytic) astrocytoma is generally removed as extensively as possible and then has a very good prognosis; life expectancy is near normal.

Meningioma

Meningioma is the most common extrinsic intracranial tumour, but is much less common than a glioma. Meningiomas arise from the meninges, commonly in the region of the arachnoid granulations, although they can arise from any part of the dura, or indeed, can occasionally arise inside the cerebral ventricles. They are almost always histologically benign.

As with other tumours, the presenting symptoms and signs will depend on possible **focal effects** (epilepsy or focal neurological deficit depending on site) or worsening oedema may lead to presentation with the symptoms of **raised ICP**. Subfrontal meningioma classically presents with progressive cognitive impairment and anosmia (although the latter can be difficult to detect, particularly in a demented patient).

Very small, incidental meningiomas can often be treated conservatively with serial imaging surveillance. However, if treatment is required, surgery is generally the best option. Meningiomas are slow growing, so they tend to be resistant to radiotherapy and to cytotoxic chemotherapy.

Surgery aims completely to remove the tumour and its origin, but this can be difficult to achieve, depending on the location. A convexity meningioma (Figure 18.4) is generally the least complicated to remove and so tends to have a lower rate of recurrence, compared to skull base meningiomas (Figure 18.5). The overall recurrence rate depends on whether atypical histological features are seen, as well as the location, but most clinical series using follow-up imaging find approximately 10% recurrence at 10 years.

Pre-operative particle embolization is often employed to reduce the blood supply to these tumours, which are often very vascular.

Despite the poor response, patients with multiple recurrent meningiomas (particularly in syndromes such as neurofibromatosis) sometimes undergo radiotherapy when repeated surgery has been unsatisfactory or is considered too high a risk. In similar circumstances, chemotherapy with hydroxyurea is sometimes tried, again with generally poor response.

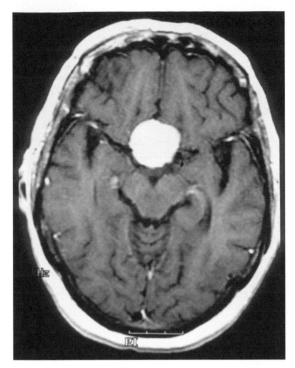

Figure 18.5 T1-weighted MRI scan, axial view, to show a suprasellar meningioma (contrast enhanced).

Pituitary region tumours

Pituitary tumours and craniopharyngiomas are often grouped together, because they both occur in the sellar region (Figure 18.6) and clinical features are often similar: neurological, visual and endocrine.

Mass effect from a tumour in this region can produce optic nerve and/or chiasmal compression, leading to progressive visual field loss, with a bitemporal hemianopia, often asymmetric or with atypical patterns. Some patients are unaware of such visual deterioration until central vision is affected.

With further expansion of the tumour there may be involvement of the cavernous sinus (leading to lesions of the cranial nerves passing through the sinus) or impingement on the medial aspect of the temporal lobe, producing epilepsy. Upwards expansion can lead to obstruction of the anterior part of the third ventricle and the foramina of Monro.

Endocrine manifestations (see p. 482) can be the result of production of excess hormones by the tumour itself (e.g. excess growth hormone leading to acromegaly), or non-productive tumour cells can gradually impair the production of hormones by the rest of the pituitary, leading to hypopituitarism. Any tumour with sufficient mass effect, may impair the function of the pituitary stalk, producing increased prolactin (although usually not of such a high level as produced by an active prolactinoma) and may also cause diabetes insipidus.

Craniopharyngiomas possibly arise from embryonic rest cells from Rathke's pouch. These form an expanding cyst in the suprasellar region. They can produce all of the features associated with mass effect in that area: all the features mentioned above, including the endocrine effects of pituitary stalk compression, but of course they do not actually produce hormones.

Investigations
- Endocrine studies (see p. 482)
- Visual fields
- Imaging – usually MRI (Figure 18.7).

Treatment of pituitary tumours

Relief of any optic nerve or chiasmal compression is urgent. Modern surgical treatment relies on a transsphenoidal approach with removal of the tumour by this route. Huge tumours may require a subfrontal craniotomy. In some patients post-operative radiotherapy may be necessary.

Bromocriptine and other prolactin inhibitors, such as octreotide, or lanreotide (analogues of somatostatin) have been used in the treatment of acromegaly and may shrink the tumour.

Following any therapy the patient will require regular follow-up with: assessment of endocrine function (with a view to any replacement therapy); measurement of the visual acuity and charting the visual fields; and often imaging.

Metastases

Metastases are very common at post mortem, but may present in neurological practice, because they often occur in the context of terminal widespread metastatic carcinoma, where palliation is the major concern. However, a cerebral metastasis can occasionally be the first presentation of carcinoma, even when the

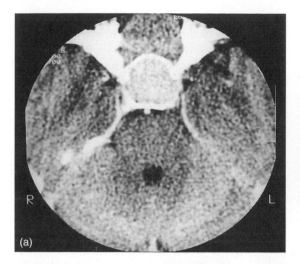
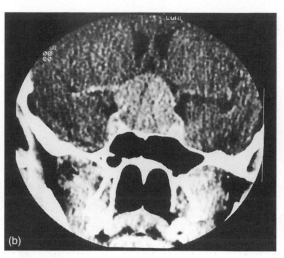
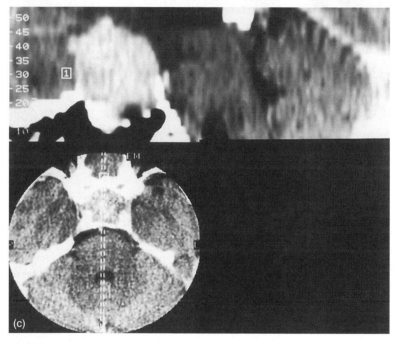

Figure 18.6 (a) Axial view of an enhanced CT brain scan to show a pituitary tumour. (b) Coronal section from the same patient to show the tumour rising well above the pituitary fossa. (c) Sagittal reconstruction from the same patient taken at the level indicated.

patient was not known to have a pre-existing primary tumour. Naturally, if the patient has a main primary tumour, the appearance of cerebral lesion is highly suspicious of metastatic disease. Also, the appearance of multiple intrinsic lesions increases the likelihood of this diagnosis (Figure 18.8). Common primary sites include the lung and breast; other sites are the kidney, gastrointestinal tract, malignant melanomas and lymphomas.

Metastatic deposits in the brain can occur in any location and can present either with mass effect or with epilepsy. Mass effect may manifest as focal neurological impairment, or with the general features of raised ICP.

Although it is not possible on imaging appearances to make the diagnosis, multiple well-defined lesions would certainly raise this possibility. Clinical examination to check for a possible primary site is

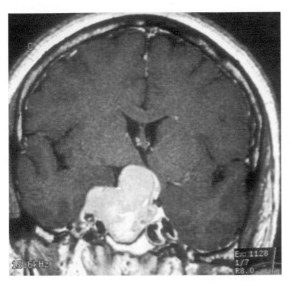

Figure 18.7 T1-weighted MRI brain scan, coronal view, to show a large pituitary tumour rising well above the sella and extending laterally on the right side (gadolinium-enhanced image).

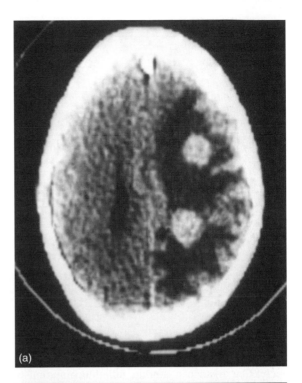

(a)

obviously important, as well as **chest X-ray**, because lung carcinoma is common (Table 18.3).

If the diagnosis cannot be made by other means, biopsy often becomes necessary to establish diagnosis. Furthermore, surgical removal of a single intracranial metastasis can often be justified, because it produces good palliation (although no increase in life-expectancy).

Further treatment will obviously depend on the underlying primary tumour, because different types of carcinoma may respond to radiotherapy and some to chemotherapy. Resection of the primary may also be indicated.

If the patient's general condition is good, cranial irradiation will usually be indicated, whether or not surgery has been performed. As always, decisions concerning further treatment will depend on the prognosis of the primary carcinoma, the degree of dissemination elsewhere and the general condition of the patient.

Lymphoma

Primary cerebral lymphoma can occur, or lymphoma deposits may appear in the context of known lymphoma elsewhere in the body. Typically, cerebral lymphoma appears diffusely in the white matter

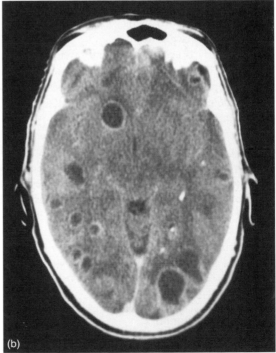

(b)

Figure 18.8 (a) Enhanced CT brain scans to show solid metastatic lesions with considerable surrounding oedema (low density). (b) Multiple cystic metastatic lesions with ring enhancement.

Table 18.3 Investigation of patients suspected of having a cerebral tumour

Blood tests	Full blood count, ESR
	Endocrine tests – pituitary lesions
	Special markers, e.g. chorionic gonadotrophin
Imaging	MRI scan (often with gadolinium enhancement) – particularly posterior fossa, craniocervical junction, parapituitary region
	CT brain scan (enhanced) – particularly if MRI is not possible
	MRA or angiography to identify vascular tumours or show blood supply
To exclude metastases or show primary	
Blood tests	Liver function, prostatic-specific antigen
Chest X-ray	
Isotope scans	Bone, liver
PET scans	

ESR, erythrocyte sedimentation rate; MRI, magnetic resonance imaging; CT, computerized tomography; MRA, magnetic resonance angiography; PET, positron emission tomography.

surrounding the ventricles. There is a marked increasing incidence among immunocompromised patients: about 5% of patients with acquired immuno-deficiency syndrome (AIDS) eventually develop cerebral lymphoma (see p. 408).

The history is usually short and often symptoms are a subtle behavioural/personality change, although focal epilepsy and progressive hemiparesis can also occur. Later, all the features of generalized raised ICP will appear.

Biopsy generally establishes the diagnosis and treatment then usually involves radiotherapy and treatment of any underlying condition. Cerebral lymphoma often has a marked short-term response to steroids, to such an extent that steroids instituted at presentation may be so effective that the lesion is hard to locate even a few days later when biopsy is attempted. It is therefore important to repeat the scan prior to biopsy to check that the lesion has not become invisible on CT scan.

Pineal region tumours

Tumours of the pineal region are very rare. They occur most commonly in males between the ages of 15 and 25 years. The most common histological type is the germinoma, which is locally malignant and may also seed through the CSF pathways.

True pinealomas, arising from the pineal tissue itself, are very rare and when they occur may be either a pineocytoma or a more malignant pineoblastoma.

Other very rare tumours in this region include chorion carcinoma (of embryonic yolk sac origin) and dermoids.

Clinical features of pineal region tumours

Tumours in the pineal region generally present by obstruction of the aqueduct, leading to hydrocephalus (Figure 18.9), or present with raised ICP. There may also be the local effects of pressure on the midbrain and tectal plate. This can present with **Parinaud's syndrome** with defects of upwards gaze and convergence (see p. 90). There may also be large poorly reacting pupils with light-near dissociation. Sometimes there is convergence nystagmus.

Treatment

Treatment is primarily the treatment of hydro-cephalus, by CSF shunting and sometimes a biopsy to establish the diagnosis. Sometimes the diagnosis can be indicated by blood and CSF tumour markers such as alpha-fetoprotein (in germinoma) and chorionic gonadotrophin (in chorion carcinomas).

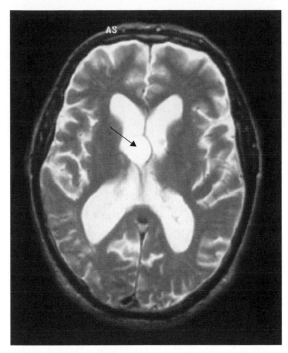

Figure 18.9 T2-weighted MRI brain scan, axial view, to show a colloid cyst slightly to the right of the midline causing an obstructive hydrocephalus.

Radiotherapy is generally useful in germinomas, whereas tumours of yolk sac origin tend to be more chemosensitive. Tumours that disseminate along CSF pathways often require full craniospinal irradiation for secondary deposits.

Posterior fossa tumours

Medulloblastoma and ependymoma

Medulloblastomas are histologically malignant tumours that are the commonest intrinsic brain tumour in children, although they can also occur in adults. Tumours typically arise in the vermis of the cerebellum, adjacent to the fourth ventricle. Thus, the presentation is often with obstructive hydrocephalus, as a result of impingement on the fourth ventricle. Occasionally, invasion of the floor of the fourth ventricle may cause vomiting as the primary symptom. If vomiting occurs in the absence of other symptoms suggesting raised ICP, the diagnosis may be difficult and the patient may often have remained undiagnosed for several months, leading to dehydration and undernutrition.

Other frequently seen features are papilloedema and truncal ataxia. Medulloblastomas may also spread along CSF pathways and so, rarely, presentation can be with secondary deposits (for example in the cauda equina).

Ependymomas also occur mainly in childhood, but are much rarer than medulloblastomas. Ependymomas also commonly arise in the region of the fourth ventricle (although they can occur anywhere there is ependyma) and so it is difficult to distinguish between medulloblastomas and ependymomas on clinical or radiological grounds. Ependymomas, however, tend to be less malignant and to have a generally better prognosis. Both types of tumour are treated by relief of any associated hydrocephalus, surgery to remove as much of the mass as possible, and then radiotherapy. Early surveillance for secondary deposits elsewhere in the craniospinal axis is essential for planning treatment.

Cerebellar astrocytoma

Cerebellar astrocytoma is another tumour of childhood, although rarer than the medulloblastoma and relatively benign. It can be either cystic or solid, and more typically is located in the cerebellar hemisphere rather than the midline. A childhood cerebellar astrocytoma, arising in a hemisphere may cause ipsilateral clumsiness or a habitual tilt of the head. Although relatively benign and slow growing, it may also eventually impede CSF drainage and so present with hydrocephalus and raised ICP. The basis of treatment is surgery: to relieve hydrocephalus, establish the histological diagnosis and to debulk the tumour mass. In the case of a cystic type, the solid nodular part is removed but the cystic wall is generally left in place.

Haemangioblastoma

Another tumour arising in the cerebellar hemisphere is a haemangioblastoma. It is generally cystic, with an enhancing nodule in the wall (Figure 18.10). It sometimes occurs as part of von Hippel–Lindau disease, where cerebellar haemangioblastoma may be associated with retinal angiomas and occasionally malignant renal and adrenal tumours. There may thus be a family history.

None of the above features can, however, be relied upon for diagnosis; surgery will be necessary

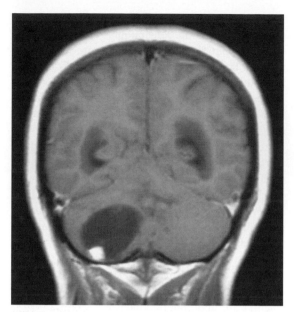

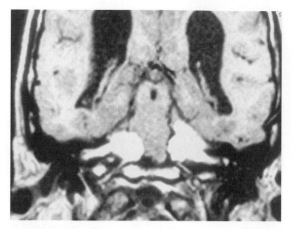

Figure 18.11 MRI brain scan, coronal view, with contrast, to show bilateral acoustic neuromas in a patient with neurofibromatosis type 2.

Figure 18.10 MRI bran scan, coronal view, to show a cystic area of low density in the right cerebellar hemisphere. Note the enhancing nodule inferiorly (gadolinium used). This was a haemangioblastoma.

to establish the diagnosis and remove the solid part, if possible. Once the diagnosis is established, the patient will require ongoing surveillance (see p. 128) for further haemangioblastomas, or the development of associated lesions. The patient and their family will also require genetic counselling.

A small, cystic lesion in the cerebellar hemisphere may be an isolated finding and relatively easy to remove at surgery. This may effectively cure the patient, if it is not part of an underlying syndrome. However, large solid lesions may be difficult to remove and extremely vascular.

Cerebellopontine angle tumours

Acoustic neuroma or schwannoma is more accurately called a vestibular neurinoma. It arises from the vestibular part of the eighth cranial nerve. True acoustic neuroma (i.e. arising from the acoustic part of the nerve) may arise in patients with hereditary type 2 neurofibromatosis, an autosomal-dominant inherited disorder. In those cases the acoustic neuroma is often bilateral.

The common sporadic type of acoustic neuroma is typically unilateral and presents with progressive

unilateral hearing impairment; often the patient will notice that they can use a telephone only on one side. The hearing impairment will eventually progress to complete **sensorineural deafness**. Other associated symptoms may include vertigo, unsteadiness, ipsilateral facial sensory symptoms and facial weakness. As the tumour further enlarges, it may cause brainstem compression, leading to rapidly worsening ataxia and eventually CSF obstruction and presentation with hydrocephalus. By this late stage headaches are typically severe and brainstem impingement may also have produced limb ataxia or even weakness. Nystagmus is often present as a result of associated peripheral vestibular disturbance. The ipsilateral corneal reflex may also be reduced with later facial sensory loss and facial weakness.

Unilateral sensorineural deafness will usually lead to an ear, nose and throat (ENT) referral assessment. The best definitive imaging is currently gadolinium-enhanced MRI (see Figure 2.14 and Figure 18.11). Where MRI is unavailable, contrast CT scanning will show most tumours over 1 cm diameter. Smaller tumours may be indirectly demonstrated on CT scan (Figure 18.12) by observing enlargement of the internal auditory meatus (although this is only present in about 60% of cases).

Large tumours with significant mass effect will require **surgery** aimed at removing the tumour if possible. The challenge is to preserve facial nerve function and any residual hearing. This is not always possible, depending on the size of the tumour. Increasingly,

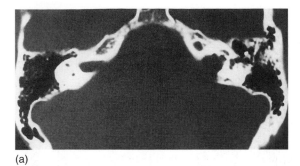

(a)

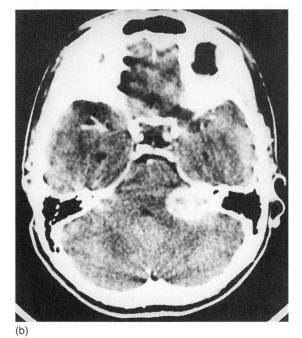

(b)

Figure 18.12 CT brain scan with adjusted window width (a), showing a very widened internal auditory meatus on the left side. (b) The enhanced view delineating the acoustic neuroma, which is displacing the fourth ventricle.

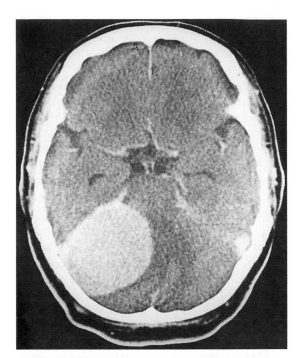

Figure 18.13 Enhanced CT brain scan to show a large posterior fossa meningioma.

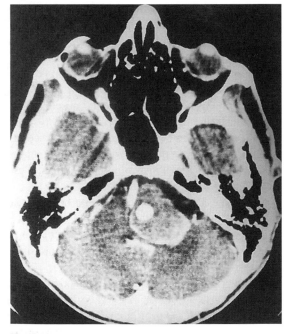

Figure 18.14 Enhanced CT brain scan showing a very large aneurysm arising from the basilar artery. This was compressing the fourth ventricle and presented as a posterior fossa mass.

small tumours can be treated by **focused radiotherapy** (e.g. gamma knife). Very small tumours may not require any immediate treatment but merely ongoing surveillance. In elderly or frail patients, it may be worth considering simple debulking or intracapsular removal to produce satisfactory relief of mass effect but with reduced risk of increasing neurological deficit.

Rarely, other tumours can arise in the cerebellopontine angle: including meningiomas, epidermoids, trigeminal neuromas or metastases (Figure 18.13 and Figure 18.14). All of these can present with local cranial nerve impairment, symptoms and signs of raised ICP and, later, brainstem impairment.

Chordoma

Chordoma is a brain tumour arising from notochordal remnants and so can occur either in the sacrococcygeal region or in the clivus. At the skull base, such tumours can present with local impingement on cranial nerves or with brainstem dysfunction. Such tumours are slow growing and so CSF obstruction and raised ICP tend to occur only very late. Scanning with CT, and sometimes plain X-ray, often show bone destruction in the skull base. The lesion will usually be defined in more detail by MRI. Subtotal removal is sometimes possible, often via the transoral route, but complete curative removal is very seldom possible.

Infection

Abscess

The two commonest forms of intracranial abscess are intracerebral and subdural (empyema). Extradural abscess is rare, although it may occur, particularly in association with skull osteomyelitis. Infection may have spread locally, for example from a chronic ear infection or air sinus disease, or it may have been blood-borne from chronic suppuration elsewhere, for example bronchiectasis or dental abscess. Subacute bacterial endocarditis may also lead to septic emboli and thus to brain abscess. Brain abscesses are more common in patients with immune compromise or in those who abuse intravenous drugs; these factors should be considered.

Any bacteria can produce abscess, because the brain is an immune privileged site, and so even low virulence organisms can establish an abscess. Sometimes even fungi or toxoplasma can be responsible, particularly in patients with AIDS.

A cerebral abscess produces an intracranial mass and so can present in any of the ways tumours present (Figure 18.15 and Figure 18.16). In addition, cerebral abscesses often produce a florid reactive oedema and so tend to be an even more potent cause of raised ICP. The rapidity of onset may mean that papilloedema has not yet developed and so the

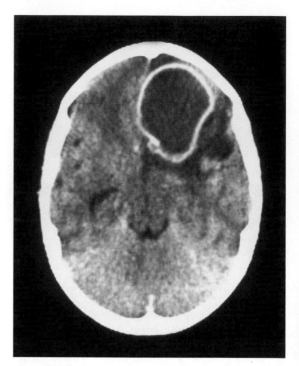

Figure 18.15 Very large ring enhancing left frontal abscess with considerable surrounding oedema (CT brain scan, axial view).

clinical pitfall is to suspect meningitis and erroneously perform a lumbar puncture, exacerbating brain shift and causing clinical deterioration.

The symptoms and signs are generally those of raised ICP with the possible addition of focal neurological effects as a result of mass effect. In general, the patient appears very ill and there are signs of infection (pyrexia, raised inflammatory markers), although clinicians should be aware that abscesses can be well 'walled-off', and the patient may therefore appear misleadingly well.

The basis of treatment is drainage of any large abscesses (to establish the microbiological diagnosis and to decrease the bacterial load) and then prolonged antibiotic therapy with serial scanning to ensure that the abscess has fully resolved before the relevant antibiotics are discontinued. Epilepsy is a common complication.

Parasitic cysts

Parasitic cysts are most commonly caused either by hydatid disease or cysticercosis.

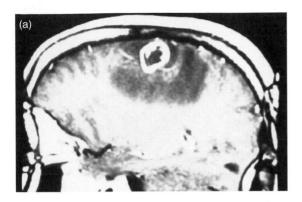

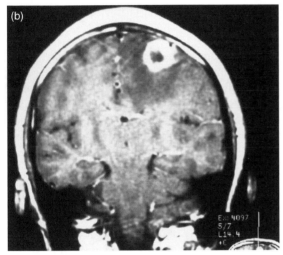

Figure 18.16 T1-weighted MRI brain scan: (a) sagittal and (b) coronal views, to show an abscess with surrounding oedema (gadolinium-enhanced scan).

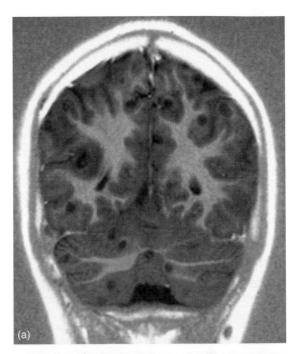

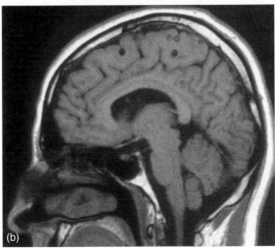

Figure 18.17 MRI brain scan, (a) coronal and (b) sagittal views, to show multiple low intensity lesions caused by cysticercosis.

Hydatid disease is the result of infection by *Echinococcus granulosus* and generally occurs in rural regions where sheep are common as intermediate hosts. Treatment of the cyst is by careful removal, avoiding spillage of the contents and then appropriate chemotherapy: praziquantel or albendazole have proved most useful.

Cysticercosis is caused by larvae from the pork tapeworm *Taenia solium* and may produce multiple encysted lesions. These often occur in the muscles, and X-ray of the thighs may reveal multiple calcified lesions. The most common presentation of cerebral cysticercosis is with epilepsy but cysts may also produce mass effect or block CSF pathways, leading to obstructive hydrocephalus. Diagnosis can often be made on specific serological tests, or good quality MRI may reveal the diagnostic appearance of the cysts (Figure 18.17). Treatment generally includes anticonvulsants and a course of specific chemotherapy with drugs such as albendazole or praziquantel with steroid cover (because treatment often exacerbates the tissue oedema as the cysts begin to necrose). The associated hydrocephalus may require treatment by removal of the obstructive cyst or a CSF shunting procedure.

Table 18.4 Causes of idiopathic intracranial hypertension

Obesity Endocrine – amenorrhoea, Cushing's disease, hypoparathyroidism Oral contraceptive pill Drugs – tetracycline, minocycline, excess vitamin A, nitrofurantoin, amiodarone, lithium, retinoids, nalidixic acid, cimetidine, tamoxifen, steroid withdrawal Severe anaemia
Always exclude venous sinus thrombosis secondary to infection, pregnancy, the oral contraceptive pill
Maximal incidence is in young overweight women, when the figure is 19:100 000 against 1:100 000 of the general population

Idiopathic intracranial hypertension

Idiopathic intracranial hypertension is of uncertain aetiology but is most frequent in young, obese females. This led to the hypothesis that the cause is endocrine, and certainly there appears to be an association with the oral contraceptive pill and with endocrine diseases supporting this link (Table 18.4).

Presentation is usually with headache, generally with the characteristics of raised ICP and often with florid papilloedema.

This condition rarely leads to brain shift, focal deficit, cognitive decline or decreased conscious level, hence the former label 'benign'. However, the condition may not be 'benign' because if the raised ICP is allowed to continue there can be progressive visual loss and, ultimately, optic atrophy.

Investigations should include imaging to exclude a mass lesion or venous sinus thrombosis, and CSF examination to exclude any 'meningitic' process and to confirm the raised pressure (>250 mm).

The basis of treatment is therefore control of headache and careful monitoring of visual acuity and fields. Any possible causative drug should be withdrawn (oral contraceptive pill, tetracycline, nitrofurantoin, excess vitamin A supplementation) and other possible causes excluded (pregnancy, venous sinus thrombosis, intracranial mass). Obese patients should be encouraged to lose weight.

Further treatment can be considered with acetazolamide (mildly effective), diuretics, or corticosteroids (although use of the last is often limited by the side-effects and subsequent withdrawal can worsen the situation). Regular lumbar punctures are sometimes sufficient, particularly as the disease is often self-limiting. However, if conservative measures fail or if the vision is threatened, surgical intervention must be considered. This may involve either optic nerve fenestration or lumboperitoneal CSF shunting.

Venous sinus thrombosis

Obstruction of any of the intracranial venous sinuses can lead to impaired venous drainage with subsequent raised ICP and even areas of venous infarction (see p. 475). This can be the result of an underlying thrombotic tendency, dehydration or may be idiopathic. It can often be diagnosed on CT imaging (producing the 'empty delta' sign on a contrast CT: the sagittal sinus in section may show contrast around its edges, but the central part of the lumen does not receive contrast, because it is obstructed by thrombus) or, more easily, on MRI. Treatment involves the correction of any underlying cause and possibly anticoagulation (although risks have to be assessed carefully in each individual case as anticoagulation may cause haemorrhage into any infarcted areas).

INTRACRANIAL PRESSURE MONITORING

Standard ICP monitoring is an invasive procedure, usually performed by passing a monitoring catheter via a hollow bolt through the skull into either the ventricle or the brain parenchyma. There are non-invasive ways of monitoring ICP: indirect techniques, such as measuring the displacement characteristics of the tympanic membrane in response to an externally applied pressure wave, or ultrasound visualization of changes in diameter of the arachnoid sheath around the optic nerve. These non-invasive methods are, however, less well-established and more difficult to calibrate.

In common with all invasive monitoring techniques used in clinical medicine, use is limited by the inherent risks of insertion, as well as the risks of infection. Therefore, in practical terms, ICP monitoring is generally used for single-event causes of raised ICP (of which head injury is by far the most frequent) that are evolving and are expected to resolve in the short term. It also tends not to be used in circumstances where clinical observation can adequately highlight any deterioration: stable, unsedated patients with a Glasgow coma score >8.

Intracranial pressure monitoring is now widely established as a standard in the intensive care of severe head injury, but would not typically be used for monitoring raised ICP caused by presence of a tumour. An exception would be, for example, where a patient is being electively ventilated overnight following surgery. In that circumstance, clinical signs in a sedated, ventilated patient tend to be very late indications of raised ICP (pupil changes, changes in pulse and blood pressure) and so short-term ICP monitoring is a useful clinical tool.

Another special circumstance is the occasional application to patients with complex shunt problems, where a period of ICP monitoring can elucidate whether symptoms (typically headache) are related to changes in ICP, even if the changes are transient or related to posture.

TREATMENT OF RAISED INTRACRANIAL PRESSURE

Apart from the specifics discussed above, the general principles of treatment include the following.

Removing or directly treating the causative lesion

The most obvious examples would be removal of the haematoma in a patient with head trauma or removal of an intracranial tumour. In severe head injury, sometimes there is a decision to remove a contused area of brain to decompress the remaining 'healthy' brain. More controversially, the bone flap can be removed to allow further space for brain expansion (i.e. changing the situation from a closed box to an open one). Although sometimes this appears helpful, there is also the danger that the cortical vessels can be included at the edge of the exposed area, leading to an area of infarction and further swelling. Further trials will be necessary to ascertain whether there is any overall benefit to the patient.

Treating oedema

The treatment of oedema depends on its causation. Cytotoxic oedema (cellular swelling) is the most common form associated with head injury and is generally thought unresponsive to steroids. Therefore, treatment involves measures to ensure continued cerebral perfusion to support metabolic demands until the oedema subsides. Vasogenic oedema, on the other hand is the type most commonly associated with tumours and is often responsive to steroids. Typically, dexamethasone 4 mg q.d.s is used in the short term to relieve peritumoural oedema, pending definitive surgical treatment. Such high doses cannot usually be sustained in the long term without encountering unacceptable side-effects.

Manipulating physiological parameters

In the intensive care environment, ICP can be treated by sedation and neuromuscular paralysis. To some extent, ICP can also be reduced by reducing temperature and PCO_2. The scope for such manipulation is, however, very limited and usually takes the form of avoiding unhelpful elevation of the above parameters: PCO_2 is generally maintained in the region of 4.0–4.5 kPa (i.e. low physiological range) and pyrexia is treated (active hypothermia is much more controversial and may even be harmful).

Infusion with hypo-osmotic fluids is avoided, because it may exacerbate oedema. Again, active dehydration may be counterproductive, because BP may fall, leading to worsening of cerebral perfusion. However, it is less controversial to say that an excessively positive fluid balance should be avoided.

Mannitol, an osmotic diuretic, is sometimes used for acute treatment of life-threatening raised ICP. Its use, however, is now much more limited than previously, since it has been realized that the fluid shifts, which are helpful in the short term, inevitably lead to 'rebound' within several hours, and furthermore the associated diuresis can produce cardiovascular instability, which is even more difficult to manage. Therefore, it is now generally restricted to a single dose to 'buy time' until a definitive procedure (such as surgery to remove a haematoma) can be performed and only in life-threatening situations. Primary teams in emergency departments are not encouraged to use mannitol routinely but to reserve its use until after the case has been discussed with the appropriate neurosurgical centre and the relative risks assessed.

Draining cerebrospinal fluid

If actual hydrocephalus exists, then CSF drainage is obviously helpful. However, in severe head injury even small amounts of remaining CSF can sometimes be drained to therapeutic advantage, if other medical means have been exhausted.

Posture

From basic principles, it should be remembered that simple elevation of the head can reduce ICP.

However, the effective BP in the carotid arteries is also reduced by head elevation. Most units agree that moderate elevation (20–30 degrees) appears to be the best compromise.

Controversies in management

Considerable controversies remain in the acute treatment of raised ICP. In particular, some clinicians believe that CPP should be maintained at all costs, whereas others believe that excessive pharmacological elevation of the BP can be counterproductive, by exacerbating cerebral oedema. Certainly, it has been shown that aiming for a CPP over 70 mmHg can lead to adult respiratory distress syndrome. Current practice is therefore to aim for a CPP in the 60–70 mmHg range.

REFERENCES AND FURTHER READING

Bret P, Guyotat J, Chazal J (2002) Is normal hydrocephalus a valid concept in 2002? A reappraisal in five questions and proposal for a new designation of the syndrome as 'chronic hydrocephalus' *Journal of Neurology, Neurosurgery and Psychiatry*, **73**:9–12.

Forsyth PA, Posner JB (1993) Headaches in patients with brain tumours: a study of 111 patients. *Neurology*, **43**:1678–1683.

McAllister LD, Ward JH, Schulman SF, DeAngelis LM (2002) *Practical Neuro-Oncology*. Boston, MA: Butterworth-Heinemann.

Pilchard JD, Czosnyka M (1993) Management of raised intracranial pressure. *Journal of Neurology, Neurosurgery and Psychiatry*, **56**:845–858.

Shakir RA, Newman PK, Posner CM (1996) *Tropical Neurology*. London, UK: WB Saunders.

Whittle IR (1996) Management of primary malignant brain tumours. *Journal of Neurology, Neurosurgery and Psychiatry*, **60**:2–5.

Wright A, Bradford R (1995) Management of acoustic neuroma. *British Medical Journal*, **311**:1141–1145.

CHAPTER 19

INFECTIONS OF THE CENTRAL NERVOUS SYSTEM

M.J. Wood

The common syndromes of central nervous system (CNS) infection are meningitis, when inflammation is confined to the subarachnoid space and meninges, and encephalitis, where the brunt of the inflammation is borne by the brain itself. Some features of the other frequently accompany either syndrome but for ease of discussion they are usually considered as separate entities.

MENINGITIS

Meningitis is divided into acute and chronic forms. The clinical features of acute meningitis develop over hours or days; those of chronic meningitis over weeks or months. One of the cornerstones of the management of meningitis is the speedy recognition of those cases that require the prompt initiation of appropriate antibiotic therapy.

Most such urgent cases are a result of acute bacterial infections and characteristically the cellular response in the cerebrospinal fluid (CSF) is predominantly polymorphs, producing purulent meningitis. The other traditional group of meningitis cases are those where the CSF pleocytosis is predominantly lymphocytes. Although most of the latter group have a viral aetiology, there are a number of other treatable causes that should always be considered.

Initial assessment of the patient

Meningitis from whatever cause is characterized by:

- Headache, often severe and described as bursting in nature, and worsened by jolt accentuation (turning the head horizontally 2–3 times/second)
- Fever
- Photophobia
- Nausea and vomiting
- Spinal muscle spasm, detected by neck stiffness and positive Kernig's sign (pain from hamstring spasm provoked by attempting to extend the knee with the hip flexed)
- In severe bacterial meningitis there may also be cerebral oedema and raised intracranial pressure leading to confusion or declining consciousness and seizures.

Some or all of such classical features of meningitis are found in nearly 90% of patients with bacterial meningitis but, in some patients, notably neonates and infants, immunocompromised patients and the very old, the signs are often much more subtle. In neonates, apathy, irritability, lethargy, a strange cry and refusal to feed may be the only features. In the elderly or immunocompromised patient, fever and confusion may develop without any specific evidence of meningeal irritation and be mistakenly ascribed to some concomitant illness or other infection.

Once the possibility of meningitis has been recognized, then the next step depends upon an assessment of the patient's condition and the speed of progression of the illness (Figure 19.1). Most patients will not have any specific clinical findings and will have experienced symptoms for more than 24 hours by the time they are first seen by a doctor. Any of the organisms listed in Table 19.1 may be responsible for the illness in this group and a decision regarding therapy depends upon the results of lumbar puncture (LP). In contrast, about 25% of patients with bacterial meningitis will have a very acute and rapidly progressive illness. In these cases, as well as in those who are semicomatose or comatose, whatever the time course of their illness, in neonates, and in those with a rash suggestive of meningococcal infection, then providing an initial brief examination fails to reveal papilloedema or focal neurological signs, an LP and blood cultures (and a coagulation screen for those with possible meningococcaemia) should be obtained and empirical therapy directed at the likely pathogens started before the CSF result is available (see below). Papilloedema and focal neurological signs are found in <1% of cases of meningitis at initial presentation and should prompt an urgent search for an intracranial space-occupying lesion by computerized tomography (CT) scan or magnetic resonance imaging (MRI) before LP can be contemplated.

The microscopic and biochemical examination of the CSF will usually give a clear indication of the type of organism causing the meningitis (Table 19.2), but there is a good deal of overlap between the findings in the various categories and a Gram's stain of the CSF is mandatory in all cases.

Acute bacterial meningitis

Epidemiology

The annual incidence of bacterial meningitis is between 3 and 5/100 000 overall population; the incidence is highest in the first month of life and nearly 75% of sporadic cases occur in children under 15 years old.

Almost any bacterium is capable of causing meningitis but, for many species, this is only as part of a generalized illness. There are, however, a few bacteria that consistently cause meningitis as a primary manifestation of disease (Table 19.1) and, in most instances, the likely aetiology of purulent meningitis can be further narrowed down by a consideration of the patient's age and previous health (Table 19.3).

Pathophysiology

In most cases of bacterial meningitis the immediate source of the pathogen is the nasopharynx; the bacteria colonize the mucosal surfaces and then cross the epithelium and spread via the bloodstream to the choroid plexus where they cross the blood–brain barrier into the subarachnoid space. The principal pathogens are capsulated bacteria and the capsule enables them to counter phagocytosis and complement-mediated bactericidal activity in the bloodstream, but the major factors that facilitate meningeal invasion are poorly understood.

The inflammatory response that begins in the subarachnoid space within a few hours of bacterial arrival has profound effects. Bacterial products trigger the release of inflammatory cytokines that upregulate adhesion molecules on endothelial cells and promote granulocyte penetration into the CSF, leading to release of further inflammatory mediators. Vascular permeability causes vasogenic cerebral oedema: cellular damage induced by toxins released from bacteria and granulocytes results in loss of cellular homeostasis and cerebral oedema worsens.

The purulent exudate obstructs the normal flow of the CSF and reduces CSF reabsorption by the arachnoid villi; hence hydrocephalus (obstructive or communicating) is produced. Vasculitis and thrombosis of the superficial meningeal vessels cause major changes in cerebral perfusion and, ultimately, infarction.

Investigations

The diagnosis of bacterial meningitis is made by culturing the blood and by examination of the CSF

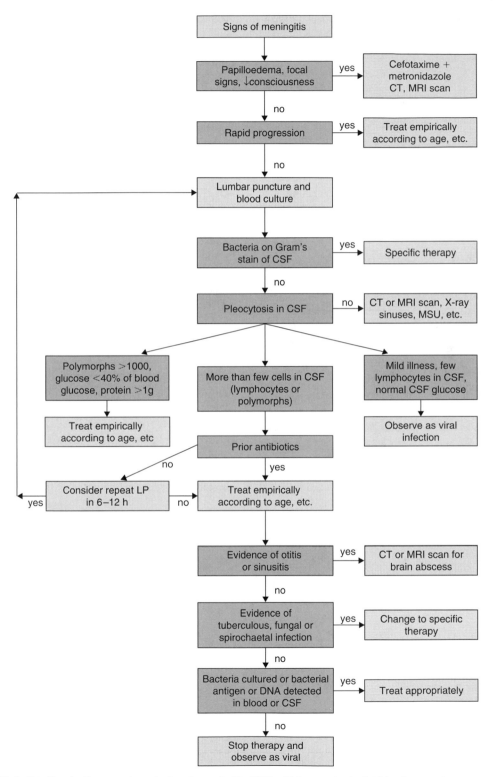

Figure 19.1 Algorithm for the management of acute meningitis. MSU, midstream urine test; LP, lumbar puncture.

Table 19.1 The predominant microbial causes of meningitis

Acute meningitis	
Common pathogens	*Neisseria meningitidis*
	Streptococcus pneumoniae
	Haemophilus influenzae
	Enteroviruses
	Herpes viruses
Rarer causes	*Listeria monocytogenes*
	Staphylococci
	Mycobacterium tuberculosis
	Gram-negative bacilli
	Leptospira
	HIV
	Other viruses
In the newborn	*Escherichia coli*
	Other Gram-negative bacilli
	Group B streptococci
	Listeria monocytogenes
Chronic meningitis	*Mycobacterium tuberculosis*
	Borrelia burgdorferi (Lyme disease)
	Brucella species
	Treponema pallidum
	Leptospira
	Cryptococcus neoformans
	Other fungi
	Parasites

HIV, human immunodeficiency virus.

(Table 19.2). **A difficult dilemma arises when the CSF examination suggests a bacterial cause (Table 19.2) but no organism can be seen on a Gram's stain.** This often results from outpatient antibiotic therapy, which has partially treated bacterial meningitis; viral meningitis, however, is also associated with polymorphs in the CSF during the first few hours of infection and occasionally it also produces a reduced glucose level. Distinguishing between the two is not always easy.

> If the patient is relatively well, then it is usually safe to observe them and repeat the LP 6–12 hours later; in viral infections, the CSF pleocytosis has often become lymphocytic by then. If the patient is obviously ill or the second LP has an increased polymorph percentage or falling glucose level, then bacterial infection must be assumed and treatment directed at the organisms most likely to be involved must be started *without delay*.

Special studies of the CSF may help: the polymerase chain reaction (PCR) may be used to amplify meningococcal DNA; bacterial antigens can be detected by counterimmunoelectrophoresis, latex agglutination or enzyme-linked immunosorbent assay; high lactate levels suggest bacterial infection; and the limulus lysate test for endotoxin indicates a Gram-negative infection. These tests may enable a more specific diagnosis to be made earlier

Table 19.2 Lumbar puncture findings in meningitis of different aetiologies

	Normal	Acute bacterial meningitis	Viral meningitis	Tuberculous meningitis
Appearance	Clear	Turbid/purulent	Clear/opalescent	Clear/opalescent
Pressure	$<20\,cmH_2O$	$>20\,cmH_2O$	$<20\,cmH_2O$	Usually $>20\,cmH_2O$
Cells	$0–5/mm^3$	$5–2000/mm^3$	$5–500/mm^3$	$5–1000/mm^3$
Polymorphs	0	$>50\%$	$<50\%$	$<50\%$
Glucose	2.2–3.3 mmol/l*	Low ($<40\%$ of blood concentration)	Normal**	Low ($<40\%$ of blood concentration)
Protein	$<400\,mg/l$	Often $>900\,mg/l$	400–900 mg/l	Often $>1\,g/l$
Other tests		Bacteria on Gram's stain	Viral nucleic acid by PCR	Bacteria on Ziehl–Neelsen or fluorescent stain
		Bacterial DNA by PCR		

*Approximately 60% of blood concentration.
**May be low in mumps meningitis.
PCR, polymerase chain reaction.

Table 19.3 Principal causes of purulent meningitis under specific circumstances

Historical data	Organism
Age	
Neonate	Group B streptococcus, *Escherichia coli*, Listeria
Under 6 years old	Meningococcus, Pneumococcus, *Haemophilus influenzae*
6–50 years old	Meningococcus, Pneumococcus
Over 50 years old	Pneumococcus, Listeria
Co-morbidity	
Diabetes mellitus	Pneumococcus, Gram-negative bacilli, Staphylococci
Alcoholism	Pneumococcus
Asplenism	Pneumococcus
Critical-care patient	Gram-negative bacilli, *Staphylococcus aureus*
Intracranial shunt	Staphylococci, Gram-negative bacilli
Immunosuppression	Listeria
Pregnancy	Listeria
Associated findings	
Petechial or purpuric rash	Meningococcus
Otitis, sinusitis	Pneumococcus, anaerobes
Pneumonia	Pneumococcus, Meningococcus
Neurosurgery	Gram-negative bacilli, staphylococci
CSF leak	Pneumococcus
Other factors	
Recurrent	Pneumococcus

than the culture results or when prior antibiotics have been used.

Treatment

The treatment of bacterial meningitis requires the prompt administration of antibiotics that achieve high levels in the CSF. This generally involves parenteral administration.

Furthermore, the penetration of most antibiotics is proportional to the degree of meningeal inflammation and therefore the dose should generally not be reduced as irritation diminishes and the patient improves.

Except in neonates and certain other special instances (see below), the vast majority of cases of bacterial meningitis are caused by pneumococci, meningococci and *Haemophilus influenzae* (the latter almost always in pre-school-age children).

A **third-generation cephalosporin** (cefotaxime, 50 mg/kg every 6 hours or ceftriaxone, 75 mg/kg every 24 hours) is suitable empirical therapy against these three pathogens. Giving more than one antibiotic in these circumstances is of no additional benefit, but if *Listeria monocytogenes* meningitis is likely then ampicillin should be added. Chloramphenicol with or without vancomycin can be given to the patient with a history of anaphylaxis from β-lactam antibiotics.

Dexamethasone, given 10–15 minutes before or shortly after antibiotics, has been shown to reduce the neurological sequelae from childhood meningitis caused by *H. influenzae* or *Streptococcus pneumoniae*, but there is as yet no convincing evidence of benefit in other forms of bacterial meningitis or in adults. Nonetheless, many would advocate the empirical administration of dexamethasone (0.15 mg/kg every 6 hours for 2 days) in all cases of presumed bacterial meningitis in children over 6 weeks of age and for adults with evidence of impaired conscious level or evidence of cerebral oedema. General supportive measures are also important and some patients will require fluid replacement, anti-emetics, anticonvulsants and treatment of raised intracranial pressure.

Fever usually settles within a few days and any recurrence of pyrexia during antibiotic therapy is likely to be caused by drug fever, subdural effusion or empyema, thrombophlebitis (cerebral or leg vein), or an unrelated infection.

Complications

Overall, there is a mortality of about 5% from bacterial meningitis and 16% of survivors have at least one major adverse outcome (severe intellectual disability, spasticity, paresis, epilepsy, deafness) when assessed 2 years later. More subtle long-term complications, particularly cognitive and behavioural impairment in childhood, are common following bacterial meningitis in infancy.

Particular forms of bacterial meningitis

Neisseria meningitidis (meningococcus)

Epidemiology
There are nine different serogroups of this Gram-negative diplococcus, which is the most common cause of bacterial meningitis in the UK, occurring most frequently in the winter months. Groups B and C are the most common serogroups seen in the UK, with smaller numbers of groups A, and W 135. Groups A and C dominate in the third world. Meningococcal disease may occur at any age but is predominantly found in children and young adults. Occasionally small clusters of cases occur in susceptible populations and in parts of sub-Saharan Africa large epidemics of type A occur annually.

Clinical features
The organism is carried asymptomatically in the nasopharynx and is transmitted by droplets. The incidence of carriage is about 10% of the general population (25–37% in those 15–24 years old) but only occasionally is acquisition followed by bacteraemia and meningitis. **There are two different forms of meningococcal disease. There is always a bacteraemic phase and in some patients this leads to fulminant meningococcal septicaemia (FMS), often without meningeal involvement, within a few hours. In others the bacteraemia is initially controlled and meningitis develops over a period of 18–36 hours.**

The bacteraemic phase is usually heralded by an abrupt onset of fever, chills and myalgia. Generalized vasculitis, resulting from disseminated intravascular coagulation and consumption coagulopathy, is a hallmark of meningococcal disease.

The visual manifestation of this is skin haemorrhages: two-thirds of patients have a rash [characteristically petechial or purpuric (Figure 19.2) but erythematous and macular in the early stages]. Widespread skin lesions, disseminated intravascular coagulation, adrenal haemorrhages, circulatory collapse and rapid progression to multi-organ failure, coma and death characterize FMS. **This is the Waterhouse–Friderichsen syndrome.** Metastatic infection in the joints, pericardium and lungs may also occur.

Mortality from FMS is 20–70% (often in the first 24 hours) and limb amputations are necessary in many survivors. The prognosis in cases of meningococcal meningitis without circulatory collapse is excellent; the mortality is 1–5% and neurological complications are infrequent. Immunologically mediated complications, notably reactive arthritis, pericarditis and fever sometimes appear 10–14 days after the onset of the disease.

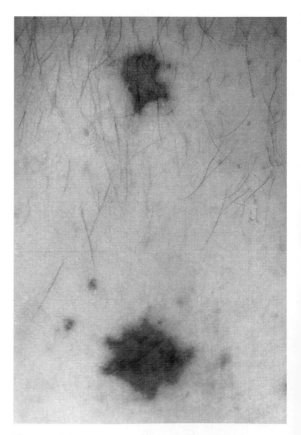

Figure 19.2 Photograph of the rash of meningococcal meningitis.

Investigations

Consideration of the possibility of meningococcal disease is required in all patients with fever and a rash and antibiotics should be administered without delay to those in whom the clinical suspicion is high. Diagnosis is made by finding *N. meningitidis* in the CSF or blood; previous antibiotics may reduce the yield and PCR testing or antigen detection may be used for confirmation.

Treatment

Treatment is with intravenous benzylpenicillin (20–30 mg/kg body weight 4-hourly) or a third-generation cephalosporin (cefotaxime or ceftriaxone) given for 5–7 days. Chloramphenicol (15–25 mg/kg body weight 6-hourly) should be used in patients with a history of an anaphylactic reaction to penicillin. There is no convincing evidence of any specific benefit from steroids, heparin, FFP (fresh frozen plasma), plasmapheresis or leukopheresis for FMS, but recent results with recombinant protein C are encouraging.

Prevention

Close contacts of the patient within the previous 7 days (household, daycare and 'kissing' contacts) are at a 1000-fold increased risk of cross-infection. As penicillin will not eradicate meningococcal carriage, the patient and all such contacts should be given rifampicin (600 mg or 10 mg/kg body weight for those aged 1–12 years and 5 mg/kg for infants) twice daily for 2 days to eliminate the organism from the nasopharynx. A single dose of ciprofloxacin (500 mg) or ofloxacin (400 mg) may be used when a large number of adolescents or adults require prophylaxis. Unconjugated polysaccharide vaccines are available against meningococci of groups A, C, W 135 and Y, but not group B. Mass vaccination of adolescents with group C vaccine has dramatically reduced the incidence of this type of disease and vaccination with the combined A, C, Y and W 135 vaccine is required for travellers to the annual Haj to Mecca.

Streptococcus pneumoniae (pneumococcus)

Epidemiology

People are at increased risk of this important form of meningitis at the two extremes of age. Other predispositions to infection include splenic dysfunction (including sickle-cell disease), alcoholism, abnormal humoral immunity (e.g. patients with multiple myeloma), and CSF leaks following skull fractures. Repeated attacks may occur. In half the cases the source of infection cannot be determined and meningitis is presumed to follow primary bacteraemia from nasopharyngeal colonization; in others, it is associated with pneumonia or infection in the middle ear or paranasal sinuses.

Symptoms and signs

Pneumococcal meningitis is often the most severe of the common forms of meningitis, with coma and seizures frequently appearing early in its course.

Neurological complications (venous sinus thrombosis, hemiplegia, ventriculitis, hydrocephalus) are frequent after pneumococcal meningitis and the mortality remains between 20 and 40%.

Treatment

Antibiotic resistance has modified recommendations for the empirical therapy of suspected pneumococcal meningitis. The frequency of penicillin-resistance in pneumococci is increasing in many countries; it is 10% in some areas of the UK, more than 25% in some US centres and Iceland and more than 50% in South Africa and Spain. Cefotaxime or ceftriaxone can be used to treat most such strains and are now recommended for empirical therapy. Vancomycin with or without rifampicin is needed for treatment of meningitis caused by a cephalosporin-resistant strain. Susceptibility testing must be performed for all isolates of *S. pneumoniae* from CSF and blood and, in areas where cephalosporin resistance is reported, all patients with presumed pneumococcal meningitis should receive high dose cefotaxime (or ceftriaxone) plus vancomycin until the isolate is proved susceptible to penicillin or cephalosporins. Treatment should be continued for 10 days or 2 weeks.

Haemophilus influenzae

Epidemiology

Bacterial meningitis caused by *Haemophilus influenzae* is almost exclusively a disease of children between the ages of 4 months and 6 years and is caused primarily by capsulated, type b strains of the small, Gram-negative bacillus. Although there has been a 90% decline in the incidence of *H. influenzae* meningitis in many countries since the introduction of conjugate *H. influenzae* type b vaccines, there are still 400 000 cases annually in the developing world.

Symptoms and signs

Meningitis is often a complication of a primary respiratory or ear infection, which is frequently acquired from another family member with a similar illness, and begins insidiously with drowsiness or irritability. Inappropriate antidiuretic hormone secretion, deafness, cortical vein thrombosis and sterile subdural effusions are common complications. The latter may require repeated aspiration or surgical drainage.

Treatment

Cefotaxime or ceftriaxone are the antibiotics of choice; ampicillin-resistance is common among *H. influenzae* and ampicillin should only be used once the organism is known to be sensitive. The duration of therapy should be for 10 days. In the developing world the mortality is nearly 30% and another 30% have major sequelae.

Prevention

The polysaccharide vaccine against *H. influenzae* type b is given to infants in the UK, many northern European countries and the USA. Unvaccinated household, playgroup or nursery school contacts under the age of 5 years are at increased risk of secondary disease and rifampicin prophylaxis [600 mg (20 mg/kg body weight) daily for 4 days] should be given to *all* family members if there is such a young child in the house, and is recommended for all attendees and staff of playgroups, etc.

Neonatal meningitis

Epidemiology

Meningitis in the newborn is a serious problem, with a high mortality and morbidity. In the UK its incidence is about 1/2500 live births and it is particularly seen in low birthweight infants (below 2.5 kg). The organisms that are responsible are chiefly group B streptococci and *Escherichia coli*, particularly strains carrying the K1 capsular antigen. Other less common organisms include *L. monocytogenes*, *Pseudomonas aeruginosa* and *Staphylococcus aureus*. Although the majority of infecting bacteria arise from the mother's genital tract and colonize the infant during birth,

others are introduced from environmental sites as a result of invasive procedures.

Symptoms and signs

The classical features of meningitis are often absent in the newborn and the signs are usually non-specific. Fever, poor feeding, lethargy, apathy and irritability may predominate. Diarrhoea, apnoea, respiratory distress or jaundice may suggest disease of another system and brief tonic spasms may not be recognized as convulsions. Neck stiffness is rare and the diagnosis of neonatal meningitis requires a high index of suspicion.

Meningitis caused by group B streptococci presents in two distinct ways, depending upon its time of onset after birth:

- **Early onset** (first week of life). This is frequently associated with prematurity or obstetric complications and the organism is from the maternal birth canal. The infant has a fulminant illness with a high mortality. Septicaemia and respiratory symptoms (often confused with respiratory distress syndrome) are prominent.
- **Late onset** (after the first week of life). This is a more insidious illness, with meningitis a prominent feature and a mortality of only about 15%. Infection is often acquired from hospital personnel or equipment.

Investigations

The diagnosis of neonatal meningitis depends upon the LP findings but it should be remembered that in the neonate normal CSF has up to 30 cells/mm^3 (often neutrophils) and a protein concentration up to 1.5 g/l.

Treatment

The treatment usually recommended for neonatal meningitis is immediate empirical administration of a combination of ampicillin and gentamicin. The penetration of aminoglycosides into the CSF is variable and levels should be measured. An alternative is to use ceftriaxone or cefotaxime, which penetrate well into the CSF and are effective against most of the likely organisms, combined with ampicillin. For premature neonates a combination of vancomycin and ceftazidime (to cover staphylococci and *P. aeruginosa*) is used empirically. Treatment can be modified upon the basis of Gram's stain or culture of the CSF.

The prognosis of neonatal meningitis remains poor with mortality up to 50% in premature infants; neurological and psychological sequelae are found in one-third of the survivors.

Other types of purulent meningitis

Shunt-associated meningitis

Up to 25% of patients with ventriculoatrial or ventriculoperitoneal shunts for hydrocephalus develop meningitis.

Most cases are caused by *Staphylococcus epidermidis*; many of the remainder are the result of infection with *Staph. aureus* or Gram-negative bacilli. The route of infection is usually by direct inoculation at the time of shunt implantation and 70% of infections occur in the 2 months after surgery. Systemic and intraventricular therapy with antibiotics (intraventricular vancomycin and systemic rifampicin for staphylococci and an aminoglycoside with or without a cephalosporin for aerobic Gram-negative bacilli) must often be combined with removal of the shunt and temporary external ventricular drainage.

Gram-negative enteric bacilli

Other than during the neonatal period, meningitis caused by Gram-negative enteric bacilli is primarily seen in patients with head injuries, alcoholics, elderly diabetics and those who have had neurosurgery. Therapy should be with a third-generation cephalosporin (e.g. cefotaxime or ceftazidime) until the responsible organism and its antibiotic sensitivity are known.

Listeria monocytogenes

Meningitis from *Listeria monocytogenes* infection is chiefly a disease of neonates or pregnant, debilitated or immunocompromised adults (especially recipients of renal transplants). Meningitis or a diffuse or focal meningoencephalitis may occur and, despite the name of the organism, polymorphs usually predominate in the CSF. Ampicillin, given for

3 weeks with or without gentamicin, is the best therapy. Co-trimoxazole should be used in penicillin-allergic patients.

Lymphocytic meningitis

Lymphocytic meningitis

If examination of the CSF shows an excessive number of lymphocytes and a raised protein but no organisms are seen on Gram's stain, then the likeliest cause is a viral infection. There are, however, other causes of this CSF picture and many of them require specific therapy. These other possibilities must, therefore, always be considered before assuming that the illness is viral in aetiology (Figure 19.1).

Tuberculous meningitis

Epidemiology

Tuberculous meningitis can occur at any age. In children or adolescents it is usually a manifestation of primary tuberculosis but in adults it is frequently the result of rupture into the subarachnoid space of a subependymal tubercle that has lain quiescent for many years.

Symptoms and signs

The clinical presentation is very variable and depends upon a number of factors: the thick meningeal exudate; vasculitis; cerebral oedema; and the presence of tuberculomas. The illness often begins with a period of general ill health and malaise which lasts for a week or two before a slowly progressive headache and signs of meningitis appear. Changes in consciousness, seizures and focal neurological signs, particularly VIth-nerve palsies, then develop.

Investigations

Diagnosis can be confirmed in 10–20% of cases by finding *Mycobacterium tuberculosis* in the CSF on Ziehl–Neelsen stains (a large quantity of CSF, up to 10 ml, should be sent for examination if tuberculosis is suspected), but treatment often has to be given on suspicion when the other CSF results, particularly the glucose level, are suggestive (Table 19.2). In children the chest X-ray often shows evidence of pulmonary tuberculosis, but in adults the X-ray is

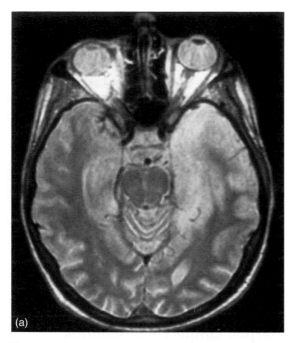
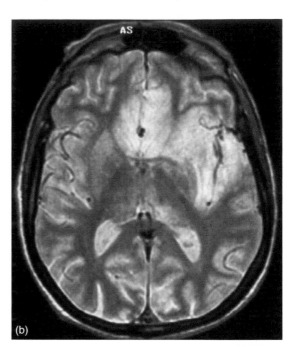

Figure 19.3 MRI brain scans, axial view, showing high signal in the right temporal lobe as a result of herpes simplex encephalitis.

CT or MRI scan (Figure 19.3). The diagnosis can be confirmed by detection of viral DNA (by PCR) or viral antigens within the CSF; CSF PCR has a sensitivity of over 95% in herpes simplex encephalitis (HSE).

Therapy

The drug of choice for the treatment of HSE is aciclovir (10 mg/kg body weight 8-hourly for 2 weeks), which is clearly beneficial providing therapy is started before severe brain necrosis has occurred. **Aciclovir should be started whenever the clinical picture suggests HSE** (i.e. any form of encephalitis for which an alternative aetiology is not evident), but investigations aimed at other treatable causes of the symptoms should be continued until the patient responds or serological proof of HSV infection is obtained.

Arbovirus encephalitis

In many parts of Asia and the Americas encephalitis is caused by various arboviruses (*arthropod-borne*

viruses) transmitted by mosquito or tick bites. Cases are only very rarely seen as importations into the UK.

Rabies

Epidemiology

Rabies is an almost inevitably fatal encephalitis, which is transmitted in the saliva of infected mammals by bites, scratches or licks of open wounds or mucous membranes. Dogs, wolves, cats and bats are the animals that most often transmit the virus to man. There are very few areas of the world where rabies is not endemic (the British Isles are, at present, a notable exception).

Symptoms and signs

The virus binds to and enters the peripheral nerves and is transported along the axons to reach the CNS. The site of the inoculation largely determines the incubation period, which can be many months following bites on the legs. The first symptoms are often non-specific but include itching or paraesthesiae at the inoculation site (often long after the wound has healed). After 2–10 days frank CNS signs of furious or paralytic rabies develop. Excitability and spasms of the pharyngeal and laryngeal muscles induced by draughts of air or the sight of water (hydrophobia) are typical of the former. The illness is rapidly progressive and, despite intensive care, paralysis, coma and death from cardiorespiratory failure are the rule. No therapy is effective.

Diagnosis

Diagnosis in life is by virus isolation from saliva, tears or CSF or by immunofluorescent detection of viral antigen in full thickness skin biopsies from hairy areas at the nape of the neck.

Prevention

Effective vaccines are available: pre-exposure prophylaxis is recommended for certain occupations or travellers, and post-exposure vaccination and immunoglobulin should be given as soon as possible after exposure to the saliva of a potentially rabid animal. Specialist advice should be sought.

Chronic and progressive viral encephalitis

In addition to these acute infections there are several chronic and progressive neurological conditions resulting from viral infections. These chronic infections are exemplified by **subacute sclerosing panencephalitis**, which is a very rare fatal infection caused by a form of measles virus and which becomes manifest as a progressive neurological deterioration only several years after an apparently uncomplicated attack of measles, and progressive multifocal leukoencephalopathy (see below).

Trypanosomiasis

Chronic African trypanosomiasis, caused by species of *Trypanosoma brucei*, may produce a myriad of neurological symptoms, including an encephalitic illness. It is acquired in areas of Africa south of the Sahara and north of the river Zambesi. Specialist advice should be sought.

CEREBRAL MALARIA

Epidemiology of malaria
Although four species of *Plasmodium* infect man, only *P. falciparum* causes cerebral malaria. Falciparum (malignant tertian) malaria is endemic in much of the tropical and subtropical world and malaria should **always** be suspected as the cause of any neurological symptoms in a patient who has returned from an endemic area within the previous 2 months. It is a medical emergency.

Symptoms and signs

Malaria is transmitted by the bite of an infected mosquito and after a short intrahepatic cycle the parasites invade red blood cells. Fever always occurs and often it is not periodic. Non-specific influenza-like symptoms are frequent. In severe disease, endothelial damage and sludging of the parasitized red cells lead to blockage of capillaries and hence ischaemia of vital organs. Cerebral malaria leads to lethargy, drowsiness, coma and almost any CNS symptoms and signs; it can progress to death with frightening rapidity. Haemolysis and disseminated intravascular coagulation compound the severity of the illness.

Investigations

The diagnostic test is examination of a peripheral blood smear. It can sometimes be difficult to differentiate between the species of *Plasmodia* but if over 1% of the red cells are parasitized or ring forms are seen then *P. falciparum* infection should be assumed.

Treatment

For cerebral malaria intravenous quinine therapy should be used and specialist advice obtained.

CENTRAL NERVOUS SYSTEM INFECTION IN THE IMMUNOCOMPROMISED PATIENT

Infections of the CNS are not uncommon in patients with compromised host defences and are often caused by pathogens that do not usually infect the normal host. Abnormalities of immune function are normally classified under one of four headings, each of which is associated with a predisposition to infection of the CNS by certain opportunistic pathogens (Table 19.5):

1 **Defects in polymorph function**. Patients with inadequate polymorph function, typically those with severe neutropenia, are prone to infection with Gram-negative aerobic bacteria (*E. coli, Klebsiella, P. aeruginosa*, etc.) and certain fungi.

2 **Defects in humoral immunity**. Defects in the ability to mount an antibody response are accompanied by an increased risk of infection by encapsulated bacteria and by a rare chronic encephalitis caused by enteroviruses. Such defects are seen in patients with B-cell lymphoma and leukaemia, or myeloma.

3 **Defects in cellular immunity**. Patients with defects in cell-mediated immunity (organ transplant recipients, patients with Hodgkin's disease and other lymphomas, those receiving steroid therapy and patients with AIDS) are highly susceptible to intracellular microorganisms.

4 **Splenic dysfunction**. Loss of splenic function, whether by disease or surgery, is associated with abnormal phagocytic function and lack of opsonizing antibodies and predisposes the individual to infection with encapsulated bacteria.

It should be appreciated that, as a result of surgery or therapy with cytotoxic or immunosuppressive drugs or corticosteroids, many patients have abnormalities of their immune system that fall into several of these categories and are thus prone to a wide range of opportunistic pathogens.

The features of meningitis caused by *Listeria* and *Cryptococcus* have already been described (see p. 391). Brief mention of some other opportunistic pathogens is given below but for all such infections specialist advice is recommended.

Candida

Meningitis from *Candida* infection is usually part of disseminated disease in a patient with neutropenia or following parenteral hyperalimentation. It is a subacute or chronic infection similar to cryptococcosis.

Table 19.5 Major opportunistic pathogens causing syndromes of central nervous system infection in immunocompromised patients

Immune defect	Meningitis	Encephalitis	Brain abscess
Polymorph defect	Gram-negative bacilli Candida	Gram-negative bacilli Candida	Aspergillus
Antibody defect	Pneumococcus *Haemophilus influenzae*	Enteroviruses	
Cellular immune defect	Listeria Cryptococcus Tuberculosis Toxoplasma	Listeria Cryptococcus Toxoplasma Varicella/zoster virus Cytomegalovirus (CMV) Papovaviruses (JC virus)	Nocardia Aspergillus
Splenic dysfunction	Pneumococcus *H. influenzae*		

CMV, cytomegalovirus.

Nocardia

The branching bacterium *Nocardia* typically causes a single brain abscess as part of a disseminated infection.

Aspergillus

Central nervous system infection with *Aspergillus* occurs in neutropenic patients and those with defects in cellular immunity. Single or multiple brain abscesses are found, often in conjunction with a CSF pleocytosis and signs of meningitis.

Toxoplasma gondii

Cerebral toxoplasmosis has become of major importance in patients with AIDS, in whom it is the most common opportunistic infection of the CNS (see p. 405).

Varicella/zoster virus

Visceral dissemination of chickenpox or shingles is not uncommon in the immunocompromised patient and encephalitis may result, usually between 1 and 6 weeks after the rash. Aciclovir should be given.

Progressive multifocal leucoencephalopathy

Progressive multifocal leukoencephalopathy is a rare progressive demyelinating disease caused by a papovavirus. It presents either as dementia or with focal signs and relentlessly progresses to death within a few weeks (see p. 407).

POLIOMYELITIS

The three strains of polioviruses are enteroviruses and, like others in this genus (see above), usually produce an asymptomatic or mild, non-specific infection. Aseptic meningitis also occurs and in a small minority of cases extensive neuronal necrosis, especially of the anterior horn cells in the spinal cord causes paralytic disease.

Epidemiology

Indigenous transmission of poliomyelitis has now been eradicated in the Western world and the World Health Organization's aim is to achieve global eradication of the disease by 2005. Polioviruses are spread by the alimentary route, either via faeces or oral secretions, and, even without vaccination, where poor sanitation and overcrowding exist almost all persons over the age of 5 years have antibodies to all three strains.

> **Symptoms and signs of poliomyelitis**
> The vast majority (90–95%) of infections are not clinically apparent. In the remainder, 2–5 days after exposure there is a 'minor illness': fever, headache, sore throat, vomiting and malaise are common complaints but resolve within a day or two. In a minority of cases (1–2% overall) the 'major illness' follows several days later. This is an unremarkable viral meningitis and in some cases there is no further progression. In about 0.15% of all poliovirus infections, however, muscle pains herald the development of frank paralysis a few days later.
> The paralysis is of the lower motor neurone type with flaccidity and absent tendon reflexes. Characteristically it is asymmetrical, proximal more than distal, affects the legs more than the arms, and progresses over 24–48 hours.

Bulbar polio

In a small number of cases the nuclei of the cranial nerves, particularly the IXth and Xth, are involved. Dysphagia, nasal speech and respiratory difficulties follow. Very rarely the respiratory and vasomotor centres in the medulla are involved.

Post-polio syndrome

Stabilization occurs after the acute phase but many patients develop new weakness, fatigue and pain

25–35 years later. These symptoms may affect muscles not obviously involved in the original attack. The syndrome results from continuing instability and denervation of the motor unit, although the cause of the symptomatic decompensation after several decades is unclear.

Investigations

In any form of neurological poliovirus infection the CSF findings are those of aseptic meningitis (see above). The virus can be cultured from the stools or throat washings (but seldom from the CSF).

Treatment

No form of treatment will affect the neurological outcome once paralysis has become established. Management consists of respiratory support if there is bulbar or respiratory muscle disturbance, prevention of contractures and rehabilitation. Contrary to the acute phase, the strength of muscles affected by the post-polio syndrome may be improved or their deterioration slowed by appropriate exercises.

Prevention

Paralytic polio can be prevented by immunization with either inactivated (IPV) or live oral (OPV) vaccines. Both forms have been widely used in infancy and there has been an increasing uptake. Occasionally vaccine-associated paralysis has been reported and OPV should not be given to immunocompromised hosts or their household contacts.

TETANUS

Epidemiology

The clinical manifestations of tetanus result from the effects of an exotoxin (tetanospasmin) produced by *Clostridium tetani*, a spore-forming, strictly anaerobic, Gram-positive rod that exists primarily in the soil. Disease results after a wound is contaminated by bacterial spores, which then vegetate and elaborate toxin. Tetanus has become rare in developed countries as a result of vaccination.

Susceptibility to tetanus

Any age group may be affected but in the UK most cases are in the elderly, who are often unprotected by vaccination. Any trivial injury may be contaminated but severe trauma with extensive tissue necrosis is particularly liable to infection. Intravenous drug abuse and the traditional practice in some societies of using animal dung on the neonatal umbilicus are other particularly hazardous practices.

Symptoms and signs

The incubation period is between 3 and 21 days (usually 5–10 days), during which tetanospasmin is transported along axons to the CNS. Tetanospasmin has its major effect upon the spinal cord, where it causes presynaptic blockade of inhibitory synapses. This produces **muscle rigidity** and **spasm**, and **sympathetic overactivity**. Many cases have masseter spasm and **trismus** as the presenting symptom. This produces the characteristic sardonic smile **(risus sardonicus)**. Stiffness of the spinal and abdominal muscles also occurs and opisthotonos can result. As the disease progresses, severe spasms of muscles occur and may result in apnoea and choking. Sweating, tachycardia and other signs of autonomic dysfunction may appear. The shorter the incubation period and the faster the progression of the disease, the more severe the illness is likely to be.

Investigations

There are no specific diagnostic tests for tetanus and diagnosis is based only upon the overt clinical signs. The CSF is normal and often there is no evidence of the original wound.

Treatment

Specific treatment should be given with a single dose of human hyperimmune immunoglobulin, 3000–6000 units intramuscularly and metronidazole, 500 mg q.d.s. intravenously for 10 days (benzylpenicillin, although traditional, is probably best avoided, because it may enhance the antagonism of γ-aminobutyric acid by tetanospasmin). Surgical excision of the injured tissue should also be contemplated.

The mainstay of treatment of tetanus is expert nursing and medical care in an intensive care unit. The number of spasms should be minimized by keeping the patient quiet and the use of benzodiazepines and, in the most mild cases, this and sedation may be all that is needed. In more severe cases paralysis and intubation are necessary. Aggressive nutritional support, control of autonomic dysfunction and prevention of pneumonia and pulmonary emboli are all vitally important.

An attack of tetanus does not confer immunity to further attacks and all patients should be given a course of vaccination.

Prevention

Everyone should receive a complete basic course of toxoid given as part of the normal childhood immunizations, with further routine boosters given every 10 years thereafter.

The use of toxoid and hyperimmune globulin should be considered in all patients with wounds and depends upon the immunization history and the type of wound (Table 19.6).

LYME DISEASE

Epidemiology

Lyme disease is caused by *Borrelia burgdorferi*, a spirochaete transmitted to humans from a reservoir in small mammals by the bite of hard-bodied ticks, common in many parts of northern Europe and North America.

Symptoms and signs

Infection may be asymptomatic, cause only the specific rash [erythema chronicum migrans (ECM)] at the site of the bite, or disseminate to many organs, including the CNS.

Primary disease

The first, and often only, manifestation of Lyme disease is ECM, an area of expanding erythema (sometimes with central clearing) at the site of a tick bite, which typically occurred 7–10 days earlier. At this stage treatment with amoxycillin (500 mg t.d.s.), oral cefuroxime axetil (500 mg b.d.) or doxycycline (100 mg b.d.) for 14 days is recommended.

Secondary disease

Some weeks or months later bacteraemic spread of the spirochaete may cause disseminated disease, including **migratory arthritis, carditis and neurological manifestations. The latter include meningoencephalitis with facial and other cranial nerve palsies, and a painful sensorimotor radiculitis.** Symptoms can

Table 19.6 Guidelines for tetanus prophylaxis in wound management

History of tetanus toxoid administration	Clean minor wounds*		All other wounds*	
	Tetanus toxoid vaccine**	Immunoglobulin	Tetanus toxoid vaccine**	Immunoglobulin
Unknown or less than 3 doses	Yes and proceed with basic immunization	No	Yes and proceed with basic immunization	Yes (250U of human tetanus immunoglobulin or 3000U equine tetanus antitoxin)
More than 3 doses	No, unless >10 years since last booster***	No	No, unless >5 years since last dose	No

*A clean minor wound is less than 6 hours old and is clean and non-penetrating. All other wounds are tetanus prone.
**Given as Td (i.e. with the low adult dose of diphtheria toxoid).
***There is little justification for boosting if the person has ever received five doses of toxoid.

be relapsing or chronic. Treatment of neurological disease is with high dose intravenous benzylpenicillin (20 megaunits daily), cefotaxime (2 g t.d.s. or q.d.s.) or ceftriaxone (2 g daily) for 14 days.

Tertiary disease

Chronic Lyme arthritis, a peripheral sensory neuritis and subacute or chronic encephalopathy may occur. The neurological symptoms are a subtle memory and cognitive dysfunction. Therapy is the same as for the secondary phase of infection but the antibiotics are generally given for up to 6 weeks.

Investigations

The diagnosis of ECM is based upon clinical judgement and a history of exposure to ticks. For extracutaneous Lyme disease laboratory support is essential. Culture of the organism is the gold standard but is insensitive. A positive enzyme-linked or immunofluorescence serological assay requires confirmation by an immunoblot for antibodies to individual *B. burgdorferi* antigens. Reliance on laboratory tests such as PCR leads to overdiagnosis in endemic areas.

SYPHILIS

Syphilis is the result of infection with *Treponema pallidum*, a slender spirochaete between 5 and 15 μm in length. It cannot be cultured on artificial media and diagnosis therefore depends upon direct visualization or serological testing.

Epidemiology

Transmission is almost always venereal, although infection can occur *in utero* or as a result of blood transfusion. The true incidence in the UK is unknown but it is more common in urban areas and has increased recently among homosexual males.

Symptoms and signs

The clinical features of syphilis reflect a complex interaction between the organism and the immune system.

Primary disease

One to six weeks after infection, a papular lesion develops at the site of inoculation. This develops into a shallow, painless, indurated ulcer (the chancre) accompanied by regional lymphadenopathy. If left untreated, it heals within 2–3 weeks.

Secondary disease

Multisystem involvement occurs 6–8 weeks later, corresponding to the time of maximal antigenic load. There is a generalized polymorphic non-itchy rash, often involving the palms and soles, moist, highly infectious, condyloma lata around the genitalia, and mucocutaneous lesions. There is a bacteraemia and the nervous system becomes infected. Central nervous system symptoms are rare but occasionally lymphocytic meningitis may develop. Secondary disease spontaneously heals after 4–6 weeks but in one-quarter of patients relapses occur at some time over the next 4 years.

Latent syphilis

During this stage there are no clinical symptoms and the infection can only be detected by positive serological tests.

Tertiary disease

Approximately one-third of patients will develop clinical evidence of late disease as a result of continuing destructive inflammation. This may only become manifest several decades after infection. The cardiovascular system (aortitis), musculoskeletal structures and the **nervous system** (20–30% of cases) are commonly involved. There are a number of varieties of neurosyphilis and more than one can occur in any individual.

Gumma

Gumma is a nodule of granulomatous inflammatory tissue, which may produce the neurological signs of a progressive space-occupying lesion.

Meningeal syphilis

Meningeal syphilis occurs 5–10 years after the primary infection and produces subacute or chronic meningitis. There may also be focal signs as a result of endarteritis of the cerebral vessels. The CSF is abnormal with a mononuclear pleocytosis, raised protein and sometimes a reduced glucose concentration.

General paralysis of the insane

Ten or more years after infection about 5% of untreated syphilitics develop general paralysis of the insane: progressive dementia, speech and thought disorders, long tract signs and exaggerated tendon reflexes.

Tabes dorsalis

The syndrome of tabes dorsalis may be delayed by 20–30 years and results from progressive demyelination of the posterior columns and dorsal nerve roots. It is characterized by ataxia, paraesthesiae, sensory loss and clusters of severe instantaneous pains in the legs or trunk (lightning pains). The loss of sensation leads to retention of urine and faeces, Charcot's joints and trophic ulceration. Optic atrophy and Argyll Robertson pupils (small, irregular pupils that react to accommodation but not to light) occur in tabes dorsalis and general paralysis of the insane.

Table 19.7 Serological tests for syphilis

Non-specific (reaginic) tests
Venereal Diseases Research Laboratory (VDRL)
Carbon Antigen test/Rapid plasma reagin test (RPR)
Specific tests
Treponemal enzyme immunoassay (EIA) for IGG, IgG and IGM, or IgM
Treponema pallidum haemagglutination assay (TPHA)
T. pallidum particle agglutination assay (TPPA)
Fluorescent treponemal antibody absorption test (FTA-abs)

Table 19.8 Treatment and follow up of syphilis

Stage	Treatment	Follow-up
Primary or secondary	Procaine penicillin* 0.6 million units (mU) IM daily for 10 days **OR** Benzathine penicillin* 2.4 mU IM on days 1 and 8	Monthly for 3, 6 and 12 months
Tertiary (cardiovascular)	Procaine penicillin* 0.6 mU IM daily for 17 days **OR** Benzathine penicillin* 2.4 mU IM on days 1, 8 and 15	As above then every 6 months for 2 years
Neurosyphilis or latent disease with abnormal CSF	Procaine penicillin* 1.8–2.4 mU IM daily plus probenecid 500 mg q.d.s. for 17 days **OR** Benzylpenicillin 3–4 mU IV every 4 hours (18–24 mU/day) for 17 days	As for tertiary disease and CSF every year for 3 years
Penicillin allergic patients		
Primary or secondary	Doxycycline 200 mg b.d. or erythromycin 500 mg q.d.s. for 14 days	
Tertiary (all types)	Doxycycline 200 mg b.d. for 28 days	

*Procaine penicillin and benzathine penicillin are not available in the UK but can be obtained by special order.

Investigations for syphilis

The demonstration of *Treponema pallidum* by dark-field microscopy is the method of choice for a suspected syphilitic chancre or condyloma lata.

In the other forms of disease diagnosis is based upon serological tests, which fall into two groups: the non-specific (reaginic) antibody tests and those for specific treponemal antibodies (Table 19.7). The reaginic antibody tests (particularly the Venereal Diseases Research Laboratory, VDRL) are useful as screening tests or for monitoring the response to treatment but false-positive results are common and any positive result in the serum therefore needs further confirmation. A positive VDRL test from the CSF is diagnostic of neurosyphilis. The specific tests recommended for screening are the enzyme immunoassay (EIA) for IgG or IgM and the fluorescent treponemal antibody absorption test (FTA-abs). The IgM EIA is recommended if primary syphilis is suspected. Once positive, the FTA-abs usually remains so for life, with or without treatment, and the test cannot therefore be used to document the adequacy of therapy.

Treatment

Penicillin remains the treatment of choice for all stages of syphilis. The recommended regimens and follow-up are summarized in Table 19.8.

REFERENCES AND FURTHER READING

Begg N, Cartwright KAV, Cohen J *et al.* (1999) Consensus statement on diagnosis, investigation, treatment and prevention of acute bacterial meningitis in immunocompetent adults. *Journal of Infection,* **39**:1–15.

Bleck TP, Greenlee JE (2000) Approach to the patient with central nervous system infection. In: Mandell GL *et al.* (eds), *Principles and Practice of Infectious Diseases*, 5th edn. New York, NY: Churchill Livingstone. pp. 950–959.

Roos KL (1996) *Meningitis: 100 Maxims.* 100 Maxims in Neurology Series. London: Edward Arnold.

Rotbart H (1995) Enteroviral infections of the central nervous system. *Clinical Infectious Diseases,* **20**:971–981.

Tunkel AR, Scheld WM (1995) Acute bacterial meningitis. *Lancet,* **346**:1675–1680.

Whitley R (1990) Viral encephalitis. *New England Journal of Medicine,* **323**:242–250.

CHAPTER 20

HIV INFECTION AND AIDS

L.A. Wilson

Twenty years ago acquired immunodeficiency syndrome (AIDS) was recognized as a distinct illness. During the subsequent pandemic, it has become essential for neurologists, as well as other physicians, to be familiar with the spectrum of associated disorders. Among these, neurological illness is common.

In those with AIDS, 10% present with neurological illness, 60% develop neurological problems, and in those coming to autopsy 85% have evidence of central nervous system (CNS) disease.

About 40 million people in the world currently are infected with the human immunodeficiency virus (HIV). Immune activation following HIV infection precipitates neurological disorders. Later, with increasing immunodeficiency, there occur a rather stereotyped group of serious opportunistic infections, lymphomas and consequences of HIV invasion of the nervous system (Table 20.1). Toxic effects of antiretroviral treatment add to the range of neurological problems needing to be addressed.

AIDS was recognized in 1981 and the causative HIV discovered 2 years later. Since then, 60 million people have been infected and over 22 million have died of AIDS. About 14 000 new infections occur every day (Table 20.2). Sub-Saharan Africa remains much the worst affected area but numbers are escalating rapidly in some other territories, notably Eastern Europe, India, China and Russia. In the UK nearly 15 000 people have died following HIV infection. Acquisition from sexual contact between men and women has come to outnumber sexual contact between men in the past few years. Intravenous drug abuse remains a small, and further declining, contributor to the UK total. Heterosexuals have tended to present with lower CD4 counts than other groups, quite often first presenting as a medical emergency with AIDS.

Table 20.1 Natural history of neurological involvement

Stage	Neurological problem
Seroconversion	Meningitis
	Encephalitis
	Myelitis
	Radiculitis
	Guillain–Barré
Seropositive but well	AIDP/CIDP
	Meningitis
	Polymyositis
Immunosuppressed	Opportunistic infection (Toxoplasma, cryptococcus, PML, CMV etc)
	Lymphoma
	HIV associated dementia
	Myelopathy
	Sensory neuropathy
	Myopathy

AIDP, acute inflammatory demyelinating polyradiculoneuropathy; CIDP, chronic inflammatory demyelinating polyneuropathy; PML, progressive multifocal leukoencephalopathy; CMV, cytomegalovirus.

The evolution of the effects of HIV infection on the body are monitored by measuring the blood CD4 lymphocyte count and the viral load (the number of 'copies' of HIV ribonucleic acid (RNA)/ml of blood). The CD4 count gives an indication of the current state of the immune system and thereby the likelihood of further problems and the appropriateness of initiating treatment, while the viral load gives an indication of the likely rate of decline in immune function and hence the proximity of further illness.

Where it has been made available, since 1996, modern combination treatment – highly active anti-retroviral treatment (HAART) – with at least three antiretroviral agents has dramatically altered the outlook for both adults and children with HIV infection. Patients feel much better, opportunistic infections (Table 20.3) are much less common, the need for

Table 20.2 Epidemiology

AIDS recognized 1981
HIV discovered 1983
HAART introduced 1996
60 million infected
22 million AIDS deaths
14 000 new infections daily
Almost half are women

HAART, highly active antiretroviral treatment.

Table 20.3 Opportunistic infections in the nervous system

CMV encephalitis
Zoster encephalitis
Herpes simplex encephalitis
Toxoplasmosis
Cryptococcal meningitis
PML
Candida/nocardia abscesses*
Histoplasmosis*
Coccidiomycosis*
Aspergillosis*
*Relatively rare

CMV, cytomegalovirus; PML, progressive multifocal leukoencephalopathy.

maintenance antimicrobial treatments has reduced, AIDS has become less common and death rates have dramatically fallen, despite an on-going steady rise in the prevalence of HIV infection. However, such therapy requires expert supervision to achieve the best results, with a need to maximize effectiveness, minimize toxicity, ensure adherence to reduce resistance, and to make appropriate changes in the context of toxicity or loss of benefit.

NEUROLOGICAL DISEASE FOLLOWING ACUTE INFECTION

Acute HIV infection is often not associated with any symptoms. Seroconversion usually occurs in 4–6 weeks. By this stage the viral load is very high, the blood CD4 count has fallen, and infectivity is high; HIV enters the CNS during this phase. With seroconversion, about half of patients develop a short-lived febrile illness with rash, malaise and lymphadenopathy. Occasionally this is complicated by a self-limiting neurological disorder with encephalitis, transverse myelitis, aseptic meningitis, peripheral neuropathy or polymyositis (Table 20.1 and Table 20.4).

As the immune response develops, antibody can be detected, the viral load falls to plateau at a 'set point' and the CD4 level recovers. The plateau viral load gives some indication of the likely time to subsequent development of AIDS. The ensuing, mostly asymptomatic, years see an increased likelihood of disorders resulting from immunostimulation, and especially Guillain–Barré syndrome in the neurological domain. Chronic inflammatory demyelinating

Table 20.4 Frequency of neurological involvement

Clinical	At seroconversion	Rare
	In asymptomatic period	Rare
	At presentation of AIDS	10%
	Symptomatic in AIDS	30–40%
Autopsy	Brain	90%
	Spinal cord	50%
	Peripheral nerve	100%
	Muscle	90%

polyneuropathy also occurs. **Minor abnormalities of the cerebrospinal fluid (CSF) constituents are common throughout this time**. Underlying HIV infection should be considered in any patient with Guillain–Barré syndrome where lymphocytes are prominent in the CSF, levels usually being of the order of 15–50 cells/mm^3. Treatment is the same as when HIV infection is not present.

Mononeuritis multiplex may present in the context of a CD4 count above 200 cells/mm^3 and is also probably then immune mediated, usually improving spontaneously or with steroid treatment. The diffuse infiltrative lymphocytosis syndrome is rare as the basis for peripheral neuropathy. A CD8 lymphocytosis and multi-organ involvement with salivary and lymph gland enlargement and sicca syndrome should raise suspicion.

OPPORTUNISTIC INFECTIONS

Cryptococcal meningitis (Table 20.5)

Cryptococcus neoformans is a fungus commonly found in soil contaminated by bird excrement. Entering the body through the lungs, it may spread via blood to the perivascular spaces and meninges of the brain. Virchow–Robin spaces can sometimes be seen on magnetic resonance imaging (MRI) to be dilated by perivascular cryptococcal infiltration, giving a pepper pot appearance in the basal ganglia. Cryptococcus is the commonest cause of meningitis in AIDS in the UK. The CD4 count is nearly always below 100. Some have developed the illness during immune reconstitution with HAART.

The illness evolves slowly over several weeks and more than half of cases do not show meningism. Headache and fever are usual, followed by increasing confusion, malaise and liability to seizures (Table 20.5). Other illnesses may present similarly, especially toxoplasmosis, tuberculous meningitis (TBM), cytomegalovirus (CMV) encephalitis and lymphoma. Changes in the CSF may be minimal or absent, although a low sugar increases suspicion. India ink staining is only positive in 75% and the most reliable test is the **cryptococcal antigen** titre in blood and **CSF**. Titres over 1:1024 are associated with a poor outcome, as are visual abnormalities, altered mental state and a positive CSF culture of cryptococcus.

Treatment (see p. 392) should be with amphotericin B by central venous line, with or without flucytosine. Oral fluconazole may suffice for less severe cases. Where the intracranial pressure is dangerously high, repeated lumbar puncture to lower pressure may be necessary to reduce symptoms and protect vision. Fluconazole has proven effective as maintenance prophylaxis but restoration of immune function by HAART allows prophylaxis to be discontinued.

Toxoplasmosis (Table 20.6)

Illness caused by activation of toxoplasmosis in the brain affects about 8% of AIDS patients in the UK. Patients may present to hospital as a medical emergency, not aware of having HIV infection. The CD4 count is usually below 200. *Toxoplasma gondii* is transmitted by eating raw or undercooked meat or from material contaminated by cat faeces. In the

Table 20.5 Symptoms of cryptococcal meningitis

Headache
Confused
Drowsy
Neck stiffness
±Papilloedema
Cryptococcal antigen in blood
Cryptococcal antigen in CSF
India ink stain ± culture CSF

Table 20.6 Symptoms of toxoplasmosis

Headache
Fever
Confusion
Drowsy
Seizures
Focal deficit
Multiple ring enhancing brain abscesses
Serum antibodies

UK, about half the population have been exposed and toxoplasmosis is very unlikely in those who are seronegative. With widespread use of HAART, rates have fallen markedly.

The sub-acute development of headache, fever and malaise is followed by increasing confusion, liability to seizures and focal neurological deficit (Table 20.6), determined by the distribution of abscess formation. Common deficits include hemiparesis, hemianopia and movement disorders such as hemiballismus.

Brain scans (Figure 20.1) usually **show ring enhancing lesions with a predilection for the basal ganglia and corticomedullary junctions**. Abscesses are often multiple and MRI may be more helpful than CT in detecting multiple lesions, which may also occur in the posterior fossa. The differential diagnosis with tuberculomas and lymphoma may be difficult.

Treatment with sulfadiazine and pyrimethamine should continue for 6 weeks where the clinical and radiological features are in keeping with the disorder. Clindamycin is an alternative to sulfadiazine if there is allergy or toxicity. **Failure of clinical improvement on treatment within 2 weeks and radiological improvement within 3 weeks, mean the diagnosis should be reviewed and biopsy of brain lesions considered**, especially in those who are seronegative. Maintenance therapy after acute treatment was essential, prior to the use of HAART, but now may be discontinued if the CD4 count rises above 200.

Cytomegalovirus infection (Table 20.7)

Cytomegalovirus (CMV) is especially common in the population at risk of HIV infection. Diagnosis is often difficult, not least given the possible coincidental presence of the virus. However, recent improvements in assaying and monitoring the virus, and in treatment regimens, have allowed better identification and management. Most patients with CMV neurological illness have advanced HIV disease with a very low CD4 count. Often there is a concurrent **CMV retinitis** (Figure 20.2). Neurological effects are diverse (Table 20.7) and include a **mononeuritis multiplex** and a

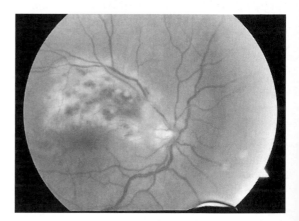

Figure 20.2 Fundus photograph showing the haemorrhagic appearances of cytomegalovirus retinitis (illustration kindly provided by Dr P Frith).

Table 20.7 Neurological effects of cytomegalovirus infection in AIDS

| Encephalitis |
| Ventriculitis |
| Myelitis |
| Radiculitis |
| Neuropathy |

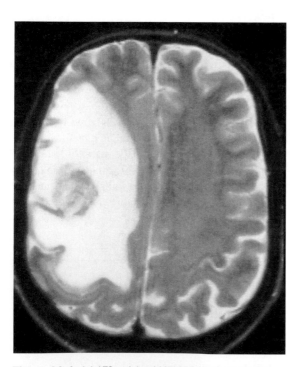

Figure 20.1 Axial T2-weighted MRI brain scan showing a toxoplasma abscess with surrounding oedema and mass effect.

progressive **radiculopathy**. The latter (see p. 165) may affect the lumbosacral roots causing severe pain with paraesthesiae in the perineum and legs, and lead to a progressive flaccid paraparesis. The CSF shows a polymorphonuclear pleocytosis and the polymerase chain reaction (PCR) for CMV DNA is usually positive. An MRI scan may show enhancement of the meninges in the conus and lumbar region.

The brain may be affected with a resulting **encephalitis**, causing effects varying from reduced attention and verbal skills to a rapidly evolving confusion and disorientation progressing to dementia, which often proves fatal. The speed of progression is usually much faster than that of primary HIV encephalopathy and the presence of a CMV retinitis further supports the diagnosis. Brainstem involvement may also occur. Pathological study shows two separate patterns, either there may be a diffuse micronodular encephalitis, with widespread microglial nodules and inclusion-bearing cells throughout the cerebral hemispheres, or invasion of the brain via the CSF with marked involvement of ependymal cells and then progressive involvement of the subependymal layers in the periventricular brain. An MRI scan reflects these findings with patchy diffuse abnormal signal in the cerebral white matter, similar to that which may be seen with HIV encephalitis, but sometimes with ventricular enhancement, which is particularly suggestive of CMV. It is exceptional to culture CMV from the CSF. However, the presence of CMV DNA by PCR helps confirm the diagnosis.

Treatment is with ganciclovir and foscarnet, and new drugs are becoming available, with on-going studies to determine the best regimen. Since the developments in antiretroviral treatment have taken place, improved CD4 levels have been associated with a substantial fall in the frequency of CMV disease and the success with this treatment has allowed cessation of CMV prophylaxis.

Progressive multifocal leukoencephalopathy (Table 20.8)

Progressive multifocal leukoencephalopathy (PML) is the result of infection of oligodendrocytes with JC virus (after initials of index patient), a papovavirus

Table 20.8 Epidemiology and symptoms of progressive multifocal leukoencephalopathy

2–3% of AIDS patients
Papovavirus causing patchy foci of demyelination
Focal presentation
Motor
Limb weakness
Hemiparesis
Facial weakness
Cognitive impairment
Visual field defect
Ataxia
Headache
Speech upset

latent in the bodies of most healthy adults. The immunosuppression of AIDS results in spread of reactivated virus or primary infection to the brain in about 4% of such patients. Destruction of oligodendrocytes leads to progressive clinical deterioration, including hemiparesis, hemianopia, mental change and ataxia.

Progressive multifocal leukoencephalopathy
In contrast to the drowsy confused patient with abscesses or lymphoma, the patient with PML is usually alert, has only modest headache and no fever. Hemiparesis and visual field defects are common and, as the disease progresses and more areas become demyelinated, cognitive impairment develops and seizures may occur.

MRI typically shows asymmetrical signal changes with little mass effect or contrast enhancement. The white matter is affected in the cerebral hemispheres (Figure 20.3), brain stem, cerebellum and occasionally the spinal cord. There is involvement of the posterior fossa in 30% of cases. However, the distinction from other processes in the brain may remain very difficult. Testing with PCR for JC DNA in the blood is of little help, as it is not much more frequently positive than in control patients; PCR in the CSF may be more helpful but may also be negative. Biopsy of the abnormal areas shows multiple asymmetric foci of demyelination with associated bizarre giant astrocytes, and abnormal oligodendrocytes

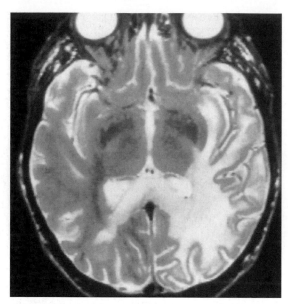

Figure 20.3 Axial T2-weighted MRI showing area of progressive multifocal leukoencephalopathy with no mass effect.

with intranuclear inclusions. The virus can be demonstrated in these cells.

Despite many reports to the contrary, there is no effective treatment. Survival before HAART was very poor, averaging 2–4 months. However, since the advent of HAART, a proportion of patients have shown clinical and radiological improvement and prolonged survival. Patients with a relatively high CD4 count, or with PML as the presentation of AIDS, tend to do better.

Tuberculosis

HIV infection increases the risk of tuberculosis, both primary and as a result of reactivation. It also increases the risk of extrapulmonary tuberculosis including meningitis (TBM) (see p. 391). About one-third of those in the world infected with HIV are co-infected with *Mycobacterium tuberculosis*. **Tuberculosis is the commonest cause of death in AIDS patients worldwide.** Control measures for tuberculosis in developed countries are associated with a much lower incidence, but increased frequency of HIV infection is found in patients screened or treated for tuberculosis.

Tuberculosis of the CNS often develops insidiously with non-specific features, including headache, lethargy, confusion and seizures. There may be cranial nerve palsies and focal signs including hemiparesis and movement disorder.

Differential diagnosis includes cryptococcosis, toxoplasmosis and lymphoma and may be difficult. Not infrequently, treatment needs to be started on a diagnosis of probability rather than certainty. Hydrocephalus and basal ganglia ischaemia are more often seen on scans in TBM, while target lesions, with a zone of low attenuation between higher central and peripheral attenuation, are more suggestive of tuberculomas than toxoplasmosis or lymphoma within the brain. Testing the CSF with PCR for tuberculosis may facilitate the diagnosis but may be falsely negative.

Treatment of tuberculosis in HIV patients depends on expert knowledge and also access to appropriate facilities. Survival is worse than with tuberculosis in immunocompetent people (see p. 392). Interactions between antituberculous therapy, especially rifampicin and antiretroviral treatment, necessitate complex decisions about management. Introduction of HAART may be associated with an exacerbation of the symptoms of tuberculosis in the initial weeks of treatment. Increasing multidrug resistance further complicates the situation.

Other infective causes need considering. The incidence of syphilis is increased, particularly causing meningitis and meningovascular disease. A non-reactive FTA-abs (fluorescent treponemal antibody absorption) serological test will help to exclude this. Recurrent and disseminated herpes zoster infections are more common.

LYMPHOMA

Cerebral lymphoma is common, developing in up to 20% of patients with AIDS (Table 20.9). The majority of cases are primary CNS lymphoma.

Systemic AIDS-related non-Hodgkin's lymphoma much less commonly involves the nervous system, showing a predilection for cranial nerves, meningeal and epidural involvement rather than the brain parenchyma.

Table 20.9 Tumours of the central nervous system

Cerebral lymphoma
Systemic lymphoma
Kaposi's sarcoma

Table 20.10 Symptoms of lymphoma

Headache
Confusion
Drowsy
Seizures
Focal deficit
Single/multiple enhancing lesions
EBV in CSF
EBV, Epstein–Barr virus; CSF, cerebrospinal fluid.

Presentation is usually with headache, confusion and lethargy (Table 20.10). Seizures may occur and focal neurological symptoms and signs are common, determined by the site of the tumours. Primary CNS lymphoma is multicentric in 50% of cases and is rarely of low grade. There is evidence that such tumours are more aggressive and respond less well to treatment than in HIV-negative people. Usually the CD4 count is low by the time lymphoma develops. Evidence of the effect of HAART on the incidence of lymphoma remains conflicting, but once lymphoma has developed survival seems improved in the context of a successful response to HAART.

Epstein–Barr virus drives increased B-cell turnover, especially in the immunosuppressed, and it is this that probably leads to the tenfold increased incidence of CNS lymphoma. Epstein–Barr virus DNA can be demonstrated in the CSF in virtually all patients with CNS lymphoma. Examination of the CSF may also reveal lymphoma cells. While it may be impossible to differentiate lymphoma from other mass lesions in the brain by scanning (Figure 20.4), periventricular spread, as shown by diffuse enhancement in this region, is particularly suggestive, as is spread across the corpus callosum. The decision whether to proceed to biopsy for confirmation of the diagnosis depends on the degree to which other aspects of the patient's illness limit chances of deriving advantage overall from any treatment.

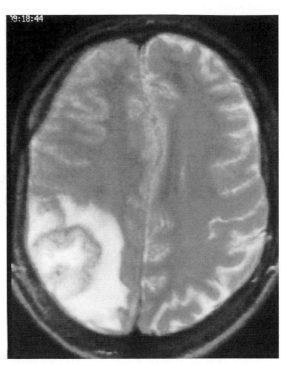

Figure 20.4 Axial T2-weighted MRI showing primary cerebral lymphoma with surrounding oedema and mass effect.

Radiotherapy remains the mainstay of treatment, usually with steroid treatment during this time to reduce associated cerebral oedema. Chemotherapy has a greater role in systemic lymphoma. Rarely, Burkitt's lymphoma and Kaposi's sarcoma may involve the nervous system.

CONDITIONS UNRELATED TO OPPORTUNISTIC INFECTION

Dementia

Dementia, resulting from HIV itself, develops in 15–30% of those with AIDS (see p. 286).

In asymptomatic people, the immune system controls viral replication in the brain and any minor cognitive impairment is unrelated to the presence of the virus. Dementia associated with HIV seldom occurs before the CD4 count has fallen below 50 and

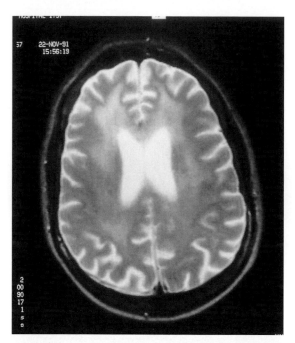

Figure 20.5 Axial T2-weighted MRI showing large ventricles (atrophy) with diffuse increase in signal from the white matter as a result of HIV encephalitis and leukoencephalopathy.

Table 20.11 Differential diagnosis in HIV-associated dementia

Depression/anxiety
Drugs
Metabolic encephalopathy
Lymphoma
Toxoplasmosis
Cryptococcosis
PML
CMV encephalitis

PML, progressive multifocal leukoencephalopathy; CMV, cytomegalovirus.

opportunistic infections have occurred. Dementia as the presentation of AIDS is most exceptional, albeit somewhat more common in children. Replication of HIV in the brain occurs predominantly in perivascular macrophages and microglia, stimulating overactivity of these cells, with the secretion of potentially neurotoxic factors, including cytokines, free oxygen radicals and HIV proteins. It is proposed that the resulting metabolic encephalopathy causes impaired development and death of neurones, leading to dementia.

Dementia associated with HIV usually develops insidiously over months. Apathy, poor concentration and slowing of thought are followed by increasing forgetfulness, neglect of usual activities and deteriorating motor skills. Neuropsychological testing helps to substantiate the presence and degree of the problem. An MRI scan (Figure 20.5) may exclude other causes such as toxoplasmosis, lymphoma and PML (Table 20.11), rather than showing any features that can specifically be attributed to HIV-associated dementia.

Dementia became less common following the introduction of zidovudine. Despite the low CNS penetrance of some of the components of HAART, the introduction of combination regimens has led to further improvements in both prevention and treatment of dementia. While this improvement has been less pronounced than the reduction in opportunistic infections, it is further in keeping with the systemic immune system playing a major role in controlling HIV activity in the brain. However, outcome is variable, some failing to respond and others relapsing after initial improvement. Numerous agents have been tried in attempts to block components of the metabolic disorder proposed to cause neuronal damage.

Spinal cord

Vacuolar myelopathy

Myelopathy with the insidious development of a spastic paraparesis, occurs in about 10% of AIDS patients.

Evidence suggests that up to 30% have spinal cord damage despite the lack of overt symptoms. Myelopathy may be seen in isolation, or in conjunction with features of an HIV-associated dementia. The mechanism remains uncertain; although disregulated cytokine release in response to the local presence of HIV is proposed. Separation of myelin sheaths leads to vacuolation in the white matter similar to a number of other metabolic disorders, including vitamin B12 deficiency. Changes are

Table 20.12 Spinal cord disease

Vacuolar myelopathy
Epidural abscess (IVDU)
Herpes virus myelitis (CMV, VZV, HSV)
Subacute combined degeneration (SACD)
Tuberculosis
Human T-cell lymphotropic virus-1
Syphilis
Lymphoma
Toxoplasma
IVDU, intravenous drug users; CMV, cytomegalovirus; VZV, varicella zoster virus; HSV, herpes simplex virus.

Table 20.13 Types of neuropathy

Lumbosacral radiculopathy (CMV)
Acute inflammatory demyelinating polyradiculoneuropathy
Chronic inflammatory demyelinating polyneuropathy
Axonal sensory (painful) neuropathy
Mononeuritis multiplex
Meralgia paraesthetica
Tarsal tunnel syndrome
Iatrogenic ('D' drugs)
CMV, cytomegalovirus.

most marked in the middle and lower thoracic cord, especially in the lateral columns and then the posterior columns.

The resulting clinical deficit varies from brisk reflexes to disabling spasticity and paraparesis requiring use of a wheelchair. Usually MRI only shows some degree of spinal cord atrophy, but any atypical feature, such as upper limb involvement, additionally requires more extensive MRI to exclude alternative causes such as compression by lymphoma (Table 20.12).

Myelopathy is substantially less frequent in the era of HAART but the efficacy of any specific treatment remains unclear.

Peripheral neuropathy

Peripheral neuropathy is the commonest disorder associated with HIV infection (see p. 165). About one-third of AIDS patients have clinical evidence of neuropathy (Table 20.13).

Inflammatory polyneuropathies occur early, as already described. The development of AIDS is followed by an increasing liability to a **symmetric, painful, distal sensory polyneuropathy**. This may be a result of a so-called primary HIV neuropathy, but is more often seen as a toxic effect of antiretroviral medication.

Painful, tingling, burning feet, often with marked exacerbation with any contact, are typical. Distal loss of pinprick and temperature sensations is present and the ankle reflexes disappear. Paradoxical exaggeration of the knee reflexes is seen when there is concurrent spinal cord disorder. Abnormalities of autonomic function are not prominent, but may occur.

While the clinical features are stereotyped, other causes of leg symptoms are often wrongly attributed to neuropathy.

Nerve conduction studies show the typical features of an axonal polyneuropathy, with increasing loss of amplitude of sensory action potentials, while nerve conduction velocities remain within normal limits or are only modestly slowed. Pathological studies have confirmed the axonal degeneration, which develops by the time of death in nearly all patients with AIDS.

Neuropathy is most often a dose-dependent effect of antiviral dideoxynucleoside analogues, the 'D drugs': didanosine (ddI), zalcitabine (ddC) and stavudine (D4T). There is a lesser liability with lamivudine (3TC). Neuropathy of identical character was commonly seen before the development of these drugs and attributed to some effect of the HIV itself, indirect or otherwise. The more acute development and rapid progression of neuropathy as a result of treatment help to distinguish the two, but only improvement following drug withdrawal may resolve the issue. This is complicated by the so-called 'coasting period', a time of up to 8 weeks following drug withdrawal when neuropathy symptoms resulting from medication may continue or increase, before improvement begins. Improvement occurs in about three-quarters of patients over a 2–4 month period. Better antiretroviral drug regimens should allow a reduction in the prevalence of neuropathy.

Table 20.14 Muscle disease

Polymyositis
HIV myopathy
Azidothymidine myopathy
Pyomyositis

Other drugs causing neuropathy in this patient group include isoniazid, vincristine and thalidomide. Pain is a common symptom of these neuropathies, and is always difficult to treat (see p. 523). Tricyclic antidepressants and gabapentin are first-line options. Many other proposed interventions usually prove disappointing for the patient.

Mononeuritis multiplex in the context of severe immunosuppression may be much more serious than the same condition developing earlier in the disease process. Sometimes there is a severe necrotizing arteritis in which CMV may be implicated. Hoarseness as a result of recurrent laryngeal nerve palsy may be a particular feature.

Muscle disease

Muscle disorders are seen throughout the course of HIV infection (Table 20.14). Clinical and biopsy features are often non-specific in this context, with several different potential mechanisms. At times it may be difficult to distinguish the contribution of spinal cord, peripheral nerve or muscle disease to the degree of any weakness.

Polymyositis may occur early, before the development of AIDS, often with associated myalgia and muscle tenderness. Results of investigations and treatment are then similar to those when the condition is not HIV related. In about one-quarter of patients developing myopathy while on **zidovudine therapy**, there is clinical improvement following drug withdrawal and there is some evidence the condition may be caused by inhibition of muscle mitochondrial function. In those patients who do not improve, the effect of the HIV itself, indirect or otherwise, is thought to be the main determining factor. Pyomyositis, with severe localized muscle pain, tenderness and swelling, is seldom seen in developed countries except in the context of HIV infection. Toxoplasmosis is rare as a cause of a

muscle disease and polymyositis is usually a result of staphylococci or Gram-negative bacteria. An MRI scan may clarify the diagnosis.

Cerebrovascular disease

Stroke resulting from both infarction and haemorrhage is recorded mostly in the late stages of AIDS. Meningovascular syphilis or a vasculitis caused by HIV or zoster infection seem the most common identifiable causes, but cardiogenic embolism (from bacterial endocarditis in IV drug users, marantic endocarditis in terminal disease, and cardiomyopathy) is an important aetiological factor.

SUMMARY

The neurological aspects of HIV infection present numerous and difficult clinical problems. It remains essential to continue to apply the principles of neurological examination, in order to avoid confusion in the localization and likely pathological basis of such problems. Added to this, knowledge of the association of particular disorders with the degree of immunosuppression usually clarifies the differential diagnosis. Coexistent disorders may confuse diagnosis and management priorities, although this has become much less of a conundrum since the introduction of HAART. Most of the neurological disorders associated with HIV infection present in stereotyped fashion, so that a basic knowledge of those described here usually enables correct diagnosis.

REFERENCES AND FURTHER READING

Berger J, Levy R (1997) *AIDS and the Nervous System.* New York, NY: Lippincott.

Carr A, Cooper DA (2000) Adverse effects of an antiretroviral therapy. *Lancet,* **356**:1423–1430.

Harrison MJG, McArthur JC (1995) *AIDS and Neurology.* Edinburgh, UK: Churchill Livingstone.

Manji H, Miller RF (2000) Progressive multifocal leukoencephalopathy: progress in the AIDS era. *Journal of Neurology, Neurosurgery and Psychiatry,* **69**:569–571.

CHAPTER 21

MULTIPLE SCLEROSIS AND RELATED CONDITIONS

R. Kapoor

INTRODUCTION

Multiple sclerosis (MS) is an inflammatory, demyelinating condition of the central nervous system (CNS). It occurs throughout the world, but is particularly common in North America, Australasia and northern Europe, affecting at least 500 000 people in the USA and 80 000 people in the UK, where it has a prevalence of approximately 1 in 800. It is a major cause of chronic disability among young adults in these populations. In recent years, there have been significant advances in management and in our understanding of the epidemiology and pathology of the condition. This new knowledge has important practical implications for diagnosis, counselling and treatment.

PRESENTATION

Multiple sclerosis usually presents with an attack of neurological dysfunction which builds up over days and then improves partially or fully over weeks or months. Following optic neuritis, for example, approximately 90% of patients recover a visual acuity of 6/9 or better, and there is electrophysiological evidence that recovery can continue for at least 2 years. Further attacks occur in time, and such patients have the so-called relapsing-remitting subtype of the illness.

Relapses are more common in early disease, with an annual frequency of 0.8–1.2 per year falling to 0.4–0.6 per year after the fifth year. Patients with relapsing-remitting disease may later develop a gradual deterioration of neurological function, often with superimposed relapses, and are then said to have **secondary progressive MS**. Approximately 40% of relapsing-remitting patients will develop secondary progressive disease 10 years after onset.

In **primary progressive MS**, which affects 10–37% of patients in different studies, disability worsens gradually from onset without true relapses and remissions. Once the progressive phase begins, primary and secondary progressive patients decline at the same rate, with disability severe enough to require aid to walk occurring after a median interval of approximately 6 years. Patients with primary progressive disease tend to present later than those with other subtypes of the illness, men and women are affected equally (as opposed to the usual 3:2 female to male preponderance), and pathological and magnetic resonance imaging (MRI) studies indicate that their illness has a less inflammatory nature.

Approximately 20% of patients, particularly those with relapsing-remitting MS, develop little disability 10 years into their illness, and the term **benign** MS is applied to this group. However, the accuracy of this term has been questioned, as the majority of these patients eventually seem to enter a progressively disabling phase of the illness.

Although most patients present between the ages of 20 and 40 years, MS can occur at either extreme of age, and patients aged below 5 years have been reported. Childhood MS may have a more acute onset, with multifocal features reminiscent of acute disseminated encephalomyelitis (see below), and may take a more progressive course than in adults. Meningeal or cranial nerve involvement can also occur.

Prognostic factors

Among patients with a **remitting course** the following suggest a more favourable long-term prognosis:

- Earlier age of onset
- Good remission from initial exacerbation
- Onset with sensory symptoms or with optic neuritis.

Five years after onset, a more favourable prognosis is associated with:

- Lower neurological deficit score
- Low relapse rate in the first 2 years after onset
- Long interval between the first two attacks.

Primary progressive MS has a poor prognosis because deterioration occurs from onset. This explains the poorer prognosis in men, who are more liable to this type of MS.

Magnetic resonance imaging studies provide additional prognostic information in patients seen during their first demyelinating episode. T2-weighted brain MRI shows lesions suggestive of MS in 50–70% of such patients with optic nerve, spinal cord or brainstem attacks. Approximately 80% of patients with several MRI lesions will develop additional attacks (i.e. MS) within 10 years (versus 10% of those without such lesions), and there is a degree of correlation between the T2 lesion load at presentation and disability after 5 or 10 years.

Less than 5% of patients experience a rapidly fulminant course, and over 80% of patients are alive 25 years after diagnosis. In a Canadian study, life table analysis revealed that life expectancy in MS patients at any given age was only reduced by 6 or 7 years compared to the general population. Severe disability, indicated by an expanded disability status scale (EDSS) of 7.5 or more, was a major risk factor for premature death, with a case fatality ratio roughly four times the rate for controls.

The **symptoms** of MS (Table 21.1) depend largely on where the pathology arises in the CNS, and because any region of the white matter can be involved, the range of presentations is very diverse. Most commonly, single lesions affect the **spinal cord (50%)**, leading to altered or lost sensation, weakness and upper motor neurone signs below the level of the lesion, and sphincter or sexual dysfunction, the **optic nerve (25%)**, giving rise to unilateral visual loss, impaired colour perception and pain on eye movement, and the **brainstem (20%)** with resulting diplopia, vertigo and ataxia.

Table 21.1 Presenting symptoms in MS

Spinal cord (50%)	
Sensory	Tingling, numbness, burning, tight bands, altered temperature sensation, Lhermitte's symptom
Motor	Weakness, heaviness, clumsiness
Sphincter	Urinary urgency, incontinence, hesitancy, constipation, faecal incontinence, impotence
Optic neuritis (25%)	
Unilateral in >90% of patients	
Blurred vision, 'patch' of visual loss, reduced colour perception, pain on eye movement, phosphenes	
Brainstem/cerebellar (20%)	
Diplopia, dysarthria, vertigo, facial numbness/weakness, deafness, paroxysmal symptoms, e.g. trigeminal neuralgia, tonic spasms	
Other (5%)	
Hemiparesis, hemianopia, dysphasia, seizures, cognitive impairment	

Some demyelinating lesions can generate excessive electrical impulse activity, and consequently about 10% of patients develop so-called **positive** or **paroxysmal** features. Again, the nature of these depends on the location of the lesion: cortical plaques can be associated with epilepsy (which occurs two to three times more commonly than in the general population), lesions of the cervical dorsal columns with Lhermitte's symptom (an electrical sensation radiating down the spine, sometimes into the arms or legs, on flexing the neck), and those in the brainstem with trigeminal neuralgia, paroxysmal limb ataxia and facial myokymia. Further manifestations include tonic spasms (painful limb contractions) and intermittent sensory disturbances.

In contrast to more focal presentations, **cognitive impairment** seems to correlate with the total T2-weighted MRI lesion load. Cognitive impairment is rare at onset but ultimately affects between 34 and 65% of patients. Recent memory, abstract thinking, attention and speed of information processing are particularly affected (and are tested only to a limited extent using standard cognitive screening), in keeping with the largely subcortical location of the pathology.

Fatigue is also a common complaint in MS, particularly during relapse, and about 40% of patients rate it as their most disabling symptom. Fatigue is sometimes related to depression, but electrophysiological studies link it more closely to excessive 'physiological' fatigue, which is central in origin. In other instances, rapid fatigability of gait or muscle contraction may relate to the well-known inability of demyelinated axons to transmit prolonged trains of action potentials without developing an intermittent conduction block.

Some patients with ADEM (Figure 21.1) have lesions in unusual sites such as the basal ganglia, or else in a typically symmetrical distribution in the cerebellar peduncles or cerebral white matter, and furthermore oligoclonal bands may only be present transiently in their cerebrospinal fluid (CSF). Nevertheless, the distinction from an initial presentation of MS can be difficult, and in rare cases there may even be one or two further relapses in the year following presentation, before the illness settles.

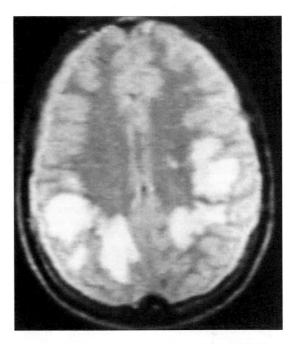

Figure 21.1 T2-weighted brain MRI, axial view, in a patient with post-mycoplasma acute disseminated encephalomyelitis revealing large multifocal cerebral white matter lesions.

Acute disseminated encephalomyelitis

In some patients, symptomatic demyelinating lesions can occur more or less simultaneously in several parts of the CNS. Such cases merge into the presentation of acute disseminated encephalomyelitis (ADEM), which often occurs after infections with agents such as *Mycoplasma pneumoniae*, Epstein–Barr virus and varicella. However, ADEM is more common in children and may be associated with features that are unusual for MS, including fever, encephalopathy and seizures.

Devic's syndrome

Another difficult presentation is that of optic neuritis and a complete myelitis, occurring either simultaneously or with an interval between the two, and without the clinical involvement of other parts of the CNS. These usually have a demyelinating aetiology, with a poor prognosis for recovery. Commonly, there are no lesions in MRI scans of the brain, nor oligoclonal immunoglobulin G bands in the CSF. Vasculitic illnesses or ADEM can also present in this way.

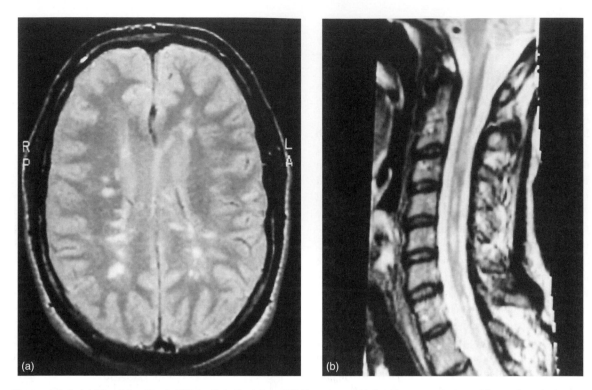

Figure 21.2 (a) T2-weighted brain MRI in clinically definite MS. There are multiple white matter lesions with a periventricular distribution, and involvement of the corpus callosum. (b) T2-weighted sagittal spinal MRI showing multiple intrinsic high signal lesions within the cervical cord.

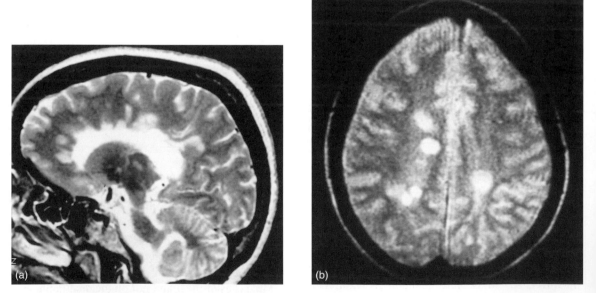

Figure 21.3 (a) T2-weighted brain MRI, sagittal view, showing multiple high signal lesions arranged along the corpus callosum (Dawson's fingers) in a patient with MS. (b) T2-weighted brain MRI, axial view, showing rather rounded prominent high signal lesions in a patient with MS.

Investigation and differential diagnosis (Figure 21.2 and Figure 21.3)

The **diagnosis of MS** depends on objective evidence that typical lesions have occurred within the CNS in different places and at different times (so-called dissemination in space and time). Frequently, this information is clear from the history and examination. If there has only been a single clinical attack, laboratory investigations may provide evidence of lesions in unrelated parts of the CNS. These tests may be particularly useful when the clinical situation is not clear, or if there is a significant possibility of an alternative diagnosis (Table 21.2).

Magnetic resonance imaging

In the absence of a second definite clinical attack, MRI may show evidence of dissemination of lesions in space and, if new or enhancing lesions appear when MRI is repeated after an interval of at least 3 months, of dissemination in time as well. Nearly all patients with MS have lesions in the brain on MRI reflecting the presence of plaques of demyelination (Figure 21.2 and 21.3). These are typically present in a periventricular distribution, within the corpus callosum, in the juxtacortical white matter (involving the subcortical u-fibres) and in the brainstem. Further evidence of ongoing disease activity is provided by the presence of lesions, which enhance with intravenous contrast (gadolinium) indicating disruption of the blood–brain barrier. Multiple MRI lesions occur in other diseases associated with intermittent neurological symptoms, including cerebrovascular disease (e.g. small vessel disease, phospholipid antibody disease and cerebral autosomal dominant arteriopathy with subcortical infarcts and leukoencephalopathy (CADASIL), neurosarcoidosis and vasculitis). In MS it is unusual for lesions to show pathological enhancement beyond 2–3 months, but sustained enhancement (as well as enhancement of the meninges) can occur in neurosarcoidosis. The interpretation of MRI abnormalities becomes complicated in older patients, as roughly 30% of normal adults aged over 50 years have small lesions of vascular origin, often distributed peripherally in the cerebral white matter. An MRI scan of the spinal cord may be helpful in such patients, as cord lesions are rare in cerebrovascular disease, but occur in 75% of patients with MS. It is also important to obtain spinal MRI in patients presenting with a progressive myelopathy, in order to exclude a compressive lesion or other pathology (Table 21.2).

Cerebrospinal fluid analysis

Lumbar puncture may be required when the clinical presentation and MRI findings are not diagnostic, and may help to show that the patient has an inflammatory disorder. An elevated CSF protein concentration or a mononuclear pleocytosis occurs in roughly 40% of patients with MS, but a cell count of more than $50/mm^3$ is unusual. In addition, at least 90% of patients have evidence of an intrathecal immune response, as indicated by the presence of immunoglobulin G oligoclonal bands in the CSF, which are not matched in the serum. However, the presence of such bands is not specific to MS, as they can arise in a number of other chronic neuroimmunological disorders including: vasculitis, infections (e.g. Lyme disease, neurosyphilis, subacute sclerosing panencephalitis and human T-cell lymphotropic virus-1), and possibly neurosarcoidosis. Such bands may disappear on repeat testing in conditions such as ADEM and systemic lupus erythematosus.

Table 21.2 Differential diagnosis of progressive spastic paraparesis

Condition	Investigations
Cord compression/AVM	Spinal MRI ($\pm$ angiography)
HTLV-1 associated myelopathy	HTLV-1 antibodies
Motor neurone disease	EMG
Adrenomyeloneuropathy	Very long-chain fatty acids, MRI (Figure 21.4)
Vitamin B12 deficiency	B12 level, blood count
Neurosyphilis	Treponemal serology
Hereditary spastic paraplegia	Family history

AVM, arteriovenous malformation; HTLV, human T-cell lymphotropic virus; EMG, electromyography.

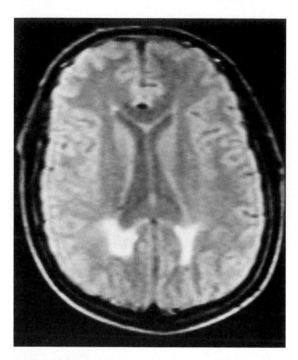

Figure 21.4 T2-weighted brain MRI, axial view, in a 40-year old male with adrenomyeloneuropathy. There are symmetrical posterior cerebral white matter lesions.

Table 21.3 Differential diagnosis of relapsing-remitting MS

Condition	Investigation
Systemic lupus erythematosus	Autoantibody screen
Sarcoidosis	Chest X-ray, SACE, liver biopsy
Behçet's disease	CRP, neuro-ophthalmology examination
Lyme disease	Borrelia serology
Neurosyphilis	Treponemal serology
MRI to exclude/confirm other pathology – also for spinal cord lesions	

SACE, serum angiotensin-converting enzyme; CRP, C reactive protein.

Evoked potentials

Slowing of axonal conduction secondary to demyelination gives rise to the characteristic delays found in visual-, auditory-, somatosensory- and motor-evoked potentials. Such abnormalities often occur in patients without a history of involvement of the relevant pathway (for example, an abnormal visual-evoked potential occurs in 70% of patients suspected to have MS and in 90% of those with definite disease) and may then be taken as evidence of dissemination of lesions in space.

Further tests

More detailed investigations may be required in some cases because of the wide differential diagnosis of MS (Figure 21.3). **Remitting disorders** include neurosarcoidosis, systemic lupus erythematosus and Behçet's disease, although the remissions in these conditions are usually incomplete. Nevertheless, an autoimmune screen, chest radiograph, serum angiotensin-converting enzyme level, and serology for specific infections, may all be indicated. **Progressive disorders** include structural lesions (although

the clinical picture can still fluctuate or occur with a stepwise progression in patients with spinal angiomas and meningiomas), vitamin B12 deficiency, and paraneoplastic syndromes. In younger patients it may be necessary to consider genetic disorders such as the leukodystrophies (Figure 21.4), spinocerebellar ataxias, and hereditary spastic paraparesis, and specific biochemical or genetic testing may be available for these (Table 21.2 and 21.3).

AETIOLOGY

Although the actual cause of MS remains unknown, the disease is thought to represent an autoimmune response to CNS antigens, possibly triggered by non-self antigens or by superantigens, in genetically susceptible individuals. Despite this autoimmune aetiology, MS only occurs in association with a limited set of immunologically determined conditions, including inflammatory bowel disease and ankylosing spondylitis.

A **genetic** susceptibility to MS is suggested by differences in its prevalence in different ethnic groups living in the same environment, and by studies of its occurrence in families; for example, the recurrence risk for monozygotic twins, is approximately 30%, compared to a dizygotic concordance of approximately 4%, a rate similar to that found in siblings. A slightly increased risk for concordance seems to exist for siblings of the same sex, with concordance rates of approximately 4% for male–male pairs and

6% for female–female pairs. The recurrence risk of developing MS for the children of affected individuals is approximately 2%. The recurrence risk in relatives is slight if they have not manifested the illness before the age of 50 years. Susceptibility to experimental autoimmune encephalomyelitis (EAE) in rodents depends on the animals' major histocompatability complex (MHC) background, indicating the importance of the trimolecular interaction (see below) in promoting T cell activation. T cell responses to autoantigens such as myelin basic protein (MBP) also show restricted or limited use of T cell receptor Vβ genes. The search for human susceptibility genes has proved less fruitful. Candidates include polymorphisms in the components of the T cell receptor, genes coding tumour necrosis factor α, and finally genes within the human leukocyte antigen complex. MS is also seen commonly in females with Leber's hereditary optic neuropathy.

An **environmental** contribution to the aetiology of MS is likely because the prevalence of the disease generally increases with increasing latitude, and because those who migrate in youth acquire much of the local risk of MS. Apparent mini-epidemics of MS have also been reported, for example in the Faeroe Islands after the arrival of British troops during the Second World War. A number of infectious agents have been linked with MS over the years, most recently herpes simplex virus 2, human herpes virus 6, and *Chlamydia pneumoniae*. However, there is still no convincing evidence for their aetiological role, and it is notable that the risk of developing MS is no higher in the spouses of patients or in their adoptees.

Effects of environmental factors and lifestyle

Patients often ask about the effects of environmental factors and of lifestyle on the course of the disease. In population studies, viral infections are associated significantly with subsequent relapse, but immunizations, anaesthesia, trauma, and stressful life events are not.

However, associations may exist in small subgroups, such as those with particularly active disease; for example, influenza vaccination does not increase gadolinium-enhanced MRI lesion activity in most patients with MS, but may do so in patients with the most active scans. Killed rather than live vaccines may be preferred if immunizations are truly indicated, and elective surgery might be avoided in an active phase of the illness.

The prevalence and severity of MS are associated with both high and low levels of **dietary fat intake** in different populations.

Pregnancy

Pregnancy was previously said to worsen the prognosis for MS, but recent studies have shown a reduction in the relapse rate during pregnancy, which is probably compensated for by a higher relapse rate in the following 3–6 months. The long-term prognosis also seems no worse in those women with MS who fall pregnant.

PATHOGENESIS

In MS the immune response appears to be triggered when MHC class 2 molecules (expressed on antigen-presenting cells such as macrophages) present antigenic peptides to the T cell receptor on Th-1 lymphocytes, forming the so-called **trimolecular complex**. Myelin basic protein and myelin oligodendrocyte glycoprotein (MOG) are major antigens in EAE, but similar myelin antigens have not been demonstrated clearly in MS. Indeed, it seems that the T cell repertoire broadens progressively in MS and in EAE (so-called epitope-spreading).

T cell homing to the CNS is promoted by adhesion to molecules of the selectin family on the venular endothelial surface of venules, but also depends on the expression there of activation-dependent adhesion molecules of the immunoglobulin and integrin superfamilies. The integrins LFA-1 and α4 β1 on T cells, and their complementary cell adhesion molecules ICAM-1 and VCAM-1 on vascular endothelial cells, may be particularly important in T cell attachment and migration.

The formation of the trimolecular complex promotes T cell activation and the production of pro-inflammatory cytokines including tumour necrosis factor α and interferon γ. An immunological cascade follows in which macrophages and B lymphocytes are recruited, and the blood-brain barrier disrupted. This pro-inflammatory response is modulated by Th-2 cells through the production of additional cytokines, particularly transforming growth factor β and interleukins 4 and 10. In addition, the immune response also generates protective neurotrophic factors.

The cellular response leads to the development of the characteristic demyelinating lesions, or plaques, which occur particularly in the CNS white matter in MS. The plaques tend to be centred on venules, and in the acute stage they are associated with a dense perivascular cuff of lymphocytes and macrophages. Chronic plaques generally contain little cellular infiltrate, and are composed of demyelinated axons and astrocytic fibrillary material. Plaques are usually quite small, but can sometimes be several centimetres in diameter, and can then be confused with tumours. The inflammatory process in MS is now also known to occur in a more diffuse manner throughout the CNS, and indeed the cerebral cortex and even the retina are commonly affected.

Immunological activation releases a number of potentially toxic pro-inflammatory compounds, including tumour necrosis factor α, and free oxygen and nitrogen radicals. These agents, along with B-cell-derived antibodies that activate complement to form membrane-attack complexes, may mediate demyelination. However, at this point it is worth noting that the pathological changes in some plaques are more in keeping with a form of primary damage to oligodendrocytes than with the more usual autoimmune picture, and indeed any given patient may only have plaques with one or other of these two forms of pathological process.

Nearly all of the clinical deficit in MS is caused by axonal conduction block, which was explained until recently by the effects of demyelination. However, inflammation can also block axonal conduction directly, through mediators such as nitric oxide. Recovery from acute relapse seems to occur when the production of these mediators declines and repair processes set in. These repair processes include remyelination, the acquisition of additional axolemmal sodium currents by persistently demyelinated

fibres, and functional readaptation in deafferented regions of the cerebral cortex.

It is likely that patients become disabled if their repair mechanisms fail, or if axons themselves degenerate. Pathological and imaging studies have shown that axons do degenerate even in early disease, and that the level of clinical disability correlates well with the extent of axonal damage. Evidence is emerging that several of the cellular and humoral components of the immune response (including cytotoxic T cells, and the direct toxicity of nitric oxide, glutamate and possibly matrix metalloproteinases) could mediate the axonal injury.

MANAGEMENT

The management of patients following an isolated demyelinating episode remains difficult. There is a natural reluctance to discuss the possibility of MS explicitly, because some of these patients will experience no further clinical relapses, and alterations of lifestyle probably have little impact on their risk of developing MS. On the other hand, the increasing availability of MRI for prognostic information after an isolated episode, and the possibility that disease-modifying treatments may have a role in this group of patients mean that MS is increasingly being discussed at an earlier stage. Either now or later, when a firm diagnosis of MS has been made, counselling should be tailored to the individual patient, and should recognize the anxiety engendered by the mention of MS. Patients often complain that sufficient information and support was not made available to them around the time of diagnosis.

The treatment of MS
The **treatment of MS** is based increasingly on the results of properly conducted clinical trials. However, the natural history of the illness and its variable expression mean that the interpretation of these studies can be difficult.

For example, Kurtzke's EDSS, the most widely accepted measure of impairment, consists of a series of separate rank-order scales requiring non-parametric statistical analysis, has a bimodal distribution in the MS population, is relatively insensitive to change of impairment, and is heavily weighted on ambulation. On the other hand, the EDSS has a reasonable inter- and intra-rater reliability. Efforts continue to identify and to validate other sensitive, reproducible and relevant clinical outcome measures, including scales of quality of life, spasticity, dexterity, and cognitive function. A surrogate, biological measure would also be very helpful.

The best of these markers is MRI for relapsing-remitting disease, although the T2-weighted lesion load does not correlate with the EDSS. The situation appears to be more hopeful with new MR techniques including MR spectroscopy assessing axonal dysfunction using the N-acetyl aspartate signal, T1-weighted lesion load, serial atrophy studies, diffusion-weighted imaging and magnetization transfer.

Symptomatic treatment

A number of clinical problems in MS respond to treatments that do not depend on a knowledge of the underlying cause of the illness. Careful use of these measures can improve quality of life considerably.

Pain and paroxysmal symptoms

Previously regarded as uncommon, pain affects at least half of patients with MS. Back pain is common, and often arises from mechanical factors associated with weakness and immobility of the lumbar spine. Nociceptive pain of this sort can be managed effectively in the same way as in cases without MS, starting with non-steroidal anti-inflammatory drugs, transcutaneous electrical nerve stimulation and physiotherapy.

Neurogenic pain

Neurogenic pain occurs in approximately 10-15% of MS patients. Once again, management is largely the same as for patients without MS, using combinations of anticonvulsants, antidepressants and transcutaneous electrical nerve stimulation, as well as pain surgery in occasional cases. However, sodium channel blocking drugs such as carbamazepine, phenytoin and lamotrigine would increase conduction block and theoretically alleviate pain at the expense of increased disability.

Trigeminal neuralgia

In MS, trigeminal neuralgia is also managed pharmacologically in the same way as the idiopathic variety, and small studies suggest that microvascular decompression and percutaneous thermocoagulation can also be successful in MS.

Paroxysmal or positive features of MS

Paroxysmal or positive features of MS, as well as true seizures, respond well to low doses of sodium channel blocking drugs, of which carbamazepine is the most widely used. A therapeutic response is often apparent using doses as low as 100 mg twice daily, although higher doses may be required, guided by measurements of blood levels.

Ataxia and tremor

Gait ataxia is best managed by physiotherapists and occupational therapists, paying particular attention to the counterproductive abnormalities of gait and posture that patients with such ataxia can adopt. Incorrect use of walking aids may contribute to these abnormalities.

Lesions of the cerebellar outflow tracts can cause a disabling upper limb tremor. Once again, occupational therapists can provide advice on coping strategies, and some patients have benefited from wearing wrist weights, which lessen the amplitude of the tremor. Small studies have suggested that isoniazid (800 mg per day, building up at weekly intervals to 1200 mg per day), clonazepam or propranolol can help some patients. Stereotactic thalamotomy or thalamic stimulation remains an option in unilateral cases, helping approximately 60% of MS patients. Unfortunately, the presence of silent, contralateral thalamic lesions means that pseudobulbar problems can complicate even unilateral thalamotomy. In addition, the initial benefits often disappear as the disease progresses, so that careful selection of patients with stable disease and unilateral signs and lesions remains important.

Fatigue

Depression should be identified, as treatment is feasible and likely to be successful. Fatigued patients with a normal mood are less easy to treat. Most learn to modify their lifestyle to cope with the problem, but in other cases graded exercise programmes can help. Pulsed steroid treatment has been advocated for episodic fatigue, assuming an inflammatory basis. Amantadine (100 mg twice daily) and modafinil (200 mg daily) have also been found to be helpful in some cases.

Bladder dysfunction

The majority of patients with MS experience bladder dysfunction during the course of their illness. This commonly arises from an interruption of the spinal pathways connecting the pontine micturition centre to the sacral spinal cord, explaining the correlation between bladder symptoms and pyramidal dysfunction in the legs, and the fact that sphincter dysfunction is rarely the sole presenting feature of MS. Detrusor hyper-reflexia results in urinary frequency and urgency, and can be treated using anticholinergic agents (**oxybutynin**, 5 mg 2–3 times daily) or **imipramine** (75–150 mg at night). These drugs can exacerbate the tendency of the bladder to empty incompletely and can precipitate urinary retention, so that the **post-micturition residual volume** should be checked after treatment has been started.

Spinal lesions can also impair the reflex mechanism of normal relaxation of the bladder neck or sphincter before the detrusor contraction, leading to simultaneous contraction of the sphincter mechanism and detrusor, and giving rise to detrusor-sphincter dyssynergia. The resulting symptoms include hesitancy, an interrupted urinary stream and a sensation of incomplete bladder emptying. Investigation with urine culture should be accompanied by a measurement of the residual bladder volume using ultrasound or bladder catheterization. Clean (rather than sterile) **intermittent self-catheterization** improves the control of continence in approximately 90% of patients with a residual bladder volume greater than 100 ml. Prophylactic antibiotics appear to be unnecessary.

Patients who complain of frequent nocturnal incontinence may be helped by the antidiuretic hormone analogue DDAVP (desmopressin) taken intranasally at night. This treatment appears to be safe and effective during long-term use as long as fluid overload is carefully avoided. In some patients where severe symptoms are not helped by these approaches, or in whom intermittent self-catheterization is not practical it may be necessary to consider a long-term suprapubic catheter.

Spasticity

Spasticity is a common and often disabling problem in MS, and is related both to an increased sensitivity of the muscle stretch reflex, and to greater muscle stiffness. Effective management is available for mild to moderate degrees of spasticity but the improvement in spasticity must be balanced against ensuing weakness and loss of function, as many patients with weak legs depend on increased tone in order to stand or to walk. There is a clear role for physiotherapy. Correction of gait abnormalities and the introduction of orthoses may be helpful, appropriate posturing and wheelchair assessment are important in more advanced cases, and passive muscle stretching twice daily may prevent contractures. There is also an increasing interest in the possibility that physical training may aid recovery by promoting the functional readaptation of distributed cortical networks in the same way that it appears to do so after stroke.

The gamma-aminobutyric acid-B receptor agonist **baclofen** has been shown to be effective in spinal spasticity and is the agent most commonly used for this in MS. Side-effects include drowsiness, muscle weakness and incoordination. **Dantrolene sodium**, which is commonly used in conjunction with baclofen, acts directly on muscle contraction and is therefore associated with muscle weakness and fatigue as well as drowsiness, weakness and bowel disturbance. Liver function tests should be monitored regularly as rare, dose-dependent hepatic toxicity can be fatal. Other anti-spasticity agents including **diazepam** and **tizanidine**, have been shown in controlled studies to be as effective as baclofen.

Severely affected patients who fail to improve with oral treatment may respond to baclofen delivered intrathecally from a subcutaneously implanted pump. The effectiveness of intrathecal baclofen has largely abolished the need to use more destructive procedures, such as intrathecal phenol installation or rhizotomy. However, selective procedures including dorsal root entry zone ablation (DREZotomy) have been introduced recently, although they still carry a risk of permanent sensory dysfunction. Some patients continue to require assessment for orthopaedic procedures for the treatment of joint deformity and contracture, for example, using tendon-lengthening procedures. Finally, there is now considerable interest in the use of **botulinum toxin** in patients with severe spasticity, either as on-going treatment or as an adjunct to physiotherapy.

Potassium channel blockers

The aminopyridines (4-aminopyridine, 4-AP, and 3,4-diaminopyridine, 3-4 DAP) inhibit potassium channels and widen the nerve action potential, reversing conduction block in experimentally demyelinated axons. These agents act similarly on synaptic potassium channels. Their ability to reverse conduction block in fibres with a critically low safety factor has led to clinical studies in patients with MS, particularly those with severe and progressive disability in whom the symptoms show temperature dependence. 4-AP crosses the blood–brain barrier more easily, and has therefore been studied more intensively than 3–4 DAP. Both agents have a small but significant beneficial effect on disability, but their widespread use has been limited by a narrow therapeutic index. They are associated with significant side-effects, including dizziness, paraesthesiae and abdominal pain. At higher doses they may precipitate an encephalopathy or seizures. 4-AP is currently available for unlicensed treatment of highly selected patients. The drug is introduced at a low dose of 5 mg given once or twice daily, and dosage increments must be titrated carefully to a maximum dose of 10 mg taken three times daily.

Management of acute relapses and isolated demyelinating episodes

Corticosteroids
Corticosteroids are the mainstay of treatment for disabling relapses. However, symptomatic treatment and prophylactic measures against deep vein thrombosis in patients with severe lower limb weakness should not be forgotten.

Corticosteroids are known to have a number of effects on immune function. They inhibit the secretion of pro-inflammatory cytokines by lymphocytes and antigen-presenting cells, and alter MHC class 2 molecule expression. Intravenous methylprednisolone reverses temporarily the breakdown of the blood–brain barrier in acute MRI lesions.

These theoretical considerations complement the evidence from controlled trials that intramuscular adrenocorticotropic hormone, as well as oral and intravenous methylprednisolone, can shorten the duration of relapse. Intramuscular adrenocorticotropic hormone given for 14 days and intravenous methylprednisolone (IV MP, 1 g daily for 3 days) have comparable efficacies. However, steroids do not seem to influence the ultimate extent of the recovery from a relapse.

The majority of relapses are treated with corticosteroids given orally, yet curiously these have been subjected to fewer controlled trials. Indeed, there is considerable uncertainty about the best regimen for acute relapse, but there is a trend towards treatment with IV MP, followed in some centres by an oral prednisolone taper. The usual precautions and contraindications applying to the use of corticosteroids should be observed. The minimum interval between courses of treatment remains unclear, although a practical lower limit of 8–12 weeks is usually adopted.

A minority of patients develop very severe disability during an acute relapse, which responds poorly to corticosteroids. Recent work suggests that some of these patients may respond favourably to a course of plasma exchange.

Disease-modifying treatments

The greatest concern of patients with MS is that their disease will progress to the point of severe disability. Treatments that offer the potential to alter the course of the disease are therefore of enormous importance. To date, there has been some success in developing treatments that reduce the rate at which relapses occur, but many of the available drugs are expensive, require parenteral administration, and have side-effects that reduce their overall impact on the quality of patients' lives. Moreover, these drugs have not been found to have a dramatic effect on the progression of disability over the relatively brief periods of only a few years during which they have been tested in clinical trials.

Azathioprine

Azathioprine is metabolised to 6-mecaptopurine, a competitive inhibitor of nucleic acid synthesis. It is known to suppress a range of T and B cell functions. In a meta-analysis of the results of all published blind, randomized controlled trials, patients on treatment were twice as likely to remain free of relapse after 3 years. Disease progression was also reduced, but only by 0.2 EDSS points. These findings have led to the use of azathioprine (2.5 mg/kg per day) in patients with frequent, disabling relapses. The treatment is associated with gastrointestinal side-effects, marrow suppression, hepatotoxicity, hyperuricaemia and skin rashes, and the blood count and liver function need to be monitored regularly. Moreover, there is concern about the potential risk of cancer in patients treated continuously for 5 or more years.

Methotrexate

The folic acid analogue methotrexate inhibits nucleotide synthesis, and interferes with the production of pro-inflammatory agents including prostaglandins and interleukin-1. It has been used successfully to treat autoimmune diseases, including rheumatoid arthritis, and appears to be well tolerated when administered chronically at doses of around 10 mg per week. In a controlled, blinded study it slowed the progression of upper limb disability, but not of other aspects of disability. These are encouraging but early results, which suggest that methotrexate could have a role in the management of progressive forms of MS.

Intravenous immunoglobulin

Intravenous immunoglobulin (IVIg) has been used successfully to treat a number of disorders with an immunological basis, including neurological conditions such as demyelinating neuropathies and myasthenia gravis. The mechanism of action is not fully understood, but IVIg may contain anti-idiotypic antibodies that modulate T and B lymphocyte activity, and down-regulate cytokine production, antigen presentation and macrophage activity. Treatment with repeated courses of IVIg has been found to reduce the rate of relapse in relapsing-remitting MS in controlled trials involving relatively small numbers of patients, and to reduce the rate at which lesions develop on MRI. Further work is under way, but the treatment is not at present licensed or in widespread use.

Mitoxantrone

The cytotoxic anthracenedione mitoxantrone has a number of actions including a DNA-intracalating ability. In various studies, including a European phase-III trial, it has been found to have significant beneficial effects on MRI activity, on relapse freqency in relapsing-remitting patients, and on the progression of disability in secondary-progressive patients. There is evidence of a dose-response effect, and the drug is commonly infused monthly (12 mg/m^2) with IV MP for 6 months. Apart from the usual cytotoxic side-effects, mitoxantrone can also cause amenorrhoea and can be cardiotoxic at cumulative doses above 140 mg/m^2. Although the drug has been licensed for relapsing and progressive MS, its use is therefore restricted in general to patients with very active disease, assessed clinically and by MRI, and to relapsing patients who do not respond to β-interferon or glatiramer acetate. The duration of treatment is limited by the potential for cardiotoxicity, and treatment protocols include regular and ongoing assessments of cardiac function.

Glatiramer acetate

Glatiramer acetate is a synthetic, random polymer of the four basic amino acids L-alanine, L-glutamic acid, L-lysine and L-tyrosine, with biophysical and antigenic properties intended to simulate those of MBP. Its synthesis and use arose from work showing that fragments of MBP could either exacerbate or attenuate the course of EAE. By mimicking MBP, glatiramer acetate could block antigen presentation competitively and could also induce antigen-specific suppressor T cells. Following encouraging work in the 1980s, glatiramer acetate was studied in a multicentre phase 3 trial involving 251 patients over 2 years, with a primary end-point of relapse frequency. Using a dose of 20 mg given by daily subcutaneous injection, treatment produced a significant, 29%, reduction of the relapse rate from 0.84 to 0.59 relapses per year. Later, it was shown that glatiramer acetate has a significant effect on MRI markers of disease activity, but interestingly this effect only became evident after 4–6 months' treatment, in contrast to β-interferon, where treatment effects are evident within a few weeks. Glatiramer acetate has been licensed for the treatment of relapsing MS. The treatment appears to be well tolerated, but side-effects include injection site reactions (usually mild and transient), and in approximately 10% of cases, a reaction following injection involving anxiety, flushing, palpitations, dyspnoea, chest pain or tightness. These symptoms appear to be transient and do not require specific treatment. Teratogenic side-effects have not been described in animal studies.

β-interferon

The first interferon to be used in MS was γ-interferon, but a trial of its use was terminated rapidly because it caused a dose-dependent increase in the rate of relapse. It is now clear, of course, that γ-interferon is a central, pro-inflammatory cytokine in the immune response during relapse. β-interferon is a glycoprotein with a single amino acid chain, which appears to antagonize the effects of γ-interferon, including the up-regulation of MHC class 2 molecules on the surfaces of antigen-presenting cells. Cytokine release by macrophages is also inhibited, and finally there is a broad enhancement of suppressor T cell function. More recently, modulatory effects on T cell migration have been reported.

In an early trial, natural β-interferon given intrathecally reduced relapse frequency. Subsequently, β-interferon 1b [**Betaferon** (Schering Health)], a non-glycosylated preparation with a serine residue instead of cystine at position 17 to improve stability, was used in a controlled, double-blind trial involving 372 patients with relapsing-remitting MS, mild disability and relatively early disease. At a dose of 8 MIU given subcutaneously on alternate days the relapse rate was reduced by approximately one-third.

MRI scans of the brain obtained at annual intervals showed that, whereas the lesion area increased by 17% compared with baseline in the placebo group, it actually decreased by 6.2% in the treated group.

β-interferon 1a (which has no amino acid substitution and is fully glycosylated) was subsequently shown to have similar beneficial effects to β-interferon 1b on the relapse rate, and on disease activity assessed using MRI, in large, controlled, double-blind trials. β-interferon 1a also increases the time to conversion to MS after isolated demyelinating episodes in patients with MRI lesions at presentation. There are two preparations, **Avonex** (Biogen) (given as a weekly intramuscular injection of 30 μg), and **Rebif** (Serono) (given as a subcutaneous injection of 22 or 44 μg three times each week). There is some indication of a dose-response effect for Betaferon and Rebif, but not for Avonex. However, detailed comparisons of the effects of the different β-interferons are difficult because of the differences in the end-points used in the various trials. All three preparations have been licensed for the treatment of relapsing MS, but despite some early optimism, they do not appear to have any major effects on the rate at which disability progresses in patients with progressive forms of MS.

The side-effect profiles of β-interferon 1a and β-interferon 1b are similar, and include influenza-like symptoms, myalgia, transient nausea, injection site reactions, fever and headache, all of which diminish during the first few months of treatment. Marrow suppression and hepatotoxicity have also occurred, but are rarely serious enough to warrant cessation of therapy. However, the drugs should not be used in patients with decompensated liver disease, poorly controlled epilepsy, severe depression, or who are pregnant. Patients may also develop cross-reacting neutralizing antibodies to β-interferon, and these may blunt its therapeutic benefits. However, the presence of antibodies does not indicate the need to switch treatment in patients who show a continuing clinical response, and indeed a significant number of patients found to be antibody-positive revert to a negative state at some point.

The indications for the use of β-interferon vary from centre to centre. Many neurologists advocate treatment for all patients with relapsing MS, particularly if serial MRI scans show an increase in disease burden. In the UK, treatment is reserved for ambulant patients with relapsing-remitting MS, when at least two severe relapses have occurred during the preceding 2 years, and in whom there is clearly no progression between relapses. Treatment is terminated if patients enter the secondary progressive phase of the illness, or if there is a marked increase in relapse frequency during follow-up, compared to baseline.

REFERENCES AND FURTHER READING

Compston A, Ebers G, Lassman H et al. (1999) McAlpine's Multiple Sclerosis, 3rd edn. London, UK: Churchill Livingstone.

Filippini G et al. (2003) Interferons in relapsing remitting multiple sclerosis: a systematic review. Lancet, 361: 545–552.

Hawkins CP, Wolinsky JS (2000) The Principles of Treatments in Multiple Sclerosis. Oxford, UK: Butterworth-Heinemann.

IFNβ Multiple Sclerosis Study Group (1993) Interferon beta-1b is effective in relapsing-remitting multiple sclerosis. Clinical results of a multicenter, randomized, double-blind, placebo-controlled trial. Neurology, 43:655–661.

Jacobs LD, Cookfair DL, Rudick RA et al. (1996) Intramuscular interferon beta-1a for disease progression in relapsing multiple sclerosis. Annals of Neurology, 39:285–294.

Johnson KP, Brooks BR, Cohen JA et al. (1995) Copolymer 1 reduces relapse rate and improves disability in relapsing-remitting multiple sclerosis: results of a phase 3 multicentre, double-blind, placebo-controlled trial. Neurology, 45:1268–1276.

Kapoor R, Miller DH, Jones SJ et al. (1998) Effects of intravenous methylprednisolone on outcome in MRI-based prognostic subgroups in acute optic neuritis. Neurology, 50:230–237.

McDonald WI, Compston A, Edan G et al. (2001) Recommended diagnostic criteria for multiple sclerosis: guidelines from the international panel on the diagnosis of multiple sclerosis. Annals of Neurology, 50:121–127.

O'Riordan JI, Thompson AJ, Kingsley DP et al. (1998) The prognostic value of brain MRI in clinically isolated syndromes of the CNS. A 10-year follow-up. Brain, 121:495–503.

PRISMS Study Group (2001) Prisms-4: long-term efficacy of interferon-β-1a in relapsing MS. Neurology, 56:1628–1636.

Runmarker B, Anderson O (1993) Prognostic factors in a multiple sclerosis incidence cohort with twenty-five years follow-up. Brain, 116:117–134.

Smith KJ, Kapoor R, Hall SM, Davies M (2001) Electrically active axons degenerate when exposed to nitric oxide. Annals of Neurology, 49:470–476.

Trapp BD, Peterson J, Ransohoff RM et al. (1998) Axonal transection in the lesions of multiple sclerosis. New England Journal of Medicine, 338:278–285.

Yudkin PB, Ellison GW, Ghezzi A et al. (1991) Overview of azathioprine treatment in multiple sclerosis. Lancet, 338:1051–1055.

Weinshenker BG, Bass B, Rice GPA et al. (1989) The natural history of multiple sclerosis: a geographically based study. 1 Clinical course and disability. Brain, 112:133–146.

PAEDIATRIC NEUROLOGY

E. Hughes and J.H. Cross

Neurological disorders in childhood fall into two broad groups: those in which there is a disorder of the central nervous system (CNS) or peripheral nervous system development, which may be genetically driven or result from an insult in fetal life; and those in which there is an acquired abnormality after initially normal development, such as occurs with neurodegenerative disorders or following brain infection or other injury. An awareness of normal processes in terms of anatomical, neurological and developmental milestones is a crucial part of paediatric practice.

DISORDERS OF CENTRAL NERVOUS SYSTEM DEVELOPMENT

Normal development	
Developmental event	*Timing (gestation)*
Primary neurulation	3–4 weeks
Secondary neurulation	4–7 weeks
Prosencephalic development	1–2 months
Proliferation	2–4 months
Migration	3–5 months
Organization	5 months–postnatal
Myelination	Mainly postnatal

In normal development, the term **primary neurulation** refers to the appearance of the neural plate and subsequent development of the neural tube, excluding the sacral segments. This process is dependent on the activity of specific surface receptors to ensure adhesion and closure of the neural tube. Interaction of the neural tube with associated mesoderm results in formation of the dura and axial skeleton. **Secondary neurulation** culminates in the gradual canalization and regression of caudal structures. The vertebral columns grow faster than the spinal cord so that the latter travels cranially in fetal life. At birth the conus is opposite L3/L4 – by adulthood it is at L1.

Prosencephalic (forebrain) development occurs in three phases: prosencephalic formation from the rostral end of the original neural tube, followed by cleavage (to divide the telencephalon from the diencephalon, to form the optic expansions and to create the paired cerebral hemispheres, lateral ventricles and basal ganglia), and then midline development. This last event results in the appearance of the commissural structures (including the corpus callosum), the optic chiasm and the hypothalamus.

Cerebral cortical development can be divided into three main stages but it is important to recognize that these overlap. **Cellular proliferation** takes place in the germinal zones of the developing prosencephalon between the 10th and 18th weeks of gestation with the full neuronal complement achieved by 20 weeks. The brain increases in size over the next 20 weeks, with the occurrence of sulcation to accommodate this. **Neuronal migration** mainly occurs in a radial fashion along microglial extensions that extend from the ventricular ependyma to the pial surface of the

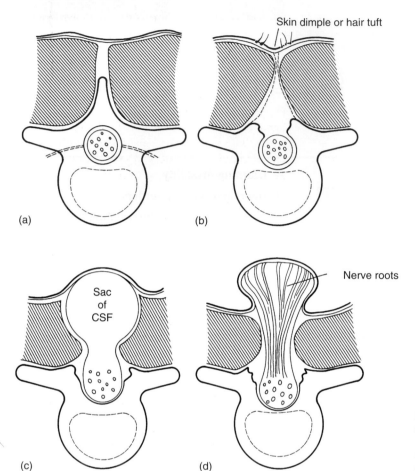

Skin dimple or hair tuft

Sac of CSF

Nerve roots

(a)   (b)   (c)   (d)

Figure 22.1 Spina bifida, transverse sections through the lumbar region: (a) normal; (b) spina bifida occulta; (c) meningocele; (d) myelomeningocele. CSF, cerebrospinal fluid.

neural tube and resulting structures. It occurs in an 'inside out' sequence with neurones destined for the deepest cortical layer migrating first, followed by those destined for more superficial layers. Migration continues as **organization** commences with formation of discrete lamina and development of synaptic connections.

Neural tube disorders (Figure 22.1)

Disorders of primary and secondary neurulation include all forms of failure of the neural tube to fuse completely, with secondarily abnormal development of related mesenchymal structures. Adequate periconceptual folate supplementation is known to reduce the risk of a further affected infant in a family, but remains difficult to achieve in low risk groups.

Specific teratogens such as sodium valproate and retinoic acid increase the risk of these defects.

Disorders of neurulation
Primary neurulation
   Anencephaly
   Myeloschisis
   Encephalocele
   Myelomeningocele
Secondary neurulation
   Occult dysraphic conditions

In **anencephaly**, there is a failure of anterior neural tube closure, which usually results in absence of the skull vault, no optic nerves (although eyes are usually present) and absent or deficient pituitary. The condition is incompatible with prolonged survival: the majority of infants are stillborn or die in the neonatal period. This is distinct from **hydranencephaly**, in which cerebrospinal fluid (CSF)-containing sacs replace most of the cerebral hemisphere structures. This is thought most probably to be the result of a vascular catastrophe in the territory supplied by the internal carotid arteries.

Encephaloceles, in turn, represent selective failure or segmental failure of anterior neural tube closure. They are most commonly seen in the occipital region, where they may be associated with other anomalies, such as brainstem and skull-base deformities and hydrocephalus. Syndromic forms exist such as the autosomal recessive condition, Meckel–Grüber syndrome, where polycystic kidneys, polydactyly, vermian agenesis and facial clefts occur with a posterior encephalocele. The swelling contains brain tissue in most cases and the outcome relates to the position of the defect and to the associated anomalies.

Whereas anterior neural tube defects have a high mortality, posterior neural tube defects, of which the classical lesion is the **myelomeningocele**, are compatible with prolonged or normal lifespan. The majority of lesions occur in the lumbar region and may be several centimetres in diameter. The axial skeleton is uniformly deficient with a variable dermal covering – typically a thin translucent membrane, or sometimes no covering at all. Management relates to the treatment of the primary lesion, detection and treatment of any associated hydrocephalus and of genitourinary, orthopaedic and neurological consequences. A multidisciplinary approach is essential. As the incidence of children being born with this condition declines with improved antenatal detection, and ideally with primary prevention, expertise in the management of these complex children may decline.

Management of myelomeningocele
- Multidisciplinary approach essential
- Early closure of primary lesion may reduce infection and improve neurological outcome
- Detection and intervention with regard to hydrocephalus: ventriculoperitoneal shunt or third ventriculostomy
- Assessment and appropriate intervention for neuropathic bladder and bowel

---

- Orthopaedic management of limb deformity, scoliosis, provision of appropriate orthotics, seating, etc.
- psychological support.

In the mildest form of **spinal dysraphism** there is a bony abnormality only – spina bifida occulta – which is usually of no functional significance. In more major forms of 'occult dysraphic disorders' the main features that may be seen are:

- Abnormally low conus
- Thickened filum terminale, tethered to a dermoid, fibrous band, lipoma or dermal sinus extension
- In 85–90% there is an associated vertebral defect and, on occasions, the cord may be split in two – **diastematomyelia** – and there may be a bony spur between
- Associated cutaneous markers may be the initial clue, typically a tuft of hair, a dimple or tract, haemangioma or superficial lipoma.

Other presenting features of spinal dysraphism (see p. 223)
- Delayed bladder control
- Gait abnormality, sometimes with asymmetric weakness or muscle deficiency
- Foot deformity such as pes cavus or talipes
- Scoliosis or back pain
- (Recurrent) meningitis.

Definitive investigation is now made using magnetic resonance imaging (MRI) and plain X-ray films as well as bladder studies (urodynamics), the latter even where overt symptoms are absent.

Hydrocephalus (Figure 22.2)

The prevalence of congenital and infantile hydrocephalus is between 0.48 and 0.81 per 1000 births. Cerebrospinal fluid is produced mainly in the choroid plexus, circulating through the foramina of Monro, via the third ventricle, through the aqueduct to the fourth ventricle. It leaves the latter to enter the

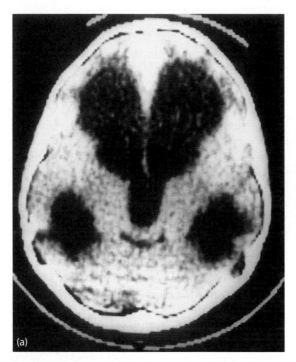 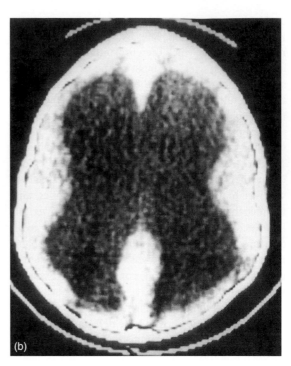

Figure 22.2 CT brain scan showing gross hydrocephalus caused by an aqueduct stenosis. Note the enlargement of the lateral and third ventricles.

subarachnoid space in the cisterna magna, which is continuous with the spinal subarachnoid space. It is generally considered that CSF is absorbed through the arachnoid villi into the venous sinuses, but there is some emerging evidence from flow studies that the main route of absorption may be through the blood capillaries.

There are three mechanisms for development of hydrocephalus:

1 obstruction of CSF pathways;
2 overproduction of CSF;
3 failure of reabsorption.

Congenital malformations resulting in obstruction include aqueduct stenosis (usually sporadic but may occur in X-linked form often with adducted thumbs), Chiari malformation often in association with myelomeningocele, and Dandy Walker association. Bony defects at the skull base may also cause obstruction, as, rarely, may a vascular aneurysm of the vein of Galen. In the pre-term infant, hydrocephalus may follow intraventricular haemorrhage. Congenital infections, or postnatally acquired infections leading to meningitis may cause adhesions and so obstruction to CSF flow or reabsorption.

A choroid plexus papilloma produces excessive CSF rather than obstruction.

In infants, hydrocephalus presents with increasing head size (head circumference deviating away from the original centile), splaying of cranial sutures and a full anterior fontanelle. Superficial scalp veins may be distended and later 'sunsetting' of the eyes is seen with failure of upgaze. There may be delayed acquisition of milestones, especially poor head control – sometimes a specific finding of 'head bobbing' may occur early with hydrocephalus secondary to a third ventricular cyst as in aqueduct stenosis. Once irritability, vomiting and other symptoms of raised intracranial pressure are evident, there is likely to have been considerable progression of the disorder. In the older child, signs are similar to those in adult patients.

The differential diagnosis of a large head in infancy is outlined in Table 22.1. Discrimination between major subgroups has been made much more straightforward by MRI.

Table 22.1 Causes of macrocephaly

Increased CSF volume
  Hydrocephalus
  Glutaric aciduria type 1
Increased cerebral volume
  Neurocutaneous syndromes, especially NF1,
    haemangiomatosis
  Dysmorphic syndromes such as Sotos, Beckwiths
  Primary megalencephaly in cortical dysgenesis
  Diffuse infiltrative tumour
  Abnormal storage as in Tay–Sachs, Sandhoff's
  Abnormal white matter in Canavan's and
    Alexander's
Of extracerebral origin
  Subdural effusions
  Vein of Galen aneurysm
  Skeletal dysplasias such as achondroplasia
Familial macrocephaly

Chiari malformation (Figure 22.3 and Table 22.2)

Abnormalities of the craniocervical junction may cause significant neurological disturbance in infants and children. In Chiari I malformations, there is caudal cerebellar tonsillar ectopia so that the tonsils are below the foramen magnum. Significant ectopia is >5 mm, although greater degrees may be normal in school-age children. This condition may be associated with congenital and acquired craniocervical anomalies.

The **Arnold–Chiari type or Chiari II** malformation involves posterior fossa structures, skull base and spinal column. There is herniation of the cerebellum through the foramen magnum, caudal descent of the brainstem with a cervicomedullary kink in more than two-thirds of patients. The low and narrowed fourth ventricle may become trapped and may herniate posteriorly and inferiorly. The majority of affected patients (>95%) have an associated myelomeningocele and presenting features are related to the primary lesion or to the associated hydrocephalus and much less often to the Chiari malformation. Occasionally, however, signs of cervical compression and lower brainstem involvement may be evident, with difficulty feeding and respiratory distress.

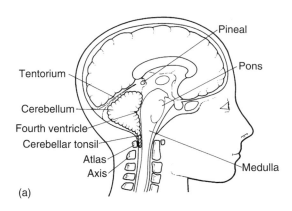

(a)

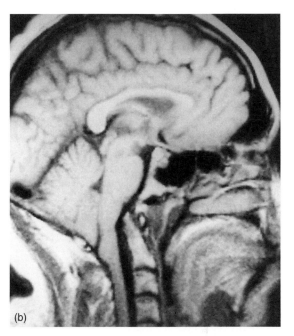

(b)

Figure 22.3 (a) Diagram of median sagittal view to show a Chiari malformation. (b) Sagittal view MRI scan of the craniocervical junction showing cerebellar ectopia.

In **basilar impression** there is upward displacement of the cervical spine, invaginating the base of the skull at the foramen magnum. This may arise as a developmental defect, or be acquired, as in osteogenesis imperfecta. A narrow foramen magnum (without basilar impression) occurs in a number of skeletal dysplasias – the best known of which is achondroplasia. Abnormalities of the odontoid peg, either congenital or acquired, may exist. In Down's syndrome and Morquio's, atlanto-axial dislocation

Table 22.2 Chiari malformation

Type/ classification	Details
Type I	Caudal displacement of cerebellar tonsils below plane of foramen magnum ($\pm$ syringomyelia in 20–75%)
Type II	Caudal displacement of cerebellar tonsils or vermis, fourth ventricle and lower brainstem ($\pm$ myelomeningocele in >95%)
Type III	Herniation of cerebellum into cervical encephalocele
Type IV	Cerebellar hypoplasia

may occur more frequently as a consequence of increased ligamentous laxity. Cervical vertebral blocks are a feature of several syndromes especially Klippel–Feil. Patients may be asymptomatic even though the deformity is a congenital one. A short neck, low hair line and restricted mobility at the neck are common. Neurologically, when deterioration occurs, characteristic features are:

- Ataxia, pyramidal signs, loss of proprioception in upper limbs, nystagmus and lower cranial nerve signs manifest as swallowing difficulties
- Occipital pain
- With or without signs of associated hydrocephalus.

Trauma may precipitate symptoms. This is a particular issue in Down's syndrome where atlanto-axial instability is very common but dangerous instability is unusual. Patients considered to be at high risk should be cautioned against activities such as trampolining or somersaulting. In symptomatic cases of basilar impression, surgical decompression of the craniocervical junction is indicated.

Disorders of cortical development

With advances in neuroimaging techniques, disorders of brain development have increasingly

been identified. They form a heterogeneous group, with clinical features ranging from severe developmental delay and epilepsy to the asymptomatic. Emerging information about the genetic basis for a number of malformations of cortical development may be of major significance when counselling patients. Current classification schemes take as their basis the stage at which cortical development was affected, combined, where available, with information from genetics, neuroimaging and pathology (Table 22.3).

Cerebral malformations will result from disruption of any part of the normal developmental process, that is ventral induction, proliferation or apoptosis, migration or organization of the cortex. Some of the disorders have been found to have a genetic basis; for example, **lissencephaly/subcortical band heterotopia** spectrum, whereas others may occur in the context of an antenatal infection or presumed vascular insult. Cerebral malformations have also been increasingly recognized as part of established syndromes and metabolic disorders.

Failure of ventral induction

Failure of ventral induction refers to the malformations that result from failure of induction involving the three germ layers. This inductive interaction not only controls forebrain development but also the formation of much of the face, so that facial abnormalities are commonly associated. The most common disorder is **holoprosencephaly**, where the anterior part of the brain is undivided, but the severity of the resulting abnormality is highly variable. In the most severe forms, death occurs in the first year of life. In less severe presentations, most infants develop seizures and have severe mental retardation.

Abnormal neuronal and glial proliferation or apoptosis

It has now been recognized that apoptosis also has an important part to play in cortical development. An abnormal brain size may therefore be a consequence

Table 22.3 Classification of cerebral malformations

Embryological event		Examples
Failure of ventral induction		Holoprosencephaly
Abnormal neuronal/glial proliferation or apoptosis	1 Decreased proliferation/increased apoptosis	Microcephaly
	2 Increased proliferation/decreased apoptosis	Megalencephaly
	3 Abnormal proliferation (abnormal cell types)	
	Non-neoplastic	Tuberous sclerosis
		Cortical dysplasia with balloon cells
		Hemimegalencephaly
	Neoplastic	Dysembryoplastic neuroepithelial tumours (see text)
		Ganglioglioma
		Gangliocytoma
Abnormal neuronal migration	1 Lissencephaly/subcortical band heterotopia	
	2 Cobblestone complex	Walker–Warburg
		Fukyama muscular dystrophy
	3 Heterotopia	Subependymal (periventricular)
		Subcortical
Abnormal cortical organization (including late neuronal migration)	1 Polymicrogyria and schizencephaly	Bilateral perisylvian syndrome
	2 Cortical dysplasia without balloon cells	
	3 Microdysgenesis	
Unclassified	1 Secondary to inborn errors of metabolism	
	2 Other unclassified malformations	

of disorders of proliferation or apoptosis. **Microcephalies** may result from reduced proliferation and/or increased apoptosis. **Megalencephalies** may be caused by increased proliferation and/or reduced apoptosis. These findings may occur in isolation or as part of a syndrome in association with other congenital anomalies. A large or small head does not invariably indicate an underlying cerebral malformation. The majority of children with large heads and normal or near normal development have genetically determined macrocephaly. This stresses the importance of measuring parental head sizes as part of the paediatric neurological examination.

Focal malformations thought to result from interference with neuronal and glial proliferation, are now most commonly encountered in children with drug-resistant epilepsy being assessed for possible surgical treatment of their epilepsy. Pathologically, balloon cells are a marker for non-neoplastic malformations resulting from abnormal proliferation. Hemimegalencephaly is an MRI and pathological diagnosis; although classified as a disorder of proliferation, abnormalities of migration and organization coexist. It may be an isolated condition or it may be associated with neurocutaneous disorders, including neurofibromatosis and tuberous sclerosis. The 'tumour' group consists of **gangliogliomas, gangliocytomas and dysembryoplastic neuroepithelial tumours**. These benign lesions have been described histologically comparatively recently and are characterized by the presence of mature neuronal and glial cells. Many will be missed or misinterpreted on CT scan and will only be fully elucidated on MRI.

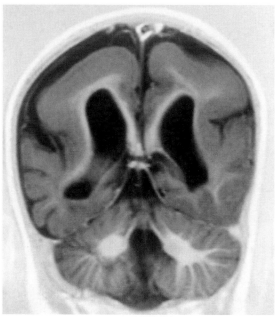

Figure 22.4 Coronal section of an MRI brain scan showing lissencephaly (lack of gyral and sulcal development).

Abnormal neuronal migration

(Figures 22.4 and 22.5)

Proteins regulating microtubule function are now known to be important for neuronal migration. Within families, the same gene mutation may give rise to a diffuse or localized malformation, whereas the gene affected influences the anatomical distribution of the malformation. **Lissencephaly** (literally 'smooth brain') refers to a disorder where there is a lack of gyral and sulcal development. Affected individuals are profoundly retarded and may have epilepsy that is difficult to treat. Several types of lissencephaly are recognized, depending on topographical distribution and presence or absence of associated anomalies, particularly of cerebellar or corpus callosum development.

In classical lissencephaly there are areas of the brain with agyria (absence of gyri) and pachygyria (few broad thick gyri). In one classical subtype **Miller–Dieker** a chromosomal deletion at 17p13.3 also produces characteristic facies with a narrow forehead, long philtrum and upturned nares, as well

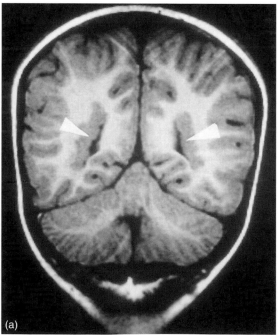

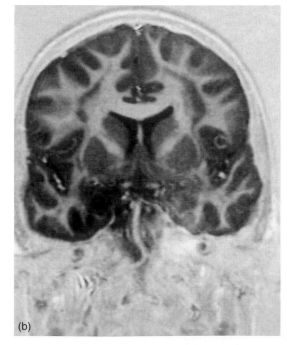

Figure 22.5 Coronal sections of MRI brain scans to show: (a) subependymal heteropias (arrowed); (b) band heterotopias.

as digital abnormalities and hypervascularization of the retina. It has now been recognized that **subcortical band heterotopia** form part of the classical lissencephaly spectrum with a common genetic basis. Other heterotopias may occur sporadically or have a familial, usually X-linked, inheritance.

In **Walker–Warburg syndrome** the cortex is thickened, sulci are shallow, meninges thickened and the cerebellum is small with an absent vermis. Hydrocephalus is commonly associated as well as eye malformations – retinal dysplasia and microphthalmia. This condition and Fukuyama congenital muscular dystrophy are members of the **cobblestone complex**, in which the glial-limiting membrane fails to prevent migration of neurones into the subpial space.

Abnormal cortical organization

Polymicrogyria and **schizencephaly** often occur together and may be a consequence of a number of genetic and environmental causes. In schizencephaly, clefts lined with grey matter extend through the cerebral hemisphere from the ependymal lining of the lateral ventricles to the pial lining of the cortex. Clefts may be unilateral or bilateral and may present with seizures, variable degree of learning difficulties or hemiparesis, depending on the extent and location of the malformation. Several bilateral polymicrogyria syndromes are now well described, of which the best known is the bilateral perisylvian syndrome. Patients present with a pseudobulbar palsy (usually with significant feeding difficulties) and epilepsy.

Associated disorders

Some developmental brain malformations may be associated with inborn errors of metabolism, in particular peroxisomal disorders such as **Zellweger's**, but also disorders of mitochondrial function, and of pyruvate metabolism as well as a number of other conditions. **Agenesis of the corpus callosum** is a common association but this is also often seen in isolation or as part of a syndrome such as that of **Aicardi**. Its true incidence is unknown as many cases are asymptomatic.

CEREBRAL PALSY

The term cerebral palsy (CP) refers to **a group of disorders of movement and posture of early onset, produced by the interaction between a static insult and the developing brain.**

The consequences for motor development will vary with the timing of the insult as well as its extent and localization, and while the underlying lesion may be non-progressive, the clinical picture is an evolving one. Conventionally, children in whom a mild motor abnormality is overwhelmed by other difficulties such as profound learning disability, tend to be excluded. In developed countries the incidence of cerebral palsy remains relatively consistent at between 1.5 and 2.5 per thousand live births. While increasingly sophisticated neonatal care has improved the outcome for many infants, it has also led to the better survival of extremely low birthweight infants (400–1000 g), in whom there is a significant incidence of major motor disability.

Almost any pathological process in the developing brain can produce a motor deficit. Aetiologically it is more helpful to look at risk factors (Table 22.4) for the development of CP. It is now clear that prenatal factors are numerically much more important than perinatal ones and in particular that 'birth asphyxia' is an uncommon cause of CP. However, a fetus that is

Table 22.4 Risk factors for cerebral palsy

Prenatal factors	Pre-term birth
	Intrauterine growth retardation
	Brain malformations
	Fetal circulatory disorder
	Genetic factors (uncommon except in ataxic form)
Perinatal factors	Hypoxic ischaemic injury
	Infections
Postnatal factors	Vascular
	Trauma including non-accidental injury
	Infections
	Prolonged seizure (very rare)

already compromised prenatally may also be more vulnerable to the process of labour. In this regard, continuous fetal monitoring with pH sampling and continuous fetal heart monitoring have proved poor predictors of outcome. Apgar scores – a theoretically objective measure of a newborn's well-being and assessment of need for intervention – are only strongly predictive of the development of CP when they remain low (<3/10) for 20 minutes or more after delivery. In the immediate neonatal period, cranial ultrasound and MRI, evoked potentials (visual and somatosensory) and electroencephalography will increase early identification of 'at risk' infants.

Classification of cerebral palsy
- Diplegia
- Tetraplegia (also called quadriplegia or double hemiplegia)
- Hemiplegia
- Dyskinetic
- Ataxic.

Conventionally, classification of CP has followed a descriptive course – with some variations in terminology acceptable, children are grouped into the following categories: spastic forms (diplegia, hemiplegia and tetraplegia), ataxic and dyskinetic forms. These categories are not mutually exclusive and during the evolution of the disorder, the predominant motor pattern may change; for example, involuntary movements may not become prominent until the second year of life. Marked hypotonia may precede the development of spasticity in the acute phase.

Hemiplegic CP is the commonest pattern in term infants in whom it is prenatally acquired in 75%, although overt structural lesions are not always apparent. Hypoperfusion events in the third trimester are most commonly implicated. It is rarely diagnosed at birth but is usually evident at around 6 months, when the child begins to show abnormally early hand preference when reaching for toys. Fisting of the affected upper limb and altered tone may then be apparent. The lower limb is less affected in term infants, so delay in walking may not be marked and is usually achieved by the age of 18 months unless there are associated learning difficulties. Hand function is most compromised. An acquired hemiplegia may occur in the context of vascular disease, migraine or status epilepticus. Facial involvement is probably present even in most cases with prenatal

onset, but is more prominent in postnatally acquired cases. In pre-term infants, leg involvement is generally more severe. 'Pre-term' hemiplegia has a non-specific association with perinatal events, such as impaired autoregulation of cerebral blood flow, acidosis and hypoglycaemia.

In **spastic diplegia (Little's disease)**, the legs are more affected than the arms, indeed upper limb function may be normal. This is the commonest pattern in children born pre-term, and while previously less often found to be associated with severe learning difficulties, this is changing. The distribution of involvement correlates with the involvement of periventricular white matter. Progressive ventricular dilatation (hydrocephalus) may follow intraventricular haemorrhage – initially secondary to impaired CSF absorption caused by blood debris, and subsequently by an obliterative arachnoiditis in the posterior fossa where blood tends to collect.

Dyskinetic CP occurs most often in term infants – motor patterns are disorganized either by superimposed unwanted movements or by fluctuating tonal abnormalities. Inability to organize or execute intended movement results in major disability, in concert with preservation of primitive infant reflex patterns. The choreoathetoid version of this condition is now less common because of a reduction in the occurrence of kernicterus (bilirubin encephalopathy), and the pattern is now seen most often following perinatal difficulties in the term baby.

True **ataxic CP** is a difficult condition to diagnose with certainty in the early stages – both progressive neurodegenerative disorders and potentially treatable conditions may present in this manner (Table 22.5).

Management

It must be recognized that for many children their motor disability is only one aspect of their special needs. Other problems that may need to be addressed include: feeding difficulties (whether as a result of posture, palatopharyngeal incoordination, oral hypersensitivity or gastro-oesophageal reflux) and respiratory difficulties, which may be a consequence of recurrent micro-aspiration. Intervention by a speech therapist may be very helpful to devise appropriate feeding strategies, but anti-reflux measures, and, in some instances, insertion of a feeding gastrostomy may be required.

Table 22.5 Differential diagnosis of cerebral palsy

Variants of normal development, e.g. bottom
  shufflers
Transient tonal abnormalities in pre-term infants
Hypotonia as apart of syndromic disorder,
  e.g. Prader–Willi, or weakness as part of congenital
  myopathy or dystrophy
Ataxia as part of a progressive disorder including
  posterior fossa and cervical cord tumours,
  leukodystrophies, DNA repair disorders such
  as ataxia telangiectasia, hereditary ataxias,
  e.g. Friedreich's
Dystonia as part of dopa-responsive dystonia
Choreoathetosis as part of decompensation of
  neurometabolic disorder, e.g. glutaric aciduria type 1
Gait disturbance secondary to poorly controlled
  epilepsy

Motor difficulties – spasms, contractures, hip dislocation, scoliosis – may be reduced or sometimes eliminated by the appropriate use of physiotherapy, provision of adequate seating and sometimes lying boards, by drug treatment including baclofen, nitrazepam and botulinum injections. Gait analysis allows more objective assessment of walking patterns, especially before considering orthopaedic or other procedures (e.g. dorsal rhizotomy).

Educationally, the need for effective communication tools cannot be overemphasized, as well as the paramount importance of appropriate positioning for the child so that they can perform to the best of their abilities. Cognitive and sensory deficits and seizures are highly relevant when determining functional outcome. A multidisciplinary approach is crucial, not only to provide an assessment of the child's condition and associated difficulties, but also to plan appropriate intervention and support.

LEARNING DISABILITY

Intellectual functioning is usually measured using a cognitive scoring system such as the Wechsler Intelligence Scale for Children or developmental tests in younger children such as the Griffith's developmental scales, which have been tested for reliability and validity on large populations. A resulting intelligence (or developmental) quotient is obtained, made up of many subscores of selected abilities. Although the overall score allows a comparison of an individual child's performance with others of the same age, it is also useful when monitoring an individual child's progress over time. Variations in scores on individual subsets may allow identification of specific areas of difficulty. It must be remembered that impaired intellectual functioning may be compounded by a delay in maturation and impaired social adjustment.

Learning disability (synonymous with mental retardation) is not a disorder but is a descriptive term, allowing grouping of individuals whose common feature is an intelligence quotient score below 70 points on a standardized test. Within this group, those with severe learning difficulties have intelligence quotients below 50. In functional terms, the presence or absence of other problems, such as epilepsy, sensory or motor impairments, or especially social communication difficulties (autism), is of major significance. Although the prevalence of severe learning disability is accepted to be 3–4/1000, the prevalence of mild learning disability is harder to define but is generally considered to be between 1 and 3% with an increased prevalence in males.

The causes of learning disability can be broadly divided based on the assumed timing of the insult into prenatal (e.g. genetic or developmental), perinatal and postnatal aetiologies. Most studies suggest that the aetiology of severe learning disability can be established in around 80%, with two-thirds of cases having a prenatal origin. However, despite advances in genetics and neuroimaging in particular, a large number of children with mild learning problems do not have a recognized cause of their difficulties. A full history, including pregnancy, delivery, developmental milestones, the presence or absence of seizures and family history is important. Examination may also give clues, especially in the form of neurocutaneous stigmata, dysmorphism, large or small head, or other congenital anomalies.

Chromosomal and other genetic disorders

Cytogenetic studies have an important role in evaluation. Clues to finding abnormalities from prior history and examination include a history of recurrent miscarriage or family history of learning difficulties, other congenital anomalies, microcephaly and other dysmorphic features.

Fragile X syndrome is characterized by the presence of a fragile site on the long arm of the X chromosome at Xq27.3, identified only when chromosomes are cultured in folate-depleted medium. It is one of the growing number of trinucleotide repeat disorders (see p. 128) and the definitive diagnosis can be made by identifying the expanded repeat trinucleotide CGG. Dysmorphic features of this condition are hard to recognize in pre-pubertal children. Evolving features apart from the learning difficulties are a normal or large head size, long face with prominent jaw, large ears and macro-orchidism. Behavioural difficulties, with hyperactivity and autistic features, are common. Women carriers do not have dysmorphic features but approximately one-third may have mild learning difficulties.

Prader–Willi syndrome is associated, in a proportion of patients, with an interstitial deletion in the region 15q11–13, which, in the majority of cases, is of paternal derivation. Other cases are a consequence of uniparental disomy for all or part of chromosome 15. In the newborn period, infants present with severe hypotonia and feeding difficulties. At this stage they are usually of low birthweight but the picture evolves to one of hyperphagia, producing marked obesity in late childhood if intake is not carefully controlled. Learning disability is generally mild. Prader–Willi and **Angelman's** syndrome are examples of imprinting, the expression of the gene being determined by parental origin. In Angelman's, a similar deletion is generally maternally derived. A percentage of patients have either no detectable deletion or a mutation of the UBE-3A gene and are at risk of recurrence. Children with Angelman's syndrome have severe learning disability, jerky ataxia (with underlying cortical myoclonus) and a cheerful disposition – hence the previous term, 'happy puppet' syndrome. Epilepsy is a feature in over 80% of cases with multiple seizure types.

Other chromosomal disorders include the **velocardio-facial syndrome** (sharing a 22q11 deletion with Di George syndrome), in which there are congenital cardiac anomalies, cleft palate and learning disability; **trisomy 21 (Down's syndrome)**, where the chromosomal complement is 47XX or 47XY; and **Klinefelter's**

syndrome (XXY), in which affected males are tall, with hypogonadism and low verbal intelligence quotient.

Metabolic causes of learning disability may easily be overlooked and may have autosomal recessive inheritance. **Phenylketonuria** is screened for in newborn infants in the UK (along with congenital hypothyroidism), and prompt diagnosis allows early dietary intervention. This has resulted in a fall in the incidence of severe learning difficulties in these children, although early treated subjects still have a mean intelligence quotient about half a standard deviation lower than their unaffected siblings.

Conditions with autosomal dominant inheritance include **neurocutaneous disorders**, such as neurofibromatosis and tuberous sclerosis. **Neurofibromatosis 1 or NF1** (formerly known as **von Recklinghausen's disease**) affects about 1 in 3000 individuals, and is characterized by multiple café-au-lait patches and neurofibromas (see Plate 2a). There is almost complete penetrance, but 30% of cases are new mutations. Neurofibromatosis 1 maps to chromosome 17. The natural history of the disorder is very variable but it may cause serious complications in some individuals, especially in relation to optic nerve gliomas, other CNS tumours, hypertension and orthopaedic problems. **Neurofibromatosis 2 or NF2** occurs in around 1 in 50 000 people and is characterized by eighth nerve tumours, but other intracranial and intraspinal tumours may occur. It maps to chromosome 22.

Diagnostic criteria for neurofibromatosis (NF1)

- Pre-puberty: >5 café-au-lait patches >5 mm
- Post-puberty: >5 café-au-lait patches >15 mm
- Two or more neurofibromas or one plexiform neurofibroma
- Axillary or inguinal freckling
- Optic gliomas
- Two or more Lisch nodules (best seen on slit-lamp examination)
- Typical bony lesion, e.g. sphenoid dysplasia
- First-degree relative with NF1

Two or more criteria needed for diagnosis.

The prevalence of learning disability in **tuberous sclerosis** is strongly linked to the presence of epilepsy under the age of 5 years and is now known to be lower than previously thought. Presentation in childhood may be with seizures, especially infantile spasms, with skin stigmata such as hypomelanotic macules, a shagreen patch, facial or periungual fibromas (see Plates IIb and IIc), or with cardiac problems or polycystic kidney disease. Behavioural disorder is common in the presence of seizures. **Incontinentia pigmenti**, an X-linked condition, is lethal in males but girls present with a blistering rash in the neonatal period, with later development of linear pigmentation. Central nervous system involvement with learning disability is seen in up to one-third of cases.

Rett's syndrome is a disorder affecting girls, associated with mutations in the *MECP2* gene but mutations are not entirely specific for this disorder. The disorder emerges after apparently normal developmental progress in the first 6 months or so of life, followed by a period of decelerating head growth, loss of previously acquired purposeful hand function accompanied by an autistic withdrawal with loss of language and the emergence of stereotypic hand movements. There is then a relatively 'stationary' phase, characterized by the appearance of pyramidal signs, scoliosis, respiratory disturbances and seizures in the majority of cases. Progressive immobility and trophic changes in the hands and feet are features of the late stages, when seizures may actually decline in frequency.

Developmental and environmental causes

Neuroimaging with MRI in children with severe learning disability in particular, has provided valuable diagnostic information through the identification of forms of cerebral dysgenesis, other structural abnormalities, evidence for exposure to in-utero infections or for metabolic disorders. Positive findings are more likely in the presence of a motor disorder, abnormal head size, seizures or neurocutaneous markers. **Congenital infection** refers to any viral infection sustained in pregnancy, but those most commonly recognized include herpes, rubella, toxoplasmosis and cytomegalovirus. The incidence of congenital rubella syndrome has declined in frequency with the success of childhood immunization programmes. However,

other viral infections may go unrecognized, and although cytomegalovirus and toxoplasma infections may have suggestive features on neuroimaging, these require confirmation with serology and this may be difficult or impossible outside the neonatal period. Exposure to **toxins** such as alcohol or drugs (both prescribed medicines and substances of abuse) puts the fetus at increased risk of an adverse outcome.

Perinatal causes

There is some epidemiological evidence that perinatal hypoxic ischaemic events are associated with later learning disability but there have been no prospective studies and there is no definite evidence to suggest that perinatal 'asphyxia' alone causes learning disability in the absence of a motor disorder.

Postnatal causes

Congenital hypothyroidism causes irreversible mental retardation if not treated within the first 3 months of life and is also associated with hypotonia, prolonged jaundice and delayed closure of the anterior fontanelle. Head injury which may be accidental or non-accidental may result in permanent sequelae, and in the case of non-accidental shaking injuries there is now evidence that learning and behavioural difficulties may become evident after an apparently 'symptom-free' interval. Meningitis in the newborn period is a major risk factor for motor, sensory and cognitive sequelae.

Miscellaneous causes

Sturge–Weber syndrome is a phacomatosis, also called encephalofacial angiomatosis because patients show an extensive angioma (port wine stain or naevus flammeus) involving one side of the face including the eye. There is an underlying pial angioma and in some cases a choroidal angioma. Early onset of seizures is commonly associated with a progressive hemiparesis and learning difficulties, probably related to ischaemia of the underlying brain. The cerebral angioma usually calcifies (Figure 22.6) but the most

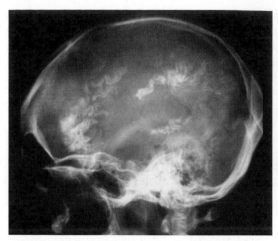

Figure 22.6 Lateral skull X-ray to show intracranial calcification. This pattern outlining the folia is typical of Sturge–Weber syndrome.

accurate way of determining extent is with gadolinium enhanced MRI.

NEUROMETABOLIC DISORDERS

Neurometabolic and other neurodegenerative disorders in children constitute a significant proportion of the paediatric neurology workload. Recognition of the progressive nature of many of these conditions is vital for accurate counselling about that child's long-term outcome, and also because of the genetic implications. The majority of the known disorders have autosomal recessive inheritance.

The evolution of progressive paediatric neurological disorders

Certain features unique to the paediatric population are relevant here:

1 The progressive nature of the disorder may not be readily apparent. This is because the progressive brain disturbance is superimposed on continuing maturational processes so that there is a period in the disease course when developmental progress outstrips the rate of deterioration. Occasionally, with disorders of prenatal onset, damage already evident at birth may be so profound that no developmental progress is observed, suggesting initially a severe static encephalopathy.

2 The age and therefore cooperation of the child may limit formal examination, and observed performance of language and fine motor tasks especially may improve markedly as confidence in the examination setting and the examiner grows. An accurate developmental history from parents is therefore crucial in determining progress.

3 Developmental maturation may unmask new problems without indicating progressive pathology – the appearance of hemiplegic posturing at around 6 months in congenital hemiplegia and of surplus or dystonic movements in the second year of life exemplifies this. A growth spurt may hinder previously acquired walking or sitting skills as may scoliosis or hip dislocation. Seizure disorders are not specific to the paediatric age group, but epileptic encephalopathies of early onset such as West syndrome or later in infancy, Lennox–Gastaut syndrome, may produce a pseudodementia. This may be exacerbated by inappropriate and often ineffective drug therapy, by behavioural disorder or occasionally by secondary damage following a prolonged seizure.

This diverse and often confusing group of disorders may be grouped according to:

1 The underlying biochemical abnormality where known;

2 Age of onset – prenatal, neonatal, infancy, childhood;

3 Predominant clinical features.

Disorders predominantly affecting muscle or nerve have been considered in other chapters so this section will concentrate on those disorders with CNS involvement. Given the large number of conditions under this heading only the major groups of disorders are considered here. While the majority of disorders described have their onset in childhood – many in the newborn period or infancy – adult phenotypes of a number of the disorders are increasingly being recognized.

Aminoacidopathies and related disorders (Table 22.6)

Disorders of intermediary metabolism do not result in storage but have a profound impact on brain development. In some cases this is already apparent at birth – evidenced by the association of callosal agenesis or hypoplasia with non-ketotic hyperglycinaemia – or of macrocephaly in glutaric aciduria type 1. For a number of conditions, neonatal screening allows early dietary or other intervention. In other conditions,

early diagnosis may allow supportive treatment until the infant is old enough for other procedures, such as liver transplantation, to be considered.

A number of clinical features are common in these conditions: vomiting, seizures, encephalopathy. Tachypnoea is a marker of either metabolic acidosis, found in the branched-chain amino acid disorders, or hyperammonaemia in the urea cycle disorders, in propionic acidaemia and methylmalonic acidaemia. Ophthalmoplegia

Table 22.6 Aminoacidopathies and related disorders (main types)

Disorder	Biochemistry	Clinical features
Urea cycle disorders: carbamyl phosphate synthetase deficiency, ornithine transcarbamylase deficiency (OTC)	Hyperammonaemia variable depending on site of block; raised orotic acid in OTC	Vomiting, drowsiness leading to coma, seizures. In late-onset forms, vomiting, anorexia, failure to thrive; later still behavioural disturbance, nocturnal restlessness and overactivity, learning difficulties, psychosis. Arginase deficiency presents with spastic diplegia
Phenylketonuria	Raised plasma phenylalanine	Learning difficulties, microcephaly
Branched-chain amino acid disorders, MSUD, propionic aciduria, methylmalonic aciduria	Raised plasma branched-chain amino acids (valine, leucine and isoleucine), raised ketoacids	Coma, ketoacidosis, hyperammonaemia (not in MSUD). Late-onset cases: recurrent encephalopathy with vomiting ataxia, drowsiness, possible cognitive decline, movement disorder
Glutaric aciduria type 1	Raised urinary glutaric acid, 3 OH glutaric acid	Macrocephaly, movement disorder often after acute illness
Homocystinuria	Raised total homocysteine + plasma methionine, reduced urinary homocystine	Learning difficulties, stroke, lens dislocation
Isolated sulphite oxidase/ molybdenum cofactor deficiency	Positive urinary sulphite, low plasma urate in combined condition	Neonatal onset: seizures, feeding difficulties, spasticity, later lens dislocation, renal stones
Tyrosinaemia	Raised succinyl acetone in urine	Hepatic failure, peripheral neuropathy, Proximal renal tubulopathy
Non-ketotic hyperglycinaemia	Raised CSF/plasma glycine ratio	Neonatal onset: encephalopathy with hiccups, respiratory insufficiency, hypotonia myoclonus, coma. EEG shows burst suppression pattern (late-onset cases with spinocerebellar degeneration)

MSUD, maple syrup urine disease.

is seen in both non-ketotic hyperglycinaemia and maple syrup urine disease. Fluctuating eye movement disorders with sparing of pupillary function should always raise suspicion about an underlying metabolic disorder – this may easily be missed and the infant labelled instead as having a hypoxic ischaemic encephalopathy.

In children presenting outside the neonatal period, intermittent drowsiness, vomiting, ataxia or psychiatric disturbance have been reported. Recurrent attacks are usually precipitated by a protein load, either dietary or catabolic, as with an intercurrent infection.

Mitochondrial and related disorders

Disorders of mitochondrial energy metabolism (Table 22.7) have a heterogeneous presentation, as in adults (see p. 147). Detection relies on a high index of clinical suspicion based on a number of recurring phenotypes, supported by biochemical evidence such as lactic acidosis, characteristic neuroimaging and tissue-specific findings, such as ragged red fibres in muscle. The latter may also be used as a source of mitochondria for DNA analysis in addition to other molecular genetic studies.

Neonatal phenotypes include a fulminant lactic acidosis with hypotonia, seizures, tachypnoea and coma. This picture may be seen in a number of respiratory chain disorders especially complex 1, as well as in disorders of pyruvate utilization. In disorders of the pyruvate dehydrogenase complex, craniofacial dysmorphism may also be evident with underlying cortical dysgenesis – callosal agenesis and subependymal heterotopias. A fatal infantile myopathy, sometimes associated with a Fanconi-type picture or with cardiomyopathy, may occur with complex 1V (cytochrome oxidase) deficiency.

In **childhood**, syndromes resemble those in adulthood and clinical features may include hypotonia, muscle weakness, ataxia, spasticity, seizures and developmental delay. Non-neurological features include failure to thrive, liver disease, renal dysfunction, short stature, cardiac defects, retinopathy or ophthalmoplegia and deafness. **Leigh's syndrome** was originally a neuropathological diagnosis based

Table 22.7 Disorders of mitochondrial energy metabolism in childhood

Transport defects	Primary carnitine deficiency
	Carnitine palmitoyl transferase deficiency
Defects of substrate utilization	Pyruvate dehydrogenase complex deficiency
	Pyruvate carboxylase complex deficiency
	Fatty acid oxidation defects: MCAD, LCAD, LCHAD, SCAD, multiple acyl CoA dehydrogenase deficiency (GA11)
Krebs cycle defects	Fumarase deficiency
	Alpha ketoglutarate decarboxylation defects
Respiratory chain disorders	Complex 1–V

M, medium; L, long; S, short; CAD, CoA dehydrogenase deficiency.

on findings of changes in the basal ganglia (especially putamen) and brainstem. It is now recognized that these changes may occur in the context of a number of different biochemical abnormalities, including respiratory chain disorders.

Other disorders of energy supply including **defects of beta-oxidation of fatty acids**, of which the best known is **MCAD** (medium chain acyl CoA dehydrogenase deficiency), tend to appear later, either as a Reye-like illness or as a cause of sudden infant death. The long-chain defects tend to be more severe and so present earlier. Later presentations may be with predominantly muscle involvement with myoglobinuria, painful muscle crises and cardiomyopathy. Transport defects may appear similarly.

Peroxisomal disorders

Peroxisomes are recently identified organelles widely distributed in the body and responsible for a number of enzyme functions. For diagnostic purposes, their main roles are in beta oxidation of **VLCFAs (very long-chain fatty acids – C24 and C26)**, bile acid and plasmalogen synthesis.

Disorders fall into two main groups, those in which peroxisome biogenesis is defective so that peroxisome numbers are reduced or absent and there is generalized enzyme dysfunction, and those in which there is a single enzyme defect.

The classical example of a generalized disturbance of peroxisomal activity is **Zellweger's syndrome**, that of a single enzyme defect, **X-linked adrenoleukodystrophy (ALD)**. In Zellweger's syndrome there is striking craniofacial dysmorphism with a large fontanelle and high forehead. Infants are profoundly hypotonic and inactive at birth. Neonatal seizures are common and there is visual failure with a pigmentary retinopathy, cataracts and sometimes glaucoma, auditory impairment, hepatomegaly, renal cysts and calcific stippling of the epiphyses, best seen at the patellae. Imaging and neuropathology reveal extensive neuronal migrational abnormalities and death occurs in the first year of life. Milder variants include infantile **Refsum's syndrome** and neonatal ALD.

X-linked ALD (gene maps to Xq 28) presents in boys with gait disturbance or school failure or occasionally with adrenal insufficiency. There is marked phenotypic variability in families – late-onset adrenomyeloneuropathy presenting as a spastic paraparesis may be seen in families with classical ALD. Women heterozygous for X-ALD may also develop a spastic paraparesis.

Confirmation of the diagnosis requires estimation of VLCFA levels, although normal levels in plasma do not preclude the diagnosis and require assay of VLCFAs in fibroblasts.

Lysosomal disorders

Lysosomal disorders are characterized by abnormal accumulation of substrate resulting from a variety of lysosomal enzyme deficiencies. They can be classified into two main groups – those in which lipid storage occurs and the mucopolysaccharidoses.

Lipid storage disorders

A number of terms are used for this group of disorders, sphingolipidoses, gangliosidoses, neurolipidoses – which may cause confusion. Sphingolipids are normal constituents of all cell membranes, the simplest consisting of a base (sphingosine) and a fatty acid. The resulting compound is called ceramide. In more complex sphingolipids, different side-chains are added to the ceramide. Gangliosides are complex sphingolipids present in high concentration in neurones. They consist of a ceramide + sugar(s) + sialic acid residue(s). Storage occurs when the normal enzymatic degradation of sphingolipids fails to occur.

Clinically, while there is wide variation in the age of onset and rate of progression, there are features in common; in particular: **ocular signs** (visual failure with a cherry red spot at the macula); **cognitive deterioration, seizures** (especially myoclonic seizures); and **motor disturbance** (with ataxia or spasticity). **Hepatosplenomegaly** and **bony changes** signal extra CNS involvement. Late-onset cases may present with an atypical phenotype with survival into adulthood.

Table 22.8 outlines features of a number of the lipid storage disorders. **Tay–Sachs disease** is the most common of the gangliosidoses. It is inherited in an autosomal recessive manner (with a marked increase in gene frequency in Ashkenazi Jews). It is characterized by loss of motor milestones from around 3–6 months of age, initially with hypotonia, then spasticity. An exaggerated startle response, progressive macrocephaly and cherry red spot at the macula are typical, but as already noted, non-specific. **Sandhoff's** syndrome is very similar in presentation, although in this case hexosaminidase A and B are deficient, just hexosaminidase A in Tay–Sachs. A 'juvenile' form exists, which is misleading terminology, because the onset is usually in the pre-school-age child with gait disturbance followed by ataxia, spasticity and dementia. A 'chronic' or 'adult' form is more often heralded by speech disturbance (dysarthria), then motor deterioration and psychiatric disorder and may simulate Friedreich's ataxia. Numerous gene mutations have been identified. The spectrum of phenotypes in GM2 gangliosidosis highlights the relevance of the disorder to paediatric and adult neurological practice.

Niemann–Pick disease refers to a group of conditions in which sphingomyelinase activity is deficient. Neurological involvement is prominent in type A but is rarely seen in type B. Type C is now considered to be a consequence of defective cholesterol esterification with normal sphingomyelinase activity in most tissues.

Table 22.8 Main lipid storage disorders

Disorder	Lipid storage (enzyme involved)	Clinical features
Disorders characterized by mainly neuronal storage		
Niemann–Pick	Ceramide phosphorylcholine = sphingomyelin (sphinogomyelinase)	Type A (classical) early onset with hepatic failure, developmental delay, then regression with spasticity, seizures, blindness
Gaucher's	Ceramide glucose = glucocerebroside (glucocerebroside β-glucosidase)	Type 1 (adult: non-neuronopathic) Type 2 (acute infantile) motor and social regression. Spasticity, bulbar involvement. Splenomegaly Type 3 (juvenile) hepatosplenomegaly, oculomotor apraxia, myoclonic epilepsy dementia, spasticity
GM1 gangliosidosis	*GM1 ganglioside (β-galactosidase)	Type 1 (generalized) hepatosplenomegaly, bony changes, dementia Type 2 (juvenile) spasticity, ataxia, dementia
GM2 gangliosidosis	GM2 ganglioside (hexosaminidase A ± B)	Type 1 (Tay–Sachs) Type 2 (Sandhoff's). Macular red spot, visual failure, macrocephaly, dementia, startle
Fabry's (X-linked)	Ceramide – trihexoside (α-galactosidase)	Skin lesions, painful crises, fevers, strokes renal involvement
Disorders involving predominantly white matter		
Metachromatic leukodystrophy	Ceramide-galactose-sulphate = sulphatide (cerebroside sulphatase, measure arylsulfatase A)	Gait disturbance, spasticity, peripheral neuropathy, dementia – late in early onset forms, prominent in late onset + psychiatric disturbance
Krabbe's	Ceramide galactose = galactocerebroside (galactocerebroside β-galactosidase)	Irritability, startle, spasticity, neuropathy seizures

*G refers to ganglioside; M,D,T to the number of attached sialic acid residues; 1,2,3 to the number of hexosides – 1 (tetra), 2 (tri), 3 (di).

In **metachromatic leukodystrophy** diagnostic assays of arylsulfatase A activity are complicated by finding a low level of activity in up to 2% of the apparently healthy population. This pseudodeficiency may also present problems for prenatal diagnosis. Other leukodystrophies exist without lipid storage but with another identified metabolic defect as in Canavan's syndrome, where acylaspartase deficiency has been found in a large proportion of cases.

Mucopolysaccharidoses (MPS)

Storage of mucopolysaccharides (glycosaminoglycans) occurs in a group of disorders characterized by dysmorphic features (coarse facies), corneal clouding, short stature with joint abnormalities and kyphoscoliosis.

Mental retardation is a feature of **MPS 1-H (Hurler's syndrome)** and **MPSIII (Sanfilippo's syndrome)**, in which it is severe, and progressive deterioration occurs. Nerve entrapment disorders especially carpal tunnel syndrome are common and craniocervical problems a feature of **type IV (Morquio's syndrome) and VI (Maroteaux–Lamy syndrome)**.

Phenotypes of the mucolipidoses and sialidoses overlap the mucopolysaccharidoses and lipid storage disorders. Myoclonus is a prominent feature of **sialidosis I** (cherry-red spot myoclonus syndrome) and **II**.

Neuronal ceroid lipofuscinoses

The **neuronal ceroid lipofuscinoses (of which Batten's disease** is the best known) are often grouped together with the lysosomal storage disorders. There are four

Table 22.9 Main subtypes of neuronal ceroid lipofuscinoses (NCL)

Name	Neurophysiology	Clinical features
Infantile NCL (Santavuori–Haltia–Hagberg disease)	ERG lost early EEG progressive loss of activity	Stereotyped hand, movements, myoclonic jerks, microcephaly, visual failure
Late infantile NCL (Jansky–Bielschowsky disease)	ERG initially normal EEG normal response to slow photic stimulation Giant VEPs initially	Myoclonic epilepsy, cognitive decline, ataxia. Visual failure late
Juvenile NCL (Spielmeyer–Vogt disease)	ERG and VEPs lost early	Visual failure early, then behavioural change, dysarthria, extrapyramidal signs
Adult NCL		Behavioural disorder and dementia in childhood. Late extrapyramidal features $\pm$ seizures

Diagnosis requires identification of characteristic neurophysiological features, and of particular inclusion bodies in skin, conjunctiva or rectal biopsy or in a blood buffy coat preparation or enzyme analysis where available.
ERG, electroretinogram; EEG, electroencephalograph; VEP, visual evoked potential.

main types of neuronal ceroid lipofuscinoses (Table 22.9) with variants of these main subtypes in addition. Progressive myoclonic epilepsy and visual failure are markers of these disorders.

REFERENCES AND FURTHER READING

Aicardi J (1998) *Diseases of the Nervous System in Childhood*. Philadelphia, PA: MacKeith Press with Cambridge University Press.

Barkovich AJ, K:uzniecky RI, Jackson GD, Guerrini R, Dobyns WB (2002) Classification system for malformations of cortical development. *Neurology*, in press, **57**:2168–2178.

Blair E, Stanley FJ (1988) Intrapartum asphyxia: a rare cause of cerebral palsy. *Journal of Paediatrics*, **112**:515–519.

Chumas P, Tyagi A, Livingston J (2001) Hydrocephalus – what's new? *Archives of Disease in Childhood*, **85**:149–154.

Gray RGF, Preece MA, Green SH, Whitehouse W, Winer J, Green A (2000) Inborn errors of metabolism as a cause of neurological disease in adults: an approach to investigation. *Journal of Neurology, Neurosurgery & Psychiatry*, **69**:5–12.

Rosenbloom L (1995) Diagnosis and management of cerebral palsy. *Archives of Disease in Childhood*, **72**:350–354.

Skeletal Dysplasia Group (1989) Instability of the upper cervical spine. *Archives of Disease in Childhood*, **64**:283–288.

CHAPTER 23

CEREBROVASCULAR DISEASE

N.A. Losseff and M.M. Brown

INTRODUCTION

Stroke can be simply defined as a focal neurological deficit resulting from a disturbance of the cerebral circulation lasting more than 24 hours (or causing early death). **Transient ischaemic attack (TIA)** is defined identically, except that the symptoms last less than 24 hours. The distinction is arbitrary. **Brain attack** is a new term to describe the acute presentation of stroke, which removes the requirement for a delay of 24 hours and emphasizes the need for urgent action to remedy the situation. It also emphasizes that at the time of presentation with symptoms suggesting stroke, other diagnoses need to be considered, such as hypoglycaemia. The term cerebrovascular accident should be abandoned, because it implies that the stroke is a chance event for which little can be done.

Stroke is usually invoked to describe events with a sudden onset. Individuals may have cerebrovascular disease without symptoms [e.g. asymptomatic carotid stenosis or infarction on computerized tomography (CT)] or acute symptoms without obvious imaging changes or focal signs (e.g. headache in some patients with subarachnoid haemorrhage or cerebral venous thrombosis). Cerebrovascular disease is an important cause of dementia, which may have an insidious onset. Often the cerebral symptoms of stroke or TIA result from cardiovascular or haematological disease arising outside the cranial circulation.

Stroke is a massive public health problem, being the third commonest cause of death in the developed world and the leading cause of adult disability. 140 000 people in the UK will have a stroke in the next year and approximately 20% of these patients will die within 30 days of onset. Above the age of 45 years, one in four men and one in five women are destined to have a stroke. For the survivors, morbidity can be considerable. Outcome following stroke varies widely from centre to centre.

It is important to recognize that the term stroke describes the clinical presentation of the patient. It is a syndrome and 'stroke' should not be regarded as a sufficient diagnosis on its own. Accurate diagnosis requires a description of the anatomical territory involved, the underlying pathology (i.e. infarction or haemorrhage), the mechanism (e.g. embolism), the underlying aetiology (e.g. atherosclerosis) and the underlying risk factors (e.g. smoking). The task of the stroke physician is to make this accurate pathophysiological diagnosis as this will then guide appropriate acute treatment and secondary preventive measures. To accomplish this requires a basic knowledge of the clinical and radiological patterns that the different stroke syndromes may produce and familiarity with the large evidence base of clinical trials, which guide stroke treatment and prevention. The stroke physician also needs to assess the functional effects of stroke on the patient and their participation in daily activities, to guide appropriate rehabilitation. The management of stroke may involve a variety of clinicians, therapists and community agencies. The stroke physician therefore needs to work as an integral part of a multidisciplinary team.

The basic subdivisions of stroke are **infarction (ischaemic stroke)** and **haemorrhage (haemorrhagic stroke)** (Table 23.1). In over 80% of cases, death of brain tissue is secondary to infarction. This may affect all or part of the territory of a large intracerebral artery, occupy the border zone between arterial supplies, or involve only a small area of white matter supplied by a penetrating vessel **(lacunar stroke)**. In 12% of cases, stroke results from primary haemorrhage within the substance of the brain. This may affect deep structures or the more superficial lobes of the brain.

In 8% of stroke cases bleeding occurs primarily within the subarachnoid space **(subarachnoid haemorrhage, SAH)**. The presentation of SAH is usually so distinct from other causes of stroke that it is not always included under this umbrella, perhaps because most patients with SAH are referred to neurosurgeons, not physicians. However, SAH is frequently complicated by cerebral infarction from vasospasm and shares underlying causes with intracerebral haemorrhage (ICH), such as cerebral aneurysm.

Table 23.1 Types of stroke

Infarction	Territorial
	Border zone
	Lacunar
Haemorrhage	Lobar
	Deep
	Posterior fossa
Subarachnoid haemorrhage	
Cerebral venous thrombosis	

Cerebral venous thrombosis is a rare cause of stroke, but can present with cerebral infarction or haemorrhage or both.

Differential diagnosis of stroke

The diagnosis of stroke and TIA requires a detailed history, which may need to be taken from a partner, carer, friend or relative, concentrating on the time course, rapidity of onset and location of the symptoms. The presence of vascular risk factors needs to be established. The **sudden onset of a focal neurological deficit** is characteristic of stroke and TIA. Most strokes reach their maximum deficit over a few minutes, but they may evolve over a few hours. If the patient survives, there is then a stable period of up to 1–2 weeks before the patient starts to recover. This long-term time course may be helpful in supporting the diagnosis of stroke when the patient has not been seen acutely or if the brain imaging is normal. In patients with large lesions, there may be an initial stable period, followed by deterioration on the second or third day caused by the development of cerebral oedema with mass effect and brainstem compression. This should always be visible on brain imaging, although magnetic resonance imaging (MRI) may be required in patients with cerebellar or brainstem infarction.

If a patient suspected of stroke has symptoms or signs that have progressed for more than a few hours, an alternative cause, such as a brain tumour, becomes increasingly likely. However, space-occupying lesions can present with the acute onset of symptoms and up to 5% of patients presenting with typical stroke-like symptoms have a subdural haematoma, tumour or cerebral abscess. The distinction is usually readily made on brain imaging, but if there is doubt, repeating the scan after 6 weeks will usually resolve the diagnosis. Occasionally, a cerebral biopsy is required.

Acute demyelination caused by multiple sclerosis or acute disseminated encephalomyelitis may present with hemiparesis, sensory impairment or brainstem symptoms that mimic stroke. Usually, the symptoms caused by inflammatory demyelination evolve over a few days. A characteristic MRI appearance and intrathecal synthesis of oligoclonal immunoglobulin may help to confirm the diagnosis. Occasionally, somatization and dissociation disorders may present with stroke-like symptoms ('hysterical' hemiparesis or sensory loss) and should be considered if there is marked fluctuation and signs inconsistent with 'organic' disease. The differential diagnosis of TIA is considered in more detail below.

> It is impossible to tell reliably the difference between infarction and ICH from the history or examination. Cranial imaging is therefore essential to make the distinction and exclude mimics of stroke.

In contrast, SAH characteristically presents with sudden, very severe headache and neck stiffness and the differential diagnosis is between other causes of acute headache and meningism.

ISCHAEMIC STROKE

Pathophysiology of ischaemic stroke

The brain is a highly metabolically active organ and even though it accounts for only 2% of body weight, it uses 20% of cardiac output when the body is at rest. Brain energy use is also dependent on the degree of neuronal activation. The brain uses glucose exclusively as a substrate for energy metabolism by oxidation to carbon dioxide and water. This metabolism allows conversion of adenosine diphosphate to adenosine triphosphate (ATP). A constant supply of ATP is essential for neuronal integrity and this process is much more efficient in the presence of oxygen. Although ATP can be formed by anaerobic glycolysis, the energy yielded by this pathway is small and also leads to the accumulation of toxic lactic acid. The brain needs and uses approximately 500 ml of oxygen and 100 mg of glucose each minute, hence the need for a rich supply of oxygenated blood containing glucose. Mean cerebral blood flow (CBF) in the cortex is normally approximately 50 ml/100 g per minute. The cerebral circulation maintains constant levels of CBF in the face of changing systemic blood pressure by a sophisticated

process termed autoregulation. However, autoregulation has upper and lower limits and in health CBF remains relatively constant over a range of mean arterial blood pressure of between 50 and 150 mmHg. The limits of autoregulation are shifted to higher values in patients with chronic uncontrolled hypertension.

> **Clinical manifestations of ischaemic stroke**
> The clinical manifestations of ischaemic stroke will depend to a large extent on the location and size of the vessel occluded, the duration of occlusion and the adequacy of collateral circulation. These will govern the location and extent of tissue ischaemia and infarction.

Severe ischaemia triggers a sequence of events, which lead to necrosis (Figure 23.1).

At the lower limit of autoregulation, further falls in perfusion pressure will lead to a reduction in CBF. However, this may be tolerated without symptoms. By increasing oxygen extraction from the blood, adequate compensation can be made even if blood flow is reduced to approximately 20–25 ml/100 g per minute. As cerebral blood flow falls further, metabolic paralysis, initially without cell disruption, ensues and this may be reversible. However if prolonged, infarction is inevitable. When CBF falls below 20 ml/100 g per minute oxygen extraction starts to fall and changes may be detected on electroencephalography. At levels below 10 ml/100 g per minute cell membrane

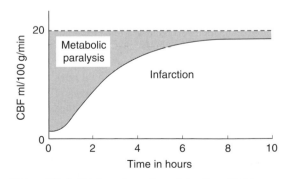

Figure 23.1 Relation of severity and duration of fall in cerebral blood flow (CBF) to effect on cerebral tissue. (Redrawn from Crowell (1982) In: *Cerebral Ischaemia Clinical and Experimental Approach.* Tokyo, Igabu-sharin.)

functions are severely disrupted and the membrane cation pumps fail to maintain cell ionic integrity. Below 5 ml/100 g per minute cell death is inevitable within a short time.

The ischaemic cascade

When neurones become ischaemic a cascade of biochemical changes potentiate cell death. These pathophysiological changes have been of considerable interest to those developing treatments to lessen the damage caused by ischaemic stroke. In the ischaemic brain as ion channels fail, K^+ moves out of the cell into the extracellular space, while Ca^{++} moves into the cell in extreme quantities, where it further compromises the ability of the cell to maintain ionic homeostasis and leads to mitochondrial failure. Hypoxia leads to the generation of free radicals, which peroxidize fatty acids in cell membranes, causing further cellular dysfunction. Anaerobic glycolysis results in lactic acidosis, further impairing cellular metabolic functions. Excitatory neurotransmitter activity (e.g. glutamate) is greatly increased in areas of brain ischaemia because of increased release and failure of uptake mechanisms. These neurotransmitters are themselves toxic at these increased levels by causing further Ca^{++} and Na^+ influx into cells through their actions on N-methyl-d-aspartate receptors. Hence ischaemia triggers a vicious cascade of events leading to cell electrical failure and then death. At some point the process becomes irreversible, even after reperfusion of tissues. Even if the severity of ischaemia is inadequate to cause necrosis it may trigger apoptosis (programmed cell death).

The ischaemic penumbra

The degree of ischaemia caused by blockage of an artery varies, partly depending on collateral supply. At the centre or core of an infarct the damage is most severe, but at the periphery collateral flow may allow continued delivery of blood, although at a lower rate. The neurones in this zone area may fail to function electrically, but remain alive and are then referred to as the **ischaemic penumbra**, by analogy with a lunar eclipse. The neurones in the penumbra are at risk of progression to infarction in the few hours after the onset of arterial occlusion, but also have the potential

to survive if the ischaemic cascade can be halted or reversed. Sophisticated neuroimaging can now be used to define areas of irreversible brain damage and areas in which perfusion is suboptimal but where irreversible infarction has not taken place. Thrombolysis and neuroprotective therapies are designed to salvage the penumbra, but it is very likely that high quality simple supportive management in the acute stage also decreases the chances of this secondary brain damage in the penumbra.

Vascular anatomy

The brain is supplied by two carotid arteries and two vertebral arteries. The internal carotid arteries begin in the neck at the carotid bifurcation and ascend intracranially. The first branch is the ophthalmic artery. The internal carotid artery then bifurcates into the anterior and middle cerebral arteries. Both anterior and middle cerebral arteries give off other branches and deep penetrating vessels. The **anterior cerebral artery** supplies amongst other structures much of the **'leg'** representation of the cortex. The **middle cerebral artery** supplies the **'arm'** representation, some of the **'leg'** representation, and the **speech** areas in the **dominant** hemisphere or the areas of **spatial awareness** in the **non-dominant** hemisphere. The **penetrating vessels** supply the **deeper** portions of the hemisphere, including the **internal capsule, basal ganglia and visual radiation**.

The **vertebral arteries** are unique in that they are the only arteries in the body to anastomose to form a larger artery, the basilar artery, which overlies the brainstem. The vertebral and basilar arteries give off three **cerebellar arteries** on each side, which supply **brainstem** and **cerebellar** structures. Perforating vessels arise from the basilar artery along its length and predominantly supply the deep areas of the brainstem, particularly the cranial nerve nuclei. At the top, the basilar artery divides to form the left and right **posterior cerebral arteries**. These supply **occipital visual cortex** and the **medial inferior temporal lobes**, containing the **hippocampus and memory** areas. The anterior, middle and posterior cerebral arteries are connected via anterior and posterior communicating vessels on both sides and all these vessels together form the Circle of Willis.

Risk factors and causes

Risk factors

Ischaemic stroke usually results from vessel occlusion from local in-situ thrombosis or embolism. Embolism can occur anywhere from a large artery (aorta, carotid or vertebral artery) to a smaller artery (30–40%) or more proximally from the heart (30–40%). Local occlusions from disease of the walls of the small penetrating blood vessels is responsible for lacunar infarction (25%). Localized reduction in blood flow distal to an occluded large artery or systemic hypotension accounts for haemodynamic infarction (<5%).

The main underlying **pathological processes** causing stroke are **atherosclerosis, cardiac embolism and hypertensive small vessel disease** (Table 23.2). Not surprisingly, the main risk factors for stroke are also the risk factors for atherosclerosis and heart disease. **Hypertension** is a particularly important risk factor because it promotes small vessel disease, atherosclerosis and heart disease, and causes both ICH, SAH and ischaemic stroke.

Risk factors contribute to the risk of developing disease of the vessel wall or enhance blood coagulability. Stroke is often associated with a combination of risk factors as the combined effect of individual risk factors on stroke incidence is much more than simply additive. The presence of one or more risk factors is insufficient to make a diagnosis of the mechanism of stroke because there is a large overlap between the syndromes associated with individual risk factors; for example, hypertension and smoking overlap as risk factors for both carotid artery stenosis and small vessel occlusion. The main value of identifying risk factors for stroke is therefore in primary prevention and secondary prevention of recurrence. Although increasing age is an important risk factor, stroke can occur at any age, including in childhood. The age of the patient should not be used as a diagnostic feature. About one-quarter of all strokes occur before the age of 65 years. Some patients who have suffered a stroke have no identifiable risk factors.

Table 23.2 Major risk factors for transient ischaemic attack or stroke

Increasing age
Hypertension
Smoking
Diabetes mellitus
Atrial fibrillation
Heart disease
Hypercholesterolaemia
Excess alcohol

Atherosclerosis of the major vessels supplying the brain is a major source of cerebral **embolism**. The emboli are usually **platelet aggregates** or **thrombus** formed on atherosclerotic plaques, but may consist of cholesterol crystals or atherosclerotic debris. It is believed that the acute occurrence of thrombosis is caused by plaque rupture, which exposes the lipid core to blood, activating the clotting cascade. Atherothrombosis may also lead to vessel occlusion, in which case stroke may result from distal propagation of thrombus, embolism or, less commonly, a reduction in distal flow (haemodynamic stroke). Symptomatic atherosclerosis is frequent at the **carotid artery bifurcation** in the neck, where it causes internal carotid artery stenosis, but also commonly affects the aorta, the carotid syphon, the common carotid artery and the vertebral and basilar arteries. Atherosclerosis may also involve the intracranial vessels, particularly the origin of the middle cerebral artery. Intracranial stenosis is more common in Asian populations.

Cardiac embolism causes stroke by promoting embolism of thrombus (or occasionally valve fragments or vegetations) from the **left hand side of the heart** to the brain, and may be divided into high risk or lower risk causes (Table 23.3). **Atrial fibrillation** remains the most important cause of cardioembolism. Careful examination of the pulse and cardiovascular system are essential in patients with stroke and TIA.

Patent foramen ovale provides a potential route for paradoxical embolism of venous thrombosis from the right to left side of the heart and thence to the brain. However, in many cases patent foramen ovale is an innocent finding and only appears

Table 23.3 Cardiac causes of ischaemic stroke and transient ischaemic attack

High risk	Atrial fibrillation (especially when combined with other risk factors) Mitral stenosis Prosthetic heart valves Bacterial endocarditis Cardiac surgery
Low risk	Myocardial infarction Ventricular/atrial aneurysm Cardiomyopathy Patent foramen ovale

Table 23.4 Haematological causes of ischaemic stroke and transient ischaemic attack

Commoner	Sickle-cell disease Polycythaemia Thrombocythaemia
Rare	Antiphospholipid antibody syndrome Thrombotic thrombocytopenic purpura Paroxysmal nocturnal haemoglobinuria Leukaemia
Common in cerebral venous thrombosis, but of uncertain relevance in arterial stroke (except in paradoxical embolism)	Inherited thrombophilia Factor V Leiden polymorphism Protein C deficiency Protein S deficiency Antithrombin III deficiency Prothrombin gene mutation

Table 23.5 Rarer non-atherosclerotic vasculopathies

Arterial dissection
Traumatic
Secondary to idiopathic connective tissue disease
Drug abuse
CADASIL
Mitochondrial cytopathies, e.g. MELAS
Vasculitis
   Systemic lupus erythematosus
   Polyarteritis nodosa
   Temporal arteritis
Sneddon's syndrome
Sussac's syndrome
Cervical or cranial irradiation
Moyamoya syndrome
Infections
Acute and chronic meningitis
Syphilis
Herpes zoster
HIV

CADASIL, cerebral autosomal dominant arteriopathy with subcortical infarcts and leukoencephalopathy; MELAS, myopathy, encephalopathy, lactic acidosis and stroke-like episodes; HIV, human immunodeficiency virus.

to be relevant if associated with an atrial septal aneurysm.

Small vessel disease: localized occlusion of arterioles, secondary to microatheroma and degenerative disease of the walls (lipohyalinosis), is the common cause of lacunar stroke (see below). Hypertension, diabetes mellitus and hypercholesterolaemia are the major risk factors. Lipohyalinosis is also one of the major causes of ICH.

Much rarer causes of infarction are haematological abnormalities (Table 23.4) and the non-atherosclerotic vasculopathies (Table 23.5). Some of the more important of these disorders are described in greater detail later in this chapter.

Haematological evidence for thrombophilia (inherited or acquired defects in thrombolytic proteins leading to thrombosis, Table 23.4) is commonly sought in younger patients but rarely proven as a cause of arterial stroke. **Cerebral venous thrombosis** is a far likelier mechanism of stroke associated with **thrombophilia**. The commonest detectable abnormality in the population is the factor V Leiden mutation, the others are rarer. Arterial stroke can occur as part of the **antiphospholipid antibody** syndrome, in which thrombosis is associated with a history of recurrent miscarriage, thrombocytopenia and sometimes serological evidence of a connective tissue disorder. **Antiphospholipid antibodies** may also be found in association with other vasculopathies, including atherosclerosis, but in most cases they do not have a pathogenic role. Other important haematological causes of stroke include sickle-cell disease, polycythaemia and thrombocythaemia.

Outcome

The average mortality within the first 7 and 30 days after stroke is approximately 12 and 19% respectively. Within the first few days, death is usually the direct result of cerebral oedema from infarction or mass effect from haemorrhage causing brainstem compression with coma and respiratory depression. Subsequently, stroke deaths are mainly caused by fatal complications of impaired swallowing and immobilization, including pneumonia and pulmonary embolism. Beyond 30 days, recurrence of stroke and myocardial infarction account for a similar proportion of late death.

Recovery from stroke is very variable. Some patients make a rapid and full recovery within a few days or weeks. In patients with more severe stroke, there is gradual spontaneous improvement. This occurs most rapidly in the first 4–6 weeks, but may continue slowly for up to a year after onset. Unfortunately, **approximately 50% of survivors remain dependant at 1 year**. Mortality figures vary from location to location. Case mix is an important determinant of outcome. Large middle cerebral artery infarcts have a 30% mortality at 1 month, while the mortality after lacunar infarction is about 5%. Even after adjustment for case mix, type of bed and use of CT scan, 3 month mortality has recently been shown to vary from as high as 42% at some units to as low as 19% at other units. Hence, even the crude indicator of death rate is enough to highlight major discrepancies between services.

Currently, clinical criteria do not predict individual outcome early after stroke with sufficient accuracy to be useful. However, many factors have been identified that may be associated with a high risk of death and poor functional outcome (Table 23.6). Prognostic scales have been developed but they explain at best only about 10% of the variance in disability at 6 months. Because clinical variables have poor predictive values in individual patients, much work has gone into developing reliable non-invasive surrogate markers of clinical outcome. These have been mostly based on imaging and biochemical markers but, like clinical factors, poorly explain the

Table 23.6 Poor prognostic factors

Increasing age
Coma at onset
Urinary incontinence at 1 week
Large lesion on neuroimaging
Severe motor impairment
Cardiac failure
Atrial fibrillation
Persistent neglect

differences in outcome; for example, although visible infarction on CT does increase the relative risk of death or dependency at 6 months, after correction for other important prognostic variables it only modestly predicts variation in impairment and disability. Hence, decisions about active management should not be based on any of these factors.

Prognosis
Individual patients may recover very well with appropriate rehabilitation despite poor prognostic factors and it is important that poor prognostic factors at onset are not allowed to become a self-fulfilling prophecy.

Clinical syndromes of cerebral ischaemia

Transient ischaemic attacks

Transient ischaemic attack (TIA) has for some time been arbitrarily distinguished from completed stroke, but the pathophysiology may be identical (e.g. severe carotid stenosis) and the difference between TIA and stroke is only one of duration. Careful history, examination and sophisticated neuroimaging often reveal that an apparent TIA has actually resulted in a permanent deficit and would be better described as a small stroke. It is nevertheless useful to distinguish between transient and persistent symptoms and signs, because the differential diagnosis of transient events includes other causes of transient focal neurological symptoms (Table 23.7).

Table 23.7 Differential diagnosis of transient ischaemic attack

Migraine
Transient global amnesia
Epilepsy
Mass lesions
Multiple sclerosis
Hypoglycaemia
Benign positional vertigo

Table 23.8 Common symptoms of transient cerebral ischaemia

Carotid territory	Monocular visual loss
	Unilateral hemiparesis
	Dysphasia
Vertebrobasilar*	Diplopia
	Dysarthria
	Vertigo/disequilibrium
	Bilateral visual loss
	Bilateral weakness or hemianopia
	Ataxia
	Sensory loss

*Various combinations of the listed symptoms.

Symptoms of TIA

The symptoms of transient ischaemia are usually negative (loss of function), maximal at onset and last from 5 to 30 minutes.

Any cause of ischaemic stroke can also cause a TIA. Very rarely a small cerebral haemorrhage may cause TIA-like symptoms. In general, TIAs are more likely to be embolic than local occlusion and high frequency attacks, for example, several per month (crescendo TIAs) are more likely to be caused by severe large artery stenosis.

Within the carotid circulation (Table 23.8) an embolus to the retinal circulation may lead to **transient monocular blindness (amaurosis fugax)**. This is usually described by the patient as like a curtain or shutter coming down over one eye and lasting only a few minutes. Occasionally, cholesterol emboli may be seen in a retinal vessel on fundoscopy during or after an attack. **Hemisphere ischaemia** is suggested by the sudden onset of **contralateral weakness or dysphasia** (if the dominant hemisphere is affected). The symptoms of hemisphere ischaemia usually last up to 30 minutes. Sensory loss in isolation is less common.

Transient ischaemic attacks within the **vertebrobasilar** circulation may cause **diplopia, facial or tongue numbness, dysarthria, vertigo and hemiparesis or quadriparesis** from brainstem involvement. If the top of the basilar artery is occluded, there may also be **hemianopia or bilateral visual loss** from ischaemia in the posterior cerebral arteries. It is very unusual for isolated vertigo or other brainstem symptoms to be caused by vertebrobasilar ischaemia. **Isolated transient vertigo** is usually the result of a **peripheral vestibulopathy**, for example, benign positional vertigo.

It has also recently become clearer that apparent transient 'ischaemic' attacks are occasionally caused by microhaemorrhages, which are not seen on conventional MRI or CT but are visible using susceptibility-weighted MRI imaging (T2* imaging). These patients usually have poorly controlled hypertension (Figure 23.2.).

Up to one-quarter of people attending specialist vascular clinics with suspected TIA turn out to have an alternative diagnosis (Table 23.7). The commonest mimic of TIA is **migraine with focal neurological symptoms**. Focal migrainous symptoms may occur as an aura preceding headache (not usually confused with TIAs) or as an isolated aura without headache (commonly confused) or occasionally after or during a headache, which is extremely rare. It should be noted that stroke and transient ischaemia of any cause are often associated with headache, while some diseases may cause both migrainous symptoms and infarction (e.g. cervical artery dissection, antiphospholipid antibody syndrome, giant cell arteritis). Transient ischaemic attack or stroke should not be attributed to migraine simply because the symptoms are associated with a migraine-like headache.

The two main features in the history which point towards migraine rather than TIA are 'positive' symptoms and spread of symptoms over time. The typical **positive symptoms of migraine** consist of zigzag lines and scintillating scotomata, while migrainous sensory aura presents as tingling in one hand, often with perioral tingling. Patients may complain of weakness but this is usually vague and

penetrating vessel occlusion takes place (Figure 23.4). These include **gait apraxia** with gait ignition failure or small-stepped gait **(marche à petit pas), postural instability** with a predisposition to falling backwards, and **vascular dementia** (see below).

Rarer causes of lacunar syndromes

Antiphospholipid antibody syndrome may present with lacunar infarction and often these patients also have a history of migrainous phenomena and headaches. **Cerebral autosomal dominant arteriopathy with subcortical infarcts and leukoencephalopathy (CADASIL)** is a rare hereditary disorder, caused by mutations in the gene coding for the notch 3 protein. Patients with CADASIL present with recurrent lacunar strokes and usually develop vascular dementia. There is often a history of migraine-like headaches. The diagnosis is suggested by a family history and florid leukoaraiosis on imaging. No effective treatment is known.

Large vessel occlusion

The pattern of infarction after **large vessel occlusion** depends on the size of the vessel occluded and the adequacy of collateral supply. Intracranial large vessel occlusion, such as middle cerebral artery or its cortical branches, is more likely to be caused by thromboembolism from the heart, aortic atherosclerosis or internal carotid artery stenosis, than by local occlusive disease, in contrast to lacunar infarction. Stenosis and occlusion are distinct. Occlusion of a vessel may occur without pre-existing atheromatous stenosis, either because of embolism to the artery, or because of local injury to the vessel wall, for example, dissection after minor trauma. Hypercoagulability of the blood rarely causes local arterial thrombosis without additional vascular pathology, but is an important cause of venous thrombosis. Alternatively occlusion may occur at the site of an atheromatous plaque or stenosis. The degree to which the brain suffers from ischaemia will depend on the duration, site of occlusion and collateral circulation. The internal carotid artery often occludes without any clinical evidence of stroke, because of the collateral supply provided by the Circle of Willis.

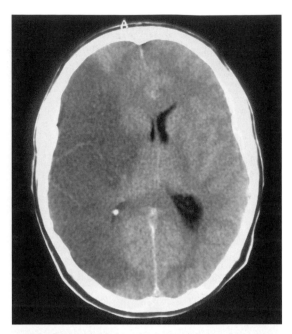

Figure 23.5 Complete middle cerebral artery territory infarction. CT at 48 hours shows infarction within the complete middle cerebral artery territory on the right with swelling of the hemisphere causing midline shift. The patient later began to develop signs of coning and decompressive surgery was carried out (see Figure 23.6).

Strokes occur after carotid occlusion only if the collateral supply is inadequate or if thrombosis spreads (or embolises) to involve the middle cerebral artery or its branches.

Middle cerebral artery territory stroke

Total occlusion

The clinical features of **occlusion of the main trunk of the middle cerebral artery** with infarction of the whole territory of the artery (Figure 23.5) include **conjugate eye deviation** (frontal lobe damage), **aphasia** (in the dominant hemisphere), **hemiplegia, hemisensory loss and hemianopia** (from involvement of **the visual radiation** in temporal and parietal lobes). In middle cerebral artery occlusion (and most lacunar syndromes) the **hemiparesis affects the arm more than the leg,** while in anterior cerebral artery occlusion the leg is characteristically much weaker than the arm because the leg area of the motor cortex is in the anterior cerebral artery

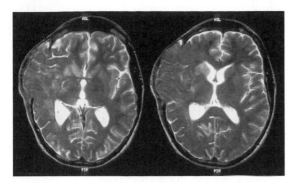

Figure 23.6 Malignant hemisphere swelling relieved by surgical decompression after complete middle cerebral artery territory infarction. MRI shows herniation of the swollen brain following decompressive craniotomy. After 2 months the defect was closed. Outcome at 6 months was excellent (patient independently ambulant, no significant cognitive deficit), although the left arm remained plegic.

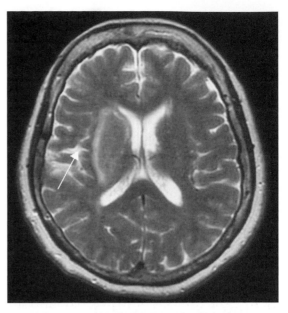

Figure 23.7 Striatocapsular infarction. This patient presented with acute right hemiplegia, neglect and dysphasia. The neglect and dysphasia resolved within a few days. The underlying aetiology was atrial fibrillation.

territory. **Neglect syndromes** in which the patient is unaware of, or ignores, the hemiplegic side occur acutely with both non-dominant and dominant hemisphere cortical damage, but generally are more severe and persistent with non-dominant parietal lobe damage.

The middle cerebral artery most commonly occludes from embolism. Occasionally atheromatous stenosis at the origin of the middle cerebral artery leads to occlusion, particularly in Asian and African races. Rarely, patients with complete middle cerebral artery territory infarction develop severe malignant oedema within 48 hours, leading to brainstem compression and death by coning. In appropriate cases, surgical decompression with hemicraniectomy is required (Figure 23.6).

Branch occlusion
Branch occlusion will produce **partial syndromes** with only some of the signs of complete territory infarction described above. **Upper branch** occlusion affecting frontal structures produces **hemiparesis, hemisensory loss, ocular deviation** and a **non–fluent expressive dysphasia** in which the patient understands speech because of an intact temporal lobe but cannot produce speech. **Lower branch** occlusions involving the temporal lobe result in **fluent receptive dysphasia**, in which the patient has difficulty

understanding language but motor production of speech is either preserved or produces a non-stop flow of nonsensical speech (jargon dysphasia).

Distal embolism
Small cortical branches are usually occluded by emboli and the patient may present only with **weakness or isolated cortical signs**, for example, dysphasia.

Deep infarction (striatocapsular infarction)
Deep infarction occurs when the trunk of the middle cerebral artery has occluded but the cortex is protected by pial collateral circulation. Deeper structures (the striatum and internal capsule) are supplied by the perforating branches, which do not have collateral supply infarct (Figure 23.7). Usually, this results from an embolus which rapidly breaks up, obstructing the **perforating lenticulostriate** arteries. The patients have **contralateral motor and sensory loss** but also exhibit **cortical signs** (unlike pure lacunar infarction). These cortical signs resolve more quickly than when the cortex itself is infarcted.

Anterior cerebral artery occlusion

The anterior cerebral artery is far less often affected than the middle cerebral artery, although the causes are similar. However, **anterior cerebral territory** infarction should raise the level of awareness for unusual aetiologies. It also occurs after SAH secondary to vasospasm. The clinical features of anterior cerebral artery occlusion are a **contralateral hemiplegia in which the leg is more affected than the arm**, because the cortical representation of the leg lies within its territory. Infarction of subfrontal cortex, especially if bilateral, may cause **frontal neuropsychological deficits**, particularly executive dysfunction, disinhibition and lack of insight, without any other signs.

Carotid artery occlusion

The picture in carotid artery occlusion is usually **identical to that of middle cerebral artery occlusion**. Infarction may be limited to a small portion of the territory or extend to involve the whole of the middle cerebral artery territory. If the carotid artery occludes from dissection, there may also be a **Horner's syndrome** on the side of the occlusion (i.e. contralateral to the limb signs). The anterior cerebral territory is often spared (via collateral flow) but may be affected in some cases. The bifurcation of the common carotid artery is the most common site of severe atheroma in the extracranial cerebral circulation and usually the internal carotid artery occludes at the origin from the common carotid. In dissection, the site of occlusion may be more distal.

Posterior cerebral artery occlusions

Occlusion of the posterior cerebral artery is commonly embolic and more patients with **posterior cerebral syndromes** are in atrial fibrillation, than with other large vessel occlusions (Figure 23.8). Emboli usually reach the posterior cerebral arteries via the vertebrobasilar system, but it should be borne in mind that in about 5% of individuals one posterior cerebral artery is supplied by a dominant

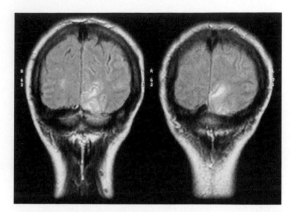

Figure 23.8 Posterior cerebral artery occlusion. Coronal MRI shows acute infarction of the left occipital pole.

posterior communicating branch of the internal carotid artery. Thus, posterior cerebral artery occlusion is occasionally caused by embolisation from carotid stenosis. The posterior cerebral artery principally supplies the occipital cortex, and occlusion usually causes an **isolated hemianopia**. This may spare the visual representation of the macular fibres when these may receive collateral supply from the middle cerebral artery. When infarction extends anteriorly to affect parieto-occipital areas, **neglect syndromes** may accompany the hemianopia. The posterior cerebral arteries also supply the **thalami** and the **medial posterior temporal lobes**. If these structures are involved, the patient may present with **confusion, or memory impairment** (thalamic or medial temporal amnesia). If both posterior cerebral artery territories are infarcted, as may happen when an embolus lodges at the **top of the basilar artery, cortical blindness and confusion** ensue. Sometimes these patients may be left with tunnel vision and may recognize small but not large objects. Memory impairment following this may be severe, especially for the acquisition of new information.

Vertebral artery occlusion

The commonest consequence of occlusion of the **distal vertebral artery** is infarction of the **dorsolateral medulla** within the territory of the **posterior inferior cerebellar artery (lateral medullary syndrome)**. This results in a **Horner's syndrome, temperature and pain sensory loss on one side of the face and the** other side of the body, **nystagmus, ataxia of the ipsilateral limbs and palatal and vocal cord paralysis**. Vertebral artery embolism or occlusion may also result in more extensive infarction of the brainstem and cerebellum and these syndromes are discussed next. The commonest site for atheroma to affect the vertebral artery is at its origin from the aorta.

Basilar artery occlusion

Whereas middle and posterior cerebral artery occlusions are more often the result of embolism, the opposite is true of the basilar artery. This is because the basilar is more commonly affected by severe atherosclerosis on which in-situ thrombus may form. **Basilar artery occlusion** also commonly occurs as a result of propagation of thrombus from an occluded vertebral artery. Basilar thrombus (Figure 23.9) may obstruct blood flow into perforating vessels supplying the central brainstem structures or the two upper cerebellar arteries. A number of clinical pictures may be encountered. In the medulla, lower cranial nerves may be affected, giving rise to a **lower motor neurone type bulbar palsy**. Upper motor neurone impairment of the same structure may cause a **pseudobulbar palsy**, with brisk facial reflexes, jaw jerk and a spastic tongue. This is often accompanied by spontaneous laughter or crying **(emotional lability)**. Above the medulla, **pontine infarction** may cause a **sixth nerve palsy, gaze paresis, internuclear ophthalmoplegia and pinpoint pupils**. Emboli may lodge at the top of the basilar causing **midbrain infarction** with **loss of vertical eye movement, pupillary abnormalities and coma**. All these syndromes will be accompanied by **quadriplegia** to some degree, which may be very asymmetric. Partial brainstem or midbrain syndromes may also be caused by localized occlusion of one of the perforating arteries from small vessel disease.

Subclavian artery occlusion

Subclavian artery occlusion is a rare cause of haemodynamic TIA and an even rarer cause of stroke. If the subclavian artery is occluded or severely stenosed before the origin of the vertebral artery, the arm may be supplied by blood flowing in

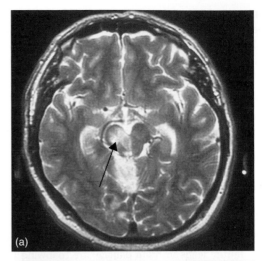

(a)

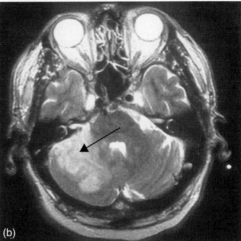

(b)

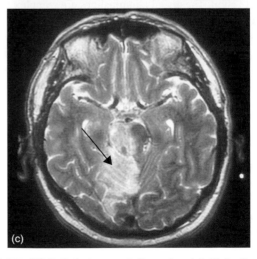

(c)

Figure 23.9 Brainstem, cerebellar and occipital infarction secondary to basilar thrombosis.

a retrograde direction down the vertebral artery at the expense of the vertebrobasilar circulation. This is known as **subclavian steal** and may occasionally result in brainstem TIAs during exercise of the arm.

Border zone ischaemia and hypoxic ischaemic encephalopathy

The brain is particularly vulnerable to a global fall in perfusion pressure. Most often this is caused by cardiac disease (arrthymia or pump failure), especially when combined with hypoxia, although hypovolaemia alone may be sufficient to cause cerebral ischaemia. The usual circumstances in which perfusion failure leads to brain damage are **following cardiac arrest, severe blood loss or cardiopulmonary bypass. Embolism** is an alternative or additional cause of focal damage during cardiopulmonary bypass. In the non-anaesthetized, non-comatose patient moderate or transient global perfusion failure results in acute reversible non-focal brain dysfunction (confusion, attention deficits, light headiness). Following a profound insult a number of syndromes are recognized, resulting from **border zone** or **'watershed' infarction** in the areas of the brain at the distal ends of the arterial supply (Figure 23.10). The parieto-occipital cortex, which lies at the border zone between the middle cerebral artery and posterior cerebral artery territories, is particularly vulnerable. Infarction of this region results in abnormalities of behaviour, memory and vision. The visual abnormalities are complex and include inability to see all the objects in a field of vision, incoordination of hand and eye movement, such that the patient cannot locate objects in the visual field, and apraxia of gaze in which the patient is unable to gaze where desired. Other areas of vulnerability are the superficial cortical and deep subcortical border zones between the anterior and middle cerebral artery, and the hippocampi, where infarction may result in an amnesic syndrome. In severe cases necrosis occurs in the basal ganglia, cerebellum and brainstem.

Vascular dementia

Vascular dementia is an umbrella term to describe the development of cognitive deficits in multiple

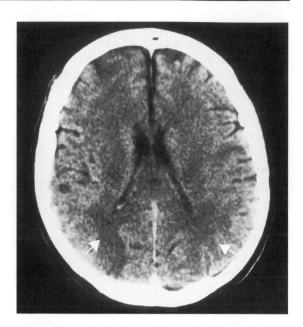

Figure 23.10 Watershed infarction following cardiac surgery. CT scan of the brain shows bilateral 'watershed' infarction more obvious on the right. This has occurred in the border zone between the middle and anterior cerebral artery territories.

domains from cerebrovascular disease (see p. 283). This is most commonly caused by multiple cortical or subcortical lacunar infarcts (Figure 23.11). Vascular dementia can also occur after multiple intracranial haemorrhages, for example: in cerebral amyloid angiopathy; after SAH; and as a result of cerebral venous thrombosis. Typically, patients have **a stepwise deterioration** associated with other features of stroke. In **diffuse subcortical small vessel disease, (Binswanger's disease (see p. 283) or subcortical arteriosclerotic encephalopathy) dementia** may be accompanied by **gait apraxia**, which results in failure to initiate gait, postural instability (often falling over backwards) and a **shuffling small-stepped, wide-based gait (marche à petit pas)**. This is often associated with diffuse periventricular demyelination secondary to ischaemia in the deep white matter, which causes patchy or diffuse changes, known as leukoaraiosis, and ventricular enlargement on CT and MRI. Urinary incontinence may occur. Characteristically, the **dementia** of small vessel disease has **subcortical features** including poor attention, slowing of mental function (bradyphrenia) and impaired executive function in excess of discrete cortical patterns of dysfunction.

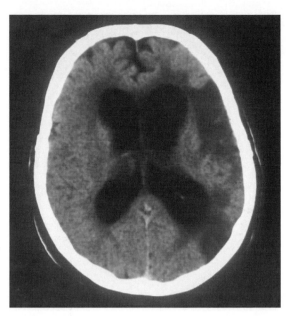

Figure 23.11 CT in vascular dementia. Atrophy, multiple lacunar infarcts and large vessel disease in a patient with vascular dementia.

Table 23.10 Causes of intracerebral haemorrhage

Hypertensive small vessel disease
Anticoagulants
Amyloid angiopathy
Arteriovenous malformation
Aneurysm
Amphetamine/cocaine ingestion
Infective endocarditis
Tumours
Disseminated intravascular coagulation
Venous thrombosis
Cerebral vasculitis

Occasionally these patients present with periods of encephalopathy associated with new infarction. Multiple cortical infarcts (from large vessel occlusions) are much rarer as causes of dementia. It is important to note that older patients with cerebrovascular disease are at increased risk of Alzheimer's disease, and **mixed dementia** caused by a combination of the two disorders is common (see p. 272).

Asymptomatic leukoaraiosis without dementia may also be found on imaging, especially in patients over 50 years of age with appropriate risk factors. There is also an increased incidence of depression in these patients.

INTRACEREBRAL HAEMORRHAGE

Approximately 10% of stroke is caused by ICH often associated with hypertension and ICH affects a wide age range.

ICH often has a sudden, devastating presentation. Patients who present in coma with vomiting and/or neck stiffness are more likely to have ICH than ischaemic stroke, but it is wrong to assume that patients with less severe stroke have ischaemia. The symptoms of small cerebral haemorrhages are indistinguishable from cerebral infarction.

This is particularly illustrated by the recognition of microhaemorrhage on T2* imaging (see p. 26), which reveals minute bleeds as the underlying cause of clinical syndromes previously thought clinically to have been caused by transient ischaemia or lacunar infarction (Figure 23.2).

The great majority of cases of ICH occur secondary to small vessel disease with rupture of small penetrating vessels in the basal ganglia, pons or cerebellum. Cerebral amyloid angiopathy is another important cause, which results in recurrent superficial lobar haematomas, usually in older patients. A ruptured cerebral aneurysm can be the reason for ICH if the bleeding occurs into the substance of the brain, rather than, or together with, SAH. Other rarer aetiologies include arteriovenous malformation and mycotic aneurysm. Non-medicinal use of cocaine and amphetamines may cause ICH, but there is often an underlying vascular malformation in these cases (Table 23.10).

One of the most important causes of ICH is anticoagulation therapy, especially when poorly controlled and combined with other risk factors.

Intracerebral haemorrhage

The rupture of a vessel results in the sudden development of a haematoma. The haematoma characteristically slowly enlarges over the first few hours, and sometimes over a few days, leading to progressive focal clinical deficit and then deterioration of conscious level secondary to mass effect. One of the most important and potentially treatable causes is anticoagulation. Any patient on an anticoagulant with new focal neurology must be assumed to have bled until proven otherwise with urgent cranial imaging. In those that have bled, anticoagulation should be immediately reversed. Neurosurgical evacuation of haematomas or shunting of associated hydrocephalus may be lifesaving.

Clinical syndromes

Haemorrhage may be divided into a number of categories depending on location. These are **deep (centred on basal ganglia structures), lobar, pontine and cerebellar**. In all sites hypertension remains the most important risk factor and, although amyloid angiopathy gives rise to lobar but not deep haemorrhage, hypertension is still the most important risk in lobar haemorrhage. Hypertension may make an underlying structural cause, such as aneurysm, more likely to rupture.

Deep haemorrhage

Subcortical haematomas may be centred on the putamen, caudate or thalamus. In **putaminal** haemorrhage the picture is of **contralateral hemiparesis and conjugate deviation of the eyes towards the side of the haematoma**. Cortical function may be impaired. If the mass becomes critical, signs of coning ensue. These haematomas may rupture into the ventricles leading to SAH. In the case of putaminal haemorrhage the presence of ventricular blood implies a very large haematoma with a poor prognosis (Figure 23.12).

Caudate haemorrhage is much rarer and small haematomas may readily rupture into the ventricles.

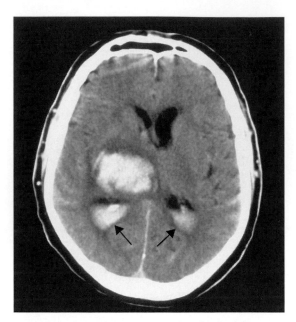

Figure 23.12 Massive deep haemorrhage. CT showing acute haemorrhage centred on the right thalamus with mass effect and intraventricular extension of blood (arrowed).

When the lesion is large, the picture is similar to putaminal haemorrhage, but if small, haematomas may present like SAH with acute headache and meningism, but little in the way of focal signs. **Thalamic** haemorrhage predominantly produces **sensory change in the contralateral limbs**. If local midbrain compression occurs, the eyes may be forced into downwards gaze with small, poorly reactive pupils. Thalamic haemorrhage in the dominant hemisphere may produce dysphasia with notable naming difficulties.

Lobar haemorrhage produces signs appropriate to the location. In the frontal lobe, eye deviation and contralateral hemiparesis is common. In the central region hemisensory loss is found associated with dysphasia in the dominant hemisphere. Parietal lobe haemorrhage causes hemisensory loss and neglect or inattention syndromes. Bleeding into the dominant temporal lobe results in a fluent dysphasia with poor comprehension, secondary to damage of Wernicke's area (Figure 23.13).

In **pontine haemorrhage** the classic presentation is **coma associated with pinpoint pupils, loss of horizontal eye movements and quadriparesis**. Hyperpyrexia

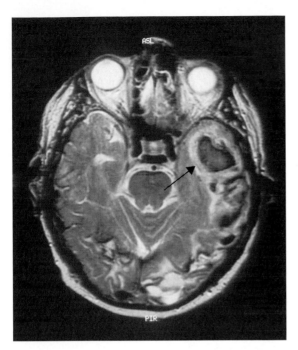

Figure 23.13 Temporal lobe haematoma secondary to poorly controlled anticoagulation. MRI shows cavitating haemorrhage in the left temporal lobe (arrowed). Previous left occipital infarction is also seen, which was secondary to posterior cerebral artery occlusion from atrial fibrillation.

and irregular respiratory patterns ensue. Although large haemorrhage here is often fatal, the outcome may be surprisingly good.

Posterior fossa cerebellar haemorrhage accounts for 10% of all primary intracerebral haematomas. It is important to recognize because it may result in secondary fatal brainstem compression and hydrocephalus (Figure 23.14). **Neurosurgical treatment can be lifesaving** and subsequently patients with cerebellar haemorrhage often make an excellent recovery. The usual presentation is with **acute headache, vomiting and unilateral ataxia**. Unilateral gaze paresis in association with ataxia or in isolation may also occur. When brainstem compression is present the clinical features are similar to those of pontine haemorrhage. This clinical picture may be present from onset or the symptoms may slowly progress over the course of hours or a few days.

Intraventricular haemorrhage mimics SAH (see below) with headache, vomiting, neck stiffness and depression of consciousness. There may be associated pyramidal signs. It may be caused by a subependymal region angioma or by extension of blood following deep haemorrhage. This is particularly the case with caudate haemorrhage, as this nucleus lies adjacent to the ventricular margin.

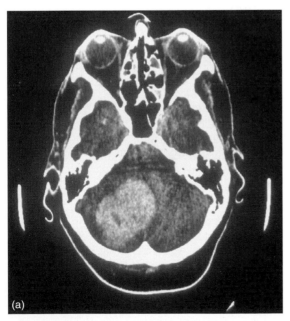

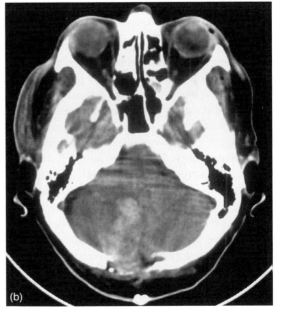

Figure 23.14 Cerebellar haematoma with secondary brainstem compression before and after surgical evacuation. Evacuation was performed in this patient because of a low conscious level associated with marked mass effect on the brainstem by the haematoma.

INVESTIGATION OF STROKE AND TRANSIENT ISCHAEMIC ATTACK

Investigation is aimed at:

- Identifying underlying pathology (haemorrhage or infarct)
- Detecting risk factors
- Establishing cause and mechanism (e.g. embolism from atheromatous carotid artery stenosis)
- Confirming or refuting the clinical diagnosis.

Investigation nearly always improves the clinician's understanding of the pathophysiology of the stroke or transient ischaemic syndrome. This then guides acute treatment and secondary preventive measures. 'Completed' stroke should not be separated from transient ischaemic syndromes when considering appropriate investigation, as the aetiological spectrum is identical, although management may be very different. Both are emergencies and should be investigated urgently to plan appropriate management and prevent further events.

Routine investigations for all patients (Table 23.11)

In all patients, routine **blood screening** should include full blood count to look for polycythaemia, thrombocythaemia or thrombocytopenia. Anaemia of chronic disease may be a marker for endocarditis or underlying cancer. Occasional haematological malignancies may be complicated by stroke. **Basic coagulation analysis** (INR, International Normalized Ratio; APTT, activated partial thromboplastin time; thrombin time and fibrinogen) should be undertaken in all patients with haemorrhagic stroke and is especially important in those receiving anticoagulants. Urea and electrolytes guide homeostatic management in the acute phase and may also reveal end-organ damage from hypertension or vasculitis. Patients suffering from significant electrolyte disturbance may present with global or focal dysfunction mimicking stroke. Plasma glucose is an essential 'triage' investigation, as hypoglycaemia must be excluded in anyone with focal signs. **Hyperglycaemia** may suggest unidentified diabetes and is also found in non-diabetics with severe stroke. Rarely, hyperosmolar non-ketotic diabetic hyperglycaemia presents as a stroke syndrome. Lipid analysis for cholesterol and fasting triglycerides should be performed. There are also arguments for performing syphilis serology in all patients. **Erythrocyte sedimentation rate (ESR)** is used as a non-specific screening test, principally for inflammatory arterial disease and endocarditis. Thyroid function tests should be performed in all patients with atrial fibrillation. In all patients **chest X-ray and electrocardiography (ECG)** should also be carried out. If they are both normal this may negate the need for echocardiography. The principal point of chest radiology is to establish the presence of a normal cardiac silhouette. The principal ECG changes of importance are left ventricular hypertrophy secondary to hypertension, previous or

Table 23.11 Investigation of stroke and transient ischaemic attack

All infarction and haemorrhage
Brain CT or MRI
Full blood count
Platelet count
ESR
Urea and electrolytes
Blood sugar
Cholesterol
Chest X-ray
Electrocardiogram (ECG)
All haemorrhage
Clotting screen
Selected patients
Neck ultrasound or MRA
Autoantibody screen
Thrombophilia screen
Syphilis serology
Drug screen
Sickle-cell test
Homocysteine
Screening for genetic causes of stroke
Echocardiography
24-hour ECG
Cerebral angiography

ESR, erythrocyte sedimentation rate; MRA, magnetic resonance angiography.

acute myocardial infarction (which may suggest cardiogenic embolus) and, most importantly, atrial fibrillation.

Neuroimaging is an essential investigation. Although MRI is greatly superior to CT at refining the pathophysiological diagnosis, it is not currently available for most patients. Scanning with **CT should be performed in all patients** to distinguish infarction from haemorrhage and to reveal mimics of the stroke syndrome, such as tumour or subdural haematoma. In the early stages, CT may be negative, depending on time to imaging, the size and severity of infarction and the skill of the interpreter. **Only 50–70% of infarcts are ever visible with CT**. It has become generally accepted that CT can 'exclude' intracranial haemorrhage in the acute phase. However, CT is not always positive in SAH and there are patients with microhaemorrhages presenting with minimal impairments, in whom CT and conventional MRI will be normal.

CT or MRI brain scan

MRI is a far more sensitive investigation for both stroke and non-stroke pathology. It is especially superior in the posterior fossa and at revealing small areas of infarction secondary to penetrating vessel occlusion. Sophisticated MRI can also be used to distinguish acute from chronic infarction using diffusion-weighted sequences (Figure 23.15a), while gradient echo sequences (T2*, see p. 26) may demonstrate microhaemorrhage. It is possible that in the future the combination of MR perfusion imaging and diffusion-weighted imaging will be used more widely to select patients for treatments such as thrombolysis or neuroprotective drugs. MRI has high sensitivity for cerebral venous thrombosis and can be used in conjunction with magnetic resonance angiography (MRA) to detect dissection of the carotid or vertebral arteries.

The information derived from imaging should be used to establish the pathophysiology and mechanism of stroke and guide management. **Most importantly the imaging abnormalities must be concordant with the clinical picture**. The presence of acute or old infarcts in more than one vascular territory should focus further investigation towards a central embolic source. Extensive asymptomatic small vessel disease is a risk factor for haemorrhage and *may* refine the decision not to give anticoagulation therapy to a

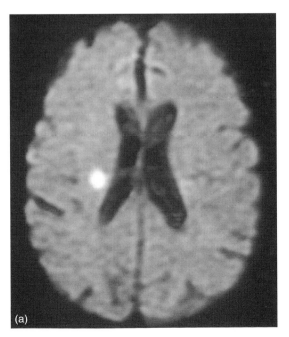 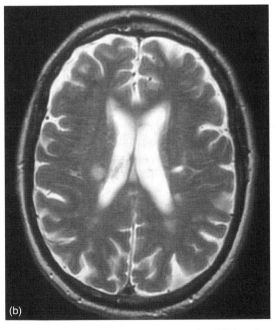

Figure 23.15 Diffusion-weighted imaging (a) shows 'light bulb' sign associated with acute infarction. On conventional T2 imaging (b) it is not as clear which area of infarction is acute.

Haematomas related to anticoagulant therapy may present as slowly evolving lesions. It is virtually always a mistake if the haematoma is small at initial imaging not immediately to reverse warfarin, as delay may have devastating consequences. This maxim includes reversing anticoagulation in patients with prosthetic valves, because the benefit/risk ratio is much in favour of anticoagulation reversal for a period of 2 weeks, after which the rebleeding rate is considerably lower. The actual rate of systemic embolism during this period is small. In appropriate patients it is necessary to exclude underlying vascular malformations with delayed MRI or angiography.

Prevention of secondary complications (Table 23.13)

Swallowing

Careful assessment of swallowing must take place in all patients with stroke; swallowing will be impaired in 50%. Ideally, a speech and language therapist should assess all patients. If this assessment is delayed, and **there is doubt about the integrity of swallowing, it is better to keep patients nil by mouth and feed them via a nasogastric tube**. The gag reflex is an insensitive screen of swallowing integrity. In general if the patient is alert and attentive, has a clear chest, normal speech and a strong, clear cough then it is safe to try sips of water, increasing to a glass and then feeding. This should be stopped if there are signs of aspiration, for example, 'wet' voice or choking, and nasogastric feeding should be instituted. If nasogastric feeding is likely to continue for more than 2 weeks, then per-endoscopic gastrostomy feeding should be considered. Per-endoscopic gastrostomy is often a better option in

Table 23.13 Important preventable and treatable secondary complications

Aspiration pneumonia
Thromboembolism
Infection
Painful shoulder
Depression

confused patients who repetitively pull out nasogastric tubes. Stroke is associated with a massive catabolic response and trials are underway comparing different feeding regimens.

> Failure to manage swallowing adequately in the early stages can result in aspiration pneumonia, which, in turn, causes fever and hypoxia, both of which are likely to exacerbate secondary brain damage.

Thromboembolism

Clinical deep vein thrombosis is rare on stroke units with active management policies because hydration, early mobilization and aspirin all contribute towards prevention. However, a small proportion of patients immobilized by stroke suffer from pulmonary embolism, usually occurring between 7 days and 6 weeks after the onset of stroke. **Compression stockings** should therefore be used routinely in **immobile** patients. **Low dose subcutaneous heparin** should be considered as an option in patients at **high risk** of venous thromboembolism; for example, those with a prior history of deep vein thrombosis. However, heparin is not recommended routinely because the benefits of heparin in preventing thromboembolism are matched by the risks of promoting cerebral haemorrhage. It should be remembered that patients in atrial fibrillation are at risk of systemic embolism to the limbs and bowel as well as recurrent stroke. However, in general, such patients should not receive anticoagulation therapy until 2 weeks after the onset of stroke, unless the patient has only had a small infarct, because the risk of causing haemorrhagic transformation negates the benefit of reduction in further embolism.

Infection

Pneumonia is common after stroke and should be vigorously treated. It is very difficult to assess prognosis at the outset in those without complicating pneumonia and even harder in those with it. Coexisting infection can make the situation appear far graver than it is. If patients are managed poorly in the acute stages because of concerns about long-term prognosis, then their poor outcome will become a self-fulfilling prophecy. Ensuring a safe swallow (see above) before allowing oral intake plays an important part in preventing aspiration pneumonia.

Painful shoulder

The complication of painful shoulder has become far rarer since the advent of correct positioning of the hemiplegic limb. This at the simplest level involves elevating the arm on a pillow when the patient is sitting to prevent partial subluxation of the shoulder joint.

Depression

Depression is common and readily treated. It should be distinguished from acute grief reactions, which are also common and nearly always self-limiting. It should be noted that organic brain disease predisposes to depression.

Early mobilization

Early mobilization on an active stroke unit, where all conscious patients are sat out of bed within a day, may well help to prevent many of the above complications.

REHABILITATION

The natural history of stroke is to improve over time, unless the patient succumbs to primary neurological death or secondary complications.

> **Aims of rehabilitation**
> Rehabilitation aims to enhance this spontaneous recovery and helps the patient to adjust to any residual deficit, as well as improving the patient's functional activity and participation.

Rehabilitation is a complicated and generally poorly understood process. It is not about 'popping down to the gym for a bit of physio'. One of the key factors in rehabilitation is that problems are addressed at three levels: impairment, limitation of activity (disability), and limitation of participation (handicap). Physicians often view problems solely at an

impairment level and are disappointed because their patient still has a weak limb, despite several weeks of therapy. They may miss the fact that despite this, participation in the activities of daily living may have changed substantially. All therapists play a crucial role. The value of **occupational therapy** and **neuropsychological input**, in addition to **physiotherapy** and **speech and language therapy**, cannot be underestimated in a population with significant cognitive impairment. Rehabilitation must be goal-oriented and combined with active discharge planning to have maximal impact. The old style maxim 'let's see what the patient is like next week' is inefficient and incompatible with efficient use of scarce resources. Effective rehabilitation is practical proof that the brain is not hardwired, but in fact has considerable capacity to reprogram itself through synaptic potentiation and dendritic sprouting.

MODELS OF SERVICE DELIVERY

TIAs and minor recovered strokes require urgent assessment to identify and treat risk factors. This can be carried out in an out-patient setting, provided the patient can be seen and investigated within a short time frame of ideally 2 weeks or less. 'One stop' clinics provide an efficient way of providing this service. Secondary prevention can be commenced in primary care at the time of referral. Patients with recurrent TIAs within a period of 1 month or less, or those with crescendo TIAs (TIAs of increasing frequency or severity) should be admitted as emergencies. There is a general trend for patients to be started liberally on antiplatelet medication but less attention is paid to the vigorous treatment of hypertension. Lowering blood pressure too much by overrigorous treatment of hypertension in acute stroke can considerably worsen outcome; it is, however, often the most important risk factor, certainly a far more common problem on a population basis than carotid stenosis. Hence, gradual control of hypertension is essential and even patients with normal blood pressure benefit from blood pressure lowering therapy after recovery from stroke or TIA.

In the past, acute stroke patients could be treated at home or in hospital; in hospital, care could be delivered within a general medical environment or a stroke unit. **Stroke units provide coordinated multidisciplinary care** within a discreet geographical area. There are now over 20 trials looking at the impact of such units compared with care on a general medical ward. Overall, stroke unit care leads to a significant reduction in the odds of death and dependency and this is seen in virtually all patient groups, irrespective of age or severity of stroke. The old maxim that aggressively managing those who seem at onset to have severe stroke syndromes is unwise, because of the likelihood that many dependent people will survive rather than die, is now untenable. While this will happen in individual cases, it will also be the case that those who would be left dependent will be shifted up a grade and leave independent. There are no reliable ways of predicting outcome at presentation with stroke, therefore all patients should be admitted to a specialized stroke service.

Stroke units may provide acute care, rehabilitation or both. All three models are effective and it seems likely that a comprehensive unit (acute care and rehabilitation) will ensure the best outcome. Acute care merges into rehabilitation and these should not be regarded as separate entities. The outcome of patients treated on general wards, for whom regular consultation has been provided by a 'mobile' expert team, or who have been cared for at home with a domiciliary stroke team, has been shown to be less effective than admission to a geographically discrete in-patient stroke unit. Geographically discrete units not only allow concentration of expertise but also allow an effective team culture to be built. As one stroke physician commented when complemented on the good outcome seen on their unit, 'it's nothing to do with me, it's the team'.

SECONDARY PREVENTION

Medical issues

The **risk of recurrence after stroke is between 5 and 15% in the first year** depending on the patient's risk factors. **After 5 years, 30% have had a recurrence.** There is also an increased risk of myocardial infarction. As well as guiding the patient through the acute phase and prospectively planning rehabilitation and

Table 23.14 Secondary prevention after stroke and transient ischaemic attack

Ischaemic and haemorrhagic stroke
Lifestyle issues
Stop smoking
Take regular exercise
Reduce excess alcohol intake
Encourage healthy diet
Medical treatment of risk factors
Lower blood pressure
ACE inhibition
Optimize diabetes treatment
Lower cholesterol with a statin
Ischaemic stroke
Prevention of thrombosis
Warfarin for atrial fibrillation
Antiplatelet therapy if not receiving
anticoagulation treatment
Treatment of severe carotid stenosis
Surgery or stenting
Cerebral haemorrhage
Clipping or coiling of aneurysm
Removal or obliteration of AVM

ACE, angiotensin-converting enzyme; AVM, arteriovenous malformation.

discharge, it is therefore vital to ensure that modifiable risk factors for recurrent stroke are addressed early after onset of TIA and stroke (Table 23.14). This will include **smoking cessation** and **antihypertensive treatment** (target >140/80 mmHg), if appropriate. There is emerging evidence that lowering even 'normal' blood pressure (using a combination of a diuretic with an ACE inhibitor) reduces the relative risk of further vascular events as much as in those with hypertension. In addition, **statins** have been shown to reduce composite vascular outcome in patients with a history of ischaemic heart or cerebrovascular disease and normal cholesterol concentrations.

Warfarin
Anticoagulation with warfarin produces highly significant reductions in vascular events for patients in atrial fibrillation and is the only proven stroke preventive treatment for this condition.

Table 23.15 Antiplatelet agents used in secondary stroke prevention

Agent	Dose	Cost/100 tablets (£)
Aspirin	Dispersible 75 mg o.d	1.30
Dipyridamole	MR 200 mg b.d.	16.25
Clopidogrel	75 mg o.d.	126.10
Ticlopidine	250 mg b.d	166.67

Table 23.16 Results of carotid endarterectomy (from North American Symptomatic Carotid Endarterectomy Trial (NASCET), *Lancet*, 2001)

% stenosis	Risk of stroke over 18 months (%)	
	Medical	Surgical
90–99	33	6
80–89	28	8
70–79	19	7

Warfarin should therefore be considered for all patients with **atrial fibrillation** after ischaemic TIA and stroke, aiming for an INR (International Normalized Ratio) of 2.5 (range 2–3). However, warfarin is not beneficial in patients with other non-cardiac causes of stroke and may be harmful in older patients or in those with hypertensive small vessel disease. In patients who are not receiving anticoagulants, antiplatelet therapy should be prescribed unless stroke has been caused by ICH (Table 23.15).

Aspirin following ischaemic stroke is definitely beneficial in doses between 75 and 300 mg o.d. Addition of modified release dipyridamole to aspirin and use of clopidogrel alone are slightly more beneficial than aspirin alone, but the differences in absolute risk reduction are small, except in those at high risk of occurrence. Ticlopidine is rarely used nowadays because of the risk of neutropenia and the need for haematological monitoring.

Carotid stenosis

There is now considerable evidence that carotid endarterectomy is beneficial in patients with recent non-disabling ischaemic stroke or TIA associated with a concordant high-grade carotid artery stenosis. If patients with **stenoses greater than 70%** (measured by the NASCET technique) are operated on by a surgeon with a resulting low morbidity and mortality rate, within a few weeks of symptoms (or months at the most), then the **stroke risk from the operation is far less than the stroke risk with medical therapy alone** (Table 23.16). Carotid angioplasty and stenting are alternatives to endarterectomy that are currently being evaluated in clinical trials. Carotid occlusion is not currently amenable to surgery.

Selecting these patients can be quite challenging and is not as simple as Table 23.16 suggests. Particular difficulties are posed by more marginal patients with a 50–70% stenosis according to the NASCET method of measurement; but this partly depends on the skill of the surgeon. This corresponds to a 70–80% stenosis by European methods. Patients with isolated transient monocular blindness are at less risk from medical treatment alone and women are at higher risk from operative complications. Hence generally, men with hemisphere ischaemia are most likely to benefit and women with transient monocular blindness least likely. The longer the period free of symptoms, the less benefit from surgery, because most recurrent strokes associated with carotid surgery occur within the first 3 months. There is unlikely to be much overall benefit if surgery is delayed for more than 6 months after symptoms.

SUBARACHNOID HAEMORRHAGE

Subarachnoid haemorrhage (SAH) is caused by **rupture of an intracranial aneurysm** in 85%, non-aneurysmal perimesencephalic haemorrhage in 10%, and arteriovenous malformation and a variety of rare conditions, in 5%. Subarachnoid haemorrhage is a devastating condition with an **overall case fatality of 50%** (including pre-hospitalization deaths). Moreover, **30% of survivors are left dependent** from major neurological deficits. The average age of onset is approximately 50 years, but SAH can occur at any age. In spite of many advances in diagnosis and treatment over the last decades the case fatality rate has not changed.

Risk factors

Considerable evidence supports the role of genetic factors in the development of intracranial aneurysms. There is strong association between intracranial aneurysms and heritable connective tissues diseases, although these only form a tiny part of any caseload. Familial occurrence is marked, with reports of up to 20% of patients with aneurysmal SAH having a first- or second-degree relative with a confirmed intracranial aneurysm. Unlike other forms of stroke, women form the majority of patients. Environmental factors have been extensively studied and cigarette smoking is the only factor consistently identified, raising the risk 3–10 times that of non-smokers. Hypertension is almost certainly also important, but to a lesser degree.

Clinical features

> **Headache in SAH**
> The cardinal clinical feature of SAH is a 'thunderclap headache'. This is a generalized headache of unique severity and sudden onset, often accompanied by nausea and vomiting.

Many patients will give a history of unusual and acute headaches predating the definite SAH by several days to weeks. It is thought that these warning headaches may be the result of aneurysmal enlargement or minor rupture. These headaches are often not diagnosed as SAH. This is not surprising given the high incidence of primary headache syndromes. Thunderclap headache, although a cardinal feature, is non-specific and only 1 in 10 of those presenting with sudden explosive headache will have SAH. However, there are no universal features to distinguish benign thunderclap headache from SAH, and cases with a typical history require investigation for SAH by CT scan, and lumbar puncture if CT is negative. However, in SAH the blood characteristically irritates the meninges soon after onset.

> Signs of meningeal irritation (stiff neck, photophobia) are found in most patients and it is a common error for these not to be elicited or to be misinterpreted in patients with acute headache.

Signs of global or focal dysfunction may also be found, depending on the severity and location of SAH. Focal deficits may be caused by intraparenchymal extension of blood, or later by vasospasm with resulting ischaemia and infarction. Patients may or may not lose consciousness briefly, or have prolonged coma at onset.

In a minority of cases, subhyaloid venous haemorrhages are visible on fundoscopy. The site of the bleeding aneurysm may be suggested by other clinical signs. A third nerve palsy suggests an aneurysm of the internal carotid or posterior communicating artery. Hemiparesis and aphasia suggests a middle cerebral artery aneurysm and leg weakness with bilateral extensor plantars, an anterior communicating artery aneurysm.

Investigation

CT scanning is mandatory in those with suspected SAH. Modern generation CT will demonstrate the presence of blood in 90–95% of patients scanned within 24 hours (Figure 23.17). However, blood is rapidly cleared from the CSF and the sensitivity

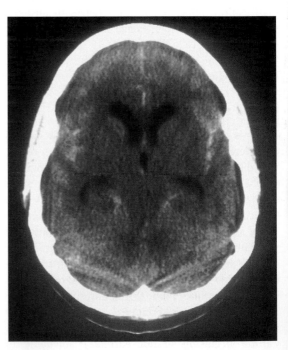

Figure 23.17 CT showing extensive subarachnoid blood and early hydrocephalus.

of **CT gradually decreases to 80% at 3 days, 50% at 1 week and 30% at 2 weeks. If clinical suspicion is strong and the CT is normal, lumbar puncture should be performed** by an experienced operator. If clinically appropriate, this should be delayed for 12 hours after the ictus to allow **xanthochromia** to be detected. Negative CSF is very helpful in excluding SAH, but bloodstained CSF may result from a traumatic tap.

A decrease in the number of red cells from bottle one to three is an unreliable way of differentiating SAH from a traumatic tap.

Xanthochromia (yellow discoloration) of the supernatant indicating haemolysed red cells is however diagnostic of SAH, as long as the patient has not had a prior traumatic lumbar puncture.

In most laboratories xanthochromia is determined by visual inspection rather than spectrophotometry, which is positive in all patients between 12 hours and 2 weeks. It should be remembered that patients may have SAH and a traumatic tap. Conventional MRI is not very sensitive to acute haemorrhage, but may be very useful after a delay when CT is negative.

In patients in whom CT or LP has confirmed the diagnosis, candidates for intervention should be referred urgently to a specialist centre for neurosurgical assessment and angiography.

Management and prognosis

General supportive care should be instituted, with particular importance being placed on the avoidance of dehydration, hypotension and hypertension. Bed-rest prior to definitive treatment is conventional but not a proven benefit. Administration of nimodipine reduces the risk of delayed ischaemia secondary to vasospasm. The **rebleeding rate from aneurysms is particularly high in the first 2 weeks** and then declines. This early high rebleeding rate, which may have devastating complications, is the reason why early intervention is favoured. In arteriovenous malformations the risk of bleeding is lower but in untreated cases persists indefinitely. In patients with a normal angiogram, in whom the haemorrhage is

often maximal in the basal cisterns (perimesencephalic SAH), the risk of recurrence is low.

If an aneurysm is identified by angiography, this can usually then be dealt with by **neurosurgical clipping of the neck or endovascular delivery of detachable coils**, which are packed into the aneurysm to prevent further rupture. It is uncertain at present which of these techniques is preferable, both in terms of immediate complications and long-term risk.

Survivors of SAH have a high incidence of cognitive problems even if there are no limb signs, and assessment for rehabilitation should address these issues.

NON-ATHEROSCLEROTIC VASCULOPATHIES AND OTHER RARE CAUSES OF STROKE

Cerebral venous thrombosis

Cerebral venous thrombosis is an important treatable, but rare, cause of stroke. It is also a condition with diverse manifestations that mimic many other neurological disorders. It is increasingly recognized because of enhanced awareness and the use of MRI. **Venous thrombosis may be septic or non-septic** (Table 23.17). Septic causes are rare but cavernous sinus thrombosis secondary to facial cellulitis, and lateral sinus thrombosis secondary to purulent otitis media or mastoiditis, are still seen from time to time. Septic thrombophlebitis of the cortical veins may also be associated with severe bacterial meningitis.

Table 23.17 Causes of cerebral venous thrombosis

Septic	Facial cellulitis
	Otitis media
	Mastoiditis
	Meningitis
Non septic	Pregnancy and the puerperium
	Contraceptive pill
	Dehydration
	Thrombophilia
	Behçet's syndrome

Aseptic thrombosis may affect the cortical veins, dural sinuses and deep veins. There are numerous potential causes. The most common include pregnancy, the puerperium, dehydration, thrombophilia and Behçet's syndrome (see p. 504). Combinations of these factors are often involved. In 20% no aetiology is uncovered.

Signs and symptoms of cerebral venous thrombosis

The clinical syndrome that manifests from cerebral venous thrombosis may be acute or subacute. The most frequent manifestations are headaches, seizures, altered consciousness, focal signs and disc swelling. Hence cerebral venous thrombosis should be considered in the differential diagnosis of those presenting with stroke, severe headache, seizure disorders, coma, acute meningoencephalitic syndromes and idiopathic intracranial hypertension.

Venous thrombosis results in venous hypertension, which leads to raised intracranial pressure. This may simply give rise to a **syndrome of headache with papilloedema and normal CT imaging**. As the venous pressure rises, lobar intracranial haemorrhage or cerebral infarction, which is often haemorrhagic, results in focal neurological deficit and depression of consciousness. Occasionally, cerebral venous thrombosis presents with SAH (Figure 23.18).

A scan using CT is often normal, but may show a filling defect in one of the venous sinuses, which is more obvious after contrast injection. The diagnosis should also be suspected if there are bilateral superficial parietal infarcts or if an infarct does not respect arterial territories. Diagnosis can be made in the vast majority of cases with **plain MRI supplemented by flow-related MR venography images**. In doubtful cases, conventional angiography may be required. The accepted treatment for cerebral venous thrombosis is anticoagulation, which has also been shown to be safe in those with haemorrhagic infarction.

Dissection

The majority of patients with stroke secondary to disease of the arterial wall will have atherosclerosis

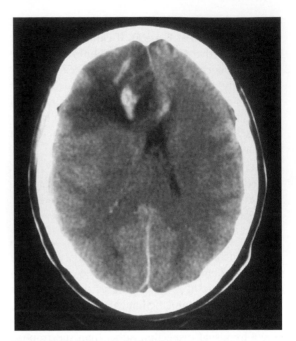

Figure 23.18 Haemorrhagic infarction secondary to cerebral venous thrombosis. The haemorrhagic infarct crosses vascular territories and is associated with generalized white matter oedema. Both these features are suggestive of venous sinus thrombosis.

or small vessel lipohyalinosis, but there are several other important non-atherosclerotic vasculopathies to consider, including **extracranial arterial dissection and cerebral vasculitis**.

Cervicocephalic arterial dissection should be especially considered in young patients. There are several connective tissue diseases that are associated with dissection including Marfan's syndrome, Ehlers–Danlos syndrome and fibromuscular dysplasia. However, the vast majority occur in apparently normal subjects, either **spontaneously** or after **trivial neck trauma or manipulation**. New evidence is emerging that some of these 'normal' subjects may, in fact, have subtle underlying collagen defects. Hyperextension of the neck during hair-washing in the salon or when painting a ceiling are common preceding events. Dissection can also result from more obvious trauma to the neck, as with penetrating injuries, or iatrogenically during catheter angiography. Dissection is produced by the subintimal penetration of blood as a result of a small tear in the intima with subsequent extension of the haematoma between the vessel layers. This may lead to occlusion of the vessel, but more often exposes a thrombogenic surface on which an intra-luminal haematoma develops. This haematoma may then embolise and produce stroke. The vast majority of cases affect the extracranial carotid and vertebral arteries. Intracranial dissection is much rarer.

Signs and symptoms of dissection [AB67]

The classic clinical scenario of dissection is a history of minor trauma to the neck followed shortly by the development of localized neck pain and headache. There is then a delay of several days (or sometimes weeks) before embolisation causes TIA or stroke. Patients usually present after stroke has occurred, but occasionally present with a painful Horner's syndrome.

In some patients, dissection may never give rise to symptomatic embolisation, but in others dissection may be instantly associated with devastating cerebral infarction. The association of **stroke with Horner's syndrome** should alert the clinician to the possibility of dissection. In the carotid circulation this results from the dissecting haematoma compressing the ascending sympathetic fibres, which surround the carotid artery. In the vertebrobasilar circulation, Horner's syndrome may also result as part of lateral medullary syndrome from occlusion of the posterior inferior cerebellar artery, with resultant infarction of the dorsolateral medulla where the descending sympathetic tracts lie, and is then not specific for dissection.

MRI provides a sensitive and non-invasive means to confirm dissection. Fine-cut axial imaging through the neck or cranium may reveal the characteristic crescentic vessel wall haematoma (Figure 23.19) and flow-related MRA may show luminal compromise. Conventional catheter angiography characteristically shows an eccentric tapering stenosis or occlusion and may also demonstrate underlying fibromuscular dysplasia. Ultrasound is less sensitive, especially if the dissection occurs in the high cervical carotid or vertebral artery.

The accepted management of dissection is to give **heparin as an anticoagulant**, followed by **warfarin for at least 3 months**. The rationale is that anticoagulation will lower the risk of embolisation. There is no clinical trial that provides solid evidence

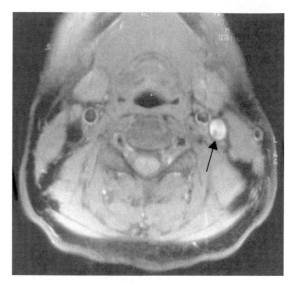

Figure 23.19 Axial MRI showing characteristic crescentic wall haematoma secondary to dissection.

for this practice, but longitudinal studies show that stroke is rare following anticoagulation. There have been no randomized-controlled trails comparing anticoagulation with antiplatelet therapy.

Vasculitis

Vasculitis is a very rare, but important cause of stroke, because of the need for urgent immunosuppression to prevent recurrence.

Vasculitis as stroke

It is exceedingly rare for vasculitis to present as stroke without other preceding features of a systemic vasculitis.

Vasculitis causing stroke may be secondary to infections, connective tissue diseases (e.g. systemic lupus erythematosus or polyarteritis nodosa; see p. 500), other systemic vasculitides, and giant cell arteritis.

Occasionally, isolated CNS vasculitis occurs without any systemic or extracranial features. In these conditions, cerebral malfunction or haemorrhage may result from true inflammation of the vessel wall, associated coagulapathies (e.g. the antiphospholipid antibody syndrome) or, more commonly, uncontrolled hypertension secondary to renal vasculitis.

Infections

Infectious vasculitis associated with **meningitis** may occur acutely in the appropriate setting of severe bacterial, fungal, tuberculous or herpes zoster infection. There is nearly always an appropriate preceding history suggestive of a meningoencephalitic syndrome. An obliterative endarteritis affecting the small vessels of the brain may occur after primary syphilis infection, with an average latency of 7 years. Headache and encephalopathy predominate in the prodrome before stroke occurs. Evidence of previous treponemal infection is easy to screen for in the blood and those with neurological involvement usually have pleocytosis and positive serology in the CSF.

Connective tissue disorders (see p. 499)

In systemic necrotizing vasculitis, stroke is most commonly seen with **polyarteritis nodosa**, usually in association with uncontrolled hypertension. Such patients have usually been unwell for a considerable time period without treatment. The systemic features include weight loss, fever and abdominal and muscle pain. Renal involvement is common and may lead to severe hypertension. Mononeuritis multiplex secondary to peripheral nerve vasculitis may also occur. The combination of infarcts and haemorrhages on CT or MR is particularly suggestive of vasculitis, but this pattern is also seen in infectious endocarditis and venous sinus thrombosis. The diagnosis of polyarteritis nodosa is suggested by positive antineutrophil cytoplasmic antibodies. Treatment with cyclophosphamide is often necessary to induce remission.

Systemic lupus erythematosus commonly causes neurological problems. These are often neuropsychiatric and are rarely a result of vasculitis. Encephalopathy, psychosis, seizures, stroke-like focal deficits, myelopathy and neuropathy are all encountered. At pathological examination the histology is often one of non-specific gliosis, although thrombosis may be observed, especially in those with antiphospholipid antibodies. Stroke may also occur secondary to embolism from Libman Sacks

endocarditis. Management may require both anticoagulation and immunosuppression.

Giant cell arteritis (see pp. 478, 500)

Temporal arteritis is the most important of the giant cell arteritides. The internal elastic lamina of the extracranial medium-sized arteries becomes fragmented and invaded by inflammatory cells. It virtually always occurs in those over 50 years and is accompanied by an elevated ESR in 90%.

Signs and symptoms of temporal arteritis
Patients with temporal arteritis complain of headache with scalp tenderness associated with malaise, depression, myalgia and sometimes claudication of the jaw muscles while eating. Examination may reveal thickened tender temporal arteries.

Stroke is a very rare complication of the disease but may occur from involvement of the extradural vertebral artery, leading to brainstem infarction. A far commoner complication at presentation is **blindness and/or an anterior ischaemic optic neuropathy** (see p. 192). Diagnosis is established by temporal artery biopsy. Treatment is with high dose prednisolone and, if the diagnosis is correct, the response of the systemic symptoms is dramatic and usually occurs within 1 day of starting treatment.

Takayasu's arteritis is much rarer. This usually affects young Asian females, and is associated with a high ESR. As well as systemic features of malaise and fever, the manifestations are a result of aortic arch inflammation, with subsequent occlusion of its branches, in particular the origin of one or both common carotid arteries.

Isolated angiitis of the central nervous system

Isolated angiitis of the CNS is a rare condition, which affects small and medium-sized intracranial vessels. It may cause a combination of infarcts and haemorrhages. The presentation is usually subacute or chronic with prominent headache, leading to encephalopathy or oedema with recurrent stroke-like focal events and the development of dementia over a few weeks or months. Angiography may reveal segmental narrowing of intracranial vessels but is neither sensitive nor specific. The CSF often shows a pleocytosis, and imaging demonstrates multiple small vessel occlusions and haemorrhages if advanced. Diagnosis is by meningeal and brain biopsy. If patients have neither headache nor CSF pleocytosis, then biopsy rarely shows vasculitis. Treatment is with steroids and cyclophosphamide.

Hypertensive encephalopathy

Hypertensive encephalopathy manifests when systemic blood pressure is sustained above the upper limit of cerebral autoregulation. Oedema develops in the hyperperfused intracerebral circulation. Patients present with headache, epileptic seizures, focal TIA or stroke-like events, and, in advanced cases, depressed consciousness. Examination may also reveal papilloedema.

> The blood pressure is often very high, for example, 250/150 mmHg.

In patients who develop hypertensive encephalopathy the rate of blood pressure elevation has often been rapid and a result of renal disease. Occasionally hypertensive encephalopathy can develop at lower blood pressure levels, particular in eclampsia associated with pregnancy.

Arteriovenous malformations

Arteriovenous malformations (AVMs) are complex tangles of abnormal arteries and veins, which lack a capillary bed but are linked by one or more direct fistulas. They are thought to arise from developmental derangements at various stages. They may present with **SAH or ICH, epilepsy or progressive focal deficit**. With the advent of MRI many are discovered coincidentally (Figure 23.20). They may be classified by size, location and their angioarchitecture. Advances in treatment modalities are occurring more rapidly than advances in our knowledge of the natural history of these lesions.

The single most important fact determining prognosis is whether the AVM has bled or not. Patients with a history of intracranial haemorrhage are at a much higher risk of **rebleeding** (up to 18% per year) than patients presenting without haemorrhage (2% per year). However, young patients without

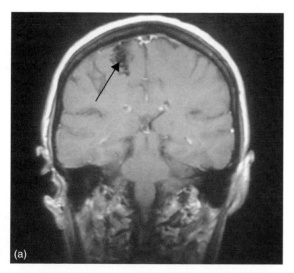
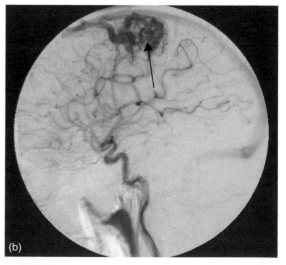

Figure 23.20 MRI and catheter angiogram showing an arteriovenous malformation. This patient presented with focal seizures and had no evidence of bleeding over prolonged follow up.

a history of haemorrhage may have a very high lifetime risk of bleeding. In any patient where treatment is considered, formal angiography in expert hands is required to define the angioarchitecture. This allows the risks of treatment or conservative management to be defined as accurately as possible. Management plans for these lesions should only be made by expert multidisciplinary teams, who can balance the risk of treatment against the risk of bleeding. Surgery is an option for treatment of accessible lesions with a single arterial supply and a single route of venous drainage. Endovascular obliteration with glue is an alternative treatment modality, which often results in partial obliteration of the AVM and may target 'high risk' elements within the malformation. It is not known whether partial obliteration is worthwhile, but it seems likely that this will reduce the bleeding risk. Radiotherapy is an option for small lesions and produces obliteration in up to 80% of lesions by 2 years, but the patient is at risk of haemorrhage during this time. Often combination therapy is necessary.

Vascular disease of the spinal cord

Spinal cord infarction is a rare disorder and is usually caused by occlusion of the anterior spinal artery, which supplies the anterior two-thirds of the cord. Most patients with anterior spinal artery occlusion have multiple risk factors, especially hypertension and diabetes. The anterior spinal artery is also vulnerable to aortic dissection. The dorsal columns are spared by anterior spinal artery occlusion thanks to a rich plexal supply. The resultant clinical picture is therefore an acute areflexic paraplegia characterized by dissociated sensory loss: that is, striking preservation of joint position and vibration sense, with marked loss of pinprick and temperature sensation in the lower limbs and trunk. No effective acute treatment is known but rehabilitation is very helpful to the patient.

REFERENCES AND FURTHER READING

Brown MM (ed.) (2000) *Stroke*. British Medical Bulletin 56.2. London, UK: RSM Press.

Caplan C (2000) *Caplan's Stroke: a clinical approach*. Boston, MA: Butterworth-Heinemann.

Warlow CP *et al.* (1998) *Stroke. A practical guide to management*. Oxford, UK: Blackwell Science Ltd.

CHAPTER 24

NEUROLOGICAL COMPLICATIONS OF MEDICAL DISORDERS

T.J. Fowler and J.W. Scadding

THE PITUITARY GLAND

Tumours are found in some 23% of pituitary glands in unselected autopsies; many of these are asymptomatic and are microadenomata, with a diameter of less than 1 cm.

Large tumours, macroadenomata, expand out from the sella as they grow. Superiorly they may compress the optic chiasm with visual symptoms, laterally they may involve the cavernous sinus (cranial nerves III, IV, Va and VI) and even damage the temporal lobe (epilepsy). They may also spread inferiorly into the sphenoid sinus or backwards into the posterior fossa. Very large pituitary tumours can result in an obstructive hydrocephalus with signs of raised intracranial pressure.

Many pituitary tumours present from excess secretion of hormone (Table 24.1). Anterior pituitary hormones are secreted in a pulsatile fashion, so serial estimations are necessary. In some 30% there may be a failure of endocrine function – panhypopituitarism. The latter may also follow ischaemic damage; for example, in post-partum haemorrhage,

Table 24.1 Pituitary hormones and associated disturbances

Excess secretion	Stimuli	Clinical condition
GH	GHRH and S+	Acromegaly*
IGF-1		Acromegaly*
ACTH	CRH	Cushing's disease*
Prolactin	PRH? TRH, VIP	Prolactinoma**
TSH	TRH	TSH-, TRH-secreting tumours
LH	GnRH	Gonadotropinoma
FSH	GnRH	Gonadotropinoma

Pituitary tumours are non-secreting in 30%.
**Common; *less common; others rare.
GH, growth hormone; GHRH, growth-hormone-releasing hormone; S +, somatostatin; IGF-1, insulin-like growth factor; ACTH, adrenocorticotropic hormone; CRH, corticotropin-releasing hormone; PRH, prolactin-releasing hormone; TRH, thyrotropin-releasing hormone; VIP, vasoactive intestinal peptide; TSH, thyroid-stimulating hormone; LH, luteinizing hormone; GnRH, gonadotropin-releasing hormone; FSH, follicle-stimulating hormone.

Table 24.2 Evaluation of basal pituitary function

Measure	Diurnal cortisol levels – midnight and 09.00 h
	Plasma ACTH
	TSH
	FT4, FT3
	LH
	FSH
	Prolactin
	GH
	IGF-1
	Plasma and urine osmolalities

ACTH, adrenocorticotropic hormone; TSH, thyroid-stimulating hormone; FT4, free thyroxine; FT3, free tri-iodothyronine; LH, luteinizing hormone; FSH, follicle-stimulating hormone; GH, growth hormone; IGF-1, insulin-like growth factor.

from pituitary apoplexy, infection, granulomas or even metastatic deposits.

Hypopituitarism

> **Hyopituitarism**
> Clinically this most commonly manifests as secondary amenorrhoea, infertility or impotence. There may be a failure of secondary sexual characteristics with loss of shaving, skin pallor, cold intolerance and slowing up [lack of thyroid-stimulating hormone (TSH) and adrenocorticotropic hormone (ACTH)]. With mass lesions, headache and visual symptoms are common.

Modern radioimmunoassays allow basal measurements of cortisol, ACTH, TSH, free tri-iodothyronine (FT3), free thyroxine (FT4), luteinizing hormone (LH), follicle-stimulating hormone (FSH), prolactin and growth hormone (GH) and insulin-like growth factor (IGF-1) levels. Plasma and urine osmolalities

assess posterior pituitary function and sometimes levels of oestradiol, progesterone and testosterone may also be appropriate (Table 24.2).

Dynamic tests of anterior pituitary function are based on the sequential administration of four hypothalamic-releasing hormones [gonadotropin-releasing hormone (GnRH), thyrotropin-releasing hormone (TRH), corticotropin-releasing hormone (CRH), growth hormone-releasing hormone (GHRH)]. These are injected intravenously (Table 24.3) and measurements of LH, FSH, TSH, ACTH, GH and prolactin levels are made at intervals. Baseline measurements are also made of oestradiol, testosterone, thyroxine, cortisol and IGF-1. An absent response suggests loss of function in the anterior pituitary cells.

To assess the pituitary gland reserve for GH and ACTH it can be stimulated by hypoglycaemia, induced by an injection of insulin (0.15 units/kg). Blood is then taken at intervals (Table 24.3) and the glucose, GH, ACTH, prolactin and cortisol levels measured. In normal patients the neuroglycopenia causes a rise in GH and ACTH (hence cortisol) but no such rise occurs in patients with hypopituitarism. The insulin stress test should not be used in patients with a history of epilepsy or ischaemic heart disease, or who are clearly hypothyroid or hypoadrenal in endocrine function. The patient should be closely monitored during the test by the doctor undertaking it.

Table 24.3 Assessment of pituitary reserve

Combined administration of four hypothalamic-releasing hormones

1	IV bolus of TRH (200 μg)	TSH response 0, 20 and 60 minutes
2	IV bolus of GnRH (100 μg)	FSH, LH response 0, 30 and 60 minutes
3	IV bolus of CRH (1 μg/kg)	ACTH response 0, 30, 60, 90, 120 minutes
4	IV bolus GHRH (1 μg/kg)	GH response 0, 30, 60, 90, 120 minutes

Insulin tolerance test – to measure ACTH and GH reserve

Hypoglycaemia used to stimulate GH and ACTH release

Inject insulin (0.15 U/Kg IV) and measure GH, ACTH, cortisol and prolactin at 0,30,45,60 and 90 minutes. Doctor in attendance throughout test.

TRH, thyrotropin-releasing hormone; TSH, thyroid-stimulating hormone; GnRH, gonadotropin-releasing hormone; FSH, follicle-stimulating hormone; LH, luteinizing hormone; CRH, corticotropin-releasing hormone; ACTH, adrenocorticotropic hormone; GHRH, growth-hormone-releasing hormone; GH, growth hormone.

Table 24.4 Causes of raised prolactin levels

Pregnancy, lactation, oestrogens
Pituitary tumours – prolactinoma
Parapituitary tumours and granulomas – gliomas, sarcoidosis
Pituitary stalk damage
Hypothalamic disease – tumours, granulomas
Drugs
    Dopamine receptor antagonists
        Phenothiazines – chlorpromazine
        Butyrophenones – haloperidol
        Anti-emetics – metoclopramide, domperidone
    Antidepressants – imipramine, amitriptyline
    Hypotensives – methyldopa, reserpine
    Cimetidine
Endocrine – acromegaly, hypothyroidism, Cushing's disease
Nipple stimulation
Stress
Major epileptic seizure

remains high and the plasma osmolality rises, often to more than 295 mosmol/kg.

Posterior pituitary function

The posterior pituitary secretes two peptides, arginine vasopressin (AVP) the antidiuretic hormone (ADH) and oxytocin. **Plasma osmolality** (normally 285–288 mosmol/kg) is maintained through AVP secretion from the osmoregulation of thirst. The AVP causes increased water reabsorption in the renal tubules, thus reducing urine output.

In diabetes insipidus there is commonly thirst with polydipsia and polyuria (urine output of >3 l/24 hours).

Diabetes insipidus is most commonly caused by posterior pituitary-hypothalamic damage from trauma, tumours, granulomas (e.g. sarcoid) or infections. If water is restricted, dehydration follows. In diabetes insipidus the water deprivation test causes the urine osmolality to rise, but the urine volume

Secreting pituitary tumours

Prolactinomas

Prolactinomas cause very high prolactin levels (Table 24.4) resulting in secondary amenorrhoea, infertility and impotence. There may also be galactorrhoea in 30–80%.

Patients may appear anxious, depressed and hostile. Many of these tumours are macroadenomata and may result in headaches and visual symptoms. They may increase in size during pregnancy. Patients show high levels of prolactin (usually greater than 3600 mIU/l), which fail to rise after TRH stimulation or after domperidone.

Dopamine agonists inhibit prolactin release and may allow some shrinkage of the gland. Bromocriptine was the first to be used but others have followed and cabergoline treatment results in some

92% of patients showing a response. Very large tumours usually require surgery.

Acromegaly

> Growth hormone excess causes gigantism before skeletal maturation and acromegaly in adults with coarsened overgrowth of facial features and in the extremities. Arthralgia and backache are common. There may be excess sweating and carpal tunnel entrapment is frequent. Patients with acromegaly have a shortened lifespan.

One-third of patients with acromegaly are hypertensive and some two-thirds have abnormal glucose tolerance. The best screening test is the serum IGF-1 level, which is significantly raised in acromegaly. Levels of GH fluctuate (there is pulsatile secretion) but some 50% of cases show a raised level. During a glucose tolerance test there is either a paradoxical rise in GH or no fall. Stimulation of TRH and GnRH may cause an elevation of GH levels.

Treatment is often surgical with a trans-sphenoidal approach. Treatment with somatostatin analogues, such as octreotide and lanreotide, is also used and will produce a clinical response in some 70% of patients, although a higher number are left with raised GH levels. Levels of IGF-1 are used to monitor the effects of treatment. These somatostatin analogues are given by injection and initially sometimes may cause some tumour expansion so the visual fields need to be monitored. Surgical treatment may be combined with radiotherapy.

Gonadotropinomas

Gonadotropinomas secrete excess GnRH, which is responsible for the pulsatile secretion of LH and FSH, so single measurements may be unreliable. They often present as large tumours with accompanying visual field defects. They may also result in hyposecretion of ACTH and TSH.

Cushing's syndrome

Cushing's syndrome is caused by adrenocortical hormonal excess. **Some 70% are caused by hypersecreting pituitary tumours**, usually microadenomas, which produce too much corticotropin (ACTH) – Cushing's disease. A few arise from the **ectopic production of ACTH**, most commonly from a **small cell lung carcinoma**. Some are ACTH independent, most often arising from an adenoma or carcinoma of the adrenal gland, or iatrogenic from corticosteroid excess. Forms of pseudo-Cushing's syndrome may arise from major depressive illness and from chronic alcoholism.

> Adrenocortical excess may cause weight gain, often central, with a moon face and buffalo hump, oedema, prominent skin striae, hypertension, glucose intolerance, oligomenorrhoea or amenorrhoea, impaired potency, hirsutism, acne, proximal muscle wasting and weakness, osteoporosis and psychiatric disturbances, such as depression, lethargy and insomnia.

Screening tests include measurements of 24-hour urinary free cortisol levels (preferably on three successive days), 09.00 h and 24.00 h plasma cortisol levels (normally plasma cortisol levels are highest in the early morning) and ACTH levels. Dexamethasone suppression, using low dose (0.5 mg 6-hourly for eight doses) or a midnight injection of 1 mg, in normal patients will suppress ACTH levels and so result in low cortisol levels. Failure of suppression indicates Cushing's syndrome and the need for more detailed tests to elucidate whether the pituitary, ectopic ACTH or adrenal excess is to blame.

In all patients with suspected pituitary tumours or disturbed pituitary function, magnetic resonance imaging (MRI), or failing that computerized tomography (CT) scanning, of the pituitary should be undertaken to establish the cause. In patients with pituitary mass lesions, the visual acuities should be recorded, the visual fields charted, and, if appropriate, the pattern evoked visual potentials measured (Table 24.5).

Table 24.5 Investigation of patients suspected of having a pituitary lesion

1	Measurement of visual acuity
2	Charting of visual fields
3	Endocrine assessment
4	Imaging of pituitary gland: MRI preferable, but CT if MR not possible

THYROID DISORDERS

Thyrotoxicosis

> **Thyrotoxicosis**
> Most patients with hyperthyroidism have evidence of a **proximal myopathy** with muscle weakness (see p. 134): a few have **bulbar weakness**. These symptoms may be the presentation. Neuropsychiatric symptoms are common and include anxiety, altered mood and behaviour, with restlessness and sympathetic overactivity. There may sometimes be a link with myasthenia gravis.

Dysthyroid eye disease particularly affects middle-aged women, and may cause ocular symptoms (see p. 195).

> Thyrotoxic patients may show proptosis (exophthalmos) with lid lag and retraction. Less often, infiltration of the external ocular muscles, particularly the medial and inferior recti, may lead to restriction of abduction and upgaze with complaints of diplopia and, commonly, pain on attempted eye movement – a restrictive ophthalmopathy (Table 24.6). The increase in volume of the extraocular muscles may lead to impaired venous drainage from the orbit, and the development of papilloedema. Optic nerve compression, with associated loss of vision may be caused by enlargement of the extraocular muscles at the orbital apex. The conjunctiva may appear oedematous and injected. The thickened and infiltrated eye muscles can be demonstrated by a forced duction test (showing the eyeball is restricted in its range of movements) or with a CT, or preferably an MRI scan of the orbital contents.

Conventional thyroid function tests, TSH levels, FT3 and FT4 assays, usually will confirm the diagnosis. Treatment is with drugs, carbimazole and propranolol, therapeutic doses of radio-iodine, or even surgery. Steroids are indicated in severe eye disease, particularly when there is papilloedema and visual impairment.

Myxoedema

> Clinically myxoedema may produce a progressive decline in mental function, with the appearance of a dementia, confusion, delusions, hallucinations and even paranoid suspicions. It is the most common treatable cause of dementia, arising in some 2–4% of elderly patients with a 3:1 female to male ratio.

There may be accompanying physical and mental slowing with a gradual decline in conscious level ending in coma. A few patients may present with an acute psychotic state, myxoedema madness.

> **Neurological manifestations of hypothyroidism**
> Hypothyroidism, in addition to dementia, may also produce a cerebellar ataxia with increasing unsteadiness. Muscle aching and fatigue are common complaints. A carpal tunnel syndrome occurs frequently in myxoedema, and a polyneuropathy may develop in a minority.

Many patients show coarse features, thinned hair, evidence of physical and mental slowing, a sensory-neural deafness, and ankle jerks with slow relaxation. There may be a bradycardia and swollen legs. There is often weight gain, cold sensitivity, constipation, a dry skin and a hoarse voice. Commonly, older women may be affected and hypothermia is a real risk in the winter.

Thyroid function tests will show a very elevated TSH level (>20 mU/l) and a low FT4 level. Treatment is with thyroxine replacement, starting with a small dose.

Table 24.6 Signs of dysthyroid eye disease

Lid lag
Lid retraction
Proptosis
Conjunctival suffusion
Restricted eye movements – particularly limited elevation and abduction (restrictive ophthalmopathy)
Papilloedema

Hashimoto's encephalopathy has been described in relation to an immune-mediated thyroiditis causing a cerebral vasculitis. Such patients may present with confusion, dementia, ataxia, seizures and myoclonus, extrapyramidal rigidity and sometimes stroke-like focal deficits.

There may be an abrupt onset and occasionally a relapsing course. The electroencephalograph (EEG) may show a diffuse abnormality and the condition initially may cause diagnostic difficulty when compared with prion disease. The presence of very high titres of thyroid peroxidase antibodies aids diagnosis. Treatment is with steroids.

ADRENAL DISTURBANCES

Addison's disease

The onset may be acute or slow and insidious depending on the cause. The adrenal gland may be destroyed by **infection (e.g. tuberculosis), a tumour (primary or secondary), or an autoimmune process**. In more chronic forms there will be excess ACTH stimulation, resulting in increased pigmentation of the skin and buccal mucosa.

> More acute crises, often precipitated by infection or surgery, may cause anorexia, vomiting, diarrhoea, abdominal pain, cramps, postural hypotension, dehydration, lethargy and weight loss.

There may be sodium and water depletion from mineralocorticoid deficiency with a low sodium, raised urea and potassium and, in a few patients, a raised calcium level. The plasma cortisol is low (<200 nmol/l) and the ACTH raised (>200 pg/l). An ACTH stimulation test with an injection of 250 μg IM of soluble ACTH (tetracosactide) normally shows a rise in cortisol level unless there is adrenal failure.

Acute treatment involves rehydration with saline, glucose and the intravenous injection of 100–200 mg of hydrocortisone with subsequent doses adjusted down until a maintenance dose is used, often hydrocortisone 20 mg mane and 10 mg nocte. Mineralocorticoid replacement with small doses of fludrocortisone 0.05–0.20 mg daily is sometimes necessary. The steroid dose will need to be increased with any intercurrent infection or proposed surgery.

HYPOGLYCAEMIA

Hypoglycaemia most often occurs in insulin-treated diabetics, less commonly from the use of oral hypoglycaemic drugs, and very rarely from insulin-secreting tumours (insulinomas). It is important that it is not missed, as prolonged uncorrected hypoglycaemia will produce irreversible brain damage.

> **Hypoglycaemia**
> Symptoms appear as the plasma glucose falls below 2.5 mmol/l and this fall will stimulate the adrenals so that pallor, sweating, tremor, tachycardia, anxiety and a light-headed feeling may appear – symptoms often recognized by diabetics so that they can heed this warning and take sugar. The low plasma glucose affects the brain, causing confusion, disordered behaviour (occasionally aggressive), slurred speech and unsteadiness. These symptoms may be mistaken for alcoholic intoxication. Continuing hypoglycaemia may cause focal neurological signs (Table 24.7) as a hemiplegia, epileptic seizures, a deteriorating conscious level and eventual coma.

> If there is clinical suspicion of hypoglycaemia, take blood for glucose estimation and immediately inject 20–30 ml of 50% glucose intravenously. The therapeutic response should be immediate unless hypoglycaemia has been prolonged or the diagnosis incorrect. Plasma glucose levels less than 2.0 mmol/l confirm the diagnosis. An insulinoma may be difficult to diagnose but a prolonged fast with estimation of glucose, insulin and plasma-C peptide levels will usually give the answer.

Table 24.7 Symptoms and signs of hypoglycaemia

Sympathetic (adrenaline)
- Anxiety
- Tremor
- Tachycardia
- Pallor
- Sweating

Neuroglycopenia (low glucose)
- Hunger
- Weakness
- Behaviour change (confusion, aggression)
- Slurred speech, unsteady
- Focal signs, e.g. hemiplegia
- Epileptic seizures
- Coma

HYPERGLYCAEMIA

Hyperglycaemia may cause a deteriorating conscious level leading to coma from:

- Diabetic ketoacidosis
- Hyperosmolar non-ketotic hyperglycaemia.

Diabetic ketoacidosis is the common cause of diabetic hyperglycaemic coma and may be precipitated by an acute infection, poor diabetic control or both. Occasionally it is the presenting symptom of diabetes but more often a known diabetic patient becomes ill over a few days with complaints of headache, weakness, vomiting and abdominal pain. There is dehydration with acidotic breathing and ketones may be present on the breath. Gradually there is increasing drowsiness, accompanied by confusion, which may lead to coma. Often the blood pressure is low and the pulse rapid.

Hyperosmolar coma arises in elderly diabetics who become haemoconcentrated with a high plasma osmolality (>350 mosmol/kg), high blood glucose (40–65 mmol/l) but no ketosis. Some patients present in shock with features of dehydration. A few present with seizures.

Investigation

Ketotic patients exhibit urinary glycosuria and ketonuria. The blood glucose is usually very high, the pH low with acidosis and a low bicarbonate, the potassium high and the sodium normal. The urea may be raised if there is considerable dehydration.

Treatment is as an emergency with intravenous rehydration with saline, intravenous insulin and correction of acidosis if severe. The electrolytes will need to be monitored regularly to maintain values, particularly potassium, within the normal range. The insulin dose will need to be titrated against the glucose value. Unconscious patients will need a nasogastric tube and aspiration of the gastric contents. Any precipitating cause for the ketosis will need correction.

Diabetes may be associated with a number of different pattern **neuropathies** (see p. 161).

HEPATIC FAILURE

Liver failure may develop acutely, for example from hepatitis or after self-poisoning with paracetamol, or more chronically, leading to a **portosystemic encephalopathy** (where substances not properly detoxified by the failing liver may be released into the circulation to disturb brain function). The latter is found most often in the cirrhotic patient, who may decompensate acutely in response to an infection, a gastric haemorrhage (often from oesophageal varices), to certain drugs, potassium loss or to protein excess.

This decompensation may be episodic so patients may show a fluctuating conscious level, irrational behaviour, delusions, hallucinations and confusion. These may be followed by a deteriorating conscious level, leading to stupor and coma. Initially there may be prominent muscle twitching and a flapping tremor of the outstretched hands (asterixis); epileptic seizures may appear. Initial mild symptoms such as restlessness, anxiety, fluctuating confusion and inverted sleep patterns may be missed.

Focal or bilateral pyramidal signs, rigidity, primitive reflexes and extensor plantar responses may be present. In coma the pupils may dilate. There may be associated stigmata from liver disease with foetor hepaticus, hepatic enlargement, spider naevi, jaundice, ascites, and oedema of the feet.

Investigations

Many patients show an elevated blood ammonia; normally this is less than 50 mmol/l but with hepatic failure it may rise to well above 100 mmol/l. In addition, there are abnormal liver function tests with elevated enzyme levels, and a prolonged prothrombin time (which may lead to bruising and haemorrhagic complications). The blood glucose may be low. The cerebrospinal fluid (CSF) may be normal or show a slight protein rise. The EEG may show paroxysmal slow wave activity mirroring the depressed conscious level; sometimes triphasic delta waves appear in stuporose patients. A CT brain scan may appear normal or show a swollen brain; it helps to exclude haemorrhagic complications.

Treatment

Treatment involves the elimination of any precipitating cause, the maintenance of a correct fluid balance with restriction of dietary protein and its replacement by intravenous glucose. Coagulation defects will need correction. Reducing nitrogenous products in the bowel may be aided by the addition of lactulose, and nitrogen-producing organisms may be treated with neomycin. In selected patients haemodialysis may be life-saving.

A progressive spastic paraparesis, portocaval encephalomyelopathy, is a rare complication, which may follow episodes of portosystemic encephalopathy or even surgery in patients with cirrhosis.

REYE'S SYNDROME

Reye's syndrome is a rare form of encephalopathy arising in children aged between 5 and 15 years, characterized by acute brain swelling with fatty infiltration of the liver. It appears often to be triggered by an acute viral infection, and in some instances perhaps by treatment with salicylates. The onset is acute with preceding symptoms of an upper respiratory tract infection, then profuse vomiting and a deteriorating conscious level ending in coma, seizures, rigidity and signs of cerebral damage. There may be a low blood and CSF glucose, abnormal liver enzymes, a prolonged prothrombin time and a raised blood ammonia. The EEG shows diffuse slow activity. The brain may become very swollen and this can be detected by imaging. The CSF is usually under increased pressure and is acellular.

Many children die but prompt recognition of the condition accompanied by treatment to lower the raised intracranial pressure, intravenous glucose and correction of any metabolic disturbances, allow some survivors, although a few may show signs of residual damage.

RENAL FAILURE

In **uraemic encephalopathy**, as the blood urea and creatinine rise, patients will become increasingly confused, drowsy and eventually comatose. Associated with the depressed conscious level may be hallucinations, twitching, tremors, asterixis, restlessness, tetany, myoclonic jerking and even tonic-clonic seizures. Very commonly such symptoms fluctuate. Patients with a depressed conscious level may show acidotic breathing, which later may wax and wane (Cheyne–Stokes). There are often associated systemic features with initial complaints of anorexia, nausea, vomiting, fatigue, pruritus, a haemorrhagic state and, in acute renal failure, oliguria.

Electrolyte disorders are common with hyperkalaemia, hyponatraemia and a rising blood urea and creatinine. There may be hypocalcaemia and hypomagnesaemia.

Treatment depends on the cause, but dialysis relieves the uraemia, and allows reversal of many of the neurological symptoms. Convulsions are usually controlled with low doses of anticonvulsants.

Hypertensive encephalopathy may also arise in patients with renal failure.

Dialysis problems

Two neurological clinical states are recognized in dialysis patients:

1 Dialysis dementia

2 Disequilibrium syndrome.

Dialysis dementia occurs in patients on long-term dialysis and may be associated with mental clouding, myoclonus, tonic-clonic seizures and speech disturbance. Initially there may be a stuttering progression resulting in intellectual decline. It is accompanied by a diffuse EEG disturbance. Aluminium toxicity from the dialysate is responsible for an acute or subacute encephalopathy.

Disequilibrium syndrome affects patients on dialysis, causing complaints of headache, nausea, agitation, irritability and even seizures. The symptoms come on within a short time, 3–4 hours, of starting dialysis and it has been suggested that they may arise from too rapid dialysis, which results in water intoxication. The symptoms usually last some hours.

Patients with uraemia may develop a peripheral sensorimotor **neuropathy** (see p. 163). After renal transplantation patients on immunosuppressive treatment are more prone to unusual infections, for example cryptococcus, listeriosis (see p. 391). Ciclosporin used as an immunosuppressant in transplant patients may provoke tremors and epileptic seizures. It may also produce 'burning' extremities, headache, weakness, ataxia and symptoms suggestive of a myopathy.

ELECTROLYTE DISTURBANCES

Hyponatraemia

Hyponatraemia is defined as a serum sodium value of <130 mmol/l. This may arise from 'water intoxication' without a sodium deficit, but sodium may also be lost from the intestines (diarrhoea and vomiting) or from renal disease. Most water intoxication

occurs in sick patients who are either being fed by nasogastric tube or intravenously. Hyponatraemia may also follow inappropriate secretion of ADH.

With a falling plasma sodium level, patients complain of anorexia and headache; they may become apathetic, drowsy and even confused. Muscle cramps, twitching and seizures may appear. Patients may pass into coma. Later, oedema of the limbs and face may appear.

A plasma sodium of less than 120 mmol/l usually causes some symptoms, commonly **confusion**, and values of less than 110 mmol/l may lead to **fits** and a significant **decline in conscious level**. It is important to measure carefully the patient's fluid input and output, the urine and plasma electrolytes and osmolalities.

Causes of inappropriate ADH secretion

These include:

1 Malignant disease – particularly carcinoma of the lung and lymphomas.

2 Nervous system disorders:
- Trauma, head injuries, subarachnoid haemorrhage
- Meningitis, tuberculous meningitis
- Strokes
- Central nervous system tumours
- Polyneuritis, e.g. Guillain-Barré, porphyria.

3 Infections – pneumonia.

4 Drugs – for example, carbamazepine, chlorpropamide, cyclophosphamide, phenothiazines, tricyclics.

In patients with inappropriate secretion of ADH there will be continuing excretion of a concentrated urine despite a hypotonic plasma with falling osmolality (often less than 270 mosmol/kg) so the urine osmolality will be greater than that of the plasma.

Recognition of the mechanism is important. Correction of dilutional fluid overload is necessary in water intoxication.

It appears there is a link with the speed of correction of hyponatraemia and the development of **central pontine myelinolysis**.

Too rapid correction may precipitate this type of brainstem damage and it has been suggested that the correction rate for hyponatraemia should not exceed 12 mEq in the first 24 hours or 20 mEq in the first 48 hours. In excess ADH states, fluid will need to be restricted to 500–1000 ml/day. Treatment of the cause is also important, such as meningitis.

Central pontine myelinolysis

In central pontine myelinolysis a focus of demyelination develops, usually within the centre of the pons. It does not show any inflammatory changes and the axons are usually preserved.

Although this was originally considered an effect of alcoholism, subsequently it has been shown to arise in the context of a severe metabolic or general medical disorder, the most common setting being hyponatraemia that is too rapidly corrected.

In addition to alcoholism it has been linked with cirrhosis, malnutrition, malignancy and hyperemesis gravidarum. Regions of extrapontine myelinolysis can also occur, for example in the basal ganglia or corpus callosum.

> The clinical spectrum varies from minimal symptoms with **ataxia to a profound tetraplegia and pseudobulbar palsy**. The signs may appear a few days after the hyponatraemia has been corrected.

MRI shows a characteristic focus of high signal on T2-weighted images and low signal on T1-weighted images in the central pons.

Hyponatraemia should always be corrected slowly (see above).

Hypokalaemia

A low serum potassium, less than 3 mmol/l, may be associated with complaints of fatigue, myalgia and muscle weakness. With values between 2.0 and 2.5 mmol/l there may be a **flaccid paralysis with depressed or absent reflexes**. There may be associated bowel involvement leading to ileus. Hypokalaemia may precipitate cardiac arrhythmias.

Sometimes there are complaints of thirst and polyuria.

> Certain medical conditions causing hypokalaemia may present with muscle weakness. These include aldosteronism (Conn's syndrome), Cushing's disease, and some forms of periodic paralysis (see p. 144). Other causes of potassium loss include diuretics, renal causes, and gastrointestinal upsets (diarrhoea and purgative abuse, pyloric stenosis and vomiting). The agents used to reduce intracranial pressure, such as mannitol or urea, by a diuresis may lead to potassium loss.

Treatment involves correction of the cause and potassium supplements.

CALCIUM METABOLISM

Hypocalcaemia

> Hypocalcaemia will produce **neuromuscular irritability** with a calcium level of less than 2.0 mmol/l, accompanied by complaints of tingling in the extremities and around the mouth, twitching, carpopedal spasm, tetany and even epileptic seizures. In many patients there may be complaints of lethargy; in a few, there may be psychotic features and even stupor.

Patients may show skin changes: a coarse, dry skin with brittle nails, cataracts, and even papilloedema. Tapping over the facial nerve will provoke twitching of the facial muscles **(Chvostek's sign)** and inflation of a pneumatic cuff around the arm above arterial blood pressure may provoke a main d'accoucheur from carpal spasm **(Trousseau's sign)**.

The serum calcium will be low and the electrocardiogram may show a prolonged QT interval. Scanning of the brain with CT may show cerebral calcification, particularly in the basal ganglia and cerebellum.

> Hypocalcaemia most often arises following surgery to the neck with the removal of the parathyroid glands (often during thyroid surgery), in

severe malabsorption, renal failure, with prolonged use of anticonvulsants, and even from primary failure of the parathyroids.

Treatment is with calcium and vitamin D supplements. In the acute situation 20–30 ml of 10% calcium gluconate injected intravenously over 10 minutes is effective.

Hypercalcaemia

Hypercalcaemia may present with 'stones, bones and abdominal groans', from renal stones (50%), bone pain and abdominal pain. Approximately one-third of patients found to have hypercalcaemia are asymptomatic.

Hypercalcaemia may cause anorexia, nausea and vomiting, constipation, polyuria and thirst. Headaches and depression are common symptoms. Fatigue, a proximal myopathy, confusion and behaviour disorders may herald neurological upsets. In a few patients, very high calcium levels may be associated with increasing confusion, drowsiness and eventual coma. Patients sometimes show a conjunctivitis from corneal calcification.

The serum calcium will be high, usually greater than 3 mmol/l, but it should be remembered that venous sampling below an inflated tourniquet may give an erroneously high calcium value.

Hypercalcaemia is most often found in primary hyperparathyroidism (where high levels of parathyroid hormone will be detected), in patients with widespread bony metastases, sarcoidosis or with vitamin D intoxication.

Treatment depends on the cause. In asymptomatic hypercalcaemia the underlying mechanism requires attention. With symptomatic patients a forced saline diuresis will increase the urinary excretion of calcium, which can be augmented by the addition of frusemide. For the hypercalcaemia of malignancy, the bisphosphonate disodium pamidronate given intravenously or sodium clodronate (which can be given orally) are effective. Calcitonin given intravenously may also result in a short-lived fall in calcium level.

VITAMIN DEFICIENCIES

Many vitamin deficiencies result from the effects of widespread malnutrition, as in cases of starvation, or from severe malabsorption. A few may reflect dietary fads or the substitution of food in the diet by alcohol.

Wernicke's encephalopathy; Wernicke-Korsakoff syndrome

Multiple small areas of necrosis and haemorrhage are found in the midbrain, the periaqueductal region, the paraventricular areas of the thalamus, the hypothalamus, the mammillary bodies and around the fourth ventricle. The cerebellum may also show neuronal loss. This damage is a result of thiamine deficiency and, if treated early, many of the clinical features can be reversed.

The condition is most commonly found in alcoholics, but also in other malnutrition states, particularly if there is protracted vomiting, which may also occur in pregnancy.

Clinical features of Korsakoff's psychosis
The presentation is usually acute with the combination of mental confusion (Korsakoff's psychosis) with an ophthalmoplegia and ataxia. The confusion includes amnesia for recent events, loss of recall and often confabulation. Many patients appear apathetic, muddled and drowsy. A few may show the more florid hallucinations of alcoholic withdrawal (delirium tremens; see p. 494).

The **ocular signs** include single or bilateral abducens palsies (54%), disturbances of conjugate gaze (44%) including an internuclear ophthalmoplegia, and often horizontal and vertical nystagmus (85%). The **ataxia** is a reflection of cerebellar damage and may be so severe as to prevent walking unaided. In over 80% there are also signs of a **peripheral neuropathy**.

Thiamine deficiency can be confirmed by a significant reduction in the red cell transketolase level. In severe cases some irreversible damage occurs and, if left untreated, the condition is fatal. Many patients are left with memory deficits (amnesic syndrome). Treatment is with intravenous thiamine 50–100 mg daily for 5 days, accompanied by the restoration of a normal diet (or adequate parenteral feeding where indicated). Glucose administration, by itself, can dramatically worsen the effects of thiamine deficiency.

Vitamin B12 deficiency

Deficiency of vitamin B12 may cause:

- A peripheral neuropathy (see p. 164)
- Spinal cord damage – subacute combined degeneration
- Optic atrophy (with centrocaecal scotomas)
- Dementia.

Commonly the presentation is with **sensory symptoms in the feet**. There may be also a spastic paresis of the legs with posterior column sensory loss. Lhermitte's sign may be positive.

The vacuolar myelopathy of human immunodeficiency virus infection may resemble subacute combined degeneration. Deficiency of vitamin B12 may arise after a total gastrectomy, in vegans, after some parasitic infestations of the intestines, and from the failure to absorb it in the stomach from a lack of intrinsic factor caused by an autoimmune-mediated atrophic gastritis, pernicious anaemia. The last may be associated with other autoimmune diseases.

Vitamin B12 deficiency is accompanied by a **macrocytic megaloblastic anaemia** and **low serum B12 level**. Anaemia may initially be absent. The CSF is normal. Nerve conduction studies usually show neuropathic changes and some patients may show abnormal visual evoked potentials. A Schilling test measuring the absorption of radioisotope-labelled B12, with and without intrinsic factor, may confirm the diagnosis and its mechanism. Antibodies to intrinsic factor are present in those with pernicious anaemia.

Treatment is with injections of hydroxocobalamin 1000 μg daily for 10 days, then monthly for the rest of the patient's life. Providing severe damage has not occurred, symptoms usually improve over the first few months of treatment.

Pellagra

Pellagra is a deficiency of nicotinic acid (niacin), which may affect the nervous system to cause fatigue, apathy, drowsiness and even confusion. It may damage the pyramidal tracts producing a spastic weakness of the legs, or more widespread neurological disturbance with extrapyramidal and peripheral nerve signs. Occasionally an acute confusional state with deteriorating conscious level arises. Many patients show skin changes with a dermatitis (often photosensitive), mucocutaneous lesions and gastrointestinal disturbances, particularly diarrhoea, and even malabsorption. A scarlet painful tongue is common.

Pellagra was originally described in vegans from poor maize-eating countries and in deprived prisoners. It is probable that many of these patients were suffering from multiple vitamin deficiencies as well as an inadequate diet.

Nutritional and toxic amblyopia

Certain deficiency states may cause optic nerve damage leading to visual failure and optic atrophy. These include vitamin B12 deficiency (see p. 192) and thiamine deficiency; the latter may have some links with the toxic effects of alcohol and/or tobacco to which many of these patients are also exposed. In many these may be nutritional neuropathies.

There is an insidiously progressive impairment of vision affecting both eyes. The acuity falls and the optic discs appear pale. Often there are centrocaecal scotomas, most easily detected by a red target. Electro-retinograms and visual evoked potentials may help to elucidate such damage. Some patients may show low red blood cell folate levels.

Abstinence from tobacco and/or alcohol is essential and most patients are also given hydroxo-cobalamin injections and folic acid, although it is equally important to ensure a good diet with thiamine and other vitamin B supplements.

Tropical amblyopia and neuropathies

> Tropical amblyopia and neuropathies arise from the combined effects of malnutrition and vita-min deficiency, most often found in deprived areas associated with starvation, or in prisoners.

Many have combinations of beriberi, pellagra and their neurological manifestations. These include a peripheral neuropathy with complaints of sensory symptoms and sometimes 'burning' in the feet, with weakness and clumsiness of the extremities: in some this may be combined with a spastic paraparesis. Other patients may show signs of a sensorimotor neuropathy with marked muscle wasting and pro-minent ataxia. There may also be signs of visual upset with blurred vision leading to optic atrophy and sometimes deafness. Many patients may show mucocutaneous lesions and some complain of abdominal pain. In some instances a toxic mecha-nism has been suggested, for example from excess ingestion of *Lathyrus sativus* or cassava.

> However, in many instances a tropical spastic paraparesis may arise from an inflammatory necrotic myelitis caused by infection with the **human T-cell lymphotropic virus (HTLV-1) virus**.

In many there are complaints of back pain, paraesthesiae, sphincter upset and leg weakness from a spastic paraparesis. Antibodies to the HTLV-1 virus can be detected by blood tests.

NEUROLOGICAL COMPLICATIONS OF GASTROINTESTINAL DISORDERS

In some 3% of patients with inflammatory bowel disease, **ulcerative colitis or Crohn's disease**, there may be neurological complications. Most often these arise from a peripheral neuropathy, usually a demyelinating polyradiculoneuropathy. Less commonly, a chronic progressive myelopathy may appear and even an inflammatory myopathy: the last two are found more often with Crohn's disease. Vascular complications include cerebral venous sinus thromboses and ischaemic strokes.

> In **coeliac disease, gluten-sensitive enteropathy**, about 10% of patients are shown to have neuro-logical complications.

The diagnosis of coeliac disease is now supported by the presence of antigliadin and anti-endomysial antibodies and anti-tissue transglutamate, although the typical villous atrophy of the intestinal mucosa on biopsy is still the histological proof. Most often the neurological features include cerebellar signs and a sensory ataxia – often linked with posterolat-eral column upset in the spinal cord. Glove-stocking sensory loss and even dementia have been described. Epileptic seizures are more common. Initially it was thought these features might all link with a degree of malabsorption, particularly of vitamin B12, folate and vitamin E, but subsequent studies and replacement therapy with such preparations have not reversed the deficits.

Whipple's disease is a very rare chronic multi-system granulomatous disease largely affecting middle-aged males. It has now been shown to be the result of a bacterial infection with *Tropheryma whippelii*. It usually presents with intestinal symp-toms – diarrhoea and steatorrhoea – accompanied by weight loss and abdominal pain. Other systemic features include fever, hyperpigmentation, lympha-denopathy and cardiac involvement. Neurological complications may appear in some 5%. Most often these include a dementia with myoclonus and a supranuclear ophthalmoplegia. A curious oculo-masticatory myorhythmia has been described where pendular oscillations of the eyes are accompanied by rhythmic contractions of the jaw muscles. Seizures, cerebellar ataxia, pyramidal and extrapyramidal signs as well as a peripheral neuropathy have been reported.

The CSF may be normal or show a mild protein rise with some inflammatory cells (lymphocytes). An MRI may show scattered high signal lesions in the brainstem, hypothalamus and cerebral hemispheres. Periodic acid–Schiff-positive macrophages may be seen in a jejunal biopsy specimen and similar periodic acid–Schiff-positive material may be present in scattered granulomatous nodules in the brain. A polymerase chain reaction test may be useful. Making the diagnosis is important, as long-term treatment with trimethoprim and sulfamethoxazole or tetracycline have proved helpful.

TOXIC EFFECTS

Alcohol and the nervous system

Most doctors are only too familiar with some of the effects of alcohol, particularly acute self-poisoning. Alcohol is an inhibitor, depressing cerebral function and this is well illustrated in acute intoxication. Alcohol is absorbed rapidly with a maximum blood concentration some 30–90 minutes after ingestion. At levels of 50 mg/100 ml there may be mild incoordination and impaired learning and by 100 mg/100 ml slurring dysarthria and obvious clumsiness. With higher levels there is depression of the conscious level resulting in coma (often 300–400 mg/100 ml). This can be fatal. There will be an accompanying peripheral vasodilation and a tachycardia.

Chronic habituation

Abstinence syndromes

Patients habituated to alcohol will develop acute withdrawal symptoms if their intake stops suddenly.

This cessation may be precipitated by injuries, an acute infection or surgical emergency leading to admission to hospital with the loss of a regular intake. These withdrawal symptoms may be the presenting features.

The first stage, **the shakes**, consists of irritability, restlessness and tremors, with an exaggerated startle response. Patients appear overactive with a tachycardia, are inattentive and sometimes febrile. Such symptoms commonly start the morning after cessation and last some 24–48 hours. They may be relieved by further alcohol.

The next stage may include **confusion** and sometimes **auditory and even visual hallucinations** accompanied by considerable **amnesia**. The **blackouts** of the alcoholic consist of gaps in memory, often lasting hours, for which they have no recall but may show some automatic behaviour. Mild hallucinatory states may be described as 'bad dreams' but when severe may merge with delirium tremens (DTs).

Withdrawal seizures, or rum fits, start 8–48 hours after cessation of drinking, most often after 12–24 hours. The seizures are usually generalized tonic-clonic attacks, either single or a cluster in series. About one-third of such patients may go on to develop DTs. Epileptic seizures may also be precipitated by binge drinking.

The final withdrawal stage is **delirium tremens (DTs)**, which has a mortality. A coexistent infective illness or injury may increase the risk of DTs. There are vivid hallucinations, often frightening (seeing animals, insects), marked confusion, anxiety and overactivity, leading to insomnia. Usually DTs start 2–4 days after stopping drinking, and usually last 2–3 days, but occasionally may last much longer.

Treatment of DTs involves adequate sedation, rehydration and usually parenteral feeding with glucose solutions and thiamine given intravenously. Any concomitant infection or injury should be treated appropriately. Sedatives used include benzodiazepines such as lorazepam, chlordiazepoxide, or diazepam. Paraldehyde may sometimes be used to sedate and control seizures.

Alcoholic damage

Alcohol may produce damage to the nervous system by its direct toxic effects.

Alcoholic damage to the nervous system

This includes:

- Peripheral neuropathy (see p. 163)
- Cerebellar degeneration with ataxia (see p. 258)
- Cerebral degeneration with dementia (see p. 288)
- Myopathy and cardiomyopathy.

Other disturbances are central pontine myelinolysis (see p. 490) and Marchiafava–Bignami disease (primary degeneration of the corpus callosum). Alcohol may also precipitate the Wernicke–Korsakoff syndrome (see p. 491).

Cerebellar degeneration

In cerebellar degeneration there is loss of cerebellar neurones leading to atrophy. This may present with clumsiness, slurred speech and ataxia, difficult to differentiate from the effects of acute intoxication, although these signs persist even after 'drying out'.

Cerebral degeneration

Chronic alcoholics may have evidence of a diffuse global dementia, with cerebral atrophy indicated by ventricular dilatation and widened cortical sulci on imaging. However, such radiological findings do not always correlate with a dementia. In older alcoholic patients (aged over 45 years) with dementia there is a much smaller chance of improvement with abstinence.

The management of alcoholic dependence is covered in Chapter 27.

Toxic effects of drugs

Many drugs may affect the nervous system. Drug toxicity includes the unwanted side-effects of those used in therapy, for example, a peripheral neuropathy (Table 24.8) or myopathic damage (Table 24.9); or those resulting from self-poisoning, for example, a depressed conscious level leading to coma as a result of overdosing with tranquillizers or antidepressants. These effects are dose-dependent. The effects of habituation to opiates and other powerful analgesics are described later (see p. 546).

Table 24.8 Drug causes of neuropathy – *common causes

Alcohol, amiodarone, amitriptyline, chloroquine, cimetidine, cisplatin, dapsone*, didanosine (ddI), disulfiram*, ethambutol, gold salts, griseofulvin, hydralazine*, indometacin, isoniazid*, lithium, metronidazole*, nitrofurantoin*, phenytoin*, propafenone, stavudine (d4T), sulfasalazine, sulphonamides, taxanes, thalidomide, tricyclic antidepressants, tryptophan, vinca alkaloids*, zalcitabine (ddc).

Table 24.9 Drug causes of myopathy – *common causes

Alcohol, amiodarone, amphetamines, beta-blockers, chloroquine*, cimetidine, cocaine, ciclosporin, emetine, fibric acid derivatives (bezafibrate, ciprofibrate, fenofibrate, gemfibrozil), heroin, HMG-CoA reductase inhibitors (atorvastatin, fluvastatin, pravastatin, simvastatin), hydralazine, isoniazid, isotretinoin, lithium, methadone, d-penicillamine, procainamide, rifampicin, salbutamol, steroids*, thyroxine, tryptophan, vincristine, zidovudine (AZT)*.

Habituation to barbiturates and other sedatives, such as benzodiazepines, may produce slowing, apathy, slurred speech, clumsiness and ataxia, like a drunk. These features may be linked with emotional lability and personal neglect. Such signs may fluctuate greatly. Withdrawal states from such habituation (see Table 27.7) may lead to restlessness, tremors, insomnia, agitation and even withdrawal seizures. Habituation may also occur to analgesics, and many chronic headache sufferers may experience a further headache unless another dose is given (medication misuse headaches).

Phenothiazines and butyrophenones, used particularly in the control of the chronic schizophrenic patient where depot injections of long-acting preparations are employed, may cause **extrapyramidal symptoms and signs** (see p. 232). These are predominantly rigidity, slowed movements and a shuffling gait. Such symptoms may be reduced by the use of anticholinergic drugs, such as benzhexol. Phenothiazines and butyrophenones may also provoke involuntary movements, dyskinesias, dystonic postures and even restlessness (akathisia). Many of these symptoms reverse with the cessation of therapy and the use of anticholinergics. However, a group of tardive dyskinesias may arise, particularly affecting the muscles of the face, mouth, neck and trunk, which may prove very resistant to treatment.

A rare complication is the **malignant neuroleptic syndrome** (see p. 244), which may occur in patients treated with a variety of psychotropic drugs, most commonly haloperidol and depot injections of fluphenazines. Here rigidity and akinesia develop relatively acutely accompanied by fever, autonomic disturbances with an unstable blood pressure and a depressed conscious level. It is associated with a massive rise in the serum creatine kinase level, a raised white count and often abnormal liver function tests. There may be a fatal outcome, although treatment with bromocriptine and dantrolene sodium has been effective together with withdrawal of the offending drug.

Drug abuse (Table 24.10)

Narcotics (see p. 546)

Alkaloid derivatives of opium, either natural opiates or synthetic analogues, act at opiate receptors concentrated in the limbic system, periaqueductal grey matter and spinal sensory pathways. These modulate central pain perception and its transmission, affording pain relief.

Diamorphine (heroin) and morphine

Diamorphine and morphine are very potent analgesics, which, in high dose, can cause euphoria, miosis, constipation, cough suppression, orthostatic hypotension and increasing cardiorespiratory depression, resulting in coma. Pulmonary oedema may develop. In acute poisoning patients will require ventilatory support and intravenous naloxone.

More **chronic use** results in drug dependence and tolerance. Drug withdrawal (see Table 27.7) results in cravings, anxiety, profuse sweating, lacrimation, rhinorrhoea, dilated pupils, goose flesh, tachycardia, abdominal cramps and limb pains, diarrhoea

and vomiting, restlessness and twitching. Such symptoms may last 7–10 days.

Addicts are more liable to suffer strokes, a vasculitis, infections (including AIDS), myelopathies, leukoencephalopathies, pressure palsies and epileptic seizures.

Cocaine (see p. 547)

Cocaine is an alkaloid derived from coca leaves that was introduced as a local anaesthetic. It is also a stimulant. It may be taken intranasally, or by intramuscular or intravenous injection. The smoking of the free alkaloid base 'crack' results in very rapid penetration into the nervous system with a resulting 'high'. Cocaine produces a rapid euphoria with sympathetic features, tachycardia, hypertension, and pupillary dilatation, which may be followed by a down phase accompanied by craving. More long-term cocaine abuse may cause hallucinations and even paranoia.

Cocaine use carries an increased risk of vascular complications – hypertension, subarachnoid haemorrhage, haemorrhagic and ischaemic stroke. There is also risk of infections, and occasional rhabdomyolysis. Epileptic seizures are particularly common. In a few patients smoking 'crack', severe cerebellar damage has occurred.

Amphetamines

Amphetamines are stimulants and have been used to overcome sleepiness and suppress appetite. In excess they may produce a sympathomimetic syndrome with delusions, paranoia, sometimes mania, hyper-reflexia, seizures, tremors and even chorea. Prolonged use may cause hypertension. They may also provoke strokes, both from intracerebral and subarachnoid haemorrhage and from a cerebral vasculitis. Ecstasy is a substituted amphetamine, 3,4 methylenedioxyamphetamine, and may cause depletion of serotonin (5-HT) and also affect dopaminergic neurones, producing a combination of a serotonin syndrome (myoclonus, agitation, hyper-reflexia, incoordination) with some features of the malignant neuroleptic syndrome (see p. 244).

Heavy metals (Table 24.10)

Heavy metals may damage the nervous system. They may be used therapeutically, for example gold

Table 24.10 Effects of some neurological toxins

Amphetamines	Insomnia, hypertension, tremor, haemorrhagic stroke
Opiates (heroin, morphine)	Cerebral infarction, rhabdomyolysis (SBE, HIV infection – dangers of IV use)
Cocaine	Hyperpyrexia, haemorrhagic stroke, vasculitis
'Drugs'	Withdrawal states
Organic solvents	Acute encephalopathy Chronic – dementia, ataxia, pyramidal signs, optic atrophy, deafness
Acrylamide	Neuropathy
Trichlorethylene	Trigeminal sensory neuropathy
Heavy metals	
Lead	Encephalopathy, motor neuropathy
Cisplatin	Sensory neuropathy, deafness
Gold	Peripheral neuropathy
Organophosphates	Peripheral neuropathy

SBE, subacute bacterial endocarditis.

injections in rheumatoid arthritis, which may cause a thrombocytopenia and bleeding resulting in peripheral and central nervous system damage. Cisplatin used in cancer treatment can cause deafness and a peripheral neuropathy.

Lead poisoning is now uncommon since its removal from paint. Previously, children were more commonly affected, presenting with irritability, confusion, clumsiness and seizures from a relatively acute encephalopathy causing a deteriorating conscious level and a grossly swollen brain. There was often anorexia, vomiting and abdominal pain. In adults a peripheral neuropathy, predominantly motor with a bilateral wrist drop, was sometimes the presentation. This was often associated with anaemia and abdominal pain.

Plasma lead levels will be raised, usually greater than 50–70 µg/dl. There will be an associated anaemia with basophilic stippling of red cells and 'lead lines' may be present on the X-rays of long bones in children.

Treatment is by the use of chelating agents.

Other metals are also toxic: **manganese poisoning** may produce an encephalopathy and extrapyramidal signs; **mercury poisoning** produces tremors, confusion and cerebellar disturbance.

Organophosphates, used as insecticides, in certain mineral oils and in sheep dip, are also toxic. They may produce a peripheral neuropathy with axonal degeneration. Acute poisoning will produce headache, vomiting, pinpoint pupils, profuse sweating and abdominal cramps (i.e. anticholinesterase effects), which may be relieved by atropine.

PHYSICAL INSULTS

Anoxia

The brain requires a rich oxygen supply. If the circulation is arrested, within 2–3 minutes the normal function fails. Consciousness may be lost even more quickly and if there is asystole the patient will become unconscious within 15 seconds. Over the next 5 seconds there may be twitching, rigidity or clonic jerks which can be mistaken for an epileptic seizure. Within 4–5 minutes of circulatory arrest cyanosis appears, the pupils dilate and become unreactive, the plantar responses become extensor and the breathing may appear stertorous. Providing oxygenation and the circulation are restored to the brain within 5 minutes, recovery usually occurs: beyond this irreversible damage may follow.

A respiratory arrest or an obstructed airway may produce acute respiratory failure, but more often the picture is a combination of hypoxia and ischaemia with concomitant circulatory failure.

The cardiopulmonary mechanisms producing acute anoxia most often follow: heart attacks with ventricular arrest or fibrillation; acute respiratory failure, for example in drowning or asthmatic crises; severe trauma; or anaesthetic mishaps. A fall in cerebral perfusion may occur during operations, particularly on the open heart, or where there is massive blood loss leading to shock. More chronic hypoxia may arise from ventilatory muscle weakness, as in Guillain-Barré syndrome, certain myopathies, and obstructive airways disease or fibrosis.

With a slower onset, hypoxic symptoms include restlessness, agitation, tremors, headache, clumsiness and confusion. Blood gases will confirm a low PO_2 and high PCO_2 (see p. 514). Ventilatory muscle weakness in the adult may be accompanied by a low vital capacity (1.0 litres or less).

Post-anoxic brain damage

Patients who have sustained anoxic brain damage, but who have survived, may show a variable picture, with depressed conscious level often with some preservation of brainstem reflexes, but commonly twitching or myoclonic jerking of the limbs, sometimes repeated seizures, decerebrate or decorticate postures and extensor plantar responses. A variety of deficits may persist in less damaged survivors. These include cognitive and behavioural disturbances, extrapyramidal and pyramidal signs, visual field defects, involuntary movements, ataxia and action myoclonus.

Electric shock

Electric shock may cause death, often from cardiac arrest. Commonly, at the site of contact, whether from an electric cable or lightning, there may be extensive burns with tissue destruction. The nervous system may be damaged directly, for example shock to the head producing a hemiplegia, or the damage may involve the spinal cord or peripheral nerves. In survivors a delayed myelopathy has been reported, with slowly progressive damage leading to muscular atrophy or even a transverse myelopathy. Instances of motor neurone disease have been described following an electric shock.

Hypothermia

Prolonged exposure to cold can cause damage, although under experimental conditions, very low body temperatures are necessary to produce a conduction block in peripheral nerves. Deep body temperatures of less than 35°C, which may follow cold exposure, particularly in the elderly, in patients with hypothyroidism, or after drug overdoses, may lead to impaired cerebral function – confusion, stupor and coma. The respiration and metabolism are slowed generally. Treatment is by gradual re-warming but there is an appreciable mortality, largely because of cardiac arrhythmias and metabolic upsets.

Heat stroke

Heat stroke most often follows vigorous exercise in very hot temperatures. It may be aggravated by impaired sweating, as in patients with Parkinson's disease on anticholinergic drugs, or in patients with tetanus and autonomic disturbance. As the body temperature rises (rectal temperature of more than 41°C), agitation and confusion may appear with later a deteriorating conscious level. Patients may convulse and status epilepticus itself may lead to hyperpyrexia with further brain damage. Death is usually caused by circulatory collapse and renal failure. Survivors may be left with cognitive deficits, spastic weakness and a severe cerebellar deficit. The latter often persists.

Malignant hyperthermia

Malignant hyperthermia is described in Chapter 6.

Decompression sickness

Decompression sickness is also termed the 'bends'. Too rapid decompression causes nitrogen under pressure in the blood to produce gas emboli and micro-infarcts, which produce acute pain in the limbs and trunk. The thoracic spinal cord is most often affected, producing a paraparesis or posterior column disturbance, but brain damage leading to a hemiplegia, vertigo or visual upset may arise. These deficits usually recover slowly. Recognition of decompression symptoms, with recompression and then much slower decompression, may help to prevent this.

Mountain sickness

Symptoms of mountain sickness develop as low-level dwellers climb to considerable heights quickly, and start some 24–48 hours after the ascent. These include headache, nausea, vomiting, lethargy, dizziness, impaired balance, irritability and insomnia. In some instances acute pulmonary oedema may develop and even cerebral oedema with papilloedema, stupor and a flaccid paralysis. The acute symptoms can be relieved by breathing oxygen. Slow acclimatization to height allows a gradual increase in the haemoglobin concentration, which will largely prevent such symptoms.

Dexamethasone and acetazolamide may help to relieve symptoms of mountain sickness.

CONNECTIVE TISSUE DISEASES

In connective tissue diseases (Table 24.11) the pathogenesis remains uncertain but they are associated with an **inflammatory disturbance of the supporting connective tissue** and often the blood vessels, with a **vasculitis**. This vessel involvement may occur in the brain, spinal cord, peripheral nerve or muscle. The vessel wall commonly shows thickening (beading) and a tendency to occlusion. All these disorders have **immunological abnormalities**, with the presence of humoral antibodies. Many may cause an aseptic meningitis with a CSF plcocytosis and mild protein rise. There is some overlap between these disorders.

Table 24.11 Connective tissue disorders affecting the nervous system

Systemic lupus erythematosus
Rheumatoid arthritis
Polyarteritis nodosa
Churg–Strauss syndrome
Giant cell arteritis – polymyalgia rheumatica
Wegener's granuloma
Scleroderma
Dermatomyositis
Sjögren's syndrome.

Systemic lupus erythematosus

In part, the pathogenesis of systemic lupus erythematosus may be vascular, including a hypercoagulable state, and in part from immunological damage. Antiphospholipid antibodies may be found linked with an increased thrombotic risk.

> Neurological manifestations occur in at least 20%; these include psychiatric symptoms; psychosis, dementia, depression; seizures, transient ischaemic attack; focal neurological signs; hemiplegia, chorea, cerebellar ataxia, cranial nerve lesions. There may be spinal cord involvement with a paraparesis; a peripheral neuropathy and a myositis.
>
> Commonly these are associated with joint and skin changes (butterfly facial rash), fever, renal and pulmonary involvement.

Immunological changes include a high erythrocyte sedimentation rate (ESR), often a normal C reactive protein (CRP), positive DNA binding (particularly double-stranded DNA) and positive antinuclear antibody (ANA).

Rheumatoid arthritis

Neurological complications (Table 24.12) most often arise from involvement of the cervical spine where atlanto-axial subluxation may cause a high cord

Table 24.12 Neurological complications of rheumatoid arthritis

Spine malalignment cord compression	Atlanto-axial subluxation, other levels particularly cervical
Peripheral nerves	Peripheral neuropathy
	Entrapment neuropathy CTS
	Mononeuropathy multiplex
	Symmetrical neuropathy
	Digital sensory
	Sensorimotor
Muscle	Myositis (rare)
Central	Cranial nerve palsies, seizures, vasculitis with stroke (rare)

CTS, carpal tunnel syndrome.

compression or there may be malalignment lower down in the cervical canal.

Peripheral nerve involvement

Peripheral nerve involvement is also common, arising from:

- Entrapment neuropathies (some 45%), e.g. carpal tunnel syndrome
- Mononeuritis multiplex
- Symmetrical neuropathy:
  (a) Digital sensory
  (b) Sensorimotor – may be severe.

There will be radiological joint changes. Scanning with MRI is the best way to show changes in the cervical canal or at the craniocervical junction. Blood tests include a raised ESR and CRP, a positive rheumatoid factor, a positive ANA (some 40%), and a normal or raised complement level. ENMG (nerve conduction and electromyographic) studies will confirm peripheral nerve involvement. Significant cord compression may require neurosurgical intervention.

Polyarteritis nodosa

Polyarteritis nodosa causes a systemic necrotizing vasculitis involving small and medium-sized arteries with irregular 'beading' leading often to occlusion and multiple aneurysm formation. Many organs are involved: the kidney in some 75% (often associated with hypertension); the lungs (asthma); the heart (80%); the skin and the nervous system. Commonly there is fever, weight loss, malaise and arthralgia.

Neurological involvement may cause a central upset (c. 50%) with headache, psychosis, confusion, dementia and an aseptic meningitis. Focal symptoms include a hemiplegia, brainstem lesions and cranial nerve involvement. There may be a peripheral neuropathy: either a distal sensorimotor pattern or a mononeuritis multiplex. Ocular involvement is also common: retinal infarcts; haemorrhages; exudates; and ischaemic optic nerve damage.

Investigations include a neutrophilia with eosinophilia in about one-third of patients, a raised

ESR and CRP, and a positive ANA. Antineutrophil cytoplasmic antibodies (pANCA, cANCA) may be present: the perinuclear pattern (pANCA) refers to the autoantigen link with myeloperoxidase, and the diffuse cytoplasmic pattern (cANCA) links with autoantigen proteinase 3. These antibodies are more likely to be present with microscopic polyarteritis. Imaging may show arterial changes. A biopsy may confirm the diagnosis and tissue may be taken from a number of possible sites.

Churg–Strauss syndrome

Churg–Strauss syndrome is a clinically distinct necrotizing vasculitis commonly affecting the lungs, with asthmatic symptoms, fever, an eosinophilia and systemic vasculitis. Nasal polyps are common. There may be purpura and skin nodules. A patchy, often painful, mononeuritis multiplex is very common and less often a polyneuropathy. Cerebral vessels may rarely be affected, resulting in memory impairment and seizures. Antineutrophil cytoplasmic antibodies are usually present. Raised serum levels of immunoglobulin E are commonly found.

Giant cell arteritis (see p. 478)

Giant cell arteritis

- Patients aged 50 years or more
- Headache in 80–90%
- Systemic upsets – fever, malaise, fatigue, weight loss, scalp ulceration
- Overlap with polymyalgia rheumatica in 40% – girdle muscle aching and weakness
- Pain on chewing – jaw claudication in c. 40%
- Visual loss in c. 20% – total loss or altitudinal defect: amaurosis fugax may precede this in 45%. If one eye is blind, there is a very high risk that the second eye will be affected
- Neurological manifestations in c. 30% – peripheral and cranial nerves, transient ischaemic attacks
- Elevated ESR 50 mm/hour or more – often near 100 mm (about 5% ESR <40 mm). CRP is

- a more sensitive index. Liver function tests abnormal in c. 30%
- Temporal artery biopsy diagnostic – may have 'skip' areas
- Treatment with steroids – 40–60 mg/day prednisolone with symptom relief.

Wegener's granuloma (see p. 205)

In Wegener's granuloma a necrotizing vasculitis with granuloma formation affects the upper and lower respiratory tract with often an aggressive spread through the sinuses, orbits and base of the skull. This may cause cranial nerve, brainstem and ocular involvement. There may be a mononeuritis multiplex. Pulmonary and renal involvement are common. There is often an associated fever, anaemia and a raised ESR and CRP. Antineutrophil cytoplasmic antibodies (cANCA) in high titre are strongly suggestive of Wegener's granulomatosis. The diagnosis may also be supported by biopsy (the highest yield being from the lung).

Scleroderma

In addition to skin and gastrointestinal tract changes, scleroderma may be associated with muscle weakness from an inflammatory polymyositis or a non-inflammatory myopathy. Rare neurological complications include a trigeminal sensory neuropathy and even stroke. Some of these patients may show the presence of extractable nuclear antigens.

Dermatomyositis

Dermatomyositis is dealt with on p. 149.

Sjögren's syndrome

The full triad of Sjögren's syndrome comprises dry eyes (keratoconjunctivitis sicca), a dry mouth (xerostomia) and a connective tissue disorder, usually rheumatoid arthritis. Perhaps as many as 40% of patients may have some neurological complications. These include a peripheral neuropathy – an axonal sensorimotor neuropathy or a sensory upset; cranial nerve palsies; a myelopathy – which may be acute, resembling a transverse myelitis or chronic more like multiple sclerosis; and cerebral involvement, most often with cognitive impairment on a subcortical basis, seizures or even focal deficits, as a hemiplegia. Such patients commonly show hyperglobulinaemia with positive non-organ-specific antibodies such as rheumatoid factor or ANA. Extractable nuclear antigens, particularly anti-Ro and anti-La are regularly found in Sjögren's syndrome. Schirmer's test (measuring the wetting of a standardized strip of filter paper inserted into the corner of the eye) will confirm the dry eyes.

Treatment

In most of these inflammatory disorders in the acute phase (apart from scleroderma), pulse methyl prednisolone may be given intravenously, followed by oral steroids. These may be reinforced by immunosuppression with cyclophosphamide, azathioprine or methotrexate. In rheumatoid arthritis, treatment also includes a number of measures to help the arthralgia and joint inflammation and ease the pain.

REMOTE EFFECTS OF CANCER ON THE NERVOUS SYSTEM – PARANEOPLASTIC SYNDROMES

Non-metastatic involvement of the nervous system including peripheral nerves, the neuromuscular junction and muscle are uncommon complications of some cancers (Table 24.13). Most commonly, small cell lung, ovarian and breast cancers, and some lymphomas including Hodgkin's disease are responsible. It is thought that these paraneoplastic neurological disorders are caused by an autoimmune reaction against an antigen expressed by tumour cells and also by different neurones. Although only approximately 1% of patients with cancer may develop such paraneoplastic nervous system involvement, about

scanning can help to distinguish between the two. Steroids may give some symptomatic relief.

Irradiation of the brachial plexus during the treatment of breast cancer is sometimes followed by progressive damage to the nerve trunks in the involved field. Usually there is a painless progressive weakness, with sensory loss in the affected arm (see p. 180) starting months to years after treatment and often associated with paraesthesiae.

Radiation may also cause **vascular damage** with an increased incidence of ischaemic damage, usually following a thrombotic lesion in the irradiated artery. This may present with a stroke-like picture.

Chemotherapy

The **drugs** used in the treatment of tumours are often **neurotoxic**. Vinca alkaloids (vincristine and vinblastine) may produce a peripheral sensorimotor neuropathy. The taxanes (paclitaxel, docetaxel) may cause a sensorimotor neuropathy. Platinum compounds (cisplatin, carboplatin, oxaliplatin) may also produce a neuropathy (often predominantly sensory) and have some ototoxicity. Procarbazine may cause ataxia from cerebellar disturbance. It is sometimes difficult to distinguish a sensory ataxia from a peripheral neuropathy with that from a cerebellar fault.

Chemotherapy may also cause some **immunosuppression** with a greater liability to opportunistic infections.

Neurological complications of organ transplantation

Often the problem is that of **opportunistic infections** in the immunocompromised patient; for example, listeriosis, fungal infections, toxoplasmosis. Cerebral emboli and bleeding may follow heart and lung transplants. Marked thrombocytopenia leading to bleeding may arise after bone marrow transplants. Post-transplantation **lymphoproliferative disorders** may occur and even result in lymphomas.

Metabolic encephalopathy may sometimes follow a transplant and be accompanied by seizures. Seizures may also be provoked by ciclosporin.

BEHÇET'S DISEASE

Behçet's disease is a **chronic relapsing multisystem vasculitis** associated with **orogenital ulceration and uveitis**. In about **one-third the nervous system** may be involved with perivascular and meningeal infiltration with lymphocytes, plasma cells and macrophages, with multiple foci of softening and necrosis in the white and grey matter often found in relation to blood vessels. Venous thromboses and thrombophlebitis are common. Skin lesions are also common with erythema nodosum and a tendency to furunculosis.

Nervous system involvement in Behçet's disease

Nervous system involvement includes:

- Brainstem focal symptoms from stroke-like episodes (29%)
- Corticospinal tract involvement (54%)
- Cerebellar disturbance (33%)
- Aseptic meningitis
- Raised intracranial pressure secondary to venous thrombosis (12%)
- Behavioural problems (12%)
- Isolated headache (60%).

Men are more commonly affected and the disease usually runs a relapsing and remitting course. In some there may be prominent visual disturbance (40–70%), which may even lead to visual loss. Some patients show aggressive disease with significant impairment of mobility in about one half after 10 years from diagnosis (requiring one-sided support to walk 100 metres). Early cerebellar signs and a progressive course with cerebellopyramidal involvement carry a poor prognosis.

The CSF may show a lymphocytic pleocytosis and in some 20% the opening pressure is raised. There may be a raised protein level and even oligoclonal bands. However, in some 30% the CSF may be normal. Inflammatory markers as the ESR and CRP are usually raised. MRI scanning with MR angiography to show the draining venous sinuses is the imaging of choice.

A pathergy test (the formation of a sterile pustule at the site of a needle puncture) has been described but is unreliable.

Treatment in the acute relapses, particularly where there has been multifocal central nervous system involvement, is usually with pulse steroids and immunosuppressive drugs, usually ciclosporin. These have only limited success. Major central venous sinus thrombosis may be treated with intravenous heparin, often combined with some steroids. Immunomodulatory treatment with thalidomide and interferon alpha have been used in treating some of the systemic manifestations in more progressive disease.

SARCOIDOSIS

Sarcoidosis

Sarcoidosis is another multisystem inflammatory disease of unknown aetiology. It results in non-caseating granulomas with infiltration of the affected tissues by T-lymphocytes and other mononuclear cells associated with macrophage aggregation. The last form either epithelioid or multinucleated giant cells. Later lesions may go on to develop fibrosis. The incidence varies between 1–40/100 000 and the disease usually presents in younger patients (<40 years old). In the USA there is a nearly threefold increased incidence in the black population.

Over 90% show respiratory system involvement, most commonly enlargement of the hilar lymph glands. Some 20–50% may present with Lofgren's syndrome – erythema nodosum, hilar lymphadenopathy and polyarthralgia. Some 25% have skin involvement (erythema nodosum, skin nodules, lupus pernio), some 25% eye involvement (uveitis, conjunctival nodules), some 40–70% show liver granulomas, and some 5–10% cardiac involvement. The salivary and lacrimal glands may be involved. Systemic symptoms may include fatigue, anorexia, weight loss, shortness of breath and fever. The clinical presentation may be protean.

Nervous system involvement in sarcoidosis

The nervous system may be involved in 5–7%. Such manifestations include:

- Cranial nerve palsies (50%) – often bilateral including cranial nerves 7, 5, 8, 9 and 10
- The optic nerves and chiasm
- Peripheral nerves – most often a mononeuritis multiplex, less commonly a symmetrical polyneuropathy
- Aseptic meningitis
- Myelopathy with intramedullary granuloma
- Hydrocephalus
- Pituitary dysfunction or hypothalamic disturbance (diabetes insipidus)
- Seizures
- Neuropsychiatric deficits
- Intracranial mass lesions from granulomas
- Proximal myopathy.

The prognosis is varied. In many patients with mild involvement there may be relapses and remissions with good recovery. However, marked pulmonary fibrosis is a bad prognostic feature and some 25% die from chronic respiratory failure. Extensive nervous system involvement also suggests a poor outcome.

The **diagnosis** is best confirmed by histological examination of tissue from a biopsy, most often from lymph glands, the skin, liver or conjunctival lesions. A chest X-ray will show enlarged hilar glands and pulmonary infiltrates. Respiratory function tests may show restricted lung volumes and abnormal gas exchange. Blood tests may confirm an inflammatory process with an elevated ESR and CRP. The serum calcium may be raised and liver function tests may be abnormal. A raised serum angiotensin-converting enzyme level is found in some 70–80% of patients but this is not specific. The CSF is commonly abnormal with a lymphocytic pleocytosis (10–200 cells mL^{-1} in 72%, an elevated protein (40–70%) and sometimes a decreased glucose. There may be increased gamma globulin levels and oligoclonal bands (some 70%). The CSF angiotensin-converting enzyme level may be raised in some 55% but again this is non-specific and raised levels have been found in other disorders. Scanning with MRI with gadolinium enhancement is the imaging of choice.

Treatment may be symptomatic but steroids remain the mainstay. With nervous system involvement prednisolone 0.5–1.0 mg/kg per day for 8–12 weeks and then tapered is one regimen that is used. Intravenous pulse methylprednisolone followed by a tapered dose of oral steroids is another. Steroids may be combined with immunosuppressive treatment, often with weekly methotrexate (10 mg), cyclophosphamide, azathioprine or even ciclosporin. Such treatments require regular blood tests to monitor the blood count, renal and liver functions.

REFERENCES AND FURTHER READING

Aminoff MJ (ed.) (1999) *Neurology and General Medicine*, 3rd edn. New York, NY: Churchill Livingstone.

Baughman RP *et al.* (2003) Sarcoidosis. *Lancet*, **361**: 1111–1118.

Hughes GRV (1994) *Connective Tissue Diseases*. Oxford: Blackwell Scientific Publications Ltd.

McAllister LD, Ward JH, Schulman SF, DeAngelis LM (2002) *Practical Neuro-Oncology*. Boston, MA: Butterworth-Heinemann.

Newman LS, Rose CS, Maier LA (1997) Sarcoidosis. *New England Journal of Medicine*, **336**:1224–1234.

Nowak DA, Widenka DC (2001) Neurosarcoidosis: a review of its intracranial manifestation. *Journal of Neurology*, **248**:363–372.

Posner JB (1995) *Neurologic Complications of Cancer*. Philadelphia, PA: FA Davis.

Siva A, Kantarci OH, Salp S *et al.* (2001) Behçet's disease: diagnostic and prognostic aspects of neurological involvement. *Journal of Neurology*, **248**:95–103.

Victor M, Adams RD, Collins GH (1971) *The Wernicke–Korsakoff Syndrome*. Philadelphia, PA: FA Davis.

CHAPTER 25

RESPIRATORY ASPECTS OF NEUROLOGICAL DISEASE

R.S. Howard and N.P. Hirsch

The care of patients with neurological critical illness may differ significantly from those with general medical disorders. In neurological units the principle areas of concern include the short-term and long-term management of coma, encephalopathy, autonomic failure and neuromuscular weakness causing ventilatory failure and impaired bulbar control. Furthermore, patients with neurological critical illness may differ from those with general medical disorders because the nature of the illness leads to an increased mean length of stay but a potentially better prognosis.

This chapter will deal mainly with neurological conditions causing respiratory insufficiency, which may require ventilatory support.

RESPIRATORY INSUFFICIENCY

Respiratory insufficiency is the inability to maintain adequate ventilation to match acid-base status and oxygenation to metabolic requirements. The initial abnormality may be intermittent nocturnal hypoventilation leading to hypercapnia and hypoxia during sleep, this eventually persists while the patient is awake and symptoms may develop concurrently. Respiratory insufficiency may develop during the course of many neurological disorders. It occurs most commonly as a consequence of neuromuscular weakness but may also accompany disturbances of brainstem function or interruption of descending respiratory pathways. Previously unsuspected respiratory insufficiency may present as failure to wean from elective, perioperative mechanical ventilation.

Symptoms

Respiratory insufficiency may develop **insidiously**. There may be exertional dyspnoea, but, in neurological disease, symptoms may be present only after the development of nocturnal hypoventilation and sleep apnoea. **Established nocturnal respiratory insufficiency is characterized by insomnia, daytime hypersomnolence and lethargy, morning headaches, reduced mental concentration, depression, anxiety or irritability.**

The symptoms of obstructive sleep apnoea are similar but the patient or their partner often complains of snoring, abnormal sleep movements and disturbed sleep with distressing dreams. Patients with progressive diaphragm weakness develop orthopnoea, which may be severe, and prevent the patient lying flat. Nocturnal orthopnoea is usually severe and can mimic paroxysmal nocturnal dyspnoea. The history is crucial in eliciting the cause of generalized weakness or failure to wean in the ITU. Evidence of pre-existing sensory and motor dysfunction should be sought by careful questioning of the patient or the patient's family. Inquiry into exposure to medications or other toxins is essential.

Clinical signs

Clinical signs are often absent in the early stages of ventilatory failure and this can lead to the condition being missed. As the condition progresses there may be an unexplained tachycardia, an accentuated second heart sound over the pulmonary valve area and signs of polycythaemia. Obesity is often present in patients with obstructive sleep apnoea. There may be increased accessory muscle activity and diaphragmatic weakness or paralysis causing paradoxical movement of the abdominal wall with inspiratory indrawing of the lower lateral rib margin when the patient is supine or near supine. As the condition progresses, the full picture of respiratory failure is present and sudden unexpected death may then occur. Coexisting bulbar dysfunction is revealed by clinical signs of lesions of the IXth and Xth cranial nerves, including loss of posterior pharyngeal wall sensation, reduced palatal movement and pharyngeal reflex, poor cough, impaired speech and ineffective swallowing. However, clinical signs of bulbar dysfunction are not always a good guide to the development of aspiration. Muscle weakness may be difficult to recognize in critically ill patients because the clinical examination is often limited by the presence of encephalopathy or sedation.

Investigations

Imaging studies (computerized tomography or magnetic resonance imaging if possible) may allow identification and characterization of CNS disorders. **Electrodiagnostic studies** are needed to define lesions of the peripheral nervous system in critically ill patients. Occasionally, **nerve or muscle biopsy** is indicated to exclude vasculitis or to distinguish an inflammatory or axonal neuropathy. Muscle biopsy may be helpful in the diagnosis of an inflammatory myopathy, vasculitis, and structurally distinct myopathies [glycogen storage disorders, acid maltase deficiency and acute quadriplegic myopathy (AQM)].

Assessment

In progressive neuromuscular disease **vital capacity (VC)** falls both because of respiratory muscle weakness and/or fatigue and reduced chest wall and lung compliance, as a result of micro-atelectasis and restriction of chest wall movement. Diaphragm weakness is associated with a marked fall (greater than one-third) in VC when sitting or lying. Regular measurements of VC (both erect and supine) allow assessment of the extent and progression of respiratory muscle weakness. Chest radiographs may show clinically unsuspected unilateral or bilateral diaphragmatic paresis, aspiration pneumonitis or bronchopneumonia. Fluoroscopic screening performed when supine may show paradoxical upward movement of the paralysed diaphragm during inspiration or, preferably, during a short, sharp submaximal sniff.

Waking **arterial blood gas tensions** are often virtually normal during the early stages of neurological respiratory insufficiency, even when significant nocturnal hypoventilation is occurring. As the condition progresses daytime $PaCO_2$ becomes elevated. Oximetry however is the measurement of choice to detect periodic sleep apnoea. However, detailed analysis of the mechanisms of sleep-induced respiratory failure requires full polysomnography.

Pathophysiology

Respiratory muscle weakness, bulbar failure or disturbance of the central control of respiration contribute to nocturnal hypoventilation and may precipitate respiratory insufficiency. Although the effects of respiratory failure as a result of neuromuscular disease can become obvious the initial abnormality is disordered breathing during sleep and this remains the critical period for respiratory compromise and sudden death.

Respiratory muscles

Adequate ventilation during rapid eye movement sleep is largely dependent on diaphragm function: episodic hypoventilation or central sleep apnoea is inevitable if the diaphragm is paralysed . The consequences of respiratory muscle weakness, which may be exacerbated by scoliosis, include widespread atelectasis, reduced compliance, ventilatory perfusion inequality and impaired airway patency. Weakness of abdominal muscles also reduces the capacity to cough as does abdominal distension caused by ileus, constipation or bladder distension. Other factors that may precipitate respiratory deterioration in patients functioning with reduced reserve include obesity, anaesthesia, sedative drugs, surgery, tracheostomy complications and general medical disorders.

Sleep apnoea and alveolar hypoventilation

Periodic apnoea is conventionally divided into obstructive sleep apnoea, central sleep apnoea and nocturnal hypoventilation. In **obstructive apnoea** there is upper airway obstruction despite normal movement of the intercostals and diaphragm. In **central apnoea** all respiratory phased movements are absent. **Alveolar hypoventilation** is characterized by a reduced ventilatory response to CO_2 and consequent CO_2 retention in the absence of primary pulmonary disease. There is progressive reduction in the tidal volume and reduced hypoxic and hypercapnic drive, which may culminate in central apnoea. These effects occur primarily during sleep but hypercapnia may persist while awake, with the development of respiratory failure.

Central control

Neural control of respiration in man may be considered to depend on three largely anatomically and functionally independent pathways, although it is clear that these systems must interact with one another.

1 **Automatic (metabolic) respiration** is the homeostatic system by which ventilation may be altered to maintain acid-base status and oxygenation to the metabolic requirements. It originates in localized areas of the dorsolateral tegmentum in the pons and medulla in the region of the nucleus tractus solitarius and retro-ambigualis, descending via pathways in the ventrolateral columns of the spinal cord. It has been suggested that the abnormal patterns associated with brainstem lesions may be of localizing value. Certainly variations in respiratory rate and rhythm may be associated with dysfunction of the automatic or voluntary system but there is considerable overlap in patterns and it is often impossible to exclude coexisting pulmonary pathology in the acutely ill.

2 **Voluntary (behavioural) respiration** operates during consciousness and allows modulation of ventilation in response to voluntary actions such as speaking, singing, breath-holding and straining. This system originates in the contralateral cortex, descending via the corticospinal tract to the segmental level. Voluntary control may be impaired by bilateral lesions affecting the descending corticospinal or corticobulbar tract and is particularly seen in association with destructive lesions of the basal pons or of the medullary pyramids and adjacent ventromedial portion, which may result in the 'locked-in' syndrome.

3 **Limbic (emotional) control** accounts for the preservation of respiratory modulation to emotional stimuli including laughing, coughing and anxiety despite loss of voluntary control. This implies that descending limbic influences on automatic respiration are anatomically and functionally independent of the voluntary respiratory system. These systems appear to be largely distinct. Destructive lesions in man have occasionally enabled the study of one or other of them functioning in isolation.

PATTERNS OF RESPIRATORY IMPAIRMENT FROM NEUROLOGICAL DISORDERS
(Tables 25.1 and 25.2)

Cortex

Periods of apnoea are common during **complex partial and generalized seizures**. They may be associated with upper airway obstruction, laryngospasm and masseter spasm leading to hypoxaemia and cyanosis. Isolated apnoea may be an ictal phenomenon requiring prolonged ventilation and may contribute to sudden unexpected death in epileptic patients. **Convulsive status epilepticus** may be associated with prolonged hypoxia, which contributes to the development of cardiac arrhythmias and secondary cerebral damage. Intubation and ventilation are mandatory to prevent the development of these complications.

Hemispheric **ischaemic strokes** influence respiratory function to a modest degree. Both reduced chest wall movement and reduced contralateral diaphragmatic excursion, particularly during voluntary breathing, contralateral to the stroke have been reported. The latter association correlates well with the localization of the diaphragm cortical representation found by transcranial magnetic stimulation and positron emission tomography scanning. Patients with bilateral hemispheric cerebrovascular disease show an increased respiratory responsiveness to CO_2 and are liable to develop Cheyne–Stokes respiration, suggesting disinhibition of lower respiratory centres. Such a response may persist months to years after the stroke. Diffuse cortical vascular disease may also lead to a selective inability of voluntary breathing (respiratory apraxia). Intermittent upper airway obstruction and apnoea as a result of periodic fluctuations in the position of the vocal cords is associated with cortical supranuclear palsy from bilateral lesions of the operculum.

Brainstem

The effects of brainstem dysfunction on respiration depend on the pathology, localization and speed of

Table 25.1 Central causes of ventilatory insufficiency or failure

Cortical
Epilepsy
Vascular
Tumour
Brainstem
Congenital (Ondine's curse) – Primary alveolar Hypoventilation
Tumour
Vascular
Multiple sclerosis and acute disseminated encephalomyelitis
Motor neurone disease
Infection:
Borrelia
Listeria
Post-varicella encephalomyelitis
Poliomyelitis
Encephalitis lethargica
Western equine encephalitis
Paraneoplastic
Leigh's disease
Reye's syndrome
Hypoxaemia
Foramen magnum and upper cervical cord
Arnold–Chiari malformation – cerebellar ectopia
Achondroplasia, osteogenesis imperfecta
Rheumatoid arthritis – odontoid peg compression
Trauma
Vascular
Disorders of the spinal cord
Acute epidural compression from neoplasm or infection
Acute transverse myelitis
Cord infarction
Other myelopathies (including traumatic)
Tetanus
Autonomic
Multisystem atrophy
Extrapyramidal
Idiopathic Parkinson's disease
Dystonia

onset of the lesion. In patients with bulbar lesions, particularly vascular or demyelinating, the combination of impaired swallow, abnormalities of the respiratory rhythm, reduced vital capacity and

Table 25.2 Peripheral causes of ventilatory insufficiency or failure

Anterior horn cell
   Motor neurone disease
   Poliomyelitis or post-polio syndromes
   Rabies

Multiple radiculopathies
   Carcinomatous meningitis
   AIDS polyradiculitis

Polyneuropathy
   Acute inflammatory demyelinating
      polyneuropathy
   Acute motor and sensory axonal neuropathy
   Acute motor axonal neuropathy
   Critical illness polyneuropathy
   Other polyneuropathies
   Hereditary motor-sensory
   Acute porphyria
   Organophosphate poisoning
   Herpes zoster/varicella
   Neuralgic amyotrophy

Neuromuscular transmission defects
   Myasthenia gravis
   Lambert–Eaton myasthenic syndrome
   Neuromuscular blocking agents
   Other:
      Botulism
      Toxins
      Hypermagnesaemia
      Organophosphate poisoning

Muscle
   Dystrophy – Duchenne, Becker, limb girdle,
      Emery–Dreifuss
   Inflammatory
   Myotonic dystrophy
   Metabolic
      Acid maltase deficiency
      Mitochondrial myopathies
   Myopathies associated with neuromuscular
      blocking agents and steroids
   Acute quadriplegic myopathy
   Myopathy and sepsis
   Cachectic myopathy
   HIV-related myopathy
   Sarcoid myopathy
   Hypokalaemic myopathy
   Rhabdomyolysis
   Periodic paralysis

reduced or absent triggering of a cough reflex all increase the risk of aspiration pneumonia. Nocturnal upper airway occlusion may also contribute to respiratory impairment.

The commonest cause of brainstem lesions that disrupt respiration is **cerebrovascular disease**. Unilateral or bilateral lateral tegmental infarcts in the pons (at or below the level of the trigeminal nucleus) lead to apneustic breathing and impairment of CO_2 responsiveness, while similar lesions in the medulla (e.g. lateral medullary syndrome) may result in acute failure of automatic respiration. Infarction of the basal pons ('locked-in syndrome') or of the pyramids and the adjacent ventromedial portion of the medulla may lead to complete loss of the voluntary system with a highly regular breathing pattern but a complete inability to initiate any spontaneous respiratory movements.

Respiratory abnormalities may be associated with **encephalitis** involving the brainstem. A variety of patterns occur during the acute phase and following recovery including alveolar hypoventilation, central sleep apnoea and respiratory dysrhythmias such as tachypnoea, myoclonic jerking of the diaphragm, apneustic, ratchet and cluster breathing. Respiratory failure has also been described as a result of **post-rubeola** and **post-varicella encephalomyelitis** and **acute disseminated encephalomyelitis**.

Brainstem tumours may lead to automatic respiratory failure or central neurogenic hyperventilation. Although aspiration and bronchopneumonia are common complications of **acute bulbar demyelination**, multiple sclerosis has only rarely been associated with central disorders of respiratory rate and rhythm. Acute loss of the automatic system has been associated with large demyelinating lesions in the region of the medial lemniscus and loss of the voluntary control system with evidence of an acute demyelinating lesion at the cervicomedullary junction.

Other clinical causes of automatic respiratory failure as a result of brainstem disorders include other central nervous system infections such as **borrelia and listeria, post-infectious encephalomyelitis, malignant disease, either primary or secondary, or as a paraneoplastic brainstem encephalitis** with anti-Hu antibodies, which may cause central alveolar hypoventilation and central sleep apnoea, culminating in respiratory failure.

Involuntary movements of the respiratory muscles

In **idiopathic Parkinson's disease** respiratory impairment is associated with upper airflow obstruction, reduced tidal volume, respiratory muscle weakness, restrictive defect as a result of respiratory muscle rigidity, abnormalities of central CO_2 sensitivity and impairment of voluntary control. Patients with primary and secondary dystonic syndromes occasionally develop severe episodes of generalized dystonia and rigidity (status dystonicus), which may be refractory to standard drug therapy. The most severe cases may develop bulbar and ventilatory failure necessitating intubation and ventilation.

Autonomic failure

Multisystem atrophy (see p. 233) is a global term, which includes many neurodegenerative disorders. A characteristic feature is paresis of the vocal cord abductors (posterior cricoarytenoids); the cords lie closely opposed leading to severe upper airway limitation during sleep and giving rise to the characteristic presenting feature of severe nocturnal stridor. Other factors also contribute to the development of respiratory insufficiency. These include abnormalities of rate, rhythm and amplitude during sleep, a reduction in central respiratory drive leading to obstructive sleep apnoea, as a result of upper airway occlusion, and central sleep apnoea, from loss of automatic control. A further important factor is the accompanying autonomic failure, which contributes to impaired cardiorespiratory control mechanisms.

Foramen magnum lesions

Lesions of the foramen magnum are an important cause of acute or subacute respiratory insufficiency. Cerebellar ectopia and syringomyelia may present with either progressive nocturnal hypoventilation, obstructive sleep apnoea or sudden respiratory arrest, usually precipitated by some intercurrent event. In patients with rheumatoid atlanto-axial dislocation, clinically unsuspected hypoventilation and sleep apnoea are common if there is severe medullary compression and this may contribute to the high mortality of the condition. Similar respiratory abnormalities may be associated with achondroplasia, osteogenesis imperfecta and foramen magnum meningioma.

Cervical cord

Traumatic, demyelinating or vascular lesions of the spinal cord, particularly at high cervical levels, may selectively affect respiratory control. Lesions of the anterior pathways, as may occur following cordotomy, lead to loss of automatic control and sudden nocturnal death from apnoea. The respiratory effects of traumatic or vascular lesions of the spinal cord depend on the timing of onset and the extent of involvement of the phrenic nerve supply (C3–C5). Complete lesions usually lead to sudden respiratory arrest and death unless immediate resuscitation is available. Patients with lesions at or above C3 and some patients with lesions at a lower level may require prolonged or even permanent ventilator support. In quadriparesis with levels below C3, there is loss of intercostal and abdominal muscle function, while diaphragm and spinal accessory muscle function is maintained. Progressive diaphragm fatigue is an important factor in predisposing to intercurrent respiratory infection. Other complications leading to respiratory problems include impaired cough effectiveness, increased physiological arteriovenous shunting and ventilation–perfusion mismatch.

Anterior horn cell

During acute poliomyelitis, respiratory insufficiency occurs as a result of respiratory muscle weakness or involvement of the central respiratory control mechanisms. Respiratory insufficiency may develop many years after poliomyelitis, even in the absence of any obvious respiratory involvement during the acute illness or convalescent phase. Respiratory insufficiency is the common terminal event in motor neurone disease either as a result of respiratory muscle or bulbar weakness leading to hypoventilation, aspiration, bronchopneumonia or pulmonary emboli. However, an important proportion of patients with motor neurone disease may develop respiratory insufficiency early in the course of the disease and may present with respiratory failure or even respiratory arrest.

Neuropathies

Acute inflammatory demyelinating polyneuropathy [Guillain–Barré syndrome (GBS)] (see p. 157) develops 1–4 weeks after an infectious illness, as a progressive weakness in the arms and legs with areflexia. The onset is relatively symmetrical and mainly motor. There may be unilateral or bilateral facial weakness. The autonomic nervous system may be affected and respiratory insufficiency requires mechanical ventilation in approximately one-third of patients. The incidence of respiratory failure requiring mechanical ventilation in GBS is approximately 20%. Ventilatory failure is primarily a result of inspiratory muscle weakness, although weakness of the abdominal and accessory muscles of respiration and retained airway secretion leading to aspiration and atelectasis are all contributory factors. The associated bulbar weakness and autonomic instability contribute to the necessity for control of the airway and ventilation. **Acute motor and sensory axonal neuropathy** is the acute axonal form of GBS, which usually presents with a rapidly developing paralysis developing over hours and rapid development of respiratory failure requiring intubation and ventilation. There may be total paralysis of all voluntary muscles of the body, including the cranial musculature, the ocular muscles and pupils. This variant of GBS may be related to precipitating enteral infection from *Campylobacter jejuni*, and probably elevation of anti-GM1 antibodies. The condition has a relatively poor outcome.

Critical illness polyneuropathy (CIP) is a sensorimotor axonal neuropathy, which develops in the setting of the systemic inflammatory response syndrome, a severe systemic response that occurs in up to 50% of those in a critical care setting in response to infection or other insults, such as burns, trauma or surgery. There is distally predominant limb weakness, atrophy and reduced reflexes. Sensory loss can be demonstrated in patients who are able to

cooperate with the examination. However the signs are variable and difficult to elicit because of sedation or coexistent encephalopathy, an even more common complication of systemic inflammatory response syndrome. Nearly half of the patients affected by CIP die from this illness. Of those who survive, recovery mirrors that seen in most axonal neuropathies: those who survive with mild to moderate neuropathy recover fully over months; those with severe neuropathy either have no recovery or a significant persistent deficit.

Phrenic neuropathies

Neuralgic amyotrophy may present with dyspnoea and orthopnoea as a result of selective or isolated involvement of the phrenic nerve, causing unilateral or bilateral diaphragm paresis. Predominant phrenic nerve involvement may occur in neuropathies associated with underlying **carcinoma, diphtheria, herpes zoster–varicella**, and following **immunization**. Acute respiratory failure is also a feature of **vasculitic, acute porphyric** and **toxic neuropathies**. Similarly, diaphragmatic weakness has also been described in **hereditary sensorimotor neuropathy** and this is associated with reduced transdiaphragmatic pressures and undetectable phrenic nerve conduction. However phrenic nerve involvement occurs most commonly as a result of **trauma during thoracic surgery, hypothermia or direct involvement by neoplasm.**

Neuromuscular junction

Respiratory failure in **myasthenia gravis** (see p. 151) often results from a myasthenic crisis (usually precipitated by infection) but is also associated with cholinergic crisis, thymectomy or steroid myopathy. Associated bulbar weakness predisposes to aspiration and acute respiratory failure, necessitating urgent intubation and ventilation. Expiratory and inspiratory intercostal and diaphragm weakness are common, even when there is only mild peripheral muscle weakness. Respiratory impairment is also an important feature in Lambert–Eaton myasthenic

patients with neuromuscular disease. *American Review of Respiratory Disease*, **135**:148–152.

Howard RS, Hirsch NP (2000) The neural control of respiratory and cardiovascular function In: Crockard A, Hayward R, Hoff JT (eds) *Neurosurgery – The Scientific Basis of Clinical Practice.* Oxford, UK: Blackwell Science Ltd. pp.289–309.

Howard RS, Wiles CM, Hirsch NP, Spencer GT (1993) Respiratory involvement in primary muscle disorders: assessment and management. *Quarterly Journal of Medicine*, **86**:175–189.

Munschauer FE, Mador MJ, Ahuja A, Jacobs L (1991) Selective paralysis of voluntary but not limbically influenced automatic respiration. *Archives of Neurology*, **48**:1190–1192.

Plum F (1970) Neurological integration of behavioural and metabolic control of breathing. In: Parker R (ed.) *Breathing*, Hering–Breuer Centenary Symposium. London: Churchill. pp.314–326.

Plum F, Posner JR (1983) *Diagnosis of Stupor and Coma.* Philadelphia, PA: F.A. Davis.

Ropper AH (1985) Guillain-Barré syndrome: management of respiratory failure. *Neurology*, **35**:1662–1665.

Smith PEM, Edwards RHT, Calverley PMA (1991) Mechanisms of sleep disordered breathing in chronic neuromuscular disease: implications for management. *Quarterly Journal of Medicine*, **81**:961–973.

Sykes MK, McNicol MW, Campbell EM (eds) (1976) Introduction. In: *Respiratory Failure.* Oxford, UK: Blackwell Scientific Publications Ltd. p.xi.

PAIN IN NEUROLOGICAL DISEASE

J.W. Scadding

Pain is a common and often severe symptom of chronic neurological disease. This is a brief survey of current thinking about definition, classification, pathophysiology and treatment.

NEUROPATHIC PAIN

The term **neuropathic pain (NP)** refers to all pains resulting from disease or damage of the peripheral or central nervous systems, and from dysfunction of the nervous system (International Association for the Study of Pain, IASP).

Confusion may arise with this definition. Formerly, NP denoted pain related to peripheral neuropathies, and **central pain** lesions of the central nervous system causing pain. **Neurogenic pain** embraced all causes, both peripheral and central, and is a term still used.

The addition of a category of 'dysfunction' in the definition of NP allows the inclusion of organic pain states, which share the clinical features of NP but which are not initiated by an identifiable injury to any part of the nervous system. The most important of these is **complex regional pain syndrome (CRPS)**, formerly known as reflex sympathetic dystrophy. However, the inclusion of 'dysfunctional' neurological pain, without further description or definition has not yet found universal acceptance.

Classification of neuropathic pain

The most straightforward classification of NP is anatomical, according to the site of initiating nervous system pathology; thus the terms peripheral neuropathic, radicular and myelopathic pain, with an aetiological subclassification (Tables 26.2 and 26.3, see below). However, this is not helpful in relation to treatment, and there is a move towards a mechanism-based classification. Unfortunately, it is not yet possible to link tightly symptoms and signs to pathophysiology, although there are some strong candidate mechanisms (see Table 26.4 below). Clearly, the development of specific and selective treatments will depend on a mechanism-based classification.

Clinical features of neuropathic pain

Neuropathic pain is qualitatively different from nociceptive (somatic) pain and does not serve the same protective function. Table 26.1 summarizes the main clinical features. Although sensory impairment is almost invariably present, it is often overshadowed by accompanying **allodynia** (all stimuli producing pain), **hyperalgesia** (enhanced pain with painful stimuli) and **hyperpathia** (delayed perception, summation and painful after-sensation).

Causes of neuropathic pain

Tables 26.2 and 26.3 list the numerous causes of NP, and serve to emphasize the magnitude of the total burden of NP in neurological disease. Precise incidence and prevalence data are not available for

Table 26.1 Clinical features of neuropathic pain

Abnormal pain quality: difficult for patients to describe
Poor localization, often diffuse
Paroxysmal pains common
Immediate or delayed onset after injury
Pain intensity markedly altered by emotion and fatigue
Sensory impairment in anatomical distribution
Associated allodynia, hyperalgesia and hyperpathia
Abnormal sympathetic function: vasomotor and sudomotor changes
Associated dystrophic change in a minority

all disease categories, but prospective studies have shown that, for example, the incidence of NP in stroke is 8%, in MS 28%, and in syringomyelia 75%.

Diagnosis of neuropathic pain

Like all pain, NP is a symptom, not a diagnosis in itself, and always has an underlying cause. Many patients with chronic pain of unknown cause are referred to neurologists and pain clinics with a putative diagnosis of NP. Such patients require the most thorough clinical evaluation, supported by appropriate investigation. Experience has shown that once attention is shifted to the difficult task of treating the pain, the diagnostic process may cease. Thus, a potentially remediable underlying cause, producing a subtle neurological deficit, may remain untreated; examples include syringomyelia and intrinsic spinal cord tumours.

Table 26.2 Peripheral causes of neuropathic pain

Mononeuropathies and multiple mononeuropathies		
Trauma including entrapment, transection, post-thoracotomy, painful scars		
Diabetic mononeuropathy and amyotrophy		
Neuralgic amyotrophy		
Connective tissue disease		
Malignant and radiation plexopathy		
Polyneuropathies		
Metabolic/nutritional	Diabetic	Cuban neuropathy
	Alcoholic	Tanzanian neuropathy
	Pellagra	Burning feet syndrome
	Beriberi	Strachan's (Jamaican neuropathy)
	Amyloid	
Drugs/toxic	Isoniazid	Thallium
	Cisplatin	Arsenic
	Vincristine	Clioquinol
	Nitrofurantoin	
	Disulfiram	
Infective	HIV	
	Acute inflammatory polyneuropathy (Guillain-Barré)	
Hereditary	Fabry's disease	
	Dominantly inherited sensory neuropathy	
Malignant	Myeloma	
	Carcinomatous	
Idiopathic neuropathy		

Many patients have pains of mixed nociceptive and neuropathic types, the commonest example in neurological practice being mechanical spinal pain associated with radicular and occasionally myelopathic pain. As nociceptive spinal pain may radiate widely, mimicking a root distribution, it can be difficult to identify the dominant pain type and treat it appropriately.

Mechanisms of neuropathic pain

The pathophysiological mechanisms of NP fall broadly into several categories: **ectopic impulse generation** in damaged primary afferent fibres, **central sensitization**, failure or reduction of normal inhibitory mechanisms **(disinhibition)**, and degenerative and regenerative changes **(plasticity)**, leading to **altered**

connectivity. These are summarized in Table 26.4. Damaged peripheral sensory neurones generate nerve impulses ectopically, in the absence of any peripheral stimulus, both at the site of the lesion and proximally, in dorsal root ganglion cells, because of the development of abnormal sodium channels in the axolemma of regenerating axons, leading to spontaneous repetitive depolarization. This abnormal sodium channel expression is modified by certain nerve growth factors, providing potential future therapeutic targets.

Following peripheral tissue, nerve or root injury, with prolonged noxious afferent input to the spinal cord, major functional changes occur in the dorsal horn of the spinal cord. These include an

Table 26.3 Central causes of neuropathic pain

Spinal root/dorsal root ganglion	
Prolapsed disc	Root avulsion
Arachnoiditis	Surgical rhizotomy
Post-herpetic neuralgia	Tumour compression
Trigeminal neuralgia	

Spinal cord	
Trauma including compression	
Syringomyelia and intrinsic tumours	
Multiple sclerosis	
Vascular, including infarction and AVM	
Dysraphism	
Vitamin B12 deficiency	
Infection including HIV and syphilitic myelopathies	
Surgery including anterolateral cordotomy	

Brainstem	
Lateral medullary syndrome	Multiple sclerosis
Tumours	Tuberculoma
Syrinx	

Thalamus	
Infarction	Tumours
Haemorrhage	Surgical lesions

Subcortical and cortical	
Infarction	Trauma
AVM	Tumour

AVM, arteriovenous malformation.

Table 26.4 Mechanisms of neuropathic pain

Peripheral nerve	
Ectopic impulse generation (EIG) (abnormal sodium channel expression)	
Increased by:	Mechanical stimulation
	Noradrenaline
	Ischaemia
	Warming myelinated fibres
	Cooling unmyelinated fibres
Decreased by:	Local anaesthetic
	Alpha receptor blockers
	Axon transport blockers
	Corticosteroid, glycerol
	Carbamazepine, phenytoin
EIG in dorsal root ganglion	

Central nervous system	
Central sensitization	
Dorsal horn neuron 'wind up': NMDA receptor mediated	
Prostaglandin and nitric oxide synthesis in dorsal horn neurones	
Disinhibition	
Deafferentation of dorsal horn cells: bursting discharge	
Reduced spinal inhibitions: surround, segmental, descending brainstem	
Reduced insular cortex inhibition in central pain	
Plasticity	
Neurotransmitter excitotoxicity: cell death	
Post-synaptic receptor upregulation	
Inappropriate regeneration, altered connectivity	

NMDA, N-methyl-d-aspartate.

N-methyl-d-aspartate-receptor-mediated 'wind-up' of dorsal horn neurones, reduction or loss of segmental, regional and descending inhibitions, neurotransmitter excitotoxicity, and degenerative changes, followed by regeneration. Regeneration may be aberrant, leading to altered, inappropriate connectivity. In certain situations, an irreversibly reorganized state may develop, the important clinical implication being that treatment aimed at the primary site of pathology will then be ineffective. In experimental preparations that model pathological situations in man, it has been shown that a lesion may produce knock-on pathophysiological effects at more rostral levels. To what extent such changes are irreversible is unknown.

COMPLEX REGIONAL PAIN SYNDROME

Complex regional pain syndrome (CRPS) is the name now given to a number of previously described conditions, including **reflex sympathetic dystrophy** and **causalgia** (Table 26.5). The reason for abandoning the term reflex sympathetic dystrophy is that it implies a crucial role of the sympathetic nervous system in the pathogenesis of the condition. This idea, and the additional previous suggestion that the condition could be defined by a therapeutic response to sympathectomy, is no longer tenable.

Characteristics of CRPS

CRPS describes a variety of painful conditions that usually:

- Follow injury
- Occur regionally
- Have a distal predominance of abnormal findings
- Exceed in both magnitude and duration the expected course of the inciting event
- Result in marked impairment of motor function
- Are associated with oedema, abnormal skin blood flow, or sudomotor activity in the region of the pain at some time during the course of the illness (IASP definition).

CRPS is divided into **type 1**, which includes all those conditions that are caused by tissue injury other than peripheral nerve (the majority of cases), and **type 2**,

which denotes the same clinical syndrome precipitated by major nerve injury. The latter corresponds to causalgia, although, strictly speaking, causalgia merely means burning pain, and thus denotes a symptom rather than a disease. For the moment, however, the IASP approved terminology makes CRPS type 2 and causalgia synonymous.

The nosology of these conditions is a matter of ongoing debate; the difficulties in finding agreed terms emphasizes the limited understanding of their pathophysiology.

The causes of CRPS are listed in Table 26.6.

Table 26.5 Complex regional pain syndrome – previously described syndromes

Reflex sympathetic dystrophy
Causalgia (major and minor)
Post-traumatic sympathetic dystrophy
Algodystrophy
Sudek's atrophy
Acute bone atrophy
Migratory osteolysis
Post-traumatic vasomotor syndrome
Shoulder-hand syndrome

Table 26.6 Causes of complex regional pain syndrome

Peripheral tissues	Fractures and dislocations
	Soft tissue injury
	Fasciitis, tendonitis, ligament strain
	Arthritis
	Deep vein thrombosis
	Prolonged immobilization of a limb
Peripheral nerve and dorsal root	Peripheral nerve trauma
	Brachial plexus lesions
	Post-herpetic neuralgia
	Spinal nerve root lesions
Central nervous system	Myelopathies, particularly trauma
	Head injury
	Cerebral infarction
	Cerebral tumour
Viscera	Abdominal disease
	Myocardial infarction
Idiopathic	

Clinical features and pathophysiology of complex regional pain syndrome

The common clinical features of CRPS are shown in Table 26.7. These may vary over time in an individual patient, with a tendency for many patients to have a warm, swollen limb in the earlier stages, becoming cold later and associated with increasing dystrophic changes. However, not all patients progress to a dystrophic phase. Attempts at staging CRPS according to signs have not proved clinically useful.

The pathogenesis of CRPS is probably heterogeneous; there is evidence of a noradrenergic sympathetic influence on the development of pain, both with and in the absence of nerve injury. Chronic inflammatory processes may contribute in CRPS type 1; microangiopathic changes have been found in limbs amputated from CRPS sufferers, and there are reports of a therapeutic effect of anti-inflammatory

Table 26.7 Clinical features of complex regional pain syndrome

Inflammatory	Pain
	Colour change
	Temperature change
	Limitation of movement
	Exacerbation by exercise
	Oedema
Neurological	Allodynia
	Hyperpathia
	Incoordination
	Tremor
	Involuntary muscle spasms
	Paresis
	Pseudoparesis
Dystrophic	Skin
	Nails
	Muscle
	Bone
Sympathetic	Hyperhidrosis
	Changed hair and nail growth
	Vasomotor abnormalities

treatment early in the course of the disease. It has also been suggested that free radical-mediated damage may be important in pathogenesis. As in the neuropathic conditions already discussed, secondary central sensitization may ensue, and form an important component of the overall pathogenesis of pain.

Psychological factors have been suggested in the pathogenesis of CRPS. It is true that patients with conversion disorder and factitious illnesses can present with symptoms closely resembling CRPS, and a diagnosis of CRPS as distinct from conversion disorder may only be clear after a series of diagnostic assessments. The severe pain of CRPS with loss of function produces anxiety and depression in many patients. Whether or not such secondary psychological factors developing early after an injury might predispose to progression to CRPS remains controversial.

Diagnosis of complex regional pain syndrome

There are no diagnostic tests for CRPS, which remains a clinical diagnosis. The cut-off point for deciding when pain is disproportionate in severity, distribution and duration to the initiating event, is a matter of subjective clinical judgement. Furthermore, a degree of oedema, vasomotor or sudomotor change following many injuries is extremely common. Three-phase isotope bone scans are frequently abnormal in CRPS, but a normal scan does not exclude the diagnosis. Prospective studies of the development of CRPS after injury are few. Estimates include 1–2% after fractures (type 1 CRPS), and 1–5% after peripheral nerve injury (CRPS type 2).

TREATMENT OF NEUROPATHIC PAIN

If NP is the result of a remediable compressive lesion, for example root compression by a prolapsed disc or benign tumour, there is a good prospect of complete relief from pain following surgery. However, even in this situation, there may be severe continuing NP with relatively minor root damage. Trigeminal neuralgia is outstandingly the example of NP most amenable to treatment (see p. 197). For the majority of patients with NP, the realistic goal of treatment is partial analgesia, combined with improvement in functional status. Patients will benefit from a multidisciplinary approach in a pain clinic setting.

Acute interventions that lead to pain relief must be accompanied by immediate efforts to rehabilitate and restore function, where possible. The different modalities of treatment used in NP are summarized in Table 26.8.

Topical and local measures

Wherever appropriate, local measures should be tried first, although many patients require combined local and systemic treatments. Patients with severe allodynia will often not tolerate any treatment in the affected area, but these local measures applied in adjacent areas may be helpful.

Topical local anaesthetic is often partially effective in allodynia. **Topical capsaicin**, which initially stimulates, then desensitizes afferent C fibres, is also beneficial in areas of allodynia and hyperalgesia.

Table 26.8 Treatment modalities for neuropathic pain

Topical	Local anaesthetic
	Capsaicin
Local	Transcutaneous electrical stimulation
	Acupuncture
	Heat, cold
	Vibration
Blocks	Somatic of nerve, plexus, root
	Sympathetic of ganglia, or regional guanethidine
Central stimulation	Spinal cord stimulation
	Deep brain stimulation
Spinal drugs	Epidural or intrathecal
Systemic drugs	
Surgery	
Psychological interventions	
Rehabilitation	

Patients with post-herpetic neuralgia form the largest group likely to benefit from these measures.

Local and regional blocks

Local anaesthetic blocks may provide temporary pain relief, and may be helpful diagnostically. **Local anaesthetic combined with corticosteroid** can increase the duration of pain relief. **Sympathetic blocks**, performed either by sympathetic plexus local anaesthetic block or **regionally, with guanethidine** in a Bier's block, are widely used for the treatment of NP of peripheral origin (scars, mononeuropathies, plexopathies, CRPS, and occasionally radiculopathies). Temporary partial analgesia lasting hours or days is commonly observed, and a small number of patients benefit from repeated blocks over long periods. Sympathetic blockade has the practical advantage of preserved motor and sensory function, compared with somatic nerve or root blocks. Thus, during the period of analgesia following the block, attempts at rehabilitation may be more successful.

The effect of sympathetic blocks is usually brief and there are many patients who show no response at all. Controlled trials have not shown significant long-term benefit from sympathetic blocks. The treatment is useful in a minority of patients, particularly in allowing the initiation of a process of rehabilitation of an otherwise exquisitely sensitive and useless limb.

Surgical sympathectomy for NP (including CRPS) is now rarely undertaken.

Spinal cord and deep brain stimulation

Antidromic **stimulation of dorsal column fibres** activating dorsal horn gating mechanisms is a likely mode of action of spinal cord stimulation, but more rostral effects at thalamic level are also possible. The technique is reserved for patients in whom all other reasonable measures have failed. It may be effective in patients with intractable pain as a result of major limb nerve injury, CRPS, plexopathies, thoracic or lumbar post-herpetic neuralgia, and, occasionally, myelopathies in the thoracic region. The commonest indication is lumbar spondylosis with radiculopathies, combined with nociceptive spinal pain in patients who have had multiple unsuccessful spinal operations (the failed back surgery syndrome).

Deep brain stimulation, targeting a number of sites in the thalamus, is rarely performed in highly selected patients. The usual indication is central post-stroke pain, resistant to all other measures. As with spinal cord stimulation, the analgesic effect may be short-lived.

Systemic drugs

Until recent years, drug trials in NP were notable for being of inadequate size and poorly controlled. A more rigorous approach has resulted in more robust data, and there have been several recent systematic surveys that now help to guide treatment. A useful statistic employed in these meta-analyses is the number needed to treat (NNT), defined as the number of patients needed to treat to produce one patient with 50% pain relief. However, this statistic hides great variability in trial design and methodology, pain measures (including quality of life measures, used only in recent studies), and duration of treatment. Table 26.9 lists systemic, local and spinally administered drugs found to have an analgesic effect in NP, with NNTs where it is possible to calculate these from the data available. Excluding **carbamazepine** for trigeminal neuralgia, the two leading drugs for NP are **amitriptyline** (and other tricyclic antidepressants), and **gabapentin**. The mode of action of both these drugs is uncertain. Amitriptyline has multiple sites of action; one possible mechanism in NP may be a facilitation of the descending serotoninergic analgesic pathway from the brainstem via the dorsolateral funiculus of the spinal cord to the dorsal horn. Gabapentin has an action on voltage-dependent calcium channels in spinal cord interneurones.

The role of **opioids** in the treatment of NP remains **uncertain**. Opioids are much less effective in NP than in nociceptive pain, but the previous view that opioids were without effect in NP must be revised in the light of new evidence from controlled trials. When all else fails in patients with severe intractable NP, a trial of opioid therapy is justified on the basis of present evidence.

Table 26.9 Drug treatment of neuropathic pain: controlled trials

Drug/route	Condition	Efficacy
Systemic:		
Tricyclic antidepressants	PHN	+NNT = 2.3
	DPN	+NNT = 3.0
	NP	+
	HIVN	−
SSRI		
Paroxetine	DPN	+NNT = 6.7
Citalopram	CPSP	−
Carbamazepine	TN	+NNT = 2.6
	DPN	+
	CPSP	−
Phenytoin	DPN	+
Gabapentin	PHN	+NNT = 3.7
	DPN	+NNT = 3.2
Mexiletine	DPN	±less than 50% analgesia
Baclofen	TN	+
Fentanyl	NP	+
Oxycodone	PHN	+
Dextromethorphan	DPN	+
	CPSP	−
Phentolamine	NP	±
Topical lidocaine	PHN	+
Topical capsaicin	PHN, DPN	+
Topical non-steroidal anti-inflammatories	PHN	+
Epidural clonidine	NP/CRPS	+
Intrathecal methyl prednisolone	PHN	+
Regional guanethidine	CRPS	−
Intranasal calcitonin	CRPS	±

PHN, post-herpetic neuralgia; DPN, painful diabetic neuropathy; NP, neuropathic pain; HIVN, painful HIV neuropathy; CPSP, central post-stroke pain; TN, trigeminal neuralgia; CRPS, complex regional pain syndrome; NNT, number needed to treat; SSRI, selective serotonin re-uptake inhibitor.

A recent trial in post-herpetic neuralgia using intrathecal methyl prednisolone has shown promising results.

Despite the various drugs now available for the treatment of NP, the therapeutic effects are all too often disappointing.

Surgical treatment

Neuropathic pain results from damage to, or disease of the nervous system, including surgical trauma, even carefully placed lesions designed to relieve pain. An example is **anterolateral cordotomy**, which interrupts the spinothalamic tract, leading to contralateral analgesia. While this achieves excellent analgesia for selected patients with cancer pain, in patients with pain from benign causes NP may develop in the distribution of the lesioned tract months to years after the procedure. The same problem has been reported with most of the surgical lesions of peripheral nerve, root or spinal cord, advocated for the relief of chronic pain, both NP and severe nociceptive pain. **Thalamotomy**, with lesions at a number of sites, has been abandoned because of the usual short duration of analgesia (often only weeks). Lesioning operations for the treatment of NP have now been largely abandoned in favour of stimulation procedures.

Psychological measures and rehabilitation

Depression in patients with intractable NP may be helped by antidepressant drug treatment, but with continuing pain, the effect is often limited. Other psychological interventions can be very helpful, including pacing and other behavioural measures. **Pain management programmes**, in which the emphasis is away from prescribed treatments towards a variety of coping strategies, are extremely helpful for many patients. They should be combined with multidisciplinary efforts at rehabilitation.

REFERENCES AND FURTHER READING

Hansson PT, Fields HL, Hill RG, Marchettini P (eds) (2001) *Neuropathic Pain: Pathophysiology and Treatment*. Progress in Pain Research and Management. Seattle, WA: IASP Press.

Kingery WS (1997) A critical review of controlled clinical trials for peripheral neuropathic pain and complex regional pain syndromes. *Pain*, **73**:123–139.

Perez RSGM, Kwakkel G, Zuurmond WWA, de Lange JJ (2001) Treatment of reflex sympathetic dystrophy (CRPS type 1): a research synthesis of 21 randomized trials. *Journal of Pain Symptom Management*, 21:511–526.

Sindrup SH, Jensen TS (1999) Efficacy of pharmacological treatments of neuropathic pain: an update and effect related to mechanism of drug action. *Pain*, **83**:389–400.

Wall PD, Melzack R (eds) (1999) *Textbook of Pain*, 4th edn. Edinburgh, UK: Churchill Livingstone.

CHAPTER 27

PSYCHIATRY AND NEUROLOGICAL DISORDERS

S. Fleminger

This chapter will discuss the overlap between neurology and psychiatry, before going on to consider psychiatric diagnosis and management, particularly where it is relevant to neurology.

NEUROLOGY AND PSYCHIATRY: BRAIN AND MIND

It has been suggested that neurologists deal with disorders of the brain, whereas psychiatrists see people with disorders of the mind. Whereas the brain may be considered like any other organ of the body, the **mind** is generally seen as indivisible from the person as an individual and is closely linked to concepts like soul and freewill. Thus a mind/person can be energetic, or lazy, or morally good or bad.

On the other hand the **brain** can become damaged and despite the person's 'best intentions' cause them to behave in an inconsiderate way; for example,

damage to the medial orbital frontal surface of the brain may result in the person becoming thoughtless and violent. Diffuse brain injury often results in problems initiating activity and a lack of drive; the patients are described as having an amotivational state.

Because behaviour may be attributed to the mind on the one hand and to disorders of the brain on the other, different words may be used to describe similar behaviours; for example, a person may be described as 'lazy' if their lack of activity is attributed to the mind, but suffering an 'amotivational state' if it is attributed to a disorder of the brain. Similarly, different words may be used to describe the same movement disorder: a *grimacing mannerism* in a treatment naive patient with schizophrenia may look very similar to an *orofacial dyskinesia* in a patient with dystonia.

Many neuropsychiatric conditions arise from an **interaction** between cerebral disease and psychological processes; for example in delusional misidentification, in which people or places are believed to have been replaced by duplicates, it is often the combined effects of both brain disease and suspiciousness that produces the symptom. Antisocial behaviour is particularly likely if there is a combination of both birth injury, causing brain damage, and poor parenting.

Therefore it is not possible to make an absolute distinction between mental symptoms, which arise from disorders of the brain, and those that arise in the absence of manifest organic brain disease. The mental symptoms of organic brain disease overlap considerably with symptoms to be found in the absence of brain disease. While it is useful to understand the importance of the cardinal symptoms of organic brain (see below), it is equally important to realize that the absence of such symptoms does not rule out brain disease; for example, a brain tumour may present with mania indistinguishable from that seen in someone with manic-depressive disorder.

BRIDGING THE GAP BETWEEN NEUROLOGY AND PSYCHIATRY

Bridging the gap
Biological psychiatry and **behavioural neurology** are bridging the gap between neurology and psychiatry. **Functional imaging techniques** enable us to see which parts of the brain may be involved in functional mental illness, for example, when a patient with schizophrenia experiences a hallucination.

These studies demonstrate how hallucinations involve the corresponding sensory association cortex, but may in addition involve areas of the cortex involved in higher order processing; for example, auditory verbal hallucinations in schizophrenia are likely to involve auditory association cortex as well as language areas and cingulate cortex. Musical hallucinations, frequently associated with acquired deafness but not with other psychotic symptoms,

tend to demonstrate a more discrete involvement of auditory processing in the right hemisphere known to be the site of music processing.

Advances in psychopharmacology
Those interested in understanding the biological foundations of psychiatry have also relied heavily on improved understanding of **neurotransmitter systems and receptors**. In the dopamine system the ventral striatal (mesolimbic) system projects to the nucleus accumbens and is involved in reward systems, whereas the dorsal striatal (nigrostriatal) system, well known for its role in movement, has been shown to influence cognitive tasks. It has been proposed that **new 'atypical'** (because they produce less extrapyramidal side-effects) **antipsychotics**, such as clozapine and risperidone, act preferentially on dopamine receptors in the ventral system and this explains their relative lack of motor side-effects. The basis for this selectivity may be that atypical antipsychotics are selective for D3 dopamine receptors, which are more abundant in ventral striatum, rather than D2 receptors, which are more likely to be involved in dorsal striatum. Neuroimaging *in vivo* of dopamine receptor blockade in the basal ganglia (largely dorsal striatum) has demonstrated that atypical drugs produce much less blockade of dopamine receptors, despite good antipsychotic effects, than, for example, haloperidol. But the antipsychotic effect of atypical drugs may, in fact, be explained by their activity at other receptors, in particular serotonin (5HT), rather than as a result of selectivity for D3.

Serotonin (5HT), in addition to any role it may play in psychotic illness, undoubtedly is involved in depression. **Selective serotonin reuptake inhibitors (SSRIs)** have become the standard treatment for depression. A more specific role for serotonin in impulse control disorders, including temper control, gambling and eating disorders, is less definite. SSRIs have now been joined by selective **noradrenaline reuptake inhibitors (NRIs)**, and while there is no good evidence of a differential effect of NRIs, it does mean that if depression has not responded to an SSRI then it may be worth trying an NRI.

Advances in the field of dementia are of interest to both neurologists and psychiatrists; **new cholinergic agents** that slow cognitive decline, and advances in molecular biology and genetics, have revitalised this area (see Chapter 14).

Transcranial magnetic stimulation (TMS) is one of several new therapeutic techniques involving direct stimulation of the central nervous system. Transcranial magnetic stimulation over the frontal lobes appears to have an antidepressant effect, and may even be an alternative to electroconvulsive therapy (ECT). There is some evidence that TMS over the left temporal lobe may inhibit auditory hallucinations. Because it can selectively interfere with cerebral cortical function, TMS is increasingly being used to study brain behaviour relationships; for example, TMS can selectively inhibit detection of visual movement when delivered over the appropriate area of visual association cortex.

LIAISON PSYCHIATRY

Up to one-third of patients attending a neurology clinic have symptoms that are largely unexplained by demonstrable neurological disease. Those with neurological disease, for example, multiple sclerosis or Parkinson' disease, have high rates of psychiatric illness, especially anxiety, depression and psychosis. Alcohol dependence may be found in up to 20% of general hospital in-patients. On average those with psychiatric disorders accompanying their medical problem utilize medical services more than those without.

Therefore there is good reason to have good liaison between a neurology service and psychiatry.

Two main models are usually described:

1 **Consultation model.** This is reactive. The medical team calls the liaison psychiatrist at times of need. At its least efficient, psychiatrists from a large rota are called at random; no single psychiatrist or team has the opportunity of developing a special liaison with any particular medical specialty.
2 **Liaison model.** The psychiatrist becomes a member of the team, taking part in ward rounds

or out-patient clinics. They may have an active role in supporting the staff, for example by facilitating staff groups. The liaison model is, however, likely to be an inefficient method of service delivery because for much of the time the psychiatrist is not actively engaged.

Most therefore favour a **consultation–liaison model.** A specific link between a psychiatrist and a medical team is developed. In this way the psychiatrist becomes known to the medical team, and easy channels of communication are created. Over time the psychiatrist is able to educate the team about the identification and management of mental illness. They themselves develop some expertise in the medical specialty. For some high risk areas, for example pain clinics, then joint clinics may be useful.

THE CARDINAL MENTAL SYMPTOMS OF DISORDERS OF THE BRAIN

Disturbances of conscious level or orientation indicate organic brain disease until proven otherwise.

It is for this reason that the neurologist concentrates on whether or not the patient is 'alert and orientated'. In addition, the presence of specific disorders of cognition and memory may indicate disruption to the normal function of the cerebral cortex.

Delirium, often called an acute confusional state, is characterized by a primary disturbance of conscious level. The patient is obtunded, or drowsy, or highly distractible. Attention and concentration are impaired. The patient is likely to be agitated and frightened. Psychotic symptoms with hallucinations, often visual, and fleeting delusions may be elicited. Delirium may also present as a hypoactive withdrawn state akin to stupor. Management consists of making the patient safe and then finding the cause. Those conditions which cause coma (see Table 4.8.) may produce delirium.

In **dementia** (see p. 270) there is generally no disturbance of conscious level, yet the patient is usually disoriented, as well as showing evidence of a global acquired impairment of cognitive function. Personality change, often with a coarsening of social behaviour, mood disturbance, particularly depression, and psychotic symptoms, both delusions and hallucinations, are also very common.

PSYCHIATRIC DIAGNOSIS

Psychiatric diagnosis, although relying often on subjective data, for example a patient describing their mental state, is nevertheless valid. Psychiatric diagnoses show good inter-rater reliability and predict outcome and treatment responsiveness. More recently, functional neuroimaging has provided objective evidence of abnormalities of brain function to match the subjective descriptions of symptoms.

It is useful to think of a **hierarchy of diagnosis** with all psychiatric diagnoses being trumped by organic mental disorders (Figure 27.1). Therefore if a patient has both depression (level 3) and schizophrenia (level 2) their course and management are determined more by the schizophrenia. Symptoms of depression may be produced by schizophrenia, but not vice versa. Organic mental disorders (level 1) may result in psychoses, neuroses (depression, anxiety, somatization disorder) or changes in personality.

Mental disorders in the absence of brain disease are crudely classified into **mental illness** (the psychoses and neuroses) and **personality disorders**. A key criterion for diagnosis of a **mental illness** is that the **normal functioning** of the person should be **impaired**.

There are many ways in which this can be manifest, most frequently difficulties working, or a decline in personal care or social relationships. On the other hand, people with a **personality disorder** may continue to function normally; the critical criterion is that they or others should **suffer** as a result of their personality traits.

PERSONALITY DISORDERS

Personality comprises the characteristic patterns of thinking and behaviour of an individual, and is made up of numerous personality traits, for example a tendency to be impulsive, or obsessional, or assertive. **Personality disorders** are distinguished by the fact that traits are present to an abnormal degree and fairly consistently from early adult life, and that suffering results. Under stress many patients with conspicuous personality traits or disorders develop a corresponding mental illness, for example somebody who is obsessional develops symptoms of obsessional compulsive disorder.

Personality disorders are classified according to the outstanding traits. In **paranoid** personality

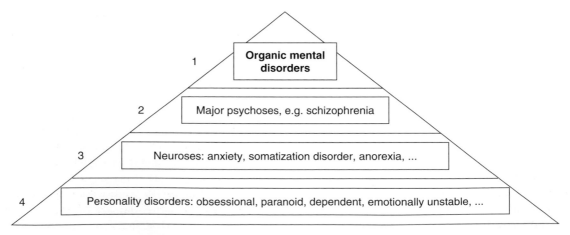

Figure 27.1 A hierarchy for psychiatric diagnosis.

disorder the person is excessively suspicious and sensitive. People with **schizoid** personality disorders are emotionally cold and distant. Indecisiveness and doubt and rigidity are typical of **anankastic** personality disorders. Other categories include **antisocial** personality disorder with aggression and lack of concern for others, and **borderline** personality disorder in which the patient tends to over-idealize, is inclined to repeated self-harm, and has periods of altered conscious level akin to dissociation (see below) with 'borderline' psychotic symptoms.

NEUROSIS

The distinction between the neuroses and psychoses has some value but it should be noted that the term neurosis has been dropped in the most recent International Classification of Diseases (ICD-10). In the neuroses insight into the disorder is maintained and symptoms tend to be reactive to life events and related to anxiety.

Anxiety disorders

The anxiety disorders consist of several conditions in which anxiety is the major problem; anxiety disorder, obsessive-compulsive disorder, and phobic disorder, including agoraphobia and social phobia.

The symptom of anxiety is common to all these conditions. Many people have problems describing their symptoms of anxiety, and will describe instead not feeling quite right, or restless. The physician needs to be alert to the possibility that strange feelings in the head may be symptoms of anxiety. Some patients describe a sense of cotton wool, or that their head is going to explode.

Anxiety is a normal human emotional response to threatening events. It can be useful and help to improve performance. On the other hand it becomes more morbid if it occurs regularly in the absence of any significant stressor, or starts to interfere with function.

Anxiety is related to fear and commonly coexists with depression. Chronic anxiety causes fatigue, irritability and poor sleep. High levels of anxiety may precipitate psychotic illness and dissociative states.

Free-floating anxiety is fairly continuous and independent of the situation or circumstance the person finds themselves in. The person is not aware of why they are feeling anxious.

Panic attacks are short-lived crescendos of anxiety such that the person experiences terror or extreme discomfort. Catastrophic thoughts, for example of impending death or going crazy, are present. Symptoms are aggravated by hyperventilation, often related to a sense of suffocation. Panic attacks tend to build up over a few minutes, may last up to 2 hours but rarely longer, and then subside. They are common, with the majority of the population experiencing a panic attack at some point.

Phobic anxiety disorders

In **agoraphobia** the patient typically feels anxious when they feel trapped and unable to return to a place of safety. Such situations are more threatening when they are alone. As a result the patient may avoid going into anxiety-provoking situations. These include crowded supermarkets, sitting in an auditorium, queuing, being in large crowds, travelling on trains or buses. In severe agoraphobia the patient avoids leaving their house.

Social phobia on the other hand is precipitated by situations in which the patient feels under scrutiny. Public speaking, or even talking in small groups, will cause anxiety. They are likely to find it difficult eating in public. The patient is very self-conscious and anxiety is reinforced by blushing or sweating. Many patients suffer both social phobia and agoraphobia.

Specific phobias include fear of spiders or thunderstorms or flying. Even thinking about the object of the phobia causes anxiety, and extreme fear may occur at the prospect of being exposed to the feared situation or object.

A key feature of all the situationally dependent anxiety disorders is **avoidance**. If the avoidance interferes with normal function, then treatment is likely to be necessary.

Obsessive-compulsive disorder

Many of us have obsessive personality traits and these are helpful in certain jobs where errors are potentially dangerous. A certain degree of perfectionism and checking is reassuring. On the other hand a person may find that recently they have had to check over and over again, or get things just right, to the extent that it interferes with their ability to function effectively; they would now be diagnosed as suffering from obsessive-compulsive disorder.

Obsessional thoughts are unwelcome, intrusive and cause anxiety. They are recognized by the person as their own thoughts, and this distinguishes them from some psychotic disorders of possession of thought. Often the obsessional thought is relieved by carrying out a **compulsion**, which is generally a motor act but can be a ritualistic thought (Table 27.1). Obsessive-compulsive disorder (OCD) is often quite responsive to life events, relapsing at times of stress. In some, however, it becomes chronically very debilitating.

There is an association between OCD and Gille de la Tourette's syndrome (see p. 241). It is necessary to distinguish between OCD and organic orderliness seen in patients with dementia.

Adjustment and bereavement reactions

After severely traumatic or distressing life events it is common to find symptoms of anxiety lasting days or weeks. In this situation benzodiazepines may be used, but physical dependence commences within days of starting their use so great care is necessary.

Psychological response to trauma

It is necessary to distinguish between events that are psychologically traumatic and those that result in physical trauma, particularly if there is head injury. If there is physical injury, then the psychological reaction has to be interpreted in the light of any physical disability and damage to the central nervous system (CNS).

> **Post-traumatic stress disorder (PTSD)** occurs following exposure to life-threatening events. In the aftermath, but sometimes after a latent interval of a few days or weeks, the characteristic syndrome appears: flashbacks, nightmares, hyper-arousal and avoidance of situations that act as reminders of the event. The syndrome may also be seen in

Table 27.1 Content of typical obsessions and compulsions

Obsession	Corresponding compulsion
Contamination e.g. My hand touched the carpet which contaminated it with faeces	Wash hands repeatedly after contact with anything that may have had contact with carpet
Physical violence e.g. I will take a knife and attack my baby	Throw away all knives, avoid being alone with baby
Anti-social behaviour e.g. I am going to swear aloud and make crude sexual jokes	Avoid public speaking, repeat a magic word in one's head to stop such thoughts, ask for reassurance that one did not swear
Orderliness/perfectionism e.g. Have to read all the books of a particular author	Avoid reading any of his books
Hall has to be painted with the same batch of paint	Repeatedly check the batch numbers, take back paint without number on
Have to drive out of the garage 'just right'	Repeatedly drives back into garage to get it just right
Accidental harm I have forgotten to turn the gas off	Repeatedly go back to check the gas tap
Visions of destruction and death Images of child being killed	

those who lost consciousness at the time of the event; implicit unconscious memories may still be activated.

Assaults are particularly likely to result in PTSD. The disorder is often complicated by depression and substance abuse, and is more common in women. Neuroendocrine studies find evidence of a chronic stress reaction, and the reduced hippocampal volume found in veterans with PTSD has been attributed to chronic high levels of corticosteroids.

The majority of those who develop PTSD will recover within a year, but a substantial proportion go on to develop chronic disabling symptoms. Selective serotonin reuptake inhibitors and cognitive behaviour therapy (CBT) have been shown to be effective, but the effect size is not large. Debriefing immediately after a trauma has not been shown to be effective and may even have deleterious effects.

Travel anxiety or phobia is a common symptom after road traffic or other transport accidents. The person experiences intense anxiety when travelling, particularly when using the same method of transport as was involved in the accident. They become hypervigilant and see danger at every opportunity.

Post-concussion syndrome is seen following head injury (see p. 359). Common symptoms include headaches, poor concentration and memory, fatigue, dizziness, noise and light sensitivity, double vision, irritability, depression and anxiety. These symptoms overlap heavily with those seen in the somatization disorders, including chronic fatigue syndrome. But, depending on the severity of the head injury, it is likely that a proportion of the symptoms are related to brain injury.

How many of the symptoms are organic is often the subject of intense debate. Some clinicians go so far as to suggest that head injury not producing loss of consciousness is nevertheless a frequent cause of brain injury. Other clinicians may assume that there are major psychological factors at play, despite the presence of good evidence of brain damage. A fair compromise is to suggest that persistent symptoms of post-concussion syndrome are often the result of **anxiety interfering with healthy recovery** from physiological damage to the brain.

The whole picture is complicated by **litigation**; many of those with surprisingly severe symptoms are seeking compensation years following a mild head injury because somebody was to blame for the injury. A reasonable estimate is that being involved in compensation increases symptoms after a head injury by 25%. The figure is greater in those with mild injuries, and probably with chronic symptoms. This excess of symptoms has been attributed to **'compensation neurosis'**. This label draws attention to the fact that symptoms may be influenced by secondary, financial gain.

Even in the absence of conscious exaggeration or fabrication of symptoms or disability, it is easy to understand that being involved in seeking compensation has a deleterious effect on outcome after injury. This may reflect the anger and bitterness experienced by patients in this situation; it is easier to come to terms with one's loss if it's an act of God, than if it is the result of somebody else's incompetence. It may reflect the process of being involved in a lengthy claim; numerous doctors are seen, each one demanding the patient goes back over the history. The normal process of recovery, involving symptoms disappearing from memory, is impeded. The process is usually stressful.

Nevertheless a more sceptical approach by the physician may be required for the patient who is involved in litigation, even if the patient is being seen for clinical management. It is possible that **secondary gain** is driving the maintenance of symptoms. **Malingering** is probably not very common, but many compensation-seeking patients give an impression that the potential for secondary gain undermines their motivation for recovery. In a proportion of patients, detective work demonstrates quite clearly that they are consciously and fraudulently fabricating the evidence.

Reporting bias complicates the picture. Patients and their family and friends overestimate the patient's health and well-being before the injury. But this rose-tinted glasses effect is not particular to those involved in compensation; it is seen in all patients with head injury, and indeed in all patients with disability. People are inclined to attribute all their problems to the illness.

The **chronic whiplash syndrome** is bedevilled by issues related to compensation.

Treatment of the anxiety disorders

Response prevention is the psychological treatment strategy that is central to treatment of the anxiety disorders. The response the patient uses to reduce anxiety is identified; this almost always involves avoiding the situation, for example by not travelling, or by getting off the train early. They are then, with negotiation, prevented from making the response. Anxiety initially increases but with treatment over a few sessions many will find that they are less anxious in the feared situation.

General **relaxation techniques** may be used. These usually involve progressive muscle relaxation techniques, along with relaxing imagery and suggestion.

Panic attacks are likely to need a specific cognitive approach in which catastrophic thoughts are challenged and replace by more realistic thoughts. The mainstay of treatment of OCD is CBT with response prevention.

Although benzodiazepines are very effective anxiolytics, they are not recommended for anxiety treatment in view of the risk of dependence. Sedative antidepressants may be of value. Over the past few years newer anxiolytic drugs have been introduced, but they are rarely the mainstay of treatment. Propranolol is effective for some patients.

The somatoform disorders: hypochondriasis, somatization and dissociative disorders

---

> **Somatoform disorders**
>
> The somatoform disorders are all conditions in which physical symptoms and complaints are not a result of organic disease. There is debate as to how the somatoform disorders should be classified. What is important is that they overlap heavily with one another and are all varieties of abnormal illness behaviour. They are associated with anxiety and depression and psychological stress.

The conditions that need to be considered are:

- Hypochondriasis: the emphasis is on *fear of illness*. The patient may or not have symptoms (most do), but they are frightened that they have a serious illness

- Somatization disorders: symptoms and signs are present in the absence of organic disease sufficient to explain them. If symptoms and signs involve the nervous system, then it is likely that they will be labelled as conversion disorder (see below)

- Dissociative disorders: this classification has recently been introduced to cover conversion disorders and dissociative states. In both conditions psychological processes are considered to be dissociated from one another. In the conversion disorders, synonymous with hysteria, typical symptoms/signs include hemiplegia, hemianaesthesia or blindness. The dissociative states consist of psychogenic amnesia, fugue and stuporose states and non-epileptic attacks.

Anxiety is a theme common to all these conditions (Table 27.2).

The diagnosis of a conversion disorder does depend on an interpretation of the mechanism involved in symptom formation; it implies a specific psychological process. However, this requires care; diagnostic classification systems in psychiatry are much more reliable and valid if they do not rely on interpretations about psychological mechanisms, but rely merely on operational criteria based on symptoms and signs.

Therefore it may be better to use the diagnosis of **unexplained medical symptoms**, or **physical symptoms not attributable to organic disease** (see below).

Hypochondriasis

The core symptom of hypochondriasis is the patient's **fear that they have a disease**; usually a life-threatening or severely disabling disease. Patients may worry that they have cancer or heart disease. Hypochondriasis is therefore a phobia, a fear of illness. Hypochondriacal concerns that may be seen by a neurologist include the fear of having a brain tumour or multiple sclerosis. Usually the fear is based on symptoms, for example headaches or visual disturbance. However, a small proportion of patients with hypochondriasis will have no physical symptoms but yet are troubled by fear of illness, and demand increasingly sophisticated investigations to rule out the possibility.

Table 27.2 Anxiety – the master mimic. Anxiety may produce symptoms through a variety of routes. The symptoms often result in referral to a neurologist

Process	Symptom
Subjective experience of anxiety	Feeling of: a pressure/ 'cotton wool' in the head Head is going to burst Tension in the body; motor restlessness
Panic	Light-headedness/sense of imminent loss of consciousness Terror of imminent death/heart attack Shortness of breath/ sense of suffocation *Globus hystericus* – difficulty swallowing
Interferes with concentration and the normal integration of conscious experience	Poor memory and cognitive impairment
Focuses attention on bodily sensations causing a sense of dysfunction	Depersonalization/ derealisation Altered feeling in body/ anaesthesia Déjà vu Altered visual or auditory sense Tinnitus, vertigo, dizziness
Muscle tension and increased excitability	Pain in the muscles Headaches Chest pains Muscle twitches/myokymia Trembling/shaking
Increased autonomic activity	Palpitations/flushing Sweating/night sweats Upper abdominal symptoms – butterflies Diarrhoea Urinary urgency and frequency Dry mouth Peripheral vascular changes
Hyperventilation	Paraesthesiae – especially perioral and hands Muscle contractions, especially muscles of hands and feet; carpo-pedal spasm Light-headedness/ epilepsy
Non-specific	Fatigue Poor sleep

Dysmorphophobia, a fear that the patient is deformed or ugly, may be regarded as a variant of hypochondriasis. Concerns about body shape tend to occur in early adult life, whereas concerns about health occur later. Correspondingly dysmorphophobia has an earlier mean age of onset than does hypochondriasis.

A key element to the diagnosis is that there is a **mismatch** between the patient's view of their health and their doctor's. As a result they may demand numerous consultations and second opinions. As with all mental illness a diagnosis is only made if the symptoms have an impact on functioning. The patient with hypochondriasis is likely to take time off work, alienate their friends and neglect themselves as a result of their constant preoccupation with their health.

They also **demand reassurance**. A model of hypochondriasis that is useful for treatment is that the patient develops increasing anxiety as they experience catastrophic thoughts of impending disease. Physical symptoms may deteriorate as the anxiety increases. Reassurance that they are alright, particularly from a doctor but also from family and friends, reduces symptoms of anxiety. A vicious cycle may be created so that the only way they can rid themselves of anxiety is by seeking reassurance.

This model is akin to other models of specific phobias in which a response alleviates anxiety (see above). **Response prevention** prohibits the patient obtaining reassurance; family and friends are taught not to reassure the patient. Cognitive therapy will focus on enabling the patient to **challenge the catastrophic thoughts** of impending illness and replace them with more appropriate thoughts (cognitions).

Some patients with hypochondriasis develop frank delusions. The diagnosis of **hypochondriacal delusions** is made when the beliefs are florid and firmly held and go beyond any evidence to support them. Enquiry may reveal a systematization of the delusional beliefs, for example, the patient may have persecutory delusions of a conspiracy involving their doctors. Hypochondriacal and dysmorphophobic delusions are classified as delusional disorders (see below)

Somatization and dissociation

Patients with physical symptoms not from organic disease

The classification of conditions in which the patient has symptoms of physical disease, with no evidence of organic disease, is clumsy. **Somatization** refers to the process whereby somatic symptoms are produced in the absence of physical disease. **Dissociation** is a more specific explanation of how somatic symptoms (conversion disorder) or altered states of conscious awareness (dissociative states) may be produced. Therefore conversion disorders are common to both somatization and dissociation.

> A significant proportion of patients who are referred to neurology clinics do not have organic disease to explain their symptoms. In one study, 10% were rated as 'not at all explained' by organic disease, with a further 20% whose symptoms were 'only somewhat explained' by organic disease. Those with lower organicity were more likely to suffer anxiety or depression.
>
> However faced with a patient with somatic symptoms but no evidence of physical disease, the physician should never close the door on the possibility that physical disease may be present or evolving. The fact that symptoms and signs cannot be explained by organic disease does not mean that organic disease is not present. Follow-up of patients diagnosed with hysteria has demonstrated that many go onto develop manifest organic illness. Multiple sclerosis, for example, is known occasionally to present with symptoms and signs that are clearly 'non-organic'. Organic illness, particularly if it involves the CNS, may predispose to hysterical reactions.

These conditions are all weakly associated with alcohol dependence and with antisocial personality disorder. Childhood experience seems to be relevant; many have poor memories of childhood, some

will have experienced illness either in themselves or others, while the dissociative states are associated with sexual abuse as a child. Women are at greater risk.

The **psychological origins** of the symptoms are suggested by observations that the symptoms are responsive to life events and other stressors, may go hand in hand with other mental symptoms, particularly anxiety and depression, and that unilateral symptoms are more often left-sided. The occasional patient may show *belle indifference*. A poor prognostic sign is a reluctance on the part of the patient to consider a psychological explanation, or part explanation, for their symptoms. Many come with fixed ideas about causation, for example, patients with chronic fatigue syndrome who believe their symptoms are caused by persistent viral infection.

Symptoms often appear in early adult life and a proportion go on to a chronic fluctuating course. Symptoms may remain restricted to one bodily system, or spread to involve many systems.

Disorders involving somatization include somatization disorder itself, as well as chronic pain syndromes, including chronic tension headache and chronic fatigue syndrome. The dissociation disorders consist of the conversion disorders and the dissociative states, as well as one or two rare conditions. Finally, it is necessary to discuss factitious disorders, in which the patient consciously fabricates symptoms.

Somatization disorder

> Somatization disorder is used to describe a condition characterized by multiple, recurrent physical symptoms involving different bodily symptoms. Patients are usually women, who often have sexual dysfunction and may have menstrual problems. Many will develop drug dependence, for example, steroids or analgesics or anti-diarrhoeal agents.

Patients with fewer symptoms, perhaps restricted to one bodily system and with symptoms that are understandable as arising from the autonomic nervous system (Table 27.2) are labelled **somatoform autonomic dysfunction**. However there is no certain value in distinguishing the various conditions, and they all overlap with chronic fatigue syndrome.

A more pragmatic approach is to acknowledge that some people are vulnerable to developing somatic symptoms, which they select from a core collection of symptoms that are common in the normal population. Whether this involves one system or many may be related to idiosyncratic factors. Somatoform syndromes are labelled cardiac neurosis, irritable bowel syndrome, gastric neurosis, atypical facial pain or chronic fatigue, depending on which are the most prominent symptoms. However, they tend to have more symptoms in common than set them apart.

Core symptoms include fatigue, muscle aches and pains and tenderness, headaches, difficulty concentrating, sleep problems, irritability, tension, dizziness, indigestion, constipation, abdominal pain, diarrhoea and regional pain.

Chronic pain syndromes

In many patients with chronic pain there is no definite organic explanation, although there may have originally been an acute cause, for example, injury. Such patients are often distressed and it can be difficult to distinguish cause and effect in the relationship between pain and depression. Analgesic abuse and dependence is often a major issue for managing these patients, with some patients demanding narcotics. Most patients do better by not taking analgesics. The worst regimen is 'as required' use of strong, quick acting, particularly intramuscular narcotics; this is likely to reinforce pain behaviour and to create dependence.

Regional pain syndromes are likely to be seen by neurologists. While there is debate about the psychological contributions to a **complex regional pain syndrome** (or reflex sympathetic dystrophy) (see p. 520), there is more of a consensus that **atypical facial pain** should be regarded as a somatoform disorder. However the low doses of **amitriptyline** that have been used successfully to treat atypical facial pain suggest that it is not acting by alleviating depression.

Chronic tension headache

Tension-type headache is specifically excluded from the somatoform disorders in ICD-10, and is classified as a neurological disorder. Nevertheless, most would accept that the psychological processes behind tension headache are similar, if not identical, to many other physical symptoms unexplained by 'organic' disease. Up to 4% of the population suffer chronic daily headaches, which tend to decline with age.

Amitriptyline, at doses of about 75 mg a day, has been shown to be effective, but no study has looked at longer term efficacy of amitriptyline. Citalopram has been shown to be effective in one study, but anecdotal evidence suggests that some SSRIs may make headache worse.

Relaxation therapy is likely to be beneficial, as is electromyographic biofeedback therapy, where the patient learns to reduce the electromyographic signal in scalp muscles.

Chronic fatigue syndrome

Chronic fatigue syndrome is characterized by severe disabling fatigue that is mental and/or physical. Other common symptoms include muscle aches and pains, concentration and memory problems and sleep disturbance. An influenza-like illness may have precipitated the syndrome, and the role of organic physical disease in maintaining symptoms is poorly understood. **Exercise avoidance** is typically seen; the patient has a marked exacerbation of symptoms after taking exercise, and as a result avoids doing so.

In ICD-10, chronic fatigue syndrome is not classified as a somatoform disorder, but as 'neurasthenia'. However the marked overlap with other somatoform disorders, in terms of shared symptomatology, suggests that this may not be a useful nosology. Myalgic encephalomyelitis is another term that is probably best avoided, suggesting as it does a definite pathophysiological process underlying the symptoms.

The focus of treatment is **graded increased moderate exercise**. Many patients have an all-or-nothing attitude to activity; when they feel a little better they do a lot, but then the next day have severe symptoms of fatigue and muscle pains and rest. The rest is then prolonged for fear of exertion, causing low levels of fitness and increased symptom following exertion. Cognitive behaviour therapy aimed at challenging assumptions, enabling the patient to feel less helpless, and problem solving, is usually incorporated into a CBT package.

Exercise programmes and **CBT** have been shown to be effective for chronic fatigue. There is less evidence to support the use of other treatments. Antidepressants should be used if depression is present, but there is no evidence of a specific effect of antidepressants on chronic fatigue syndrome.

Dissociation: conversion disorders

Conversion disorders, a specific form of somatization disorder, usually present to the neurologist who may label the symptoms and signs as **hysterical**. Typical symptoms include hysterical blindness, hemianaesthesia, and paralysis. Problems with balance may be seen; astasia-abasia describes the extravagant wobble that is seen on standing and walking.

> It is dangerous to assume that because a neurological symptom is bizarre or unusual or situationally dependent, it is caused by a conversion disorder; for example, patients with Huntington's chorea may have a bizarre gait disturbance, and be better able to walk backwards than forwards. It would be easy to label paroxysmal kinesigenic choreoathetosis as hysterical.

On the other hand, certain patterns of symptoms are almost pathognomonic of conversion disorder. Tunnel vision, in which the same physical area, perhaps a circle 2 feet in diameter, is the limit of the visual field, whether at 3 feet or 10 feet from the patient, is almost certainly a result of conversion disorder; likewise hemianaesthesia, which involves the whole body from head to toe right down the middle.

The conversion disorders may be understood as an attempt to relieve the mind of anxiety by production of a physical symptom. For this reason 'belle indifference' may be seen; the patient, rather than being upset and distressed by their symptoms, has found relief from their anxiety. Some patients on the other hand will complain of anxiety symptoms or be upset by their disability.

Once an organic illness has been reasonably confidently ruled out, the mainstay of treatment is to encourage return of normal activity. Some clinicians advocate enabling the patient to have an 'excuse' for recovery without ever confronting the patient with their diagnosis. This may involve enrolling the patient in a rehabilitation programme, for example, alongside patients with stroke. Suggestion during hypnosis or an interview while under the influence of Amytal (amobarbital) may be tried for more stubborn symptoms.

Patients may be labelled 'hysterical' if they are attention seeking and emotionally labile or theatrical. It is probably better to use the less pejorative term **histrionic**.

Dissociation: dissociative states

In the dissociative states there is a failure to integrate conscious life, particularly with autobiographical memory.

> In **psychogenic amnesia** autobiographical memories for a period of time, lasting seconds to years, are lost without any organic disease to explain the amnesia. Often there is a psychologically traumatic event related to the amnesic gap. Reported loss of memory for criminal offending may be factitious and for secondary gain, but many people without obvious secondary gain do report loss of memory at times of extreme arousal. Personal identity is retained, so that at no stage does the patient not know who they are. Prolonged retrograde amnesia, for example, for years leading up to the injury, after a minor head injury raises the suspicion of psychogenic amnesia, but has been described following bilateral temporal lobe damage. Psychogenic amnesia needs to be distinguished from transient global amnesia.

In **fugue states** personal identity is lost. As the name implies, the person in a fugue state is typically found some distance from home, having been missing for a day or two, and is taken to a police station not being able to say who they are. During the fugue the person is usually able to interact normally with others. Precipitants include psychosocial stressors, for example, a marriage that is breaking down or serious financial debt. Fugue states are also precipitated by alcohol and depression and probably altered brain function, for example, an incipient dementia. Occasionally they occur repeatedly.

Psychogenic **stupor** is diagnosed when there is no physical cause found for a reduced level of consciousness. There appears to be a constriction of conscious awareness and unresponsiveness to external stimuli. The patient may lie motionless and mute and it may only be the presence of tracking eye movements that indicates that the patient is neither asleep nor unconscious. A normal sleep–wake cycle is usually maintained. There is usually a psychological stress triggering the stupor. The differential diagnosis includes severe catatonic states associated with manic-depressive illness or schizophrenia.

> **Non-epileptic attack disorder (NEAD),** also described as pseudoseizures, involves brief ictal episodes with altered conscious level not as a result of epilepsy or other recognized causes of syncope. Many patients have both epilepsy and NEAD (Table 27.3). Other evidence of abnormal illness behaviour may well be present with evidence of a propensity to seek medical help. There is an association with a history of sexual abuse in childhood (see p. 306).

The seizures themselves may be so florid, for example with gyratory movements of the arms and legs, as to immediately suggest a non-organic cause. However, epileptic seizures arising from medial orbital frontal lobe can have a bizarre appearance.

In the accident and emergency department **'pseudo status epilepticus'** is occasionally seen in patients who abuse benzodiazepines; they have learnt that a prolonged pseudoseizure is a quick way to obtain diazepam.

In many patients doubt about the diagnosis remains, until a seizure, obtained during an electroencephalography recording, shows a normal background rhythm. This may require telemetry, with continuous recording of a video of the patient and their electroencephalography over several days (see p. 308).

Because a significant proportion of patients who present with epileptic-like symptoms do not have epilepsy, it is important to diagnose NEAD early. However, even if only the occasional seizure is a result of epilepsy, then the patient may benefit from anti-epileptic drugs. Therefore a cautious approach is necessary. Non-epileptic attack disorder should

be treated with CBT, which will enable the patient to look for psychological precipitants and manage anxiety symptoms that may play a role. An important part of management is to help the patient accept that the seizures may not all be caused by epilepsy. Reattribution techniques are useful (see below).

Other conditions involving dissociation

Ganser syndrome and multiple personality disorder are generally regarded as dissociative states. In the Ganser syndrome the patient offers 'approximate answers' that are so nearly correct, or so exactly opposite to being correct, as to imply an underlying knowledge of the correct answer. The syndrome is typically seen in forensic settings, where secondary gain may be present and sometimes conscious fabrication or malingering is suspected.

Multiple personality disorder is another condition in which there may be uncertainty about how genuine the patient is. Some suggest that it is iatrogenic and only occurs in response to overzealous questioning by the clinician in a suggestible patient. The patient behaves as though they are more than one person. The two or more personalities usually are unaware of each other's existence. Quite often the personality change is triggered by a psychologically traumatic event. They sometimes occur in forensic settings, raising the possibility of fabrication for secondary gain.

Factitious disorders

Some patients, usually with evidence of other personality disorder, particularly narcissistic personality disorder, make up stories of ill health, or make themselves ill. This is associated with *pseudologia fantastica*, a tendency to tell big stories, lies, about one's own prowess, for example dramatic athletic feats or connections with royalty. Probably the most important management task in the factitious disorders is to prevent unnecessary operations and other interventions.

Management of the somatoform disorders

Patients with somatoform disorders usually attribute their problems to physical illness, and are therefore

Table 27.3 Characteristics of epilepsy and non-epileptic attack disorder (NEAD)

Characteristics	Epilepsy	NEAD
Semiology	Full range of seizure disorders with distinctive patterns, e.g. petit mal, partial complex fits with an aura tonic-clonic pattern tend to be highly stereotyped	Highly variable both across patients, and even within an individual patient may vary from one fit to the next
Cyanosis	May be seen	Very rare
Incontinence	May be seen	Rare
Tongue biting	May be seen	Rare
Burns	May be seen	Rare
Other injuries	May be seen	Rare
Plantar reflexes	Extensor after tonic-clonic	Flexor
Eyes shut	Easy to open	Flicker and may be held firmly
Duration	Seconds to minutes	Very variable, may last up to 1 hour
Arise from sleep as demonstrated using EEG	Frequently	Never
Ictal EEG	Abnormal	Normal
Post-ictal EEG	Quite often shows alteration of amplitude and rhythm	Unchanged by seizure
Blood prolactin	>1000 U/l	May be slightly raised
Responsive to psychological events	Frequently	Very frequently

expecting physical treatments. Given that the treatment is going to be psychological, it is important that they are enabled to reattribute their symptoms to psychological causes. This is particularly important if the general physician is going to refer them to a psychiatric clinic for treatment.

> The first important principle in management is to ensure confidence in the diagnosis. Rule out possible organic causes even if there may be functional overlay. Investigations need to include, as a minimum, a full blood count, U&Es and thyroid function. Explain what investigations have been undertaken and the findings obtained.

This is then the foundation for working on the **reattribution** of physical symptoms. The reattribution model consists of three stages:

1 **Feeling understood.** The doctor is much more likely to be successful in helping a patient to change their attribution about the cause of their symptoms if the patient feels understood. This cause is helped by taking a take a full history and examination and not relying on others for the diagnosis. It is also helpful during the interview to respond to mood cues, for example the patient saying 'I was really troubled by that', and to explore family and social factors, and the patient's health beliefs.

2 **Changing the agenda.** Acknowledge the reality of the physical symptoms, but feed back the negative findings. Introduce into the discussion the psychological factors that the patient has described, for example life events and mood changes.

3 **Making the link.** This stage enables the patient to understand how psychological stress or disorder may result in their physical symptoms or concerns. Therefore, in a patient with tension headache, one might describe how anxiety and depression can produce muscle tension and

therefore pain. In a patient with a NEAD with episodes of loss of awareness one might draw their attention to observations of people having no recollection of an extremely frightening event. If possible, illustrate the theme with observations the patient has made about the psychological responsiveness of their own symptoms.

The reattribution model is likely to be complemented by **anxiety management**, for example, relaxation therapy, and **CBT** targeted at the particular symptom. Cognitive behaviour therapy will usually begin with a detailed diary of symptoms, noting antecedent events or situations that may act as triggers, as well as the consequences of the behaviour. This will be used to drive a behavioural programme, while cognitive therapy will help the patient identify and challenge negative thoughts as well as increase a sense of control. General measures may be necessary to improve quality of life and reduce disability, possibly through a rehabilitation programme.

Clinically significant anxiety and depression should be treated with psychotropic drugs if necessary.

Some incorrigible patients remain fixed in their beliefs about the physical origin of their symptoms and refuse, or fail to respond to, psychological treatments. In some cases the target will be to reduce the patient's consumption of medical services by good liaison with their general practitioner and the local hospitals.

Anorexia nervosa

Anorexia nervosa is characterized by an intense **fear of gaining weight** or becoming fat, dieting such that weight is maintained at 15% less than normal healthy weight, and a disturbed body image, feeling themselves to be fat. Other characteristics include abnormal eating behaviour, for example eating only very low calorie food, not eating with others, excessive exercise or laxative use to curb weight gain, and amenorrhoea. The median age of onset is 17 years, and over 90% of sufferers are female.

Body changes include thin hair and skin with easy bruising. Complications of dietary restriction have been described, including Wernicke's encephalopathy from thiamine depletion. Mild cerebral atrophy may be seen.

Treatment includes re-feeding to reach normal weight as well as family support. Associated mental symptoms, in particular OCD, may need treatment with SSRIs.

Prognosis is poor if the illness extends in to the 20s and 30s with a significant percentage of patients dying from suicide or complications of anorexia.

In **bulimia nervosa**, dieting alternates with binge eating. After bingeing the person usually induces vomiting. Weight is likely to be in the normal range, and the patient is sometimes overweight. Compared with anorexia nervosa, bulimia tends to have a later onset, late teens to 20s, and a worse prognosis. It is associated with other impulse control disorders, for example shop lifting.

PSYCHOSES

The psychoses are those conditions in which some aspect of reality testing is disturbed as a result of delusions, hallucinations or thought disorder. Insight into the condition is generally lacking.

Delusions are false beliefs that are held with conviction. Empirical evidence or argument against the belief is dismissed. To be regarded as a delusion, the belief must be outside cultural and religious norms. It may be difficult to distinguish from an overvalued idea or confabulation.

Overvalued ideas are, for example, seen in anorexia nervosa, where the patient is convinced that they are fat; this is a value judgement and not open to verification. Hypochondriasis is often associated with overvalued ideas; for example, the conviction that a particular diet is essential to health. **Confabulations** involve false memories and are seen in confusional states. They are generally fleeting and changeable, but if persistent and firmly held are indistinguishable from delusions.

Delusions in mental illness are usually paranoid, that is, self-referential; the patient may believe they themselves have special powers, or believe that someone is trying to kill them. Such delusions often have to be distinguished from ideas of reference. This is the common experience of thinking that things happening around one refer to oneself, for example, hearing a car hooting and thinking it is hooting at you. More pathological are **sensitive ideas of reference** in which the person is convinced that somebody is taking the 'Mickey' or criticizing them.

Hallucinations are false perceptions in the absence of a sensory stimulus. All sensory modalities may be involved but the commonest are auditory verbal hallucinations. Visual hallucinations are more often found in the organic psychoses.

It is important to determine whether insight is preserved. Insight is likely to be preserved in elderly patients with poor eyesight who develop visual hallucinations; the patient will realize that their mind is playing tricks on them.

Thought disorder describes the disorganized language of some patients with schizophrenia. It is not easy or possible to follow their train of thought. Sometimes the language is so disorganized that the grammatical construction of sentences and therefore any meaning, is lost. Thought disorder is indistinguishable from what is observed in some patients in delirium, and is easy to confuse with the word-salad that may be produced by patients with a severe dysphasia, particularly if fluent (Wernicke's). Thought disorder may involve expression of language more than comprehension, but when severe it is very likely that the patient will have little understanding of what is going on around them.

The major psychoses are **schizophrenia** and **manic–depressive psychosis**.

Schizophrenia

Schizophrenia is characterized by a chronic illness which is usually relapsing-remitting. Onset is early in adult life, particularly in men; as a result it is rare for a patient with schizophrenia to obtain a university degree. The lifetime risk is about 1%, and is much greater, 10–15%, in first-degree relatives of a patient with schizophrenia.

Symptoms

Symptoms of schizophrenia
Delusions, hallucinations and thought disorder, in the absence of affective disorder sufficient to explain the psychosis, are the core symptoms. Some depressive symptoms are not uncommon, particularly after treatment of an acute relapse.

It is important to determine the mood congruence of any delusions or hallucinations, for example derogatory auditory verbal hallucinations in somebody who is severely depressed suggest the diagnosis may be a psychotic depression, rather than schizophrenia. But if the patient is fatuously describing how somebody is trying to kill them, then this suggests schizophrenia.

A lack of emotional responsiveness and expression are characteristic of schizophrenia. At interview patients lack emotional warmth or rapport.

Some 'first-rank' symptoms are particularly important for the diagnosis of schizophrenia, although they are not diagnostic. They include auditory verbal hallucinations that talk about the patient in the third person, or provide a running commentary. Disorders of the ownership of one's thoughts, for example the experience that one's thoughts are broadcast and can be received at a distance, and passivity phenomena, that one's actions or thoughts are under another person's control.

Motor symptoms
Catatonia is used to describe disorders of movement in the absence of any obvious neurological explanation. A variety of motor symptoms are seen. General activity may be increased or reduced. Mutism is common. Unusual postures may be adopted and waxy flexibility occurs when patients maintain a posture that they have been placed in by the examiner. The patients may be negativistic; gegenhalten describes the sense that the harder the examiner pushes or

pulls, the harder the patient pushes or pulls to stop a limb being moved. Mannerisms and stereotypies, movements without a purpose, are seen.

Over the past few decades catatonic symptoms are seen less frequently, perhaps because they are particularly sensitive to antipsychotic drugs. They are seen in schizophrenia and affective disorder, but importantly may herald a neurological disease, particularly if it involves the basal ganglia.

Negative symptoms

Most of the symptoms described above are 'positive'. They are usually fairly sensitive to antipsychotic medication. However, perhaps more disabling in the long run are negative symptoms including **lack of ambition and drive**, social withdrawal and lack of emotional warmth.

Treatment of schizophrenia

Antipsychotics are effective both in treating an acute psychotic episode and in preventing relapse. Long-term treatment is recommended if there is a history of relapses off treatment. There is some evidence that delay in treating the first episode of schizophrenia results in a worse outcome in the long term, but the evidence is not conclusive.

Depot antipsychotics, which are given by intramuscular injection once every 1–4 weeks, have the advantage of ensuring compliance. However they should only be started after a small test dose has been given and when the diagnosis is reasonably firm.

Over the past few years **atypical antipsychotics**, with less likelihood of producing extrapyramidal side-effects (EPSE) (see p. 232) have been introduced; for example, **risperidone, olanzapine and quetiapine**. Almost all are restricted to oral preparations but some suggest that because they are better tolerated by patients, compliance is improved. However, a recent review has cast a little doubt on the benefits of new atypical drugs, suggesting that if classical drugs are given at equivalent low dose they too produce few EPSEs.

Clozapine, an atypical antipsychotic, is recommended for treatment-resistant schizophrenia, as well as seeming to produce less EPSE. However, its potential to cause agranulocytosis, particularly in the elderly, means that its use has to be closely monitored, with frequent blood counts. Side-effects include sedation, hypersalivation, hypotension, as well as myoclonus and epilepsy.

Psychological therapies may be effective, but should never be given in isolation in the absence of antipsychotic medication. **Family therapy** aiming at reducing expressed emotion, for example, overt criticism of the patient by their family, may be effective. Recently, **cognitive techniques** to help patients challenge delusions or cope with hallucinations are being studied. **Compliance therapy**, helping the patient to take their medication regularly, probably has a role for some patients.

Psychosocial measures aimed at reducing social isolation and other stressors that result from the illness are essential. Patients with severe chronic schizophrenia are likely to need residential care.

Prognosis

Insidious onset, lack of acute psychotic attacks with affective symptoms, negative symptoms, and poor treatment compliance predict a poor prognosis. Many will end up in residential care. A proportion, perhaps 10%, of patients with chronic schizophrenia, develop dementia. More than 10% of patients with schizophrenia commit suicide. Homicide is very rare.

Delusional disorders

Delusional disorders differ from schizophrenia in as much as the only symptom of psychosis is **paranoid delusions**. These are invariably well **systematized**, that is, all related to the same theme; for example, a patient may become convinced that they are at the mercy of some huge international conspiracy against them, which started as a result of a small argument at work many years ago. Chronic grandiose delusions may be seen. **Erotomania** is an example in which the patient is convinced that another person, usually famous, loves them. As a result they may stalk and pester the subject of the delusion. Hypochondriacal and dysmorphophobic (belief that one's body is ugly or misshapen) delusions are also seen (see above).

Personality tends to be well preserved, unlike in schizophrenia, and some patients function quite well despite their delusions. Antipsychotic medication is not always successful, partly because of poor compliance.

Hallucinoses

Chronic auditory verbal hallucinosis, in the absence of other psychotic symptoms suggesting schizophrenia, is occasionally seen. **Alcohol dependence** is the commonest cause, in which case the voices are often derogatory, for example swearing obscenities at the patient. **Deafness or impairment of sight** may be associated with auditory and visual hallucinations, respectively. In the elderly, delusions of infestation may appear to arise from somatic hallucinations of insects crawling over the skin.

Organic psychoses

Chronic epilepsy, particularly temporal lobe epilepsy, may result in a psychotic illness that is indistinguishable from schizophrenia.

The natural history of the illness may be different with a later age of onset, relative preservation of personality and a failure to develop negative symptoms over time.

Psychotic symptoms occur in about one-third of patients with **Alzheimer's disease**, and in **Lewy body dementia** (see p. 281) they are even more common.

Of particular interest is the observation that psychotic symptoms in these dementias may be responsive to **donepezil** or **rivastigmine**, drugs that increase cholinergic transmission. This is particularly useful, given that antipsychotics are likely to produce severe EPSEs in Lewy body dementia.

Psychotic symptoms may be seen in **Parkinson's disease**, particularly when dopaminergic treatment is increased.

Visual hallucinations are common but often with preserved insight and not particularly troublesome. However persecutory delusions may demand treatment. Very low doses of the atypical antipsychotic drugs **clozapine** or **olanzapine** may treat the psychosis without exacerbating the parkinsonism.

Drug dependence may result in psychosis (see below).

AFFECTIVE DISORDERS: MANIC-DEPRESSIVE PSYCHOSIS

Manic depressive psychosis

When somebody suffers episodes of depression and episodes of mania they are described as suffering **bipolar affective disorder**, or manic-depressive psychosis. The word psychosis is used even though they may never have suffered psychotic symptoms. Such illnesses are usually classified together with depression that tends to relapse and remit without obvious psychological precipitants, in which biological symptoms and severe mood disturbance are prominent. The classification acknowledges the fact that they are at high risk of suffering a manic illness in the future, and may well have a first-degree relative with bipolar disorder.

In the absence of a history of mania, depression is diagnosed as **major, moderate or minor depression**, and this is qualified by saying whether the depression is recurrent or associated with psychotic symptoms.

Brief-lived depression, which occurs only in response to a major stressor, is usually classified as an **adjustment disorder** (see above).

Depression involves subjective and objective evidence of mood disturbance, with alterations in behaviour, thought content and cognition, and biological symptoms (Table 27.4). Psychotic symptoms are seen in more severe depressive illness, and are mood congruent.

The words **mania** and **hypomania** are interchangeable. Numerous symptoms may be found,

Table 27.4 Symptoms and signs of affective disorder

Symptom	Depression	Mania
Appearance and behaviour and objective mood symptoms	Psychomotor retardation/poverty of speech, poor self-care, poor eye contact, tearfulness, agitation	Increased motor and mental activity. Jocular. Irritated by what they perceive as attempts to frustrate their plans. Spends money, promiscuous, family and work ignored, thoughtless. Pressure of speech, loosening of associations. Overfamiliar
Subjective mood symptoms and thought content	Low mood, hopelessness, low self-esteem, helplessness, worthlessness. Self-blame, guilt, feelings that life is not worth living. Suicidal thoughts. Anxiety symptoms common	Cheerful, elated or euphoric. A sense of having lots of things to do and lots of energy. A sense of well being. Grandiose and full of themselves. Irritable and angry if demands not met
Biological/somatic symptoms of mood disturbance	Anhedonia (reduced ability to experience pleasure), fatigue, diurnal variation of mood, sleep disturbance usually with insomnia and early morning wakening but occasionally excessive sleep, appetite disturbance, reduced libido and very occasionally constipation and amenorrhoea	Does not need sleep, lots of energy, increased libido
Psychotic symptoms	Delusions of guilt or persecution, and auditory hallucinations, often derogatory or command hallucinations to injure themselves. Nihilistic delusions of rotting or being dead	Delusions, usually of a grandiose theme
Cognitive	Poor concentration and complaints of poor memory especially in elderly	Attention and concentration are usually disrupted
Insight	May be preserved till late	Insight is lost early

with a core elevation of mood and sense of well-being and energy. Insight is lost early and this, along with the tendency to irritability and aggression, makes management difficult. The patient often refuses medication and continues to put themselves at risk and jeopardise their social and vocational network. They are quite likely to need to be admitted under a section of the Mental Health Act.

Often there is a mixture of manic and depressive symptoms present in the same episode: a mixed affective state. Irritability is common to both depression and mania, but usually more troublesome in manic patients. Mania is often immediately followed by depression as insight returns.

The major risk of depression is suicide (Table 27.5), while patients with mania place themselves in the way of all sorts of untoward events, including injury.

Causes of manic-depressive illness and differential diagnosis

Depression is common, especially in women; some community surveys have identified clinically significant depression in over 20% of the population.

Table 27.5 Suicide assessment and management

High risk	Previous attempts, family history, suffers depression, schizophrenia or drug dependence, recent loss, recent diagnosis of physical illness, access to method (guns – farmers; drugs – anaesthetists), recent discharge from psychiatric hospital
Immediate risk requiring urgent management	Threats to commit suicide especially if recent attempt (i.e. within weeks or months), especially if dangerous method and good evidence of intent, especially if at present they are confused, distressed or psychotic. Command hallucinations to harm
Management	Assess for risk factors above, get history from notes and informants
	Don't be afraid to ask for suicidal thoughts – start by asking about mood generally, then inquire about feelings of life not being worth living, then ask directly if they are having/have had suicidal thoughts. If 'yes' then explore frequency and whether they feel they will act on their thoughts
	Never assume a threat to commit suicide is an idle threat
	Make safe: Is there a carer? Are they reliable? Who will look after medication? Admission to hospital required? If in hospital, observe with 1:1 nursing? Access to open windows, balconies, knives, other methods of self-injury?
	Keep others informed of concerns, e.g. GP
	Get psychiatric opinion urgently if any uncertainty
	Consider detention under Mental Health Act
	Document what you have done and why

It tends to increase with age and is associated with a family history of depression, having a physical illness, and recent life events, especially 'loss events', for example, death of spouse, loss of job.

Depression needs to be distinguished from disorders of the brain that can produce similar biological symptoms, but without any core mood disturbance, for example Parkinson's disease or brain injury. Metabolic conditions, in particular hypothyroidism, may mimic depression. Anorexia may be part of anorexia nervosa, or the result of a neoplasm. If the latter is the case, the general lethargy and malaise may be mistakenly regarded as confirming the diagnosis of depression.

Most neurological disorders are associated with depression; for example, there are increased rates of depression in multiple sclerosis, Parkinson's disease, epilepsy and traumatic brain injury. A recent systematic review of **depression after stroke** concluded that although stroke is associated with depression, there is no evidence for an effect of lesion location; the review strongly refuted previous suggestions that depression is particularly associated with frontal left-sided strokes. For all these neurological conditions the increased prevalence of depression is not simply caused by a psychological reaction to disability; patients with non-CNS disorders, but with equivalent disability, tend to show less depression.

Some drugs may induce depression, particularly older antihypertensive agents. **Alcohol abuse** and **steroids** may lead to mania or depression.

Mania is much less common than depression. A family history of affective disorder is quite likely to be found. Manic illness may be precipitated by life events, including those that would be expected to be followed by depression.

Brain injury and infections may precipitate mania. It is now rare to see general paresis of the insane as a result of syphilis, which sometimes presented with mania, on the other hand mania may be observed in brain lesions, particularly if in the right hemisphere or involving the frontal lobes.

Some patients with damage to the frontal lobes look very similar to manic patients; they may be overfamiliar, jocular, thoughtless, irritable and slightly pressured in their speech. They are more likely to be fatuous, rather than distinctly elated. Euphoria with lack of insight and concern about their illness, is found in some patients with severe damage to the CNS, for example as a result of multiple sclerosis. Patients after traumatic brain injury may well show frequent dramatic shifts of mood, lasting a day or two, and therefore be described as showing 'rapid cycling' mood disorder.

Drugs, particularly amphetamines, can produce mania. In some patients antidepressants precipitate mania.

Treatment of affective disorders

Antidepressants, antipsychotics and mood stabilizers are used to manage the affective disorders.

Newer antidepressants have the advantage of having fewer cholinergic and sedative side-effects. They are much safer in overdose than older tricyclic antidepressants and are therefore the first line of treatment. There are several different classes (Table 27.6) related to selective pharmacological effects. There is little good evidence that drugs of different classes have selective clinical profiles. One important feature when selecting an antidepressant is its potential toxicity in overdose. Another is whether or not it is sedative; if so it is likely to be useful for insomnia or anxiety symptoms, but not if fatigue is a prominent symptom.

Table 27.6 Antidepressant drugs

Antidepressant class	Examples	Comments
Tricyclic antidepressants (all have increased risk of cardiac toxicity in overdose)	Amitriptyline	Standard highly effective drug quite sedative
	Imipramine	Ditto, but less sedative
	Dothiepin	Sedative with less cardiac side-effects
	Trazodone	Less anticholinergic side-effects, sedative, quite selective for serotonin, good in the elderly
	Lofepramine	Less sedation and anticholinergic side-effects
Monoamine oxidase inhibitors (MAOI)	Phenelzine	Potentially dangerous, dietary (tyramine) and drug interactions produce hypertensive crisis
	Moclobemide	Reversible inhibitor of MAOA (RIMA) little if any dietary restrictions
Selective serotonin reuptake inhibitors (SSRI)	Fluoxetine	Not sedative, quite alerting
	Citalopram	Both quite 'neutral' and with little
	Sertraline	enzyme induction
Serotonin and noradrenaline reuptake inhibitors (SNRI)	Venlafaxine	
Selective noradrenaline reuptake inhibitors (NRI)	Reboxetine	
Presynaptic alpha$_2$ antagonist	Mirtazapine	Increases central noradrenergic and serotoninergic transmission

If one antidepressant has not worked, then it is better to choose a drug from another class as the next line of treatment. First ensure that the patient has been compliant and has achieved adequate dosage for long enough (at least 6 weeks). For severe treatment-resistant depression, adjuvant therapy with lithium may be necessary, though this may run the risk of producing a serotoninergic crisis. Combinations of antidepressants need expert management.

Electroconvulsive therapy may be useful to treat severe depression, particularly if a quick response is needed, for example if somebody is refusing food and drink. **Predictors of a good response to ECT** include psychomotor symptoms, including agitation or retardation, or other biological symptoms, and psychotic depression. Disease of the CNS is generally not a contraindication because the main risk of the ECT is the brief anaesthetic. Use of ECT may be particularly effective in Parkinson's disease; it has been shown to improve both the depression and the parkinsonism.

Mood stabilizers are used for the management of manic-depression. **Lithium** will be recommended if somebody has had more than two relapses in the space of 5 years. Thyroid and renal function need to be monitored, as do lithium blood levels; the therapeutic window is quite narrow. **Carbamazepine** and **valproate** are increasingly being used as alternatives to lithium.

Antipsychotics are used to manage mania but are usually stopped once the mania is in remission.

ALCOHOL AND OTHER DRUG ADDICTIONS

Drug dependence, addiction and abuse are, for all intents and purposes, synonymous. It is of course possible to abuse a drug without becoming dependent, but this is rare.

Drug dependence is both **physical**, that is, the body becomes physiologically dependent on the drug, and **psychological**. For some drugs, for example cocaine, ecstasy and cannabis, there is very little physical dependence. For others, such as benzodiazepines, physical dependence may develop long before psychological dependence.

Table 27.7 Drug-dependence withdrawal syndromes

Alcohol (delirium tremens)	1–4 days after stopping, delirium with visual hallucinations, other psychotic symptoms and fear, epileptic seizures
Opiates ('Cold turkey')	Piloerection (goose flesh), rhinorrhoea/lacrimation, sweating, stomach cramps, diarrhoea, dilated pupils, shivering, yawning, fatigue
Benzodiazepines	Muscle tension and twitching, anxiety/panic/depersonalization, rebound REM (nightmares) hyperacuity, metallic taste in mouth, other abnormal sensations, convulsions
Amphetamines	Fatigue, dysphoria, anhedonia, hyperphagia

REM, rapid eye movement.

Physical dependence is demonstrated by tolerance, increased doses of drug are needed to produce the same effect, and withdrawal symptoms (Table 27.7). Cross-tolerance to benzodiazepines, alcohol and barbiturates occurs, probably largely explained by their common agonist effects on the gamma-aminobutyric acid receptor.

Psychological dependence consists of craving and an increased **saliency** for drug taking; drug taking becomes more important than anything else in the person's life and as a result, work, family, leisure and social life suffer.

Fast-acting, short-life **opiates** are highly addictive. The opiate withdrawal syndrome, although very unpleasant, is not dangerous. Of much greater danger is overdose producing coma with pinpoint pupils. The other great danger is infection from intravenous drug use, ranging from local abscesses to systemic and CNS infection with opportunistic organisms. Intravenous drug users are at high risk of contracting human immunodeficiency virus and hepatitis.

Amphetamine produces a sense of well-being and energy, as well as anorexia and lack of sleep. Long-term use will often induce paranoia and hallucinations (see p. 541).

Cocaine produces a sense of euphoria as a result of its effects on reuptake of catecholamines, including dopamine and serotonin. It is highly addictive, partly because of its very quick onset if taken intranasally or by smoking the free alkaloid base 'Crack'. Dangerous effects are related to sympathetic overdrive and possible direct effects on cerebral blood vessels. Cardiac, pulmonary and cerebrovascular problems are seen (see p. 547).

Methylenedioxymethamphetamine (MDMA) ('Ecstasy') promotes release of brain monoamines. However, it is probably also directly neurotoxic for serotoninergic cells. Chronic use is associated with cognitive impairment.

The mode of action of **cannabis** is a little uncertain, although endogenous cannabis receptors have recently been identified. Its main effect is to induce a sense of calm, but in a significant minority its effects are directly opposite, with panic attacks, depersonalization, and sometimes persecutory delusions with hallucinations. Chronic use may be associated with increased risk of schizophrenia, but it is difficult distinguishing cause and effect; patients with schizophrenia may be more likely to take cannabis. There is no physical dependence syndrome.

Volatile substance abuse ('glue sniffing') is more common in teenagers. It rapidly induces an altered state of consciousness, often with euphoric mood, but death from cardiac arrhythmias and respiratory depression are seen. Long-term use is associated with cerebellar atrophy and probably results in some cognitive impairment.

Alcohol dependence

Alcohol dependence is of great importance to the neurologist; it is common and alcohol is toxic to the central and peripheral nervous systems and to muscle. A high index of suspicion is needed and the CAGE is a useful screening test: have you ever felt the need to Cut down your drinking, felt Annoyed by criticism of your drinking, felt Guilty about how much you drink, or needed an Eye-opener. Blood tests may suggest the diagnosis with a high gamma-GT (glutamyl transpeptidase), or mean corpuscular volume. High risk professions include publicans, doctors and journalists.

Healthy drinking limits are 21 units of alcohol per week (1 unit = 10 ml pure alcohol) for men, and 14 for women, that is, about a pint of normal-strength beer a day for a woman.

Depression and **anxiety** are commonly associated with alcohol dependence. Some patients develop **persecutory delusions**. **Reduced anger control**, particularly when drunk, is a very troublesome effect. **Suicide and alcoholic hallucinosis**, chronic auditory verbal hallucinations that usually consist of a voice hurling abuse at the patient, are less frequent psychiatric complications.

Patients who are alcohol-dependent often present to the accident and emergency department, where they may be difficult to assess if drunk or agitated. It is important to be alert for other causes of impairment of conscious level over and above intoxication. Subdural haematomas and other intracranial space-occupying lesions, post-ictal states, Wernicke's encephalopathy, delirium tremens, hepatic encephalopathy, hypoglycaemia, and infection, both systemic and intracranial, are all easy to miss. Routinely give thiamine, remembering that alcohol-dependent patients are at particular risk of developing Wernicke's encephalopathy when glucose or another source of carbohydrate is given.

Cognitive impairment is common. Classical Wernicke–Korsakoff syndrome with a selective anterograde amnesia, is rarely seen. It is more usual to find a gradual cognitive decline, selective for memory. Early signs may be the appearance of 'memory blackouts'; the person has no recollection of events that happened while they were drunk, but were nevertheless conscious of at the time (see p. 494).

Treatment for alcohol dependence is largely aimed at education about the harmful effects of alcohol, with support to reduce and stop drinking. However success rates are not good. Brief interventions, for example given by GPs, are almost as effective as intensive programmes of detoxification followed by psychotherapy. Detoxification programmes involve substitution of alcohol with a benzodiazepine, and then weaning off the benzodiazepine over the course of a few days. This is unlikely to be successful at home because of the risk of abusing both the prescribed benzodiazepine and alcohol.

MANAGEMENT OF AGGRESSION AND AGITATION

Aggression in the accident and emergency department is usually caused by **intoxication** with alcohol and other drugs, often in somebody with a **personality disorder**. On the other hand, most agitation and aggression on hospital wards is related to **drug withdrawal**, especially alcohol, and/or **fear** and acute confusional states **(delirium)**. Agitation is also associated with anxiety and akathisia. Poor sleep, pain, constipation, systemic illness, and side-effects of prescribed drugs, may be playing a part. Unexplained agitation may be a prodrome to delirium.

Therefore the first priority, after making sure of the immediate safety of the patient and others, is to consider what physical illness may be present, in particular one involving the CNS.

Safety, for a patient with severe agitation or physical aggression, requires **plenty of staff**, preferably men. The security staff should be called and, if necessary, the police. One to one and sometimes two to one nursing may be required once the acute situation is settled.

Some patients will settle with reassurance and explanation. Relatives may be able to help. Others will need medication and the psychiatry liaison team should be called. The standard regimen consists of **haloperidol and lorazepam**. The patient should be placed on regular nursing observations, monitoring respirations and neurological state. If sedation is required for more than one or two days, it is worth starting regular atypical antipsychotic medication, for example, **olanzapine**, which has less chance of producing extrapyramidal side-effects. Every opportunity should be taken to review evidence of physical illness.

Much of the management is common to that of delirium. Nursing should be in a side room with consistent staff and plenty of light and things to occupy the patient. On the other hand it should be a calm environment with opportunities for rest.

CAPACITY, CONSENT, THE MENTAL HEALTH ACT AND COURT OF PROTECTION

'Capacity for what?' is the retort when you are asked to assess a patient's capacity. Patients may be quite capable in one area of decision making, but entirely incompetent in another.

Consent to treatment

Capacity to consent to treatment requires a person to:

- Understand that they are ill and may benefit from treatment
- Understand the treatments that may be beneficial and their risks
- Be able to choose between options without their choice being distorted by a mental illness, for example a delusion about a treatment or a fear of needles.

In British law nobody can consent to treatment on behalf of another adult. If an adult patient lacks capacity to consent, then **medical/surgical treatment decisions** rest with the clinical team, acting in the patient's **best interests** under **common law**. This, for example, allows emergency treatment of an unconscious patient. Moreover, people are assumed to have capacity until proved otherwise; in a patient with cognitive impairment, their capacity to consent to treatment should be explicitly assessed.

When a patient who has been assumed capable of consenting then **refuses essential treatment**, their capacity should be assessed. This should be undertaken by a psychiatrist because if they are found to be lacking capacity it is likely to be because refusal was the result of mental illness. However, if found incapable of consenting as a result of a mental illness, yet the treatment itself is for a *medical/surgical* condition, then the treatment can go ahead in the patient's best interests under *common law*. An example would be where a patient refuses operation on a burst appendix, believing that the pain in their stomach is caused by rats gnawing their intestines.

> **Consent to treatment for mental disorders**, at least in England and Wales, falls under the remit of the **Mental Health Act**. Patients with mental disorders can be detained in hospital under the Mental Health Act for treatment of their mental disorder.

Compulsory detention

Compulsory detention requires:

- They must have a mental disorder of such severity as to warrant detention
- They must be at risk of harm to themselves or others if they were not detained
- There is no suitable alternative to hospital treatment.

Two doctors must recommend detention, at least one of whom is a specialist in mental disorders. A social worker then makes the application if they agree detention is warranted. The patient's next of kin must be consulted. Patients can be detained to a general hospital as well as a mental hospital, and do not need to be under the care of a psychiatrist to be detained. Emergency powers to detain for up to 3 days can be authorized by a doctor or nurse.

Mental symptoms resulting from intoxication with alcohol or other drugs do not constitute grounds for detaining someone. But mental disorders caused by alcohol or drugs, for example, delirium tremens, are grounds for detention.

In England and Wales the **Mental Health Act Commission** oversees the running of the Mental Health Act and regularly visits hospitals where patients are detained to ensure good practice. The **Mental Health Review Tribunal**, a court within the legal system, acts to enable patients who wish to appeal against their detention to have their case heard by an independent tribunal. Tribunals consist of a lawyer in the chair, an independent psychiatrist and a lay person.

It has been standard practice not to detain patients with dementia who do not resist treatment or demand to leave, despite the fact that they lack capacity to consent and that if they did try to leave they would be kept on the ward for their own safety. The argument is that their consent can be inferred from their behaviour. This practice is being questioned and some argue that if a patient lacks capacity to consent to treatment, for example, because of dementia, then they should be detained under the Mental Health Act in order to ensure that they have the right to an independent review of their treatment, regardless of whether they appear to consent to the treatment.

Capacity to administer one's finances and affairs

Power of Attorney enables a person, the donor, to authorize another, the attorney, to act on their behalf to administer their financial affairs. The limits of the attorney's authority are defined in the Power of Attorney; for example, it might be to collect rent and manage a property while the donor is travelling. Should the donor become incapable of managing their affairs the Power of Attorney is immediately annulled.

If a person wants a Power of Attorney to extend beyond the time that they lose capacity, then they can set up an **Enduring Power of Attorney**. This is typically for patients who have recently been diagnosed with a dementing illness. To set up an Enduring Power of Attorney the patient must have capacity to authorize the Power; that is they must understand the implications of handing over authority to another person to act on their behalf. They *do not* have to have the capacity to administer and manage their own finances and affairs at the time they make the Enduring Power of Attorney; this latter faculty is generally regarded as more cognitively demanding. But once they have lost the power to administer and manage their finances and affairs then the Court of Protection has to be notified.

The **Court of Protection** is usually called in when it becomes apparent that somebody is not capable of administering and managing their own finances and affairs, for example, after a severe brain injury. To be registered with the Court of Protection, the patient must suffer a mental disorder as defined by the Mental Health Act. The Court of Protection will appoint a receiver, for example, the spouse, who will be accountable to them. In British law the spouse/next of kin is not able to administer a patient's finances on their behalf without the authority to do so.

REFERENCES AND FURTHER READING

Carson AJ, Ringbauer B, Stone J, McKenzie L, Warlow C, Sharpe M (2000) Do medically unexplained symptoms matter? A prospective cohort study of 300 new referrals to neurology outpatient clinics. *Journal of Neurology, Neurosurgery, and Psychiatry*, **68**:207–210.

Creed F, Mayou R, Hopkins A (1992) *Medical Symptoms Not Explained by Organic Disease*. London, UK: Royal College of Psychiatrists and Royal College of Physicians of London.

Gelder MG, López-Ibor JJ, Andreasen NC (2000) *New Oxford Textbook of Psychiatry*. Oxford, UK: Oxford University Press.

Lishman WA (1998) *Organic Psychiatry: The Psychological consequences of Cerebral Disorder*, 3rd edn. Oxford, UK: Blackwell Science Ltd.

Moore DP (2001) *Textbook of Clinical Neuropsychiatry*. London, UK: Arnold.

Rogers D (1985) The motor disorders of severe psychiatric illness: a conflict of paradigms. *British Journal of Psychiatry*, **147**:221–232.

Ron MA, David AS (1998) *Disorders of Brain and Mind*. Cambridge, UK: Cambridge University Press.

Wessely S, Nimnuan C, Sharpe M (1999) Functional somatic symptoms: one or many? *Lancet*, **354**:936–939.

CHAPTER 28

NEUROLOGICAL REHABILITATION

A.J. Thompson

INTRODUCTION

Improving the management of neurological disorders requires an understanding of their pathology and in particular the mechanisms underlying disability and recovery. Imaging tools such as structural magnetic resonance imaging, are providing new insights into mechanisms of disability in a range of neurological disorders, while functional magnetic resonance imaging, particularly when used with neurophysiological techniques, is providing complementary information relating to recovery, notably the role of plasticity in stroke, head injury and multiple sclerosis (MS). Thus the neurologist in collaboration with the neuroscientist is well placed to play a key role in the management of these disorders. Indeed the active management of neurological disorders is a natural and logical next step following their investigation and accurate diagnosis. This represents a welcome extension of the role of the neurologist.

DEFINITION

Rehabilitation may be defined as an active process of change by which a person, who has become disabled, acquires and uses the knowledge and skills necessary for optimal physical, psychological and social function.

The key components of rehabilitation are therefore:

- Educational
- Patient centred
- Facilitation of self-management.

It may also be defined as a process that minimizes the impact of disease by **reducing disability and handicap and maximizing independence and quality of life**. This definition introduces the World Health Organization Illness Model (Figure 28.1). This is exemplified by a patient with a spastic paraparesis; the impairments would include weakness and spasticity of their lower limbs, the disability might include difficulty with mobility, which could include walking, transferring and even turning in bed, and handicap might include difficulty with using public transport, driving and even continuing in employment.

Recently, the term disability has been changed to **ability** and handicap to **participation**, which are considered to have a more positive connotation and also serve to emphasize the fact that there is

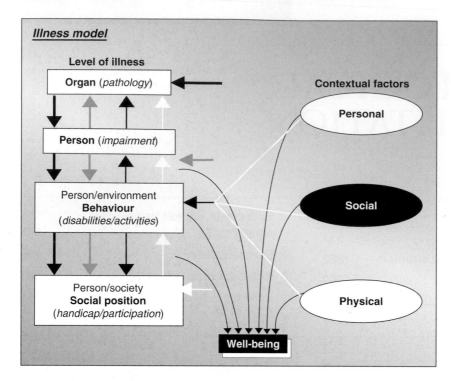

Figure 28.1 Illness model incorporating levels of impact based on WHO, contextual factors and their complex interactions. (Courtesy of Professor D. Wade.)

a complex, two-way interaction between these concepts and a number of contextual factors, including physical (environment), personal and social.

Over and above these levels lies the multidimensional concept of **Health Related Quality of Life**. This concept is particularly important in rehabilitation, as it has at its heart, the patient's perspective of disease impact, and incorporates issues such as coping skills, mood and adaptation, which are fundamental to the rehabilitation process.

RELEVANCE TO NEUROLOGICAL DISORDERS

With this background, it is not difficult to see that the overwhelming majority of neurological disorders have a major impact on patients. This is easy to appreciate in acute events such as stroke, be it ischaemic or haemorrhagic, and trauma to brain and spinal cord. These are the conditions that have led the way in establishing rehabilitation services. However, the philosophy of rehabilitation is equally appropriate to the many neurological conditions that result in progressive disability of varying severity, such as MS, Parkinson's disease, amyotrophic, lateral sclerosis, non-traumatic myelopathy and neuromuscular disorders ranging from the acute Guillain-Barré syndrome to the slowly progressive muscular dystrophies. Static conditions such as poliomyelitis and cerebral palsy may also produce a changing pattern of needs during adult life, either as a result of musculoskeletal problems or neurological change. Finally, common neurological disorders, such as epilepsy and headache, also have a considerable impact on patients, which, although sometimes less obvious, is equally important to manage.

Neurological disorders account for about 40% of those people most severely disabled, who require daily help, and the majority of individuals with complex disabilities involving physical, cognitive and behavioural impairments.

Rehabilitation has three separate facets: **Process, Structure** (characteristics of a rehabilitation service) and **Outcome** (aims of rehabilitation). These can be further broken down as follows.

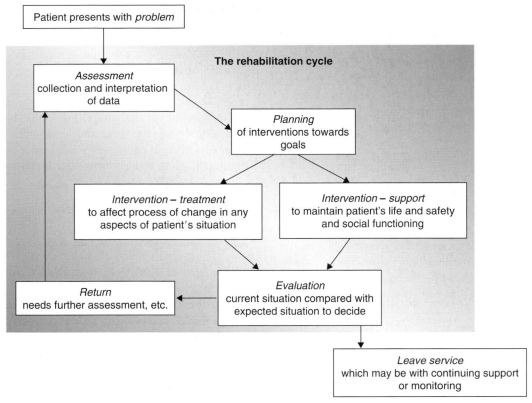

Figure 28.2 The rehabilitation process. (Reproduced with permission from D. Wade from *A study of services for Multiple Sclerosis*, Wade D, Green Q (2001) Royal College of Physicians.)

Process (Figure 28.2)

- Assessment
- Goal setting
- Intervention (treatment and or support)
- Evaluation.

Structure

The structure is based on a multidisciplinary team who:

- Work together with patient towards common goals
- Involve and educate the patient and family in the process
- Have relevant expertise and experience (knowledge and skills)
- Resolve most of the problems faced by the patient.

Outcome (aims of rehabilitation)

The aims of rehabilitation are to:

- Maximize patient's participation in chosen social setting
- Minimize the pain and distress experienced by the patient
- Minimize the distress of, and stress on, the patient's family and/carers.

Some of these areas require further explanation, particularly those relating to the process of rehabilitation.

ASSESSMENT

Assessment

Assessment is the first and most important step in the rehabilitation process and has a number of clear objectives:

- To clarify and quantify the functional deficit
- To identify areas of potential functional improvement
- To determine the input required to maximize functional independence
- To estimate the likely duration of such input.

In order to achieve the assessment objectives it is essential that the assessing team has the appropriate range and level of expertise. A number of disciplines working together is inevitably required, in a **multidisciplinary or interdisciplinary team**. The disciplines involved will depend on the neurological condition being managed but will usually include **medical input** (either a neurologist with an interest in rehabilitation or a physician in rehabilitation medicine), **nursing** (clinical nurse specialist in rehabilitation), **physiotherapy, occupational therapy, speech and language therapy, psychology and social services.** Input may also be required from a **dietician, continence advisor, counsellor and orthotist.**

The ability of the team to work as an interactive unit is crucial as it strives to solve complex, multi-faceted problems. A useful example is the management of bladder dysfunction with clean intermittent self-catheterization. This depends on reasonable cognitive function (to plan and execute task), reasonable upper limb function (tremor or weakness will be problematic) and manageable lower limb tone (severe adductor spasm will prevent access). All these issues will need to be considered if treatment is to be successful.

The disciplines involved have individual but complementary areas of expertise. **Physiotherapy** is concerned with restoring normal patterns of movement and teaching control of tone, improving posture and seating and maximizing transfers and bed mobility, where appropriate. The **occupational therapist** is concerned with enabling optimal function in aspects of daily living that are important to the patient (self-care, work and leisure). The **speech and language therapist** covers the related areas of speech (dysarthria and dysphasia) and swallowing (dysphagia) but usually specializes in either one or the other.

The **psychologist** has a particularly important role in identifying and quantifying cognitive deficit, which informs the patient, carer and treating team, and forms the basis of a cognitive rehabilitation programme. Apart from the traditional nursing expertise in continence, nutrition and skin care, the **nurse specialist** can ensure that the rehabilitation process moves from the therapy area to the ward. The team is usually, though not invariably, lead by the **physician**, who helps to coordinate the expertise and has an understanding of the underlying pathophysiology.

Goal setting – long term/ short term

Based on expert assessment, the process of goal setting determines the anticipated achievement for the proposed period of rehabilitation. The long-term goal must be realistic and achievable and must incorporate the patient's perspective. This is then broken down into short-term goals, which must be easily measurable.

Evaluation

It is essential to **evaluate** all aspects of the rehabilitation process, including benefit to the patient, efficacy of the process and service delivery. Benefit to the patient can be evaluated using measures of disability (ability), handicap (participation) and quality of life. These measures can either be generic such as the Barthel Index or Functional Independence Measure, two well-established disability scales or disease-specific. They must be scientifically sound, that is, they must be reliable, valid and responsive and clinically useful. Using such measures in randomized, controlled trials, benefits have been demonstrated from rehabilitation in conditions as diverse as stroke and MS.

The rehabilitation process itself may be evaluated using integrated care pathways, which document all expected interventions and can identify when the planned processes do not happen or goals fail to be achieved. The reasons for these failures are documented (variances), thus providing an excellent audit tool (Figure 28.3).

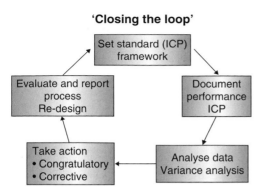

'Closing the loop'

Figure 28.3 Role of integrated care pathways as an audit tool – closing the loop.

AIDS, APPLIANCES AND SPECIALIST SERVICES

Aids and appliances may usefully reduce the impact of conditions such as stroke and MS. These range from simple devices, such as adapted cutlery and pens for upper limb dysfunction and ankle-foot orthoses to support weak ankle dorsiflexion and thereby improve gait. Providing an appropriate wheelchair, which may seem quite straightforward, often requires detailed assessment, particularly when there are specific needs. Failure to address these issues may result in failure to prevent secondary complications, such as worsening posture, kyphoscoliosis and tissue shortening. Communication aids may be a useful support for patients with severe dysarthria or expressive dysphasia, provided they are provided following expert assessment and it has been established that the patient will find it sufficiently useful to continue using it.

EVIDENCE TO SUPPORT NEUROLOGICAL REHABILITATION

The past decade has seen a number of studies **evaluating** the effect of rehabilitation in a range of neurological disorders. In the field of stroke, it is now established that **Stroke Units result in better outcome** in terms of survival, level of disability and reintegration back into the community. These benefits are independent of the severity of the stroke and the site of the lesion. Studies of physiotherapy in stroke have also indicated benefit, which relates to both the amount of therapy and the target (upper or lower limb). **Benefit** from both in-patient and out-patient rehabilitation has been **shown in MS**, although studies are small and there is a need for a better evidence base. Benefit from various therapies in **Parkinson's disease** has been evaluated in a series of Cochrane reviews, and again further studies have been suggested. Duration of benefit is more difficult to demonstrate and there is an inevitable 'wearing off' of effect, arguing for a more 'continuous service'.

SERVICE DELIVERY

Meeting the needs of patients who have either suffered a single episode, such as stroke or head injury, or have a chronic neurological condition, such as MS or Parkinson's disease, is extremely difficult and requires a responsive, flexible service, which can provide continuity of care. Such a seamless service simply does not exist, and recent evaluation of the models of care available for patients with stroke or MS demonstrates that services are patchy, fragmented and unresponsive. It is perhaps as a response to this unmet need that there are plans to establish a national service framework to address services for disability, particularly those related to neurological disorders.

RIGHTS FOR THOSE WITH DISABILITY

Employment is regarded as a basic human right and efforts have been made to prevent discrimination in this or other areas on the basis of disability.

> The Disability Discrimination Act (1995) defines a disabled person as anyone with a physical or mental impairment that has a substantial and long-term effect (usually greater than one year) on his or her ability to carry out normal day-to-day activities.

Discrimination occurs when an individual has been treated less favourably than a non-disabled person simply because of his/her disability. The Disability Rights Commission, an independent organization, was set up in April 2000 by Act of Parliament to work towards the elimination of discrimination and to build a society where all disabled people can participate fully as equal citizens.

REFERENCES AND FURTHER READING

British Society of Rehabilitation Medicine (2000) *Vocational rehabilitation – the way forward.* Report of a working party (Chair: Frank, A.O.) London, UK: British Society of Rehabilitation Medicine.

Drug and Therapeutics Bulletin (2002) MS, Parkinson's disease and physiotherapy. *Drug and Therapeutics Bulletin*, **5**:38–40.

Edwards S (ed.) (2002) *Neurological Physiotherapy*, 2nd edn. London, UK: Churchill Livingstone.

Intercollegiate Working Party for Stroke (2000) *National Clinical Guidelines for Stroke.* London, UK: Royal College of Physicians.

Langhorne P, Dennis M (eds) (1998) *Stroke Units: an evidence based approach.* London, UK: BMJ Books.

Royal College of Physicians (2000) *Medical rehabilitation for people with physical and complex disabilities.* London, UK: Royal College of Physicians.

Thompson AJ (2000) Neurological Rehabilitation: from mechanisms to management. *Journal of Neurology, Neurosurgery, and Psychiatry*, **69**:718–722.

Wade DT, Green Q (2001) *A study of services for multiple sclerosis. Lessons for managing chronic disability.* London, UK: Royal College of Physicians.

Wade DT, Bareld A de Jong (2000) Recent advances in rehabilitation. *British Medical Journal*, **320**:1385–1388.

APPENDICES

Fluvastatin	Lescol	Nevirapine	Viramune
Foscarnet	Foscavir	Nifedipine	Adalat, Adipine
Fosphenytoin sodium	Pro-epanutin	Nitrofurantoin	Furadantin
Furosemide/Frusemide	Lasix	Nortriptyline	Allegron
Gabapentin	Neurontin	Olanzapine	Zyprexa
Galantamine	Reminyl	Ondansetron	Zofran
Ganciclovir	Cymevene	Orphenadrine	Disipal
Gentamicin	Genticin	Oxcarbazepine	Trileptal
Glatiramer acetate	Copaxone		
Griseofulvin	Fucin, Grisovin	Paroxetine	Seroxat
		Penicillamine	Distamine
Haem arginate	Normosang	Pergolide	Celance
Haloperidol	Haldol, Serenace	Phenelzine	Nardil
Hydralazine	Apresoline	Phenobarbitone	Luminal
Hydroxocobalamin	Neocytamen	Phenytoin	Epanutin, Dilantin
Hyoscine	Scopaderm	Pimozide	Orap
		Piracetam	Nootropil
Ibuprofen	Brufen	Pizotifen	Sanomigran
Indinavir	Crixivan	Pramipexole	Mirapexin
Indometacin	Indocid	Pravastatin	Lipostat
Interferon alpha	Intron, Roferon A	Prazosin	Hypovase
Interferon beta 1a	Avonex, Rebif	Prednisolone	Deltacortril, Prednesol
Interferon beta 1b	Betaferon	Primidone	Mysoline
Isoniazid	Isoniazid	Procainamide	Pronestyl
Isotretinoin	Roaccutane	Prochlorperazine	Stemetil, Buccastem
		Propofol	Diprivan
Lamivudine (3TC)	Epivir	Propranolol	Inderal
Lamotrigine	Lamictal	Pyrazinamide	Zinamide
Levetiracetam	Keppra	Pyridostigmine	Mestinon
Lithium carbonate	Camcolit, Priadel	Pyrimethamine	Daraprim
Lorazepam	Ativan		
		Quetiapine	Seroquel
Medroxyprogesterone	Provera, Depo Provera		
Mefenamic acid	Ponstan	Rifampicin	Rifadin
Mefloquine	Lariam	Riluzole	Rilutek
Memantine	Ebixa	Risperidone	Risperdal
Methotrexate	Methotrexate	Ritonavir	Norvir
Methylphenidate	Ritalin	Rivastigmine	Exelon
Methylprednisolone	Medrone	Rizatriptan	Maxalt
Methysergide	Deseril	Ropinirole	Requip
Metoclopramide	Maxolon		
Metoprolol	Betaloc	Saquinavir	Invirase, Fortovase
Metronidazole	Flagyl	Selegiline	Eldepryl, Zelapar
Midazolam	Hypnovel	Sertraline	Lustral
Moclobemide	Manerix	Sodium fusidate	Fucidin
Modafinil	Provigil	Sodium Valproate	Epilim
		Stavudine (d4T)	Zerit
Nadolol	Corgard	Sulfadiazine	Sulphadiazine
Nalidixic acid	Negram	Sulphalsalazine	Salazopyrin
Naproxen	Naprosyn, Synflex	Sulpiride	Dolmatil
Naratriptan	Naramig		

Sumatriptan	Imigran	Trimethoprim	Monotrim
		Trimipramine	Surmontil
Tetrabenazine	Nitoman		
Tetracycline	Deteclo	Vancomycin	Vancocin
Thiopental sodium	Thiopental	Venlafaxine	Efexor
Thioridazine	Melleril	Vigabatrin	Sabril
Tiagabine	Gabitril	Vinblastine	Velbe
Timolol	Betim, Blocadren	Vincristine	Oncovin
Tizanidine	Zanaflex		
Topiramate	Topamax	Warfarin	Marevan
Tramadol	Zydol		
Tranylcypromine	Parnate	Zalcitabine (ddC)	Hivid
Trihexyphenidyl	Broflex	Zidovudine (AZT)	Retrovir
(Benzhexol)		Zolmitriptan	Zomig

RECOGNIZED GENETIC DEFECTS IN SOME SELECTED NEUROLOGICAL DISORDERS

N. Wood

Chromosome	Gene location	Test
Chromosome 1		
Infantile Batten's disease, ceroid lipofuscinosis	1p32	AR
HMSN (II) CMT (II)	1p35–36	AD
Carnitine palmitoyl transferase deficiency	1p32–12	AR
Gaucher's disease	1q21	AR
HMSN1b (CMT)	1q22–23	AD +
Nemaline myopathy	1q21–23	AD
Hypokalaemic periodic paralysis	1q31	AD +
Chromosome 2		
Limb girdle dystrophy	2p	AR
Familial spastic paraplegia (younger onset)	2p21–24	AD
Cerebrotendinous xanthomatosis	2q	AR
Familial motor neurone disease	2q33–35	AR
Chromosome 3		
Spinocerebellar ataxia (SCA7)	3p14–21	AD
GM 1 gangliosidosis	3pter–21	AR
Von Hippel–Lindau disease	3p26–25	AD
Retinitis pigmentosa	3q	AD
Chromosome 4		
Huntington's disease	4p16.3	AD *
Facioscapulohumeral dystrophy (some only)	4q35–ter	AD
Chromosome 5		
Infantile spinal muscular atrophy	5q11–13	AR *

Sandhoff's disease (Hexosaminidase B)	5q13	AR
Hyperekplexia (startle disease)	5q	AD
Limb girdle dystrophy (dominant)	5q22–24	AD

Chromosome 6

Spinocerebellar ataxia (SCA1)	6p22–23	AD *
Juvenile myoclonic epilepsy	6p24	AD +
Retinitis pigmentosa (peripheral)	6p21	AD

Chromosome 7

Myotonia congenita	7q35	AD +

Chromosome 8

Familial spastic paraplegia (HSP)(recessive)	8q	AR
Ataxia with vitamin E deficiency	8q	AR +

Chromosome 9

Friedreich's ataxia	9q13–21.1	AR *
Familial dysautonomia	9q31–33	AR
Torsion dystonia (some families)	9q34	AD
Tuberous sclerosis	9q34.1–34.2	AD

Chromosome 10

Ataxia, infantile onset	10q23–24	AR

Chromosome 11

Spinocerebellar ataxia (SCA5)	11cen	AD
Niemann–Pick disease	11p15	AR
Tuberous sclerosis (some families)	11q14–23	AD
Ataxia telangiectasia	11q23	AR +
Acute intermittent porphyria	11q23.2	AR
McArdle's disease	11q13	AR

Chromosome 12

Dentatorubropallidoluysian atrophy (DPLA)	12p12ter	AD *
Episodic ataxia/myokymia	12p13	AD
Spinocerebellar ataxia (SCA2)	12q23–24.1	AD *

Chromosome 13

Wilson's disease	13q14.2–21	AR +

Chromosome 14

Familial Alzheimer's disease (early onset)	14	AD +
Krabbe's leukodystrophy	14q24.3–32	AR
Spinocerebellar ataxia (SCA3) Machado–Joseph disease	14q24.3–32	AD *
Familial spastic paraplegia (HSP) (older onset)	14q	AD
Dopa-responsive dystonia	14q	AD +

Chromosome 15

Prader–Willi/Angelmann's syndrome	15q11–12	–
Limb girdle dystrophy (recessive)	15q15	AR
Tay-Sachs disease (Hexosaminidase A)	15q23–24	AR
Familial spastic paraplegia (HSP) (early onset)	15q	AD

Chromosome 16

Juvenile Batten's disease	16p12	AR
Tuberous sclerosis (some families)	16p13.3	AD
Spinocerebellar ataxia (SCA4)	16q24- ter	AD

Chromosome 17

HMSN1a (CMT)	17p11.2	AD *
Neuropathy with liability to pressure palsies	17p11.2	AD *
Miller-Dieker syndrome	17p13.3	–
Sjögren–Larsson syndrome	17q	AR
Neurofibromatosis I	17q11.2	AD
Limb girdle dystrophy	17q	AR
Muscle sodium channel disorders (hyperkalaemic periodic paralysis)	17q22–24	AD +

Chromosome 18

Familial amyloid neuropathy (transthyretin) (common mutations only)	18q11.2–12.1	AD *

Chromosome 19

Periodic ataxia without myokymia	19p13	AD
Familial hemiplegic migraine (some families)	19p	AD +
Malignant hyperthermia	19q13.1	AD +
Central core disease	19q13.1	AD +
Myotonic dystrophy	19q13.2	AD *
Familial Alzheimer's disease (ApoE) (late onset)	19q	AD

Chromosome 20

Familial prion dementias	20pter-12	AD +
Familial benign neonatal convulsions	20q	AD

Chromosome 21

Familial Alzheimer's disease (APP gene)	21q11–22	AD +
Familial motor neurone disease	1q22.1–22.2	AD +

Chromosome 22

Unverricht–Lundborg disease myoclonic epilepsy (Baltic)	22q22.3	AD
Metachromatic leukodystrophy	22q13.3ter	AR
Neurofibromatosis II	22q11–13.1	AD *

AR, autosomal recessive; AD, autosomal dominant.
p,q represent the short and long arms on chromosome; numbers bands.
*Direct simple gene test available.
+ gene known, limited screening often research based.

X Chromosome	Gene location	
Rett's syndrome	Xp22	
Duchenne dystrophy	Xp21.2	*
Becker muscular dystrophy	Xp21.2	*
Ornithine transcarbamylase deficiency	Xp21.1	
HMSN (CMT)	Xq13–21	
Spastic paraplegia (HSP-X-linked)	Xq13–22	

Allan–Herndon syndrome	Xq21	
Bulbospinal neuronopathy (Kennedy's disease)	Xq21.3–12	*
Fabry's disease	Xq22	
Pelizaeus–Merzbacher disease	Xq22	
Lesch–Nyhan disease	Xq26	
Fragile X/mental retardation	Xq27.3	*
Adrenoleukodystrophy	Xq28	
Emery–Dreifuss muscular dystrophy	Xq28	

*Simple direct gene test available.

Some Common Mitochondrial Disorders

KSS	Sporadic	Deletion of mitochondrial DNA (3243)
CPEO	Sporadic	Deletion of tandem duplication
	Maternal	point mutation tRNA leucine (3243)
MELAS	Maternal	Point mutation tRNA leucine (commonly 3243)
MERRF	Maternal	Point mutation tRNA lysine (commonly 8344)
Myopathy	Maternal	Point mutation tRNA leucine (commonly 3250)
LHON	Maternal	Point mutation
	ND4 11778	
	ND1 3460	
	ND6 14484	

LHON, recognition pattern of point mutation linked with prognosis.

KSS, Kearns–Sayre syndrome; PEO, progressive external ophthalmoplegia; MELAS, mitochondrial myopathy, encephalomyelopathy, lactic acidosis and stroke-like episodes; MERRF, myoclonic epilepsy with ragged red fibres; LHON, Leber's hereditary optic neuropathy.

Note – deletion/duplications are found commonly in muscle DNA from a biopsy sample and can be missed in a blood sample.

Reference

Rosenberg R, Pruisner SB, Dimauro S, Barchi RL (1997) *The Molecular and Genetic Basis of Neurological Diseases*, 2nd edn. London, UK: Butterworth-Heinemann.

Websites of interest

http://www.geneclinics.org/
http://www.ncbi.nlm.nih.gov/omim
http://www.gig.org.uk/
http://www.genome.gov/

INDEX